ETIOLOGY AND PATHOPHYSIOLOGY OF PARKINSON'S DISEASE

Edited by **Abdul Qayyum Rana**

Etiology and Pathophysiology of Parkinson's Disease

Edited by Abdul Qayyum Rana

Published by InTech

Janeza Trdine 9, 51000 Rijeka, Croatia

Technical Editor Silvia Vlase

Cover Designer InTech Design Team

Additional hard copies can be obtained from orders@intechopen.com

Etiology and Pathophysiology of Parkinson's Disease,
Edited by Abdul Qayyum Rana
p. cm.
ISBN 978-953-307-462-7

For EU product safety concerns:
IN TECH d.o.o., Prolaz Marije Krucifikse Kozulić 3, 51000 Rijeka, Croatia,
info@intechopen.com or visit our website at intechopen.com.

Meet the editor

Dr. Abdul Qayyum Rana is a Canadian neurologist who specializes in the field of Parkinson's disease and Movement Disorders. He is a fellow of the Royal College of Physicians and Surgeons of Canada. After completing his neurology residency training, Dr. Rana undertook a clinical fellowship in Parkinson's disease and Movement Disorders at the University of Ottawa, Canada. He is currently the director of the Parkinson's Clinic of Eastern Toronto and Movement Disorders Centre located in Toronto, Canada. He is also founder of World Parkinson's Education Program. He is the author of "Frequently Asked Questions About Parkinson's Disease", which is a series of thirteen brochures about Parkinson's disease, translated in many languages and used in several countries around the world. Dr. Rana has also written the following books: "A Synopsis of Neurological Emergencies", "An Aid to Neuro-ophthalmology", "An introduction to Essential Tremor", "50 Ways Parkinson's Could Affect You", and "What is Parkinson's disease in Arabic?".

Contents

Preface

Parkinson's disease is a complex neurological condition which is quite disabling and interfering with one's activities of daily life. The exact etiology of Parkinson's disease remains unknown. Currently it is believed that Parkinson's disease occurs due to interaction of environmental and genetic factors. Recently, there have been many significant developments in understanding the genetic mechanisms involved in Parkinson's disease. This book not only provides a good review of the genetics of Parkinson's disease but also gives a detail of other molecular pathways involved in the pathological process responsible for causation of Parkinson's disease.

A great focus has been given to pathophysiology of Parkinson's disease, role of basal ganglia and other parts of brain involved in Parkinson's disease. Every effort has been made to present correct and up to date information in this book, but medicine is a field with ongoing research and development, therefore readers may use other sources if the content of this book is found to be insufficient. Information presented in this book is considered generally accepted practice; however the authors, editor, and publisher are not responsible for any errors, omissions, or consequences from the application of this information.

Dr. Abdul Qayyum Rana
Parkinson's Clinic of Eastern Toronto & Movement Disorders Center, Toronto, Canada

1

Etiology and Pathogenesis of Parkinson's Disease

Taku Hatano and Nobutaka Hattori
Department of Neurology, Juntendo University School of Medicine, Tokyo, Japan

1. Introduction

The pathological hallmarks of Parkinson's disease (PD) are marked loss of dopaminergic neurons in the substantia nigra pars compacta (SNc), which causes dopamine depletion in the striatum, and the presence of intracytoplasmic inclusions known as Lewy bodies in the remaining cells. It remains unclear why dopaminergic neuronal cell death and Lewy body formation occur in PD. The pathological changes in PD are seen not only in the SNc but also in the locus coeruleus, pedunculo pontine nucleus, raphe nucleus, dorsal motor nucleus of the vagal nerve, olfactory bulb, parasympathetic as well as sympathetic post-ganglionic neurons, Mynert nucleus, and the cerebral cortex (Braak et al. 2003). Widespread neuropathology in the brainstem and cortical regions are responsible for various motor and non-motor symptoms of PD. Although dopamine replacement therapy improves the functional prognosis of PD, there is currently no treatment that prevents the progression of this disease.

Previous studies provided possible evidence that the pathogenesis of PD involves complex interactions between environmental and multiple genetic factors. Exposure to the environmental toxin MPTP was identified as one cause of parkinsonism in 1983 (Langston & Ballard 1983). In addition to MPTP, other environmental toxins, such as the herbicide paraquat and the pesticide rotenone have been shown to contribute to dopaminergic neuronal cell loss and parkinsonism. In contrast, cigarette smoking, caffeine use, and high normal plasma urate levels are associated with lower risk of PD (Hernan et al. 2002). Recently, Braak and coworkers proposed the "Dual Hit" theory, which postulated an unknown pathogen accesses the brain through two pathways, the nose and the gut (Hawkes et al. 2007). Subsequently, a prion-like mechanism might contribute to the propagation of α-synuclein from the peripheral nerve to the central nervous system (Angot et al. 2010).

Approximately 5% of patients with clinical features of PD have clear familial etiology. Therefore, genetic factors clearly contribute to the pathogenesis of PD. Over the decade, more than 16 loci and 11 causative genes have been identified, and many studies have shed light on their implication in, not only monogenic, but also sporadic forms of PD. Recent studies revealed that PD-associated genes play important roles in cellular functions, such as mitochondrial functions, the ubiquitin-proteasomal system, autophagy-lysosomal pathway, and membrane trafficking (Hatano et al. 2009). In this chapter, we review the investigations of environmental and genetic factors of PD (Figure 1).

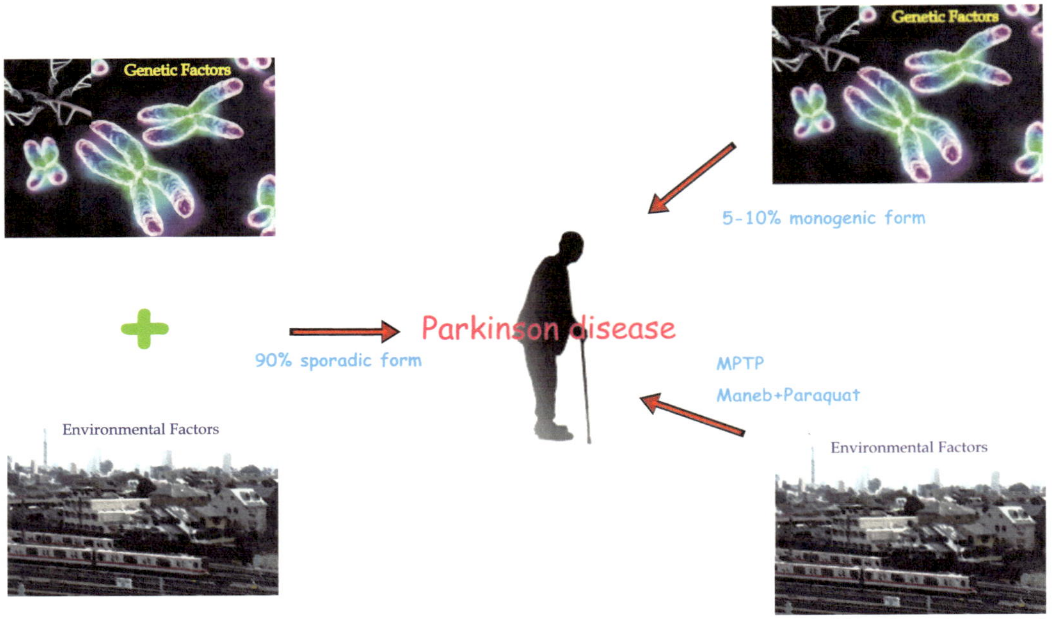

Fig. 1. Although the etiology of Parkinson disease (PD) remains unknown, 5-10% of patients have clear familial etiology, which show a classical recessive or dominant Mendelian mode of inheritance. On the other hand, MPTP or a combination of maneb and paraquat are environmental risk factors for PD. Several PD-related genetic factors (e.g., SNPs in α-synuclein) have been discovered, and the interaction between genetic and environmental factors might contribute to sporadic PD.

2. Environmental factors and PD

2.1 1-methyl-4phenyl-1,2,3,6-tetrahydro-pyridine (MPTP)

Langston et al reported on four patients who developed typical parkinsonism after repeated injection of MPTP intravenously (Langston & Ballard 1983). Furthermore, these patients responded to treatment with levodopa and bromocriptine and experienced motor fluctuations, similar to patients with idiopathic PD. Interestingly, fluorodopa positron emission tomography (FD-PET) study of subjects exposed to MPTP demonstrated that transient exposure to this toxin could lead to progressive nigral degeneration (Vingerhoets et al. 1994). Neuropathological findings of 3 subjects with MPTP-induced parkinsonism showed moderate to severe dopaminergic neuronal degeneration without Lewy bodies in the substantia nigra. Interestingly, there was gliosis; clustering microglia around nerve cells and extraneural melanin. These findings indicated active and continuing neuronal cell degeneration (Langston et al. 1999). PET and neuropathological studies suggested that an active neuronal cell death process was persistent for years after these subjects were exposed to MPTP. MPTP is a by-product of the chemical synthesis of a narcotic meperidine analog. This chemical agent is highly lypophilic, therefore it quickly crosses the blood-brain barrier and converts to 1-methyl-4-phenyl-2,3-dihydropyridinium ion (MPP+), which is the active toxic compound, via monoamine oxidase B within nondopaminergic cells, such as glial cells and serotonergic neurons. MPP+ is transported into dopamine neurons by the dopamine transporter, and therefore exhibits selective toxicity to dopaminergic neurons. Furthermore, MPP+ accumulates in mitochondria, where it inhibits the mitochondrial electron transport chain component complex I (Przedborski & Vila 2003). Mizuno et al reported that MPP+ inhibited the α-ketoglutarate dehydrogenase complex of the mitochondrial tricarboxylic acid cycle, which synthesizes succinate from α–ketoglutarate (Mizuno et al. 1987). In SNc of sporadic PD subjects, decreased activity and protein levels of complex I have also been reported (Schapira et al. 1989). Thus biochemical changes in dopaminergic neuronal degeneration in sporadic PD were essentially similar to those of subjects exposed to MPTP.

2.2 Pesticides

Epidemiological studies have suggested the association between PD and exposure of pesticides such as rotenone and paraquat. Rotenone is a potent and high-affinity specific inhibitor of complex I. In rodents, continuous infusion of these toxic agents induced dopaminergic neuronal cell death and inclusion bodies, which were similar to Lewy bodies in PD patients (Betarbet et al. 2000). Therefore, both MPTP and rotenone disrupt mitochondrial function and play important roles in the nigral cell degeneration in PD.

Paraquat, which is a member of a chemical class known as bipyridyl derivatives, is one of the most commonly used pesticides, and leads to oxidative and nitrative stress (Berry et al.). The chemical structure of paraquat is similar to MPP+. Epidemiologic studies implicate the association between exposure to this toxin and the development of PD. Interestingly, recent studies revealed that exposure to a combination of paraquat and maneb, which is also widely used as an agricultural pesticide, exacerbate dopaminergic degeneration in the rodent model and cause an increased incidence of PD in humans (Costello et al. 2009). In this context, exposure to a combination of several toxins could lead to greater risk of developing PD than a single toxin.

2.3 Caffeine, cigarette

Smokers and coffee drinkers have been associated with a lower risk of PD in several epidemiological studies. Hernan et al. conducted a meta-analytic review for the association between caffeine intake, smoking, and the risk of PD. Interestingly the cigarette smokers had 60% lower risk for the development of PD than people without a history of smoking (Hernan et al. 2002). Some experiments suggested that chronic nicotine treatment could have protective effects against the nigrostriatal neuronal cell death in MPTP-treated animal models. Several studies revealed that cigarette smoking inhibited monoamine oxidase (MAO) activity and nicotine stimulated dopamine release. As a result, cigarette smoking may suppress free radical generation via MAO-B-associated metabolism of dopamine, and be able to protect against dopaminergic cell death (Miller et al. 2007). Similar to cigarette smoking, coffee drinking could result in a 30% decreased risk of PD compared with non-coffee drinkers (Hernan et al. 2002). Chen et al reported that caffeine had similar effects as A_{2A} antagonists, and attenuated MPTP toxicity via A_{2A} receptor blockade (Chen et al. 2001).

2.4 Disease process and dual hit theory

Braak and colleagues proposed neuropathological staging in PD. They reported that the dorsal motor nucleus of the glossopharyngeal and vagal nerves and the anterior olfactory nucleus were initially affected, and subsequently the substantia nigra and locus coeruleus became involved. Cortical areas showed less vulnerability, gradually becoming affected (Braak et al. 2003). These pathological findings suggest that the neuronal degeneration in PD may extend from peripheral systems, such as olfactory and autonomic systems to cortices. They also proposed the so-called "Dual-Hit" hypothesis, which suggests that neurotropic pathogens may enter the nervous system via both nasal and intestinal epithelium (Hawkes et al. 2007). These events may promote α-synuclein aggregation and subsequently misfolded α-synuclein may propagate between cells in a prion-like manner (Angot et al. 2010). By using cultured cell models and α-synuclein transgenic mice models, Desplats et al demonstrated direct neuron to neuron transmission of α-synuclein aggregates (Desplats et al. 2009). Actually, in the brains of PD patients who received fetal ventral mesencephalic transplants, grafted nigral neurons contained Lewy body-like inclusions (Li et al. 2008, Kordower et al. 2008). These results corroborate the hypothesis that progression of α-synuclein aggregation relies on the same mechanisms of prion propagation. In conclusion, environmental factors could play important roles in the pathomechanisms of neuronal degeneration in sporadic PD

3. Genetic factors and PD

3.1 α-synuclein

α-synuclein is a 140-amino acid protein that is abundantly expressed throughout the brain, and especially in presynaptic nerve terminals. In 1997, an α-synuclein A53T mutation was isolated from an autosomal dominant PD case. Cases of sporadic PD and A53T-associated patients displayed similar clinical phenotypes, with the exception of a relatively earlier age of onset and atypical features such as cognitive decline, severe central hypoventilation, orthostatic hypotension, myoclonus and urinary incontinence (Polymeropoulos et al. 1997, Spira et al. 2001). In addition, A30P (Kruger et al. 1998) and E46K (Zarranz et al. 2004) mutations were also identified. Following the identification of mutations in the α-synuclein gene, multiplication of *SNCA* has also been identified to cause autosomal dominant familial PD (Ibanez et al. 2004, Chartier-Harlin et al. 2004, Nishioka et al. 2006, Ahn et al. 2008). Considering that α-synuclein protein is the major component of Lewy bodies (Spillantini et al. 1997), aggregation of α-synuclein is thought to be a key event in dopaminergic neuronal cell death in both *SNCA*-linked and sporadic PD (Lee & Trojanowski 2006). α-synuclein has a high propensity to aggregate, just like other proteins associated with neurodegenerative disease, such as tau, amyloid precursor protein, and poly Q proteins (Bossy-Wetzel et al. 2004, Cookson 2005). α-synuclein exists in solution as an unstructured monomer, however, monomeric α-synuclein can form insoluble fibrillar aggregates with an antiparallel β-sheet structure through the formation of oligomeric forms (protofibrils). The fibrils assemble in vitro, and these filaments closely aggregate just like pathologic inclusions in PD or MSA (Cookson 2005). Fibril formation by pathogenic mutations is accelerated in vitro compared with the wild type (Narhi et al. 1999, Conway et al. 2000, Greenbaum et al. 2005). In several experimental models, including cultured cells, rodent, *Drosophilae* and *Caenorhabditis elegans*, pathogenic mutants also promote self-aggregation and oligomerization into protofibrils, compared with the wild-type protein. Some studies suggest that α-synuclein could participate in a protein degradation pathway such as the ubiquitin-proteasomal system (UPS) (Rideout et al. 2001, Zhang et al. 2008), and chaperone-mediated autophagy(Cuervo et al. 2004).

The functions of α-synuclein under normal physiological conditions remain unknown. However, several studies have shown that α-synuclein associates with synaptic vesicles and modulates neurotransmitter release (Jensen et al. 1998, Li et al. 2004). Electrophysiological study in α-synuclein knockout mice revealed that α-synuclein could act as an activity-negative regulator of DA neurotransmission at synaptic terminals (Abeliovich et al. 2000). α-synuclein is also speculated to have various other functions, such as modulation of tyrosine hydroxylase (TH) activation (Perez et al. 2002), inhibition of vesicular monoamine transporter-2 (VMAT2) activity (Guo et al. 2008), and interaction with septin4, which have been implicated in exocytosis (Ihara et al. 2007). Recently, Cooper and colleagues reported that α-synuclein blocked endoplasmic reticulum (ER)-to-Golgi vesicular trafficking, and induced ER stress followed by cell death (Cooper et al. 2006). In addition, α-synuclein may interact with the synaptic membrane through lipid rafts (Fortin et al. 2004, Kubo et al. 2005), which are known to be a signaling platform for cellular functions such as signal transduction, membrane trafficking and cytoskeletal organization. These data indicate that α-synuclein plays important roles in vesicle sorting and regulation of catecholamine metabolism in dopaminergic neurons.

3.2 LRRK2

LRRK2 mutations were identified as the causative gene for PARK8-linked familial PD (Paisan-Ruiz et al. 2004), (Zimprich et al. 2004). Some screening studies reported that *LRRK2* mutations were identified not only in familial PD but also in sporadic PD. Since then, *LRRK2* mutations seem to be the most frequent cause of autosomal dominantly-inherited familial PD (Lesage et al. 2006, Ozelius et al. 2006). R1628P and G2385R are polymorphic mutations and have been demonstrated as risk factors for sporadic PD in Asian populations (Di Fonzo et al. 2006, Funayama et al. 2007). The clinical features of patients with *LRRK2* mutations essentially resemble sporadic PD with good response to levodopa. Pathological studies of autopsy cases with I1371V, A1441C, Y1699C, G2019S, and I2020T mutations have revealed neuronal cell loss accompanied by Lewy bodies indistinguishable from those of sporadic PD. Some individuals display pleomorphic pathologies, including synucleinopathy, tauopathy, TDP-43 proteinopathy, substantia nigral neuronal loss alone, and neuronal loss with nuclear ubiquitin inclusions (Zimprich et al. 2004, Covy et al. 2009). Although some antibodies against the functional domain fail to detect Lewy bodies, other antibodies directed against the N-terminal and C-terminal residues are able to stain Lewy bodies. Thus, there is controversy as to whether LRRK2 is a component of Lewy bodies. LRRK2 also colocalizes with tau-positive inclusions in fronto-temporal dementia with MAPT N279K mutation (Miklossy et al. 2007). Considering this pleomorphic pathology, LRRK2 seems to be involved in disease-modifying pathways in various neurodegenerative diseases.

The LRRK2 protein is a 2527 amino acid polypeptide (~280 kDa), consisting of leucine-rich repeats (LRR), Ras of complex proteins (Roc) followed by the C-terminal of Roc (COR), mitogen-activated protein kinase kinase kinase (MAPKKK) and WD40 domains (Mata et al. 2006). LRRK2 protein belongs to the ROCO protein family. LRRK2 proteins localize in the cytoplasm and membranous organelles, including ER, Golgi apparatus, early endosomes, lysosomes, synaptic vesicles, mitochondria, and the plasma membrane (Hatano et al. 2007). We found LRRK2 bound to lipid rafts within the synaptosomes (Hatano et al. 2007). Several results suggest that LRRK2 also interacts with the Rab family and presynaptic proteins, and modulates the membrane trafficking system.

An in vitro phosphorylation assay using thin-layer chromatography revealed that LRRK2 might also function as a serine/threonine kinase (West et al. 2007). The frequent LRRK2 G2019S and adjacent I2020T mutations are located within the kinase domain and exhibit increased activity (West et al. 2005, Gloeckner et al. 2006). The kinase activity could be regulated by GTP via the intrinsic GTPase Roc domain (Smith et al. 2006, West et al. 2007). Considering that at least some of the mutations alter the kinase activity and are neurotoxic, misregulated kinase activity may explain the core damaging effect of LRRK2 in neurons. Actually, several groups reported that LRKK2 is able to modulate several signal transduction pathways, such as the ERK1/2, TNFα/FasL and Wnt signaling pathways (Berwick & Harvey 2011), and the microRNA pathway, which regulates protein synthesis (Gehrke et al. 2010). The interaction between LRRK2 and parkin is also reported, but there is no evidence to associate LRRK2 with other genes, such as α-synuclein, tau, and DJ-1 (Smith et al. 2005). Further investigations may reveal how LRRK2 participates in pathways of other PARK gene-related dopaminergic neuronal degeneration.

3.3 PINK1/Parkin pathway

Mutations in parkin were identified as the cause of autosomal recessive early onset PD (EOPD) (Kitada et al. 1998), followed by mutations in DJ-1 (Bonifati et al. 2003), and PINK1 (Valente et al. 2004, Hatano et al. 2004). PARK2-linked EOPD is characterized by a spontaneous improvement after sleep or a nap, diurnal fluctuation, some dystonic features which are predominantly in the foot, good response to levodopa, early onset (average age of onset is in the twenties), no dementia, no autonomic failure, and lack of Lewy bodies (Yamamura et al. 1973, Mori et al. 1998). The clinical features of PARK2-linked EOPD are distinguishable from those of patients with the common form of PD. Pathological studies in patients with PARK2-linked EOPD have shown that the substantia nigra and locus coeruleus exhibit selective degeneration with gliosis (Mori et al. 1998). Other pigmented neurons in these regions contain traces of melanin pigments, and the cell cytoplasm is scanty compared with that of normal individuals without neurodegenerative disorders. Although the brain tissue of two cases, which were positive for parkin mutation showed the presence of Lewy bodies (Farrer et al. 2001, Pramstaller et al. 2005), they are generally absent in PARK2-mutation brains.

Parkin protein is linked to the ubiquitin-proteasome pathway as a ubiquitin ligase (E3) (Shimura et al. 2000). Most Lewy bodies also stain strongly for ubiquitin, which is highly involved in the protein degradation system. Furthermore, the collaboration between parkin and PINK1 could be associated with mitochondrial quality control systems (Geisler et al. 2010, Vives-Bauza et al. 2010, Narendra et al. 2010, Kawajiri et al. 2010, Matsuda et al. 2010). *Parkin*-deficient *Drosophila* exhibit mitochondrial structural alterations in testes and muscle tissue (Greene et al. 2003). *PINK1*-deficient *Drosophila* also exhibited degeneration of flight muscles and dopaminergic neuronal cells accompanied by mitochondrial abnormality, and share phenotypic similarity with *parkin*-deficient *Drosophila*. Overexpression of parkin reversed the muscle damage in *PINK1*-deficient *Drosophila*, but PINK1 overexpression could not reverse the *parkin*-null-linked damage (Clark et al. 2006, Park et al. 2006). Furthermore, mitochondrial abnormalities in *PINK1*- or *parkin*-deficient *Drosophila* were reversed by knockdown of *Mitofusin* (*Mfn*), *Optic atrophy 1* (*Opa1*), or overexpression of Dynamin-related protein1 (Drp1), which participate in mitochondrial fusion and fission (Deng et al. 2008). These findings suggest that PINK1 might associate upstream of parkin to regulate mitochondrial dynamics. The interaction between PINK1 and parkin was also analyzed by using a cultured cell system (Shiba et al. 2009). Narendra and colleagues (2010) reported accumulation of parkin in mitochondria impaired by carbonyl cyanide m-chlorophenylhydrazone. Such accumulation promotes the selective autophagy of damaged mitochondria (mitophagy). Several groups have recently shown that PINK1 might be required for parkin-mediated mitophagy (Geisler et al. 2010; Vives-Bauza et al. 2010; Narendra et al. 2010; Kawajiri et al. 2010; Matsuda et al. 2010). We reported that parkin relocates cytoplasm to damaged mitochondria in a membrane potential-dependent manner (Matsuda et al.2010). PINK1 plays a critical role in recruiting parkin to mitochondria with low membrane potential to initiate the autophagic degradation of damaged mitochondria. Pathogenic parkin mutations affect mitochondrial localization. Therefore, loss of the association between parkin and damaged mitochondria could lead to nigral cell death in *PARK2-linked* EOPD. Immunoprecipitation using anti-LC3 antibodies revealed the direct interaction between PINK1 and endogenous LC3 (Kawajiri et al. 2010). These results suggest that mitochondrial degradation by the PINK1/Parkin pathway is dependent on mitochondrial autophagic activity. Geisler et al. (2010) also reported that the kinase activity of PINK1 in mitochondria might be needed to induce translocation of parkin to depolarized mitochondria. Parkin modified VDAC1 via Lys27 poly-ubiquitylation, and promoted autophagic degradation of damaged mitochondria. Interestingly, they also revealed that the autophagic adaptor p62/SQSTM1 is recruited to mitochondrial clusters and could be associated with PINK1/Parkin-mediated mitophagy. Funayama et al. identified PD patients carrying both *parkin* and *PINK1* mutations, whose onset age was younger than that of patients with the same *parkin* mutation alone. The presence of digenic mutations, such as *parkin* plus *PINK1* mutations, suggests that a *PINK1* mutation could influence the clinical symptoms of parkin-linked PD (Funayama et al. 2008). However, Kitada and colleagues (Kitada et al. 2009) reported that triple knockout of Parkin, PINK1, and DJ-1 resulted in normal morphology and numbers of dopaminergic and noradrenergic neurons in the substantia nigra and locus coeruleus. Therefore, understanding the PINK1/Parkin pathway underlying the mitochondrial dynamics helps clarify the pathomechanics in PD.

4. Conclusion

The pathological mechanisms and causes of PD remain largely unknown. Most PD patients have not been associated with a particular genetic background or certain exposure of environmental toxins. However, Japanese and European groups performed genome-wide association studies and revealed that the α-synuclein locus, the MAPT locus, the LRRK2 locus, the BST1 locus, and 1q32 (PARK16) may be genetic risk factors for PD (Satake et al. 2009, Simon-Sanchez et al. 2009). Although the α-synuclein locus, LRRK2 locus, and PARK16 are confirmed as genetic risk factors for PD across populations, BST1 and MAPT may be risk loci correlated with ethnic differences. Conversely, α-synuclein is involved in the virulent effects of the environmental toxin MPTP. High mRNA and protein levels of α-synuclein have been described in the brains of MPTP-treated mice (Vila et al. 2000). Although α-synuclein-deficient mice exhibited marked resistance to MPTP-induced degeneration of dopamine neurons (Dauer et al. 2002), some lines of α-synuclein transgenic mice have exhibited increased sensitivity to MPTP (Nieto et al. 2006, Yu et al. 2008). These results also suggest that various genetic-environmental interactions may have influences on dopaminergic neuronal metabolism and kinetics, such as signal transduction, vesicle transport, autophagy (mitophagy), and mitochondrial stress (Figure 2). In addition, a prion-like transmission of α-synuclein may trigger the development of nigral degeneration in PD. Taken together, the new findings based on the interaction between familial PD-related proteins and environmental factors could shed light on the pathomechanisms for PD.

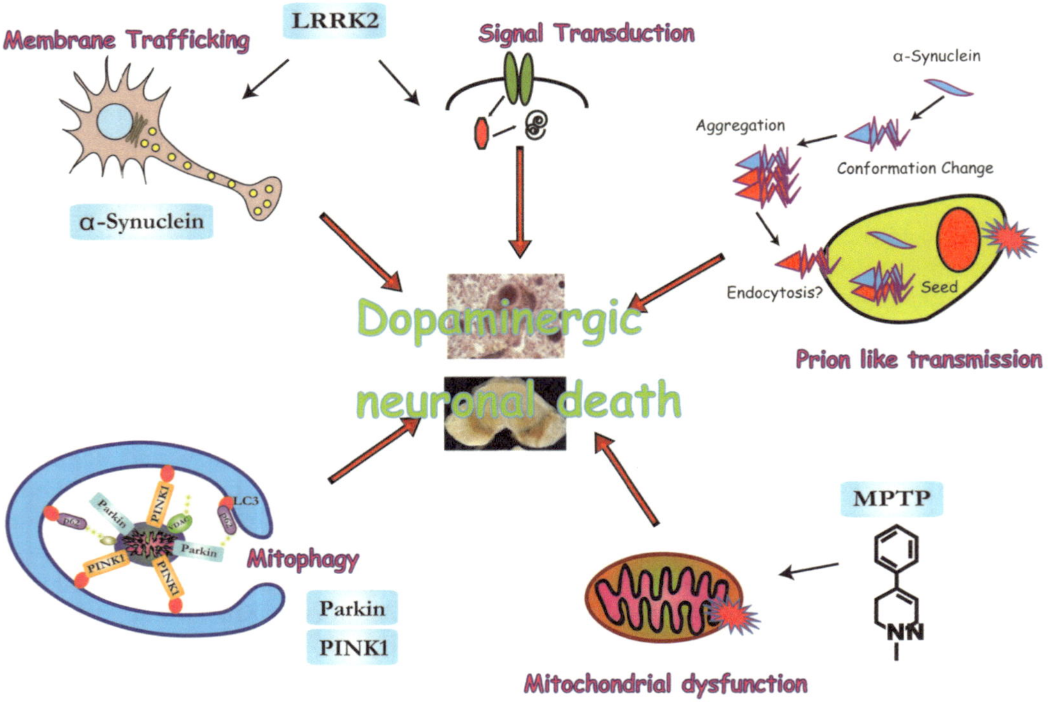

Fig. 2. Summary of pathogenetic factors involved in Parkinson's disease (PD). Recent evidence indicated that the PINK1/Parkin pathway participates in mitochondrial removal via autophagy (mitophagy). LRRK2 may associate with cell signaling pathways and the membrane trafficking system. Several environmental factors, such as MPTP, paraquat, and rotenone are known as mitochondrial toxins. In addition, a prion-like transmission of α-synuclein may trigger the development of nigral degeneration in PD.

5. Acknowledgments

This study was supported in part by grants for research on diseases of the brain from the Ministry of Education, Science and Sports in Japan.

6. References

Abeliovich, A., Schmitz, Y., Farinas, I. et al. (2000) Mice lacking alpha-synuclein display functional deficits in the nigrostriatal dopamine system. *Neuron,* 25, 239-252.

Ahn, T. B., Kim, S. Y., Kim, J. Y. et al. (2008) alpha-Synuclein gene duplication is present in sporadic Parkinson disease. *Neurology,* 70, 43-49.

Angot, E., Steiner, J. A., Hansen, C., Li, J. Y. and Brundin, P. (2010) Are synucleinopathies prion-like disorders? *Lancet Neurol,* 9, 1128-1138.

Berry, C., La Vecchia, C. and Nicotera, P. (2010) Paraquat and Parkinson's disease. *Cell Death Differ,* 17, 1115-1125.

Berwick, D. C. and Harvey, K. (2011) LRRK2 signaling pathways: the key to unlocking neurodegeneration? *Trends Cell Biol,* 21, 254-265.

Betarbet, R., Sherer, T. B., MacKenzie, G., Garcia-Osuna, M., Panov, A. V. and Greenamyre, J. T. (2000) Chronic systemic pesticide exposure reproduces features of Parkinson's disease. *Nat Neurosci,* 3, 1301-1306.

Bonifati, V., Rizzu, P., van Baren, M. J. et al. (2003) Mutations in the DJ-1 gene associated with autosomal recessive early-onset parkinsonism. *Science,* 299, 256-259.

Bossy-Wetzel, E., Schwarzenbacher, R. and Lipton, S. A. (2004) Molecular pathways to neurodegeneration. *Nat Med,* 10 Suppl, S2-9.

Braak, H., Del Tredici, K., Rub, U., de Vos, R. A., Jansen Steur, E. N. and Braak, E. (2003) Staging of brain pathology related to sporadic Parkinson's disease. *Neurobiol Aging,* 24, 197-211.

Chartier-Harlin, M. C., Kachergus, J., Roumier, C. et al. (2004) Alpha-synuclein locus duplication as a cause of familial Parkinson's disease. *Lancet,* 364, 1167-1169.

Chen, J. F., Xu, K., Petzer, J. P. et al. (2001) Neuroprotection by caffeine and A(2A) adenosine receptor inactivation in a model of Parkinson's disease. *J Neurosci,* 21, RC143.

Clark, I. E., Dodson, M. W., Jiang, C., Cao, J. H., Huh, J. R., Seol, J. H., Yoo, S. J., Hay, B. A. and Guo, M. (2006) Drosophila pink1 is required for mitochondrial function and interacts genetically with parkin. *Nature,* 441, 1162-1166.

Conway, K. A., Lee, S. J., Rochet, J. C., Ding, T. T., Williamson, R. E. and Lansbury, P. T., Jr. (2000) Acceleration of oligomerization, not fibrillization, is a shared property of both alpha-synuclein mutations linked to early-onset Parkinson's disease: implications for pathogenesis and therapy. *Proc Natl Acad Sci U S A,* 97, 571-576.

Cookson, M. R. (2005) The biochemistry of Parkinson's disease. *Annu Rev Biochem,* 74, 29-52.

Cooper, A. A., Gitler, A. D., Cashikar, A. et al. (2006) Alpha-synuclein blocks ER-Golgi traffic and Rab1 rescues neuron loss in Parkinson's models. *Science,* 313, 324-328.

Costello, S., Cockburn, M., Bronstein, J., Zhang, X. and Ritz, B. (2009) Parkinson's disease and residential exposure to maneb and paraquat from agricultural applications in the central valley of California. *Am J Epidemiol,* 169, 919-926.

Covy, J. P., Yuan, W., Waxman, E. A., Hurtig, H. I., Van Deerlin, V. M. and Giasson, B. I. (2009) Clinical and pathological characteristics of patients with leucine-rich repeat kinase-2 mutations. *Mov Disord,* 24, 32-39.

Cuervo, A. M., Stefanis, L., Fredenburg, R., Lansbury, P. T. and Sulzer, D. (2004) Impaired degradation of mutant alpha-synuclein by chaperone-mediated autophagy. *Science,* 305, 1292-1295.

Dauer, W., Kholodilov, N., Vila, M. et al. (2002) Resistance of alpha -synuclein null mice to the parkinsonian neurotoxin MPTP. *Proc Natl Acad Sci U S A,* 99, 14524-14529.

Deng, H., Dodson, M. W., Huang, H. and Guo, M. (2008) The Parkinson's disease genes pink1 and parkin promote mitochondrial fission and/or inhibit fusion in Drosophila. *Proc Natl Acad Sci U S A,* 105, 14503-14508.

Desplats, P., Lee, H. J., Bae, E. J., Patrick, C., Rockenstein, E., Crews, L., Spencer, B., Masliah, E. and Lee, S. J. (2009) Inclusion formation and neuronal cell death through neuron-to-neuron transmission of alpha-synuclein. *Proc Natl Acad Sci U S A,* 106, 13010-13015.

Di Fonzo, A., Wu-Chou, Y. H., Lu, C. S. et al. (2006) A common missense variant in the LRRK2 gene, Gly2385Arg, associated with Parkinson's disease risk in Taiwan. *Neurogenetics,* 7, 133-138.

Farrer, M., Chan, P., Chen, R. et al. (2001) Lewy bodies and parkinsonism in families with parkin mutations. *Ann Neurol,* 50, 293-300.

Fortin, D. L., Troyer, M. D., Nakamura, K., Kubo, S., Anthony, M. D. and Edwards, R. H. (2004) Lipid rafts mediate the synaptic localization of alpha-synuclein. *J Neurosci,* 24, 6715-6723.

Funayama, M., Li, Y., Tomiyama, H. et al. (2007) Leucine-rich repeat kinase 2 G2385R variant is a risk factor for Parkinson disease in Asian population. *Neuroreport,* 18, 273-275.

Funayama, M., Li, Y., Tsoi, T. H. et al. (2008) Familial Parkinsonism with digenic parkin and PINK1 mutations. *Mov Disord,* 23, 1461-1465.

Gehrke, S., Imai, Y., Sokol, N. and Lu, B. (2010) Pathogenic LRRK2 negatively regulates microRNA-mediated translational repression. *Nature,* 466, 637-641.

Geisler, S., Holmstrom, K. M., Skujat, D., Fiesel, F. C., Rothfuss, O. C., Kahle, P. J. and Springer, W. (2010) PINK1/Parkin-mediated mitophagy is dependent on VDAC1 and p62/SQSTM1. *Nat Cell Biol,* 12, 119-131.

Gloeckner, C. J., Kinkl, N., Schumacher, A., Braun, R. J., O'Neill, E., Meitinger, T., Kolch, W., Prokisch, H. and Ueffing, M. (2006) The Parkinson disease causing LRRK2 mutation I2020T is associated with increased kinase activity. *Hum Mol Genet,* 15, 223-232.

Greenbaum, E. A., Graves, C. L., Mishizen-Eberz, A. J., Lupoli, M. A., Lynch, D. R., Englander, S. W., Axelsen, P. H. and Giasson, B. I. (2005) The E46K mutation in alpha-synuclein increases amyloid fibril formation. *J Biol Chem,* 280, 7800-7807.

Greene, J. C., Whitworth, A. J., Kuo, I., Andrews, L. A., Feany, M. B. and Pallanck, L. J. (2003) Mitochondrial pathology and apoptotic muscle degeneration in Drosophila parkin mutants. *Proc Natl Acad Sci U S A,* 100, 4078-4083.

Guo, J. T., Chen, A. Q., Kong, Q., Zhu, H., Ma, C. M. and Qin, C. (2008) Inhibition of vesicular monoamine transporter-2 activity in alpha-synuclein stably transfected SH-SY5Y cells. *Cell Mol Neurobiol,* 28, 35-47.

Hatano, T., Kubo, S., Imai, S., Maeda, M., Ishikawa, K., Mizuno, Y. and Hattori, N. (2007) Leucine-rich repeat kinase 2 associates with lipid rafts. *Hum Mol Genet,* 16, 678-690.

Hatano, T., Kubo, S., Sato, S. and Hattori, N. (2009) Pathogenesis of familial Parkinson's disease: new insights based on monogenic forms of Parkinson's disease. *J Neurochem,* 111, 1075-1093.

Hatano, Y., Sato, K., Elibol, B. et al. (2004) PARK6-linked autosomal recessive early-onset parkinsonism in Asian populations. *Neurology,* 63, 1482-1485.

Hawkes, C. H., Del Tredici, K. and Braak, H. (2007) Parkinson's disease: a dual-hit hypothesis. *Neuropathol Appl Neurobiol,* 33, 599-614.

Hernan, M. A., Takkouche, B., Caamano-Isorna, F. and Gestal-Otero, J. J. (2002) A meta-analysis of coffee drinking, cigarette smoking, and the risk of Parkinson's disease. *Ann Neurol,* 52, 276-284.

Ibanez, P., Bonnet, A. M., Debarges, B., Lohmann, E., Tison, F., Pollak, P., Agid, Y., Durr, A. and Brice, A. (2004) Causal relation between alpha-synuclein gene duplication and familial Parkinson's disease. *Lancet,* 364, 1169-1171.

Ihara, M., Yamasaki, N., Hagiwara, A. et al. (2007) Sept4, a component of presynaptic scaffold and Lewy bodies, is required for the suppression of alpha-synuclein neurotoxicity. *Neuron,* 53, 519-533.

Jensen, P. H., Nielsen, M. S., Jakes, R., Dotti, C. G. and Goedert, M. (1998) Binding of alpha-synuclein to brain vesicles is abolished by familial Parkinson's disease mutation. *J Biol Chem,* 273, 26292-26294.

Kawajiri, S., Saiki, S., Sato, S., Sato, F., Hatano, T., Eguchi, H. and Hattori, N. (2010) PINK1 is recruited to mitochondria with parkin and associates with LC3 in mitophagy. *FEBS Lett,* 584, 1073-1079.

Kitada, T., Asakawa, S., Hattori, N., Matsumine, H., Yamamura, Y., Minoshima, S., Yokochi, M., Mizuno, Y. and Shimizu, N. (1998) Mutations in the parkin gene cause autosomal recessive juvenile parkinsonism. *Nature,* 392, 605-608.

Kitada, T., Tong, Y., Gautier, C. A. and Shen, J. (2009) Absence of nigral degeneration in aged parkin/DJ-1/PINK1 triple knockout mice. *J Neurochem,* 111, 696-702.

Kordower, J. H., Chu, Y., Hauser, R. A., Freeman, T. B. and Olanow, C. W. (2008) Lewy body-like pathology in long-term embryonic nigral transplants in Parkinson's disease. *Nat Med,* 14, 504-506.

Kruger, R., Kuhn, W., Muller, T. et al. (1998) Ala30Pro mutation in the gene encoding alpha-synuclein in Parkinson's disease. *Nat Genet,* 18, 106-108.

Kubo, S., Nemani, V. M., Chalkley, R. J., Anthony, M. D., Hattori, N., Mizuno, Y., Edwards, R. H. and Fortin, D. L. (2005) A combinatorial code for the interaction of alpha-synuclein with membranes. *J Biol Chem,* 280, 31664-31672.

Langston, J. W. and Ballard, P. A., Jr. (1983) Parkinson's disease in a chemist working with 1-methyl-4-phenyl-1,2,5,6-tetrahydropyridine. *N Engl J Med,* 309, 310.

Langston, J. W., Forno, L. S., Tetrud, J., Reeves, A. G., Kaplan, J. A. and Karluk, D. (1999) Evidence of active nerve cell degeneration in the substantia nigra of humans years after 1-methyl-4-phenyl-1,2,3,6-tetrahydropyridine exposure. *Ann Neurol,* 46, 598-605.

Lee, V. M. and Trojanowski, J. Q. (2006) Mechanisms of Parkinson's disease linked to pathological alpha-synuclein: new targets for drug discovery. *Neuron,* 52, 33-38.

Lesage, S., Durr, A., Tazir, M., Lohmann, E., Leutenegger, A. L., Janin, S., Pollak, P. and Brice, A. (2006) LRRK2 G2019S as a cause of Parkinson's disease in North African Arabs. *N Engl J Med,* 354, 422-423.

Li, J. Y., Englund, E., Holton, J. L. et al. (2008) Lewy bodies in grafted neurons in subjects with Parkinson's disease suggest host-to-graft disease propagation. *Nat Med,* 14, 501-503.

Li, W., Hoffman, P. N., Stirling, W., Price, D. L. and Lee, M. K. (2004) Axonal transport of human alpha-synuclein slows with aging but is not affected by familial Parkinson's disease-linked mutations. *J Neurochem,* 88, 401-410.

Mata, I. F., Wedemeyer, W. J., Farrer, M. J., Taylor, J. P. and Gallo, K. A. (2006) LRRK2 in Parkinson's disease: protein domains and functional insights. *Trends Neurosci,* 29, 286-293.

Matsuda, N., Sato, S., Shiba, K. et al. (2010) PINK1 stabilized by mitochondrial depolarization recruits Parkin to damaged mitochondria and activates latent Parkin for mitophagy. *J Cell Biol,* 189, 211-221.

Miklossy, J., Qing, H., Guo, J. P., Yu, S., Wszolek, Z. K., Calne, D., McGeer, E. G. and McGeer, P. L. (2007) Lrrk2 and chronic inflammation are linked to pallido-ponto-nigral degeneration caused by the N279K tau mutation. *Acta Neuropathol,* 114, 243-254.

Miller, L. R., Mukherjee, S., Ansah, T. A. and Das, S. K. (2007) Cigarette smoke and dopaminergic system. *J Biochem Mol Toxicol,* 21, 325-335.

Mizuno, Y., Saitoh, T. and Sone, N. (1987) Inhibition of mitochondrial alpha-ketoglutarate dehydrogenase by 1-methyl-4-phenylpyridinium ion. *Biochem Biophys Res Commun,* 143, 971-976.

Mori, H., Kondo, T., Yokochi, M., Matsumine, H., Nakagawa-Hattori, Y., Miyake, T., Suda, K. and Mizuno, Y. (1998) Pathologic and biochemical studies of juvenile parkinsonism linked to chromosome 6q. *Neurology,* 51, 890-892.

Narendra, D. P., Jin, S. M., Tanaka, A., Suen, D. F., Gautier, C. A., Shen, J., Cookson, M. R. and Youle, R. J. (2010) PINK1 is selectively stabilized on impaired mitochondria to activate Parkin. *PLoS Biol,* 8, e1000298.

Narhi, L., Wood, S. J., Steavenson, S. et al. (1999) Both familial Parkinson's disease mutations accelerate alpha-synuclein aggregation. *J Biol Chem,* 274, 9843-9846.

Nieto, M., Gil-Bea, F. J., Dalfo, E. et al. (2006) Increased sensitivity to MPTP in human alpha-synuclein A30P transgenic mice. *Neurobiol Aging,* 27, 848-856.

Nishioka, K., Hayashi, S., Farrer, M. J. et al. (2006) Clinical heterogeneity of alpha-synuclein gene duplication in Parkinson's disease. *Ann Neurol,* 59, 298-309.

Ozelius, L. J., Senthil, G., Saunders-Pullman, R. et al. (2006) LRRK2 G2019S as a cause of Parkinson's disease in Ashkenazi Jews. *N Engl J Med,* 354, 424-425.

Paisan-Ruiz, C., Jain, S., Evans, E. W. et al. (2004) Cloning of the gene containing mutations that cause PARK8-linked Parkinson's disease. *Neuron,* 44, 595-600.

Park, J., Lee, S. B., Lee, S. et al. (2006) Mitochondrial dysfunction in Drosophila PINK1 mutants is complemented by parkin. *Nature,* 441, 1157-1161.

Perez, R. G., Waymire, J. C., Lin, E., Liu, J. J., Guo, F. and Zigmond, M. J. (2002) A role for alpha-synuclein in the regulation of dopamine biosynthesis. *J Neurosci,* 22, 3090-3099.

Polymeropoulos, M. H., Lavedan, C., Leroy, E. et al. (1997) Mutation in the alpha-synuclein gene identified in families with Parkinson's disease. *Science,* 276, 2045-2047.

Pramstaller, P. P., Schlossmacher, M. G., Jacques, T. S. et al. (2005) Lewy body Parkinson's disease in a large pedigree with 77 Parkin mutation carriers. *Ann Neurol,* 58, 411-422.

Przedborski, S. and Vila, M. (2003) The 1-methyl-4-phenyl-1,2,3,6-tetrahydropyridine mouse model: a tool to explore the pathogenesis of Parkinson's disease. *Ann N Y Acad Sci,* 991, 189-198.

Rideout, H. J., Larsen, K. E., Sulzer, D. and Stefanis, L. (2001) Proteasomal inhibition leads to formation of ubiquitin/alpha-synuclein-immunoreactive inclusions in PC12 cells. *J Neurochem,* 78, 899-908.

Satake, W., Nakabayashi, Y., Mizuta, I. et al. (2009) Genome-wide association study identifies common variants at four loci as genetic risk factors for Parkinson's disease. *Nat Genet,* 41, 1303-1307.

Schapira, A. H., Cooper, J. M., Dexter, D., Jenner, P., Clark, J. B. and Marsden, C. D. (1989) Mitochondrial complex I deficiency in Parkinson's disease. *Lancet,* 1, 1269.

Shiba, K., Arai, T., Sato, S., Kubo, S. I., Ohba, Y., Mizuno, Y. and Hattori, N. (2009) Parkin stabilizes PINK1 through direct interaction. *Biochem Biophys Res Commun.*

Shimura, H., Hattori, N., Kubo, S. et al. (2000) Familial Parkinson disease gene product, parkin, is a ubiquitin-protein ligase. *Nat Genet,* 25, 302-305.

Simon-Sanchez, J., Schulte, C., Bras, J. M. et al. (2009) Genome-wide association study reveals genetic risk underlying Parkinson's disease. *Nat Genet,* 41, 1308-1312.

Smith, W. W., Pei, Z., Jiang, H., Dawson, V. L., Dawson, T. M. and Ross, C. A. (2006) Kinase activity of mutant LRRK2 mediates neuronal toxicity. *Nat Neurosci,* 9, 1231-1233.

Smith, W. W., Pei, Z., Jiang, H., Moore, D. J., Liang, Y., West, A. B., Dawson, V. L., Dawson, T. M. and Ross, C. A. (2005) Leucine-rich repeat kinase 2 (LRRK2) interacts with parkin, and mutant LRRK2 induces neuronal degeneration. *Proc Natl Acad Sci U S A,* 102, 18676-18681.

Spillantini, M. G., Schmidt, M. L., Lee, V. M., Trojanowski, J. Q., Jakes, R. and Goedert, M. (1997) Alpha-synuclein in Lewy bodies. *Nature,* 388, 839-840.

Spira, P. J., Sharpe, D. M., Halliday, G., Cavanagh, J. and Nicholson, G. A. (2001) Clinical and pathological features of a Parkinsonian syndrome in a family with an Ala53Thr alpha-synuclein mutation. *Ann Neurol,* 49, 313-319.

Valente, E. M., Abou-Sleiman, P. M., Caputo, V. et al. (2004) Hereditary early-onset Parkinson's disease caused by mutations in PINK1. *Science,* 304, 1158-1160.

Vila, M., Vukosavic, S., Jackson-Lewis, V., Neystat, M., Jakowec, M. and Przedborski, S. (2000) Alpha-synuclein up-regulation in substantia nigra dopaminergic neurons following administration of the parkinsonian toxin MPTP. *J Neurochem,* 74, 721-729.

Vingerhoets, F. J., Snow, B. J., Tetrud, J. W., Langston, J. W., Schulzer, M. and Calne, D. B. (1994) Positron emission tomographic evidence for progression of human MPTP-induced dopaminergic lesions. *Ann Neurol,* 36, 765-770.

Vives-Bauza, C., Zhou, C., Huang, Y. et al. (2010) PINK1-dependent recruitment of Parkin to mitochondria in mitophagy. *Proc Natl Acad Sci U S A,* 107, 378-383.

West, A. B., Moore, D. J., Biskup, S., Bugayenko, A., Smith, W. W., Ross, C. A., Dawson, V. L. and Dawson, T. M. (2005) Parkinson's disease-associated mutations in leucine-rich repeat kinase 2 augment kinase activity. *Proc Natl Acad Sci U S A,* 102, 16842-16847.

West, A. B., Moore, D. J., Choi, C. et al. (2007) Parkinson's disease-associated mutations in LRRK2 link enhanced GTP-binding and kinase activities to neuronal toxicity. *Hum Mol Genet,* 16, 223-232.

Yamamura, Y., Sobue, I., Ando, K., Iida, M. and Yanagi, T. (1973) Paralysis agitans of early onset with marked diurnal fluctuation of symptoms. *Neurology,* 23, 239-244.

Yu, W. H., Matsuoka, Y., Sziraki, I., Hashim, A., Lafrancois, J., Sershen, H. and Duff, K. E. (2008) Increased dopaminergic neuron sensitivity to 1-methyl-4-phenyl-1,2,3,6-tetrahydropyridine (MPTP) in transgenic mice expressing mutant A53T alpha-synuclein. *Neurochem Res,* 33, 902-911.

Zarranz, J. J., Alegre, J., Gomez-Esteban, J. C. et al. (2004) The new mutation, E46K, of alpha-synuclein causes Parkinson and Lewy body dementia. *Ann Neurol,* 55, 164-173.

Zhang, N. Y., Tang, Z. and Liu, C. W. (2008) alpha-Synuclein protofibrils inhibit 26 S proteasome-mediated protein degradation: understanding the cytotoxicity of protein protofibrils in neurodegenerative disease pathogenesis. *J Biol Chem,* 283, 20288-20298.

Zimprich, A., Biskup, S., Leitner, P. et al. (2004) Mutations in LRRK2 cause autosomal-dominant parkinsonism with pleomorphic pathology. *Neuron,* 44, 601-607.

2

Genetics of Parkinson Disease

Celeste Sassi
[1]Laboratory of Neurogenetics, National Institute on Aging, National Institutes of Health, Bethesda,
[2]Department of Molecular Neuroscience and Reta Lila Weston Institute, UCL Institute of Neurology, London,
[1]USA
[2]UK

1. Introduction

Parkinson's disease (PD) is the second most common progressive neurodegenerative disorder second to Alzheimer's disease, affecting 1-2% of individuals over 60 years of age, with a risk that increases with age.

Its phenotypic complexity, characterized by motor (resting tremor, bradikinesia, rigidity and postural instability) and non-motor (autonomic dysfunction and cognitive impairment) symptoms lead to the description of this disorder as a syndrome rather than a monolithic disease. Genetic research in the past 10 years, in particular mapping and cloning of genes which cause the inherited form of the disease, has shown that "Parkinson syndrome" is not one disease entity but rather an atherogeneous group of disorders that are associated with a spectrum of clinical and pathological changes. It is believed to be caused by the interaction of environmental factors and genetic variants acting on the stage of an aging brain.

There is a growing body of evidence that genetic risk factors are of major importance in PD. So far 16 loci have been identified involved in PD.

PD can be referred mostly as sporadic (90-95%) and to a lesser extent as familial (5%)

Familial PD is caused by very rare highly age penetrant mutations, inherited in a Mendelian way (autosomal recessive or dominant). The biological effect of these mutations is sufficient alone for the development of the disease.

Sporadic PD is a complex multifactorial disease in which very common genetic variants play a very modest role singularly while taken all together, interacting with other genes and environmental factors, they can exert an important cumulative effect leading to the development of the disease.

In the last decade pathogenic mutations in five genes (*SNCA, LRRK2, PRKN, DJ-1* and *PINK1*) have been linked to familial PD. Recently genome wide association studies, GWAS, across different populations identified other 6 loci involved in the sporadic disease (*MAPT, SNCA, HLA-DRB5, BST1, GAK* and *LRRK2*). Finally a meta-analysis of the 5 previous GWAS discovered 5 new loci in association with the idiopatic disease (*ACMSD, STK39, MCCC1/LAMP3, SYT11* and *CCDC62/HIP1R*) (International Parkinson Disease Genomics Consortium, 2011)

2. Familial PD

Familial PD is monogenic and caused by rare highly age-dependent penetrant mutations, which follow a Mendelial pattern of inheritance (autosomal dominant or recessive).

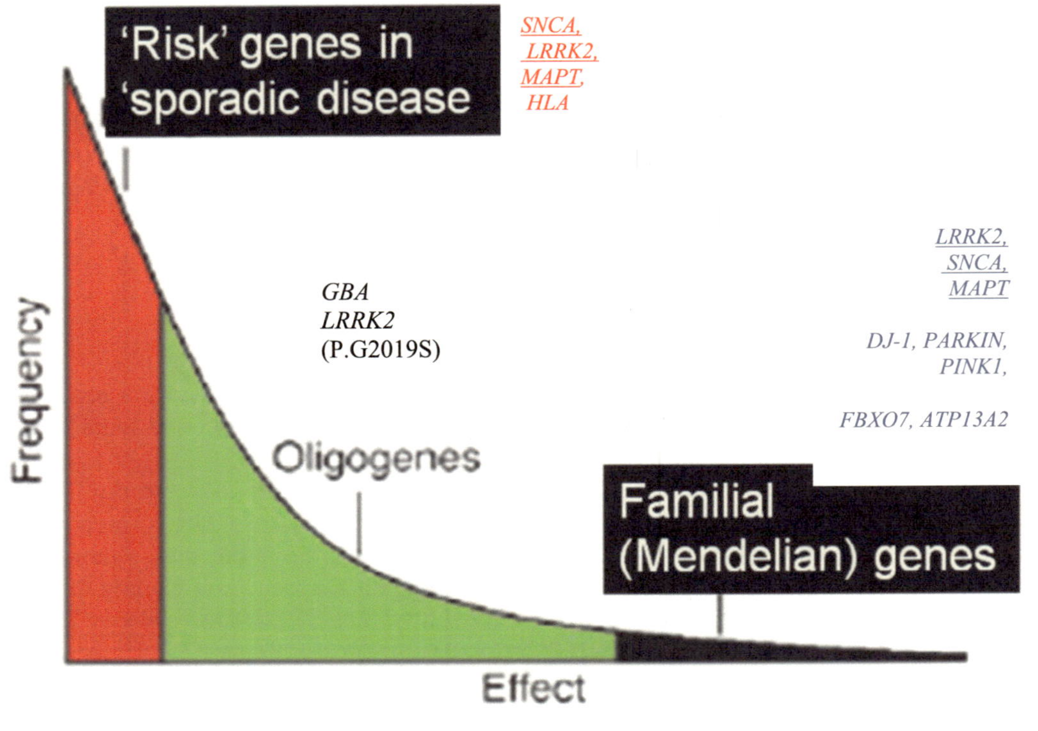

Fig. 1. The hyperbole descrives the relationship between the allelic frequency and the biological effect in the complex traits. The monogenic Mendelian forms are responsible for the familial Parkinson's disease, in which rare mutations can cause, independently from other factors, the disease, with a probability which increases with the age, due to the penetrance. The complex, poligenic, sporadic form is linked to risk factors which can be very common in the population but unable alone to determine the disease without interacting with other factors like genetic or environmental ones. Mutations in several familial (Mendelian) genes have been identified as causal factors for PD. Mutations in *LRRK2, SNCA, MAPT, UCHL1* determine the autosomal dominant disease while the recessive form is caused by mutations in *PARKIN, PINK1, DJ-1* and to a lesser extent *FBXO7* and *ATP 13A2*. Common variants in *SNCA, LRRK2, MAPT, HLA*, contribute to the development of the idiopatic disease. High-risk factors for the sporadic disease are mutations in *GBA* and *LRRK2* genes, especially among isolated populations like Ashkenazi Jews. Interestingly rare highly penetrant dominant mutations in *SNCA, LRRK2* and *MAPT* cause familial parkinsonian syndromes and common variants at the same loci increase susceptibility for PD in the general population.

Locus (chromosomal position)	Gene	inheritance, mutations	age at onset	mutations	clinical phenotype	pathology	comment
PARK1 and PARK4 4q21	Alpha-synuclein SNCA	Autosomal dominant	38-65 years (duplications) 28-48 years (triplications)	Ala30Pro, Gly46Lys and Ala53Thr substitutions; genomic duplications and triplications.	Progressive levo-dopa responsive parkinsonism, associated with cognitive decline, autonomic dysfunction and dementia: progression is more rapid in SNCA triplication cases	Diffuse Lewy bodies disease with prominent nigral and hippocampal (CA2-3) neuronal loss	Genetic and functional data indicated that common promoter and intronic variability are associated with sporadic PD
PARK2, 6q25.2-q27	parkin	Autosomal recessive	30 years on average (range 16-72)	Homozygous and compound heterozygous missense (>57) and exonic deletion/duplication/ triplication mutations	Parkinsonism often presenting with dystonia, with diurnal fluctuations and sleep benefit; typically responsive to very low doses of L-DOPA	Predominantly nigral neural loss, although compound heterozygotes with Lewy bodies and tau pathology are described	Mutations account for 50% of familial juvenile and early-onset parkinsonism, and 18% of sporadic disease (<50 years at onset)
PARK3, 2p13	unknown	Autosomal dominant	60 years			Nigral degeneration with Lewy bodies, plaques and tangles	
PARK5, 4p14	UCHL1	Autosomal dominant and sporadic PD	55-58 years (Ile93Met) Late onset	Linkage for the Ile93Met substitution is equivocal Susceptibility to sporadic PD is associated with a Ser18Tyr polimorphism	Sporadic PD	Indetermined for Ile93Met cases; UCHL1 protein is a prominent component of Lewy bodies	The Ser18Tyr association is supported by meta-analysis and functional data
PARK6, 1p35-p36	PINK1	Autosomal recessive	20-40 years	Missense and exon-deletion mutation	Parkinsonism that progresses slowly and is responsive to low doses of L-DOPA	Undetermined	Rare cause (1-2%) Haploisufficiency might predispose to the disease

Locus (chromosomal position)	Gene	inheritance, mutations	age at onset	mutations	clinical phenotype	pathology	comment
PARK7, 1p36	DJ1	Autosomal recessive	20-40 years	Homozygous missense (Leu166Pro) and deletion (del Ex1-5) mutations, and compound heterozygotes	Slowly progressive Parkinsonism, occasionally with behavioural or psychiatric disturbance; rare compound heterozygotes documented with parkinsonism with dementia or amyotrophy	Undetermined	Rare cause (<1%) of cases with onset at <50
PARK8, 12p12	LRRK2	Autosomal dominant and sporadic disease	Between 50 and 70 years (range 32-79)	Many domimant substitutions, notably Arg1441Cys/Gly/His, Tyr1699Cys, Ile2012Thr, Gly2019Ser and Ile2020Thr	Parkinsonism consistent with sporadic PD; dystonia, amyotrophy, gaze palsy and dementia occasionally develop	Heterogeneous pathologic findings: predominantly Lewy body disease; rare cases have also neurofibrillary tangles and/or nigral neural loss	Common coding variation might affect risk in sporadic PD
PARK9, 1p36	ATP13A2			unknown			
PARK10, 1p32	Unknown	Autosomal dominant	50-60 years			No pathology reported	
PARK11, 2q37.1	GIGYF2	Autosomal dominant	late		Parkinsonism consistent with sporadic PD	No pathology reported	
PARK12, Xq21-q25							
PARK13, 2p13	HTRA2						
PARK14, 22q13.1	PLA2G6						
PARK15, 22q12-q13	FBXO7	Autosomal recessive	20-40 years		Parkinsonian-pyramidal syndrome		
PARK16, 1q32	NUCKS1, RAB7L1 SLC41A1						

The classic approaches of linkage analysis and positional cloning have been very successful strategies to identify genes causing the autosomal-dominantly inherited diseases including the major forms of familial PD.
This strategy relies on the availability of large and clinically well-characterized families, usually with at least 8–10 affected family members. By studying the co-segregation of genetic (DNA)markers, the genetic locus of the disease-causing gene in a given family can be narrowed down to a region of several million base pairs (megabases, Mb) of DNA. The statistical method to estimate the likelihood that a particular set of neighbouring DNA markers (a so-called haplotype) are co-inherited with a disease gene as a result of its physical proximity on the chromosome (i.e. that DNA markers and disease gene are 'linked') is called linkage analysis. The most important prerequisite for this type of study, in addition to the availability of sufficiently large families, is the unequivocal classification of affected and unaffected family members. Erroneous classification, which in many age-related complex diseases is a real possibility, will lead to false linkage results (Gasser, 2008). When a disease locus is identified with sufficient confidence (a so-called lod score of >3 is equivalent to a genome-wide p.value of 0.05 and is considered to be significant evidence), all the genes in the identified region have to be sequenced and analysed for potentially disease-causing mutations. Of course, not all of the identified sequence variants in a linked region are pathogenic. This means that either the demonstration of mutations in several independent families co-segregating with a disease is necessary (amounting in effect to a replication of the initial finding) or the careful functional studies in model systems are required to prove pathogenicity.
Mutations in the genes *LRRK2* and *SNCA* are responsible for the autosomal dominant form of the disease through a gain of toxic function. Mutations in *PARKIN, PINK1* and *DJ-1* are the most common cause of the autosomal recessive form through a loss of protective function.

3. Autosomal dominant PD

3.1 SNCA (PARK1 and 4, 4p21)

It was the first gene to be inequivocally associated with familial autosomal dominant PD. It encodes for α-synuclein, a small protein, which is aboundantly expressed in the brain and localized mostly to presynaptic nerve terminals. This protein has a central role in the learning process, brain plasticity, vescicular trafficking and dopamine synthesis but many aspects of the normal function of alpha-synuclein are still unknown. There is still no good explanation for the selectivity of neural damage in PD, which is prominent in dopaminergic cells whereas α-synuclein is expressed in many areas of the brain.
Alpha synuclein plays a role in both familial and sporadic form of PD and for this reason can be an interesting target for the development of new therapies.
The protein is linked to the phospolipid membrane strate through the N-terminal edge and to a lesser extent it is free in the cytoplasm. It is hypothesized that a possible pathological role derives from a conformational change that lead to an imbalance between the protein linked to the membrane and that free in the cytoplasm, with a consequent aggregation and fibril formation.
Three missense mutations are causal factor for the familial autosomic dominant form of the disease

- A53T, identified within an Italian family and three Greek families (Polymeropoulous et al., 1997)
- A30P, identified in a German family (Krüger et al.,1998)
- E56K, identified within a Spanish family (Zarranz et al., 2004)

The pathogenic mechanism is supposed to be a conformational change due to the amminoacid substitution in the protein chain, which facilitates α-synuclein aggregation. Clinically, the phenotype is more aggressive with an higher incidence of cognitive impairment and autonomic disfunction. *SNCA* point mutations have so far been found only in large, multigenerational PD families, never in sporadic PD. The phenotype of patients with *SNCA* point mutations is that of L-dopa responsive parkinsonism with a relatively early age at onset, rapid progression, and high prevalence of dementia, psychiatric and autonomic disturbances, reminiscent of Lewy body dementia. Several family members from these kindreds have come to autopsy and they invariably showed cell loss of dopaminergic neurons of the substantia nigra, and severe and widespread Lewy pathology, particularly in the form of Lewy neuritis. The identification of *SNCA* point mutations as a cause of PD soon led to the discovery that the encoded protein, a-synuclein, is the major fibrillar component of Lewy bodies and Lewy neuritis in familial as well as sporadic cases. The currently favoured hypothesis settles that the ammoniacid changes within alpha-synuclein lead to an increased tendency of the protein to form oligomers and later on fibrillar aggregates, representing a 'toxic gain of function'. However, the precise sequence of events which lead from aggregation to cellular dysfunction and cell death is still not obvious. Some studies favour the hypothesis that the mature aggregates (Lewy bodies) are not themselves the toxic moiety, but rather an attempt to the cell to clear small toxic oligomers. A direct link between α-synuclein and PD was further supported by the discovery that multiplications of the wild-type sequence of *SNCA* (duplications and triplications) (Singleton et al., 2003) cause PD with or without dementia in some families. This finding was of major mechanicistic importance because indicates that an increase in wild-type a-synuclein protein expression appears to be toxic to neurons. A dose dependency of this effect is demonstrated by the fact that patients with *SNCA* triplications (4 copies of the gene) have an early age of onset (mean of around 35 years) and high prevalence of dementia, while patients with *SNCA* duplications (3 copies) have a more typical late-onset PD phenotype.

The presence of α-synuclein-containing aggregates in the absence of coding *SNCA* mutations in sporadic disease suggest that other α-synuclein modifications, such as alternative splicing, phosporylation,, alterations in gene expression, or additional interacting genes may contribute to sporadic PD.

Then interaction of α-synuclein with proteins aggregating in other neurodegenerative diseases is coming increasingly into focus. 'Cross-seeding' of α-synuclein and tau has been hypothesized by a recent study. Interestingly this molecular mechanism may turn out to be the biological basis of the recently confirmed and refined association of *MAPT* haplotypes with PD and of an interaction of genetic variants in the *SNCA* and *MAPT* genes.

3.2 LRRK2 (PARK8, 12p21)

The gene spans a genomic region of 144 Kb, with 51 exons encoding LRRK2 or Dardarin, a 2527 amino acids protein, with various conserved domains recognized in its primary ammino-acid sequence. More than 40 variants have been identified in the gene and at least 16 of them are recognized as pathogenic ones. Missense mutations in this gene were found

to cosegregate with the disease in several families and are the most common cause of mendelian PD identified so far. In studies across several populations, 5–15% of autosomal dominant PD families carried mutations in *LRRK2*. One particularly common mutation, a base pair change at position 6055,better known as the 'G2019S-mutation', is responsible for familial PD in up to 7% of cases in different Caucasian populations , but was found, somewhat surprisingly, also in 1–2% of sporadic patients. Even higher G2019S prevalence rates of up to 40%were found in genetically isolated populations,such as the Ashkenazi Jewish and the North-African Arab populations, both in sporadic and familial cases. P.G2019S is the most common mutation among Caucasian patients and it is responsible for the 0.5-2% of the cases of the sporadic disease and for the 5% of the familial cases. This mutation is particularly frequent among the Askenazi Jews and the Arabs from North Africa, where it is responsible for 18-30% of the cases. The substitution has been identified also in the Iberian Peninsula, where it is involved in the 2.5-65% of the cases of the sporadic disease. It seems that the mutation has been originated in North Africa or in the Middle East and probably later it has been spread to Europe and Northern America. It has also been hypothesized a common founder for the p.G2019S substitution probably dated back to the 13th Century. The presence of the mutation in the Middle East and in North Africa lead to guess that the mutation should be even more older. The Fenices were known to be the principal merchants of the ancient world and probably they were responsible for the diffusion of this substitution.
Due to its relatively high frequency, the p.G2019S mutation offers for the first time the possibility of looking at gene-gene interactions. Three Spanish patients simultaneously harbouring heterozygous mutations in *LRRK2* and in the parkin gene did not present with an earlier age at onset or a more severe disease. The G2019S mutation also seems to be fully dominant, as homozygous mutation carriers have been identified who also do not differ from heterozygotes with respect to disease severity or age of onset.
Another, even more common *LRRK2* variant, G2385R, has been found in the Asian population in 6–10% of sporadic PD patients, as opposed to 3–5% of controls. Consequently, this variant confers a relative risk of about 2 to 3 of developing PD,suggesting that different alterations in one and the same gene may act as a high-penetrance disease-causing mutation or as a genetic risk variant in sporadic populations.To date, more than 20 potentially pathogenic mutations in *LRRK2* have been identified, but in only six of them pathogenicity can be considered to be highly likely (R1441C, R1441G,R1441H, Y1699C, G2019S and I2020T), because of firm evidence of cosegregation in affected families and functional data suggesting an alteration of kinase activity.The most extensive clinicogenetic study so far estimated the overall frequency of *LRRK2* mutations in the European population to be 1.5%in sporadic and 4%in familial cases, with a geographic gradient decreasing from Mediterranean countries (Spain, Portugal, Italy) to northern countries. The average age of onset was 58 years, with a wide range from the mid-20s (rarely) to over 90 years. The clinical picture was that of typical asymmetric L-dopa responsive parkinsonism that was indistinguishable by any single criterion from PD in individuals without *LRRK2* mutations. As a group, the disease appeared to be somewhat more benign in patients with mutations in *LRRK2*, with slower progression and a lower frequency of dementia and psychiatric complications.
In contrast to the finding that α-synuclein stains Lewy bodies and tau stains neurofibrillary tangles and grains, LRRK2 immunocytochemistry has so far failed to highlight any specific,

neurodegenerative lesion , and it is unclear how LRRK2 substitutions result in neuropathology. *LRRK2* mutations may therefore be an upstream event in the cascade leading to neurodegeneration with different pathologies.

LRRK2 is widely expressed in the brain, with highest levels in the striatum and the hippocampus but a relatively low abundance in the substantia nigra; it can also be detected in other organs, such as the spleen, the lung and the liver. It has been found in the cytoplasm as well as associated with membranes. Its function and the mechanism by which LRRK2 mutations cause neuronal degeneration are unknown. By sequence homology, LRRK2 can be assigned to the group of recently identified ROCO proteins and contains a protein kinase domain of the mitogen-activated kinase class, suggesting a role in intracellular signalling pathways. Although the natural substrate of LRRK2 is unknown, cell culture studies using generic substrates or LRRK2 autophosphorylation paradigms suggested that at least some pathogenic mutations seem to be associated with an increase, rather than a loss, of kinase activity, and that kinase activity appears to be necessary for neurotoxicity in vitro. This discovery raises the interesting possibility that kinase inhibition may be a potential therapeutic strategy. An interesting aspect of LRRK2-associated PD is its heterogeneous pathology. Post-mortem changes in patients with *LRRK2* mutations are those of typical Lewy-body PD in most cases, but also include diffuse Lewy-body disease, nigral degeneration without distinctive histopathology and, rarely, even aggregates of the microtubule-associated protein tau, suggestive of progressive supranuclear palsy or frontotemporal dementia. Different pathological findings were even reported in a single family with an R1441C mutation. *LRRK2* mutations may therefore be an upstream event in the cascade leading to neurodegeneration with different pathologies. However, the vast majority of patients with a G2019S mutation, in whom pathology has been reported, seem to conform to the typical α-synuclein Lewy-body type of PD. No direct link between LRRK2 and α-synuclein has so far been demonstrated. α-synuclein does not seem to be phosphorylated by LRRK2.

Despite its still poorly understood role in pathogenesis, LRRK2-associated PD is of particular interest since it is the first example of a mendelian form of PD that is common enough to provide the opportunity to study the development of the disease in a sizeable population. Longitudinal studies in presymptomatic mutation carriers may reveal premotor changes by clinical, biochemical or imaging methods, indicating the very early phases of the neurodegenerative process. It is in this population that studies exploring neuroprotective or preventive measures are most promising to yield first results

3.3 UCHL1 (Park 5, 4p14)

The ubiquitin C-terminal hydrolase-L1 (*UCH-L1*) was first identified as an abundant (1–2% of total brain protein), neuronspecific protein encoded by a 9.5 kb gene product (Day and Thompson, 1987; Doran et al., 1983). UCH-L1 is a de-ubiquitinating enzyme that removes carboxy-terminal ubiquitin *UCH-L1* from substrates but does not break bonds within polyubiquitin complexes and results in the recycling of ubiquitin. In addition,UCHL1 protein is found in several pathological structures including Lewy bodies and some Alzheimer's neurofibrillary tangles (Lowe et al., 1990). Furthermore, recent studies have identified a single dominant mutant (I93M) in two members of a PD-affected family. Inversely, a polymorphism in *UCH-L1* (S18Y) has

been suggested to reduce the risk of developing sporadic PD. Interestingly, another study hypothesizes that UCHL1 may possess two enzymatic activities, hydrolase and ligase activity. Overexpression of UCH-L1 variant I93M resulted in an accumulation of α-synuclein. Furthermore, they suggest that this accumulation is due to an ubiquitination of α-synuclein by dimerized UCH-L1. However, the S18Y polymorphic variant of UCH-L1 has reduced ligase activity but normal hydrolase activity,
which may explain the 'protective' effect of the S18Y polymorphism. With evidence of UCH-L1 and parkin being involved in certain forms of familial PD, this gives credence to the involvement of the UPS in PD. However, it is unclear how UCH-L1 can promote the specific neurodegeneration of dopaminergic neurons in familial PD and what role it plays in the sporadic form.

4. Autosomal recessive PD

The strategies of linkage mapping and positional cloning can also be used to identify loci in genes responsible for autosomal-recessive monogenic diseases. This mode of inheritance is characterized typically by the occurrence of the disease in siblings while the parents are obligatory heterozygous mutation carriers and usually remain healthy. Autosomal-recessive PD has clinically been first recognized and characterized in Japan (Ishikawa and Tsuji, 1996). Sibling pairs with PD often have much earlier age of onset compared with patients with the sporadic disease, which is why the term 'autosomal-recessive juvenile parkinsonism'(AR-JP): has been coined. Since families with a recessive disease are usually much smaller than multigenerational dominant pedigrees, linkage analysis is only successful if several families mapping to the same locus are included into a study.
So far, mutations in three genes have been identified in clinically 'pure' forms of autosomal recessive PD: *PARKIN* (PRKN, or PARK2), *PINK1* (PARK6) and *DJ-1*(PARK7). *PRKN* encodes for parkin, a cytoplasmatic protein which functions in the cellular ubiquitination/protein degradation pathway as an ubiquitin ligase. *DJ-1* and *PINK1* encode for mitochondrial proteins. Genetics mutations in these genes cause PD through the loss of the wild-type protein neuroprotective function, leading to oxidative stress, iron accumulation and mitochondrial dysfunction.
They cause PD with earlier onset (<45 years) and slower progression compared to idiopatic PD. Three additional recessive genes have been added to the list more recently-*ATP13A2*, *PLA2G6* and *FBXO7*- which all also cause, when mutated, an early-onset disease with parkinsonism, but also with additional features such as dystonia, which often is seen as the first symptom, dementia, oculomotor disturbances and spasticity.

4.1 PARKIN (PARK2, 6q25.2-q27)

Juvenile cases of parkinsonism in siblings were first recognized in Japan. The first genetic locus for autosomal- recessive juvenile parkinsonism (AR-JP), as this form of PD was called, was mapped to chromosome 6.
Mutations were then identified in a large gene in that region that was called parkin. Clinically, these patients suffer from L-dopa-responsive parkinsonism and often develop early and severe L-dopa-induced motor fluctuations and dyskinesias. Some show diurnal fluctuations, with symptoms becoming worse later in the day. Dystonia at onset of the disease is common. *Parkin* mutations turned out to be a common cause of parkinsonism

with early onset, particularly in individuals with evidence of recessive inheritance. Nearly 50% of families from a population of sibling pairs with PD had *parkin* mutations. Also, *parkin* mutations are responsible for the majority of sporadic cases with very early onset (before age 20), and are still common (25%) when onset is between 20 and 35. Prevalence is almost certainly well below 5% in those with onset later than 45. Several studies have described the clinical spectrum of *parkin*-associated parkinsonism. Mean age at onset in a European population was 32 years; progression of the disease was usually relatively slow, but L-dopa-associated fluctuations and dyskinesias occurred frequently. Dystonia (usually in a lower extremity) at disease onset was found in about 40% of patients, and brisk reflexes of the lower limbs were present in 44%. Psychiatric abnormalities have been recognized in PD patients with *parkin* mutations but there are no systematic studies to determine whether this is a characteristic feature associated with *parkin*-mutations. Phenotype– genotype studies implicate that the type of mutation may influence the clinical phenotype to a certain degree: patients with at least one missense mutation showed a faster progression of the disease with a higher UPDRS (United Parkinson's Disease Rating Scale) motor score than carriers of truncating mutations. Missense mutations in functional domains of the *parkin* gene resulted in earlier onset. It is still controversial whether heterozygous mutations in the *parkin* gene can cause parkinsonism or can confer an increased susceptibility for typical late-onset PD. There is evidence from imaging studies that heterozygous carriers of *parkin* mutations have reduced uptake of fluorodopa in the basal ganglia. Furthermore, families with heterozygous mutation carriers manifesting symptoms of PD have been described. On the other hand, the frequency of heterozygous mutations in the *parkin* gene was found to be similar in elderly healthy individuals, as compared to a cohort with late-onset typical PD and in a large family reported recently, 12 heterozygous carriers of a particular *parkin* mutation (ex3delta40) were asymptomatic. Also, in a group of families with PD showing anticipation (late-onset PD in the parent generation and early-onset PD in the offspring) genotyping results did not support the explanation that the presence of single or compound heterozygous *parkin*-mutations contribute to this phenomenon. Therefore, at present the data are still insufficient to confidently judge the role of single heterozygous *parkin* mutations in the development of PD. Knowledge on the neuropathology of molecularly confirmed cases of AR-JP is still based on only a few cases. Severe and rather selective degeneration of neurons in the substantia nigra and the locus coeruleus, usually with absence of Lewy bodies, has been described.

As mutations in *parkin* cause parkinsonism, in all likelihood by a loss-of-function mechanism, the study of the normal function of parkin provides insight into the molecular pathogenesis of the disorder. Several groups have now shown that parkin, a protein found in the cytosol but also associated with membranes, functions in the cellular ubiquitination/protein degradation pathway as a ubiquitin ligase. It has been hypothesized that the loss of parkin function may lead to the accumulation of a nonubiquitinated substrate that is deleterious to the dopaminergic cell but, due to its nonubiquitinated nature, does not accumulate in typical Lewy bodies. Several proteins have been shown to interact with parkin. However, the putative toxic protein, which has been hypothesized to accumulate due to the lack of *parkin* in patients (or in knock-out animals) has not yet been identified. However, novel functions of *parkin* are being identified, and it is possible that they may be of equal or even greater relevance to the pathogenesis of PD. For example, it has been shown that parkin does not only mediate the well-studied ubiquitinylation via lysin48 (K48), which directs ubiquitinylated proteins for proteasomal degradation, but also via lysin63 (K63), which may play a role intracellular signaling processes and also in Lewy body formation. A recent study revealed a decreased abundance of a number of proteins involved in mitochondrial function or oxidative stress, accompanied by a reduction in respiratory capacity of striatal mitochondria, a decreased serum antioxidant capacity and increased protein and lipid peroxidation These novel findings indicate that proteasomal dysfunction, although supported by several lines of evidence, might not be the sole mechanism contributing to neurodegeneration in *parkin*-related disease. Whatever the mechanism, increasing evidence suggests an important role of *parkin* for dopamine neuron survival. Overexpression of wildtype rat parkin could protect against the toxicity of mutated human A30P α-*SYN* in a rat lentiviral model of PD. The *parkin* mediated neuroprotection was associated with an increase in hyperphosphorylated α-*SYN* inclusions, suggesting a key role for parkin in the genesis of Lewy bodies. Recently, two biochemical modifications of Parkin (*S*-nitrosylation and dopamine quinine-adduct formation) were identified in cellular studies and human brain specimens. These data indicated that reduced E3-ligase activity of the wild-type Parkin protein (rather than an autosomal recessive mutation in the two *Parkin* alleles) could also occur as a result of the principal pathogenetic process that is responsible for the development of sporadic PD.

4.2 PINK1 (PARK6, chr.1p35-1p36)

The new locus was identified in a large Italian family and it causes familial recessive PD in 1-9% of the cases. The phenotype was similar to that seen with *PRKN* mutations and characterised by early-onset parkinsonism (range 32 to 48 years), with slow progression and sustained response to L-dopa. In this and two other consanguineous PARK6- linked families, two different mutations in the gene *PINK1* (encoding PTEN-induced putative kinase 1) were identified. Several studies confirmed the presence of *PINK1* mutations in patients with early-onset PD. Most mutations were missense mutations in conserved regions, but whole-gene deletions have also been described. Almost all described patients with *PINK1* mutations have slow disease progression and a good response to L-dopa. As in *PRKN* related disease, except for the earlier average age of onset, no single feature can separate *PINK1*-related disease from idiopathic PD. There are some indications that *PINK1*-mutated patients have a higher prevalence of psychiatric disturbances, particularly anxiety and depression, which is only relatively rarely observed in *PRKN*-related cases . Wild-type PINK1 is thought to function as a protein kinase with possible activity inside the mitochondria, thereby strengthening the hypothesized link between mitochondrial dysfunction and oxidative stress in PD pathogenesis.

4.3 DJ-1 (PARK7, chr.1p36)

The third locus for AR-JP, PARK7, was mapped also to chromosome 1p36, in a Dutch family, and the gene was identified as the oncogene *DJ-1*. Again, the phenotype closely resembles that found in patients with *PRKN* and *PINK1* mutations, but this statement is based on a small number of identified patients.Mutations in the gene are responsible for 1-2% of the AR-JP. However, one recessive family, which carries two homozygous mutations in the *DJ-1* gene, has been described with early-onset parkinsonism, dementia and amyotrophic lateral sclerosis, suggesting that the clinical phenotype associated with mutations in this gene, although rare, may be rather wide.

There are now eight recessive loci, which can lead to EOPD syndromes. These are the classical recessive loci, *PRKN* (PARK2), *PINK1* (PARK6), *DJ-1* (PARK7). Loss of function mutations at *PRKN, PINK1,* and *DJ-1* nearly always give rise to a pure parkinsonian phenotype which has an early onset, a benign course, sleep benefit and a good and prolonged response to L-dopa. The lifespan of mutation carriers is only marginally reduced and there have been no reports of brain iron accumulation. All three proteins have functions related to mitochondrial biology and *PRKN* mutations are usually not associated with Lewy bodies. More recently, five other genes, *ATP13A2* (PARK9), *PLA2G6* (PARK14), *FBX07* (PARK15) and *SPG11* and the *PANK2*, have been identified that cause early-onset forms of parkinsonism associated with a variety of other signs and symptoms, including, in variable combinations, dystonia, ataxia, spasticity and dementia.

4.4 ATP13A2 (PARK9, 1p36)

It was the first of these genes to be characterized, encoding a predominantly neuronal P-type ATPase, in a recessively inherited early-onset parkinsonian syndrome described as 'Kufor- Rakeb syndrome' . Patients with this disease have rapidly progressive parkinsonism, spasticity, vertical upgaze palsy and dementia. The substrate and function of the protein is unknown. The wild-type protein was found to be located in the lysosome of transiently transfected cells, while the unstable truncated mutant proteins were retained in the endoplasmic reticulum and degraded by the proteasome. It can be speculated that either overload of the proteasomal protein degradation machinery or lysosomal dysfunction due to the absence of sufficient levels of ATP13A2 protein might lead to neurodegeneration. In fact, there is increasing evidence for an important role of the lysosome in the aetiology of PD: α-synuclein is degraded by chaperone mediated autophagy, and mutations in the gene encoding lysosomal glucocerebrosidase are an important cause of PD. Nevertheless, a direct involvement of the lysosome in the neurodegenerative process in Kufor-Rakeb syndrome and its potential bearing for PD remains speculative at this time

4.5 PLA2G6 (PARK14, 22q13.1)

Another interesting addition to the recessive genes causing parkinsonian syndromes that may give important insight into underlying pathogenetic processes is the gene for phospholipase A2 group VI (*PLA2G6*). Mutations in this gene have been identified in two recessive childhood-onset disorders: infantile neuroaxonal dystrophy (INAD) and neurodegeneration with brain iron accumulation (NBIA). There is brain iron accumulation in some patients with INAD, so when gene mapping identified a common locus in families with these disorders on chromosome 22, it was reasonable to suspect that the disorders may be allelic. In fact, a large number of mutations were identified, including missense changes, small deletions with and without frameshift, nonsense mutations and large deletions. As patients with two null mutations tended to have the most severe phenotype, a loss of function mechanism can be assumed. Interestingly, in addition to axonal swellings throughout the cortex, striatum, cerebellum, brainstem and spinal cord, the pathological picture also includes a-synuclein positive Lewy bodies, and thus these disorders share this important pathological feature with PD. Lewy bodies are also found in another form of neurodegeneration with brain iron accumulation (NBIA type 1; formerly called Hallervorden–Spatz disease), caused by mutations in the gene for pantothenate kinase 2 (*PANK2*). Therefore, there seems to be an interesting but still little understood link between iron accumulation (which is also found in PD proper), a-synuclein aggregation, and neurodegeneration with parkinsonian symptoms.While the 'classic' phenotype of NBIA types 1 and 2 is that of a young-onset progressive extrapyramidal-pyramidal syndrome with visual disturbance through optic atrophy or pigmentary retinopathy, mutations in both genes can be associated with a parkinsonian syndrome of later onset. Recently, *PLA2G6* mutations have been identified in patients with adult-onset L-dopa-responsive dystonia–parkinsonism, pyramidal signs and cognitive/psychiatric features, and cerebral and cerebellar atrophy on magnetic resonance imaging but lack of iron in the basal ganglia.

4.6 FBXO7 (PARK15, 22q12-q13)

Finally, mutations in a novel and still poorly characterised gene, *FBXO7*, have been found in members of two families with early-onset, progressive parkinsonism and pyramidal tract signs, a phenotype that had been described clinically as the pallidopyramidal syndrome. Loss of function mutations in *FBX07* appear to give a phenotype which resembles *PRKN* mutation associated phenotype but the disease is generally less benign and has a reduced life expectancy, pyramidal signs and late cognitive problems. This overlap of phenotypes related to *FBX07* and *PRKN* mutations is consistent with the related functions of these two genes and their likely common disease pathway. Like PRKN, F-box proteins, such as FBXO7, are components of the modular E3 ubiquitin protein ligases. The genetic heterogeneity was surprising given their initially common clinical features

5. Role of heterozygous mutations in 'recessive' genes

A considerable percentage of patients with PD was shown to carry a single heterozygous mutation in the *Parkin*, *DJ1* or *PINK1* genes, raising the intriguing question of whether the much more frequent heterozygous mutations in 'recessive' genes might act as susceptibility factors for PD. Several ways lead to explore the potential role of these mutations. First, the frequency of single heterozygous mutations in ethnically matched PD cases and controls could be compared. According to recent reports, heterozygosity for *Parkin* mutations was similar between patients and controls, whereas heterozygous *PINK1* mutations were rarer in controls. Lincoln *et al.* indicated that there was no elevation in PD risk for people who carry a single mutant *Parkin* allele. In most studies, however, healthy controls are not subjected to detailed neurological and neuroimaging examinations, leaving open the possibility that mild clinical (or preclinical) changes could have been present but were not screened for. As recently shown for *Parkin* and *PINK1* families, subtle, but unequivocal, clinical signs of possible or probable PD can be found on careful motor examination in a considerable number of the heterozygous mutation carriers who consider themselves asymptomatic. Furthermore, it could be argued that at least some of the controls had not yet reached the age of their disease onset. Second, the heterozygous offspring of homozygous or compound heterozygous mutation carriers could be examined in a prospective manner, an approach that is currently being used in several cohorts. The probability that a second mutation might have been overlooked in these carriers is much lower than the probability of a mutation being missed in sporadic cases of PD. Last, further functional studies of the affected allele carriers would be highly valuable. Haploinsufficiency, leading to a functional loss of heterozygosity or a dominant-negative effect of some mutant alleles, could explain why a second mutation cannot (and need not) be found for some mutations in the above-mentioned recessive genes. Although the role of heterozygous mutations in the development of clinical signs currently remains a matter for debate, there is growing evidence that they are associated with pre clinical changes. PET studies have revealed reduced [18F]fluoro-dopa uptake by nerve terminals in the striatum of heterozygotes; there are also structural neuroimaging changes that indicate an increased deposition of metals in the substantia nigra, and there is reorganization of striatocortical motor loops with detectable changes in connectivity patterns.These collective data have important implications. Some carriers of heterozygous mutations might be in the preclinical period of PD, thereby affording unique opportunities to examine the relative risk associated with the affected allele and to study the natural history of the disease. This group also represents an ideal study population to be used not only to investigate compensatory mechanisms, facilitating the development of a sensitive surrogate marker, but also to detect the earliest PD-specific changes, allowing the development of urgently needed clinical biomarkers. Finally, these individuals could provide a small, but important, target population in which to evaluate the 'proof of principle' of a therapeutic intervention in future neuroprotection trials.

6. Sporadic PD

Sporadic PD is multifactorial, complex and polygenic, generally determined by several common non-coding genetic variants, each of them play a role as a very modest risk factor singularly but with an important cumulative effect taken all together, interacting with environmental factors, other genes or functional variants, controlling the expression, splicing, phosphorylation, influencing the age at onset, severity and progression of the syndrome.
Association studies have been widely used in an attempt to identify common genetic variations that carry a mild to moderately increased risk to develop a disease. Over the years, literally hundreds of studies have been published, but unfortunately, only very few of them have produced robust and reproducible results. Several are the reasons which can justify the failure of this approach: most studies were greatly underpowered in relation to the small increases in the relative risk that today are known to be conferred by common genetic variants (usually the odds ratios are in the range of 1.2–2, with some exceptions, for example apolipoprotein E for AD). Then the choice of candidate genes was often based on rather arbitrary rationales with very weak experimental or epidemiologic evidence. As the gene-mapping studies in monogenic diseases have shown, newly identified genes most often could not have been predicted based on the current knowledge of pathogenesis. Furthermore in most studies only arbitrarily chosen individual genetic variants were investigated, thus it was a priori unlikely that the causative variant or a variant in high linkage disequilibrium, tagging the risk-conferring variant, would be among those studied. Finally, it is not easy to match patient and control cohorts with respect to their genetic background. Often, due to different recruiting strategies, these cohorts differ in their genetic composition (a problem called undetected population stratification, which today can be easily resolved in GWAS, see below). Due to different allele frequencies in different populations, spurious associations can be detected.
In the idiopatic cases an attempt is made to evaluate the PD population as a whole, using association studies and non parametric linkage methodology and trying to define risk alleles that contribute to the sporadic form of the disease.

Common genetic variants in *SNCA* can increase the susceptibility for idiopatic PD, while the *LRRK2* p.G2019S mutation can cause sporadic PD. Recently GWAS discovered new genes associated with PD: *GBA, MAPT, GAK, BST1, HLA, LONGO1*and *LONGO2, PARK16, SYNPHILIN.*

6.1 SNCA (PARK1-4, 4q21)

Previous studies have found associations between Parkinson's disease and polymorphisms located within both the α-synuclein gene promoter and other gene regions. Particularly interesting is a complex polymorphic dinucleotide repeat polymorphism (NACP-REP1), located 10 kb upstream of the transcriptional start site of *SNCA*. In this case the number of dinucleotide repeats are directly linked to an higher risk to develop PD. Indeed the 263 haplotype is associated to the disease while the 259 one has a protective effect.
The *SNCA* gene consists in two haplotype blocks (genetic regions usually inherited as a single block, with a high degree of Linkage disequilibrium). The first block ranges from the promoter region to intron 4 while the second block includes exons 5 and 6 and the 3'-untraslated region. The second block gives the strongest association signal with PD. Becasuse the SNP variability is noncoding and not within a region of species-conserved sequence identity or a miRNA binding site, the biologic mechanism remain unclear. Alternative splicing, phosporilation, expression modification or even linkage disequilibrium with another functional variant within the gene have been hypothesized as possible mechanisms. Gene expression may also be influenced by epigenetic interactions, including methylation, recently implicated in the downregulation of *SNCA* gene expression, which may warrant further investigation.

6.2 LRRK2 (PARK8,12q12)

Even if mutation in *LRRK2* are the most common cause of familial autosomal dominant PD, the p.G2019S substitution is of special significance as it is frequently identified not only in autosomal dominant, but also sporadic PD. Thus, being the most common cause of PD. The mutation is particularly frequent in PD patients residing in, or having genealogical ties to North Africa or the Middle East. This phenomenon can be explained by the fact that most *LRRK2* p.G2019S substitution carriers originate from a common founder.

6.2.1 The LRRK2 c.6055G>A (p.G2019S) mutation

P.G2019S is located in the mitogen-activated protein kinase (MAP) domain of the LRRK2 protein. The identification of p.G2019S substitutions as the most common cause of both familial and sporadic PD has been a major breakthrough. The frequency of p.G2019S substitutions differ remarkably throughout the world. This is due to a common founder for most p.G2019S carriers, originating from the Middle East or North Africa. Two large studies on Lrrk2 p.G2019S parkinsonism conclude that the phenotype of Lrrk2 p.G2019S can not be distinguished from idiopathic PD. There are some indications of a more benign course of p.G2019S parkinsonism compared to idiopathic PD with a slower disease progression and less cognitive impairment. However, methodological issues may have contributed to these observations. The penetrance of Lrrk2 p.G2019S has been much debated over the last years. Hulihan et al. investigated sporadic PD in Tunisia and found a lifetime penetrance of 45% (95% CI: 20–100%) for p.G2019S substitution carriers. Healy et al. additionally included hereditary patients and estimated that 74% had PD by age 79 years. Interestingly, homozygous p.G2019S carriers do not have more severe disease than heterozygous carriers, this lack of gene-dose effect is consistent with the hypothesis that the p.G2019S substitution increases kinase activity. The pathology of p.G2019S parkinsonism is consistent with LBD in most, but not all cases.

6.3 GBA (1q21)

GBA is responsible to cause Gaucher Disease, GD, when the mutation is present in homozigosity. Patients with GD and relatives have an increased susceptibility for PD (2-3 fold), susceptibility which can increase among different populations like Ashkenazi Jews (5-6 fold), when the mutation in the gene is present in heterozigosity. *GBA* encodes a lysosomal enzyme that cleaves glucocerebroside. As α-synuclein is in part degraded by chaperone-mediated lysosomal pathway, it is conceivable that *GBA* mutations may increase the risk for PD by altering cellular α-synuclein homeostasis. It is supposed that the pathologic effect is due to the lack of the physiologic function or gain of a toxic one. Neuropathologically, Lewy bodies are present in the hippocampal region, corresponding to Braak stages 5 and 6, indicating that the dementia can be very similar to Lewy bodies dementia. Phenotipically GBA mutations carriers present the clinical features of sporadic PD with an higher and more severe incidence of dementia, olphactory disfunction, bradikinesia and a lower frequency of rigidity.

6.4 MAPT (17q21.1)

MAPT, encodes for the microtubule associated protein tau. Risk alleles of the associated SNPs are in LD with the H1 haplotype. An association between *MAPT* locus and PD could seem surprising, given the classic separation of synucleinopathies and tauopathies but the role of *MAPT* in neurodegenerative diseases is well established and this association is biologically plausible, despite the lack of neuropathology in PD. The combination of risk variants in *MAPT* and *SNCA* doubles the risk of developing PD, supporting the idea that related pathways contribute to neurodegenerative diseases. Finally, although we do not understand the relationship between the *MAPT* locus and Parkinson disease, it is worth remembering that while *LRRK2* mutations usually give rise to a-synuclein pathology, they sometimes give rise to tangle pathology (Zimprich et al., 2004) and that, while *MAPT* mutations usually give rise to tangle pathology, they sometimes give rise to Lewy body pathology.

An association to *MAPT* is absent in the Asian population.

6.5 GAK (4p16)

GAK (cyclin G associated kinase, a cell cycle regulator) is a serine thereonine kinase. It is a particularly promising candidate because it is one of 137 genes shown to be differentially espressed in PD, with an 1.56 fold change in expression in the substantia nigra pars compacta of PD patients compared to controls. Protective role postulated: decreased in expression or depletion enhance alpha-synuclein toxicity.

6.6 BST1 (4p15)

BST1(bone marrow stromal cell antigen) catalyses the formation of cyclic ADP-ribose (cADPR). cADPR mobilizes calcium (Ca2+) from ryanodine sensitive intracellular Ca2+, stored in the endoplasmic reticulum. Distruption of the Ca2+ homeostasis has recently been proposed of a possible cause of selective vulnerability of dopaminergic neurons in PD. Associated SNPs in the *BST1* region may modify ADP-ribosylcyclase activity, thus leading to Ca2+ dyshomeostasis in dopaminergic neurons.

6.7 HLA (HLA-DRA; HLA-DQ;HLA-DR (6p21.3)

The *HLA* variant that displayed the strongest statistical association with Parkinson's disease, rs3129882, is a noncoding polymorphism in intron 1 of *HLA-DRA*. The protein chains encoded by the closely linked *HLA-DRA* and *HLA-DRB* form the class II HLA-DR antigens that are expressed by antigen-presenting cells, including microglia in the brain, and which interact with T-cell receptors. HLA-DRB chains are highly variable and have been associated with numerous disorders, including multiple sclerosis, which, like Parkinson's disease, is a progressive neurodegenerative disorder. HLA-DRA, on the other hand, is practically monomorphic and therefore has not been investigated for disease association. The conventional explanation for this finding is that PD is associated with a classical polymorphic HLA antigen and that rs3129882 is a proxy for this antigen. Alternatively, the association of Parkinson's disease with an intronic *DRA* variant may reflect involvement of regulatory elements, which would be in line with Parkinson's disease–specific overexpression of DR antigens in substantia nigra. The evidence for genetic association of PD with HLA region, particularly when obtained from a hypothesis free-GWAS, where the entire genome is scanned without pre-existing bias towards any particular genes, lends strong and independent support to the involvement of neuroinflammation and humoral immunity in Parkinson's disease pathogenesis. Studies have shown elevated DR expression in the brain and cerebrospinal fluid of individual with PD. The sustained presence of reactive DR positive microglia has been observed in the substantia nigra of individuals with PD, as well as animals and humans affected with 1-methyl-4-phenyl-1,2,3,6,-tetrahydropiridine-induced (MPTP) parkinsonism. It is postulated that chronic immune activation and neuroinflammation occurs in response to an initial trigger, possibly related to alpha-synuclein accumulation, and produces neurotoxins and oxidative damage that could kill neurons. From a therapeutic perspective, vaccination aimed neutralizing neuroimmune dysfunction was recently shown to attenuate neurodegeneration in a Parkinson's disease model: further, NSAID use is associated with reduced reduced risk of developing PD in humans. The newly discovered association of PD with HLA region highlights the involvement of an important biological pathway in the etiology of the disease and point to a potential drug target that will stimulate research toward new therapies.

6.8 LINGO1 and LINGO2 (15q24.3)(9p21.2)

A significant overlap between the diagnoses of PD and essential tremor (ET) is frequently observed. In retrospective analyses, 6-20% of ET patients have been described to exhibit signs of Parkinsonism. A recent prospective study demonstrated that patients with ET have a four-fold elevated risk to develop PD over an observational period of 3.3 years. Conversely, a diagnosis of ET was proposed to be 5 to 10 times more likely in subjects with PD than in controls. Furthermore it has been demonstrated that the risk of ET in first-degree relatives of patients with PD is significantly elevated. A neuropatholgical study demonstrated the occurrence of Lewy bodies in the brainstem in an older subset of ET patients. Genetic variation in the leucine-rich repeat and Ig domain containing Nogo receptor interacting protein1, (LINGO1) and its paralog (LINGO2) was recently associated with an increased risk of developing essential tremor (ET) and Parkinson's disease (PD). LINGO1 plays a role in early brain development and oligodendrocyte differentiation. Because of its presumed role in neural survival and myelination, LINGO1 has been targeted in vivo and in vitro in model of spinal cord injury, autoimmune encephalitis and PD.

6.9 PARK16(1q32)

The PARK16 region contains five functionally interesting candidate genes for PD etiology. *SLC41A1* is a magnesium (Mg2+) transporter. It is of interest that Mg2+ deficiency is thought to be an environmental risk factor for the amyotrophic lateral sclerosis (ALS)-parkinsonism/dementia complex. Furthermore, *RAB7L1* is a small GTP-binding protein that plays an important role in regulation of exo-and endocytotic pathways, and *NUCKS1* is a nuclear protein containing several consensus phosphorylation sites for casein kinase II and cyclin-dependent kinases of unknown function.

Although pathogenic mutations and risk alleles within the PARK16 locus seem to be rare in European ancestry populations, further molecular analyses within different populations are required to examine its biochemical role in PD.

6.10 Synphilin

The presynaptic protein synphilin 1 and its isoform 1A have been associated with PD. Synphilin is an interactor of α-synuclein and is modulated by parkin. Synphilin is widely expressed with highest levels in brain, heart and placenta.

6.11 Omi/HtrA2 (PARK 13, 2p12)

In vitro and *in vivo* studies strongly implicate loss of Omi/HtrA2 protein in disrupted mitochondrial homeostasis and subsequent cell death. Moreover, recent pathoanatomical studies indicate that Omi/HtrA2 represents a consistent pathological marker for neurodegeneration in different α-synucleinopathies (Kawamoto et al.,2008). Loss of Omi/HtrA2 function may contribute to a broader spectrum of neurodegeneration, as decreased levels of Omi/HtrA2 were demonstrated in brains of Huntington's disease patients. Therefore, while some genetic association studies provide no consistent support for an association of *Omi/HtrA2* and PD, functional studies suggest that further study of this gene in the context of neurodegenerative disorders is justified. We cannot exclude the possibility that other neurodegenerative diseases besides PD may be influenced by *Omi/HtrA2* variations.

Recent discoveries from meta-analysis study of previous GWAS, identified 11 loci that surpassed the threshold for genome-wide significance (p<5x10(-8)). Six were already known loci (*MAPT, SNCA, HLA-DRB5, BST1, GAK* and *LRRK2*) and 5 were newly identified loci (*ACMSD, STK39, MCCC1/LAMP3, SYT11* and *CCDC62/HIP1R*) (International Parkinson's Disease Genomic Consortium, 2011)

ACMSD is involved in picolinic and quinolinic acid homoeostasis and is a possible therapeutic target for several disorders that affect the CNS. The locus identified near *STK39* has been associated with autism and infl ammatory status, although there have been no reports of this locus contributing to neurodegenerative phenotypes. The *LAMP3* locus might modulate neurosecretory function in PC12 cell lines.

HLA-DRB5 is involved in multiple sclerosis, immunocompetence, and histocompatibility. The association with Parkinson's disease at *HLA-DRB5* supports the theory that inflammatory factors are associated with the pathogenesis of PD.

7. Pathogenic pathways

Familial and sporadic PD present similar clinical features, which reinforce the hypothesis that common pathways might be at the basis of a so analogous phenotype. Generally dystonia appears as the first symptom in the familial cases, while gait impairment and postural instability are one of the first manifestation for the sporadic ones. Evidence is emerging that some of the pathways covered in the rare monogenic forms of PD: dysfunction or impairment of the ubiquitin-proteosome system and/or mytochondria, may play a direct role in the etiology of the common sporadic disorder and genetic variation contribute to the risk of developing PD.

So far, the proteins that have been linked to parkinsonism by genetic studies have roles in:

- mitochondrial function (α-synuclein, *PARKIN, PINK1, DJ-1, FBXO7, Omi/HtrA2, POLG1*)
- lysosome (*GBA, ATP13A2*)
- the ubiquitin–proteosome system (*PARKIN* and *UCHL1*)
- vescicle dynamics (α-synuclein),
- MAPKKK signaling (*LRRK2*),
- oxidative stress
- microtubule stability (*MAPT*)
- embryonic development (α-synuclein, *PARKIN, UCHL1, LRRK2, Omi/HtrA2, NURR1, PITX3*)

These disparate functions might overlap as they all lead to the age-associated dysfunction and death of dopaminergic neurons that characterize PD. However, the relationships between these functions are not direct and the connections between them are not immediately evident.

7.1 Mitochondrial dysfunction (α-synuclein, *PARKIN*, *PINK1*, *DJ-1*, *FBXO7*, *POLG1*, *Omi/HtrA2*)

The pathway that has come most clearly out of the analysis of the Mendelian genes is a mitochondrial damage repair pathway. α-synuclein has long been known to modulate mitochondrial function, but the mechanism remains unknown. A possible role in mitochondrial signaling has been hypothesized. Parkin enhances transcription and replication of mitochondrial DNA in proliferating cells. Furthermore, Parkin, an E3 ubiquitin ligase, and PINK1, a mitochondrial kinase, are involved in the elimination of damaged mitochondria. DJ-1, and possibly FBX07, another ubiquitin ligase, are also likely to play a role in the mitochondrial pathway. DJ-1 can protect the cell against oxidative stress and can also translocate to the mitochondria. (Cookson 2010). The similar phenotype can confirm a common role of these genes in the mitochondrial pathway (Paisan-Ruiz et al., 2010; Valente et al., 2004;Yamamura 2010).

POLG1 is a mitochondrial DNA polymerase (Polymerase gamma 1) of the inner membrane that synthesizes, replicates and repairs mitochondrial DNA. Several mutations within POLG1 have been associated with parkinsonism in addition to other clinical phenotypes.

HtrA2 also known as Omi (HtrA2/Omi) is serine protease localized to the inner membrane space of mitochondria. A variation within Omi (G399S) was found in four patients with late-

onset PD and a polymorphism (A141S) has been suggested to be a risk factor in Germans. Furthermore, a possible implication has been demonstrated by animal models: knocking out Omi in mice leads to neurodegeneration with features of motor neuron dysfunction, ataxia and parkinsonism with striatal damage.
In addition MPTP can damage in a selective way dopamine neurons and mitochondria causing parkinsonism. (Langston 1989).

7.2 Lysosome pathway (*GBA*, *ATP13A2*)

A second pathway that is likely to be involved in Parkinson disease clearly involves the lysosomes. Proteins with short half-lives are mostly degraded by the proteasome whereas most cytosolic proteins with half lives longer than 10 hours are degraded by the autophagy- lysosome pathway. Glucosecerebrosidase, GBA, and ATP13A2 are lysosomal enzymes. A role of GBA protein in PD is suggested by the clinical observation of association of PD with Gaucher's disease. Patients with this well characterized recessive neurometabolic disease, caused by mutation in the glucocerebrosidase gene (*GBA*) have a high prevalence of PD. Screening of PD patients for *GBA* mutations found a higher number of heterozygous mutations carriers as compared to healthy controls. *GBA* encodes a lysosomal enzyme that cleaves glucocerebroside. As α-synuclein is in part degraded by chaperone-mediated lysosomal pathway, it is possible that *GBA* mutations may increase the risk for PD by altering cellular α -synuclein homeostasis. Within the chaperone-mediated lysosomal uptake pathway α-synuclein binds lysosomal membrane receptors before being selectively translocated into the lysosome. Mutant α-synuclein also binds to receptors, but instead of being translocated sufficiently blocks not only its own uptake but also uptake of other substrates. Mutations in ATP13A2, a lysosomal ATPase, cause autosomal-recessive early onset PD further linking lysosomes to neurodegeneration

7.3 Ubiquitin proteosome pathway (*PARKIN*, *UCHL1*)

The ubiquitin proteasome pathway has been strongly implicated in PD pathogenesis. *Parkin* functions as an E3 ubiquitin ligase. Some disease causing mutations within parkin impair its ligase activity leading to intracellular accumulation of parkin substrates. Accumulation of potentially toxic proteins might be especially detrimental for vulnerable neurons like dopaminergic neurons. Furthermore a missense mutation has been described in *UCHL1*, a deubiquitylating enzyme. The I93M substitution decreases UCHL1 enzymatic activity in vitro. Deubiquitylation is an important process to recycle ubiquitin monomers from proteins that have been targeted to the proteasome. In addition overexpressed wildtype or mutant α-synuclein has been shown to inhibit proteasome function in vitro and in vivo, even if not directly involved in the proteosomal pathway.

7.4 Embryonic development (α-synuclein, *PARKIN*, *UCHL1*, *LRRK2*, *Omi/HtrA2*, *NURR1*, *PITX3*)

α-synuclein is important not only in brain but also in peripheral tissues during normal human prenatal development. From 15 to 23 gestational weeks α-synuclein is expressed in almost all fetal human organs while in adult human tissues an high alpha-synuclein expression can be observed only in the brain.

Parkin expression is correlated with cell maturation and implicates a physiological role of parkin in various types of neurons. *UCHL1* is highly expressed in cultured NPCs (neural progenitor cells) as well as in embryonic brain in general. UCHL1 has been shown to be involved in regulating morphology of NPCs and in mediating neurogenesis. Involvement of *LRRK2* in neurite outgrowth might explain high expression levels in the first two or three weeks after birth. *Omi/HtrA2* is found in various fetal tissues. Loss of Omi/HtrA2 (mouse mutant mnd2, motor neuron degeneration2) leads to muscle wasting, neurodegeneration, involution of the spleen and thymus, and death by 40 days of age. Since dopaminergic neurons have long been central to PD research and genes involved in development of these cells deserve special attention. Dominant mutations in *Nurr1* have been reported in families with late onset PD. Nurr1, a member of the nuclear receptor superfamily of transcription factors is critically involved in the development of ventral midbrain dopaminergic neurons. Mutations within *Nurr1* have not been found again, association studies turned out to be negative in most studies. In addition (mice deficient for *PITX3*), a homeobox transcription factor, which is expressed from E11 to adulthood, fail to develop dopaminergic neurons of the substantia nigra . Taken together several PD associated genes are expressed during development. The potential involvement of these genes in early stages of the disease remains to be determined. Additionally PD is by no means restricted to dopaminergic neurons. It will be of great interest to identify genes with involvement in developmental stages of several cell types affected in PD.

Numerous working models have been proposed to integrate the complexities of environmental, biochemical, genetic and neuropathological evidence. However, a more simplicistic model of PD pathogenesis depicts a progressive imbalance between the forces that promote degeneration of at risk neurons by increasing mitochondrial dysfunction and oxidative stress during the aging process, and those that encompass individual or integrated cellular-defense mechanism.

Genetic therapy should move forward, aiming to restabilize the balance between these antagonist forces: enhancing the neuroprotective ones (*PRKN, DJ-1, PINK1*) and/or stopping and silencing potentiallty harmful effects ones (*SNCA, LRRK2*)

8. Pathological mechanisms in neurodegenerative diseases

Parkinson's disease is a progressive neurodegenerative disease which shares genetic influences and pathways with other neurodegenerative diseases like Alzheimer's disease (AD). Specifically, common pathways involve protein aggregation and neuroinflammatory process.

Several lines of investigation have now converged to show that the etiologies of AD and PD share common mechanisms (Bossy-Wetzel et al., 2004). One of the commonalities between AD and PD is the extra and intracellular accumulation of protein aggregates rich in β-pleated sheet conformation, representing the hallmarks of these two slowly progressive neurodegenerative disorders. Such protein aggregates might arise, in part, as a consequence of impaired proteasomal and/or autophagic removal of the damaged proteins (Taylor et al., 2002; Bence et al., 2001). The conformational change that results in the accumulation of misfolded proteins – amyloid-β (Aβ) and tau in AD and α-synuclein in PD – is associated with progressive dysfunction and death of cells in selected brain areas, determining clinical presentation. The intermediate forms of pathogenic proteins such as oligomers and protofibrils are thought to have cytotoxic effects on neurons. There is considerable overlap in the mechanisms by which oligomeric Aβ and α-synuclein damage and kill neurons that may include: oxidative stress and free radical formation, impaired bioenergetics and mitochondrial dysfunction, disruption of neuronal Golgi apparatus and transport, molecular chaperones, neurotrophins and "neuroinflammatory" processes.

While variability in several genes may influence the risk for developing one disease, single genes often affect the risk for more than one trait. This diversity is best exemplified by variability in the tau and alpha-synuclein (*SNCA*) proteins, which alter risk of PD (*MAPT* and *SNCA*), progressive sopranuclear palsy corticobasal degeneration (*MAPT*), and multiple system atrophy (*SNCA*).

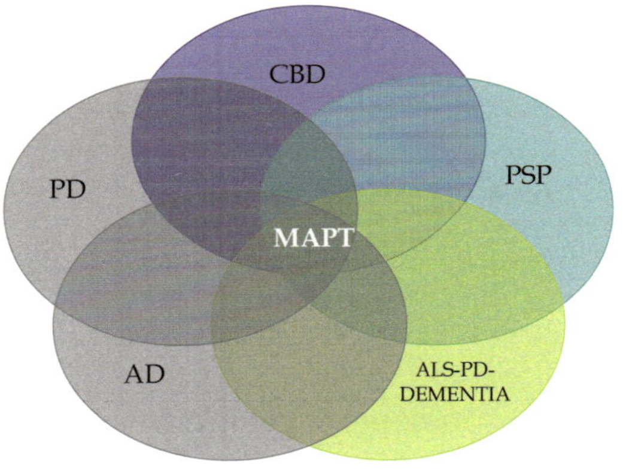

Fig. 2. Mutations and variants in the *MAPT* gene, encoding for tau protein, are involved in several neurodegenerative diseases, tauopathies: progressive sopranuclear palsy, PSP, corticobasal degeneration, CBD, Alzheimer disease, AD, Als-PD-dementia complex of Guam and Parkinson's disease.

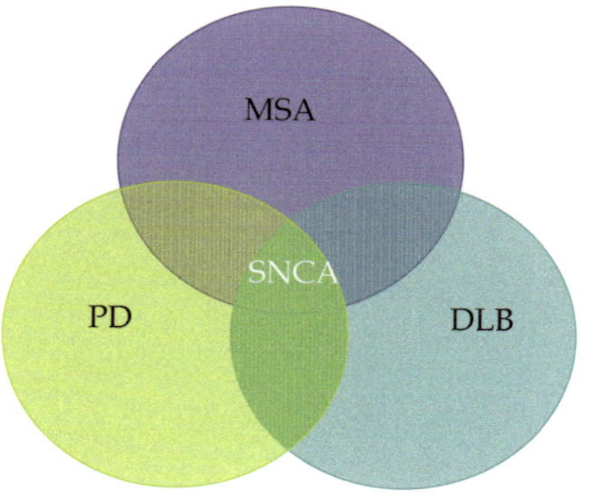

Fig. 3. Mutations and variations in the *SNCA* gene, encoding for α-synuclein, are involved in several neurodegenerative diseases, synucleinopathies: Parkinson's disease, PD, Multi system atrophy, MSA, Dementia with Lewy Bodies, DLB

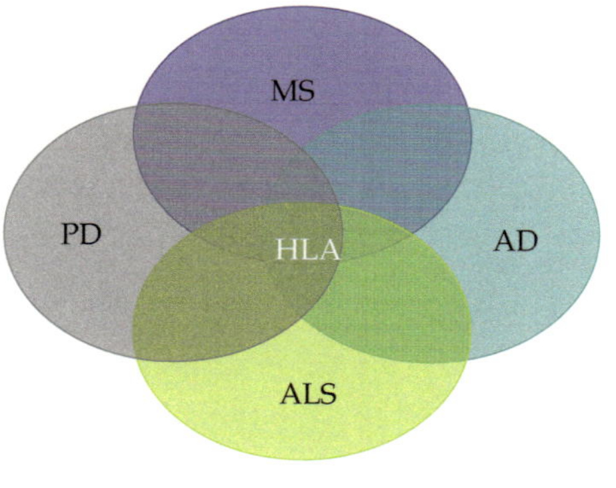

Fig. 4. Variations in the *HLA*, the major histocompatibility complex gene, are involved in several neurodegenerative diseases: Parkinson's disease, PD, Alzheimer disease, AD, Multiple sclerosis, MS, Amiotrofic Lateral Sclerosis, ALS.

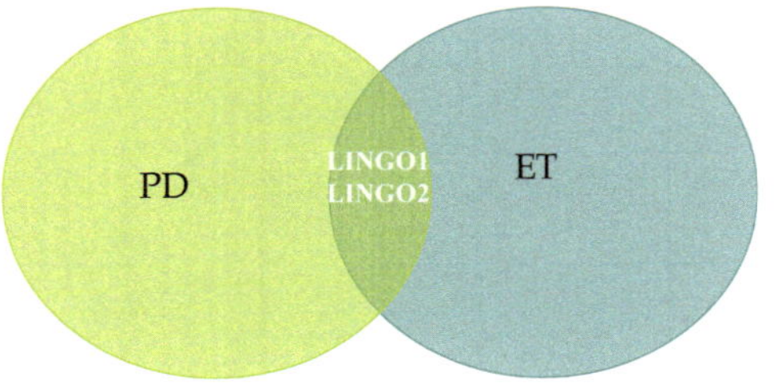

Fig. 5. Variations in *LINGO1* and *LINGO2* are risk factors for Parkinson's disease, PD, and essential tremor, ET.

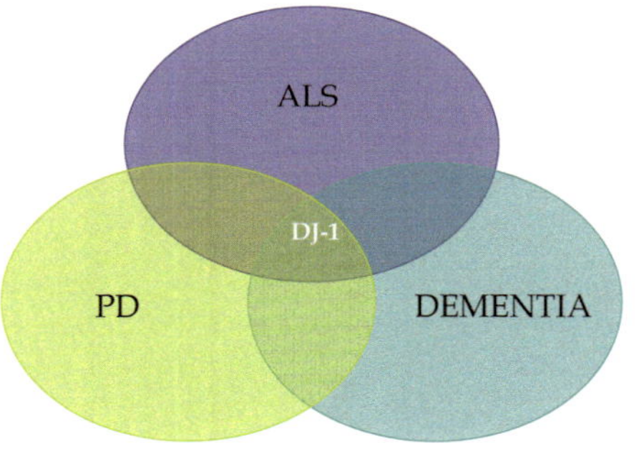

Fig. 6. Mutations in *DJ-1* can be involved in several neurodegenerative diseases: Parkinson's disease, PD, dementia and Amyotrophic Lateral Sclerosis, ALS.

Ultimately, a joint GWA study of a pooled population of individuals with Alzheimer's disease and Parkinson's disease might be a powerful approach to identify common genetic susceptibility factors for these diseases. One interesting model is that tau acts as a downstream factor involved in both β-amyloid and α-synuclein toxicity, with neurofibrillary tangles only forming in the presence of amyloid. Therefore, β-amyloid and α-synuclein might reinforce each other's effect on neurodegeneration in the aging population, and the relative proportions of each pathology could correlate with the extent of dementia or parkinsonism, respectively. Recent studies suggest that environmental factors may contribute to neurodegeneration through the induction of epigenetic modifications, such as DNA methylation, and chromatin remodeling, which may induce alterations in gene expression programs. Epigenetics, which refers to any process that modifies gene activity without changing the actual DNA sequence, and leads to modifications that can be transmitted to daughter cells, is a relatively novel area of research that is currently attracting a high level of interest. Epigenetic modulation is present since the prenatal stages, and the aging process is now accepted to be associated with a loss of phenotypic plasticity to epigenetic modifications. Since aging is the most important risk factor for idiopathic AD and PD, it is expected that epigenetic alterations on DNA and/or chromatin structure may also accumulate during neurodegeneration, explaining to some extent the etiology of these chronic and progressive disorders.

9. References

Abou-Sleiman, P. M., Healy, D. G., Quinn, N., Lees, A. J., & Wood, N. W. (2003). The role of pathogenic DJ-1 mutations in Parkinson's disease. Annals of Neurology, 54(3), 283-286.

Aharon-Peretz, J., Rosenbaum, H., & Gershoni-Baruch, R. (2004). Mutations in the glucocerebrosidase gene and Parkinson's disease in Ashkenazi Jews. The New England Journal of Medicine, 351(19), 1972-1977.

Berg, D., Niwar, M., Maass, S., Zimprich, A., Moller, J. C., Wuellner, U., et al. (2005). Alpha-synuclein and Parkinson's disease: Implications from the screening of more than 1900 patients. Movement Disorders, 20(9), 1191-1194.

Berg, D., Schweitzer, K., Leitner, P., Zimprich, A., Lichtner, P., Belcredi, P., et al. (2005). Type and frequency of mutations in the LRRK2 gene in familial and sporadic Parkinson's disease. Brain, 128(Pt 12), 3000-3011.

Bonifati, V., Rizzu, P., Van Baren, M. J., Schaap, O., Breedveld, G. J., Krieger, E., et al. (2002). Mutations in the DJ-1 gene associated with autosomal recessive early-onset parkinsonism. Science, 299, 256-259.

Conrad, C., Andreadis, A., Trojanowski, J. Q., Dickson, D. W., Kang, D., Chen, X., et al. (1997). Genetic evidence for the involvement of tau in progressive supranuclear palsy. Annals of Neurology, 41(2), 277-281.

Conway, K. A., Lee, S. J., Rochet, J. C., Ding, T. T., Williamson, R. E., & Lansbury, P. T.Jr, (2000). Acceleration of oligomerization, not fibrillization, is a shared property of both alpha-synuclein mutations linked to early-onset Parkinson's disease: Implications for pathogenesis and therapy. Proceedings of the National Academy of Sciences of the United States of America, 97(2), 571-576.

Cookson, M. R., & van der Brug, M. (2007). Cell systems and the toxic mechanism(s) of alpha-synuclein. Experimental Neurology, 290(1), 5–11.

Dehghan, A., Kottgen, A., Yang, Q., Hwang, S. J., Kao, W. L., Rivadeneira, F., et al. (2008). Association of three genetic loci with uric acid concentration and risk of gout: A genomewide association study. Lancet, 372(9654), 1953–1961.

De Marco, E. V., Annesi, G., Tarantino, P., Rocca, F. E., Provenzano, G., Civitelli, D., et al. (2008). Glucocerebrosidase gene mutations are associated with Parkinson's disease in southern Italy. Movement Disorders, 23(3), 460–463.

Denson, M. A., & Wszolek, Z. K. (1995). Familial parkinsonism: Our experience and a review of the literature. Parkinsonism & Related Disorders, 1(1), 35–46.

Derkatch, I. L., Uptain, S. M., Outeiro, T. F., Krishnan, R., Lindquist, S. L., & Liebman, S. W. (2004). Effects of Q/Nrich, polyQ, and non-polyQ amyloids on the de novo formation of the [PSIþ] prion in yeast and aggregation of Sup35 in vitro. Proceedings of the National Academy of Sciences of the United States of America, 101(35), 12934–12939.

Dickson, D. W., Lin, W., Liu, W. K., & Yen, S. H. (1999). Multiple system atrophy: A sporadic synucleinopathy. Brain Pathology, 9(4), 721–732.

Di Fonzo, A., Rohe, C. F., Ferreira, J., Chien, H. F., Vacca, L., Stocchi, F., et al. (2005). A frequent LRRK2 gene mutation associated with autosomal dominant Parkinson's disease. Lancet, 365(9457), 412–415.

Dodson, M. W., & Guo, M. (2007). Pink1, Parkin, DJ-1 and mitochondrial dysfunction in Parkinson's disease. Current Opinion in Neurobiology, 17(3), 331–337.

Duda, J. E., Giasson, B. I., Mabon, M. E., Miller, D. C., Golbe, L. I., Lee, V. M., et al. (2002). Concurrence of alpha-synuclein and tau brain pathology in the Contursi kindred. Acta Neuropathologica (Berl), 104(1), 7–11.

Elstner, M., Morris, C. M., Heim, K., Lichtner, P., Bender, A., Mehta, D., et al. (2009). Single-cell expression profiling of dopaminergic neurons combined with association analysis identifies pyridoxal kinase as Parkinson's disease gene. Annals of Neurology, 66(6), 792–798.

Farrer, M., Gwinn, K., Muenter, M., DeVrieze, F. W., Crook, R., Perez Tur, J., et al. (1999). 4p haplotype segregating with familial Lewy body parkinsonism. Movement Disorders, 13 (Suppl. 2), 253–253.

Farrer, M. J., Stone, J. T., Lin, C. H., Dachsel, J. C., Hulihan, M. M., Haugarvoll, K., et al. (2007). Lrrk2 G2385R is an ancestral risk factor for Parkinson's disease in Asia. Parkinsonism & Related Disorders, 13(2), 89–92.

Fuchs, J., Nilsson, C., Kachergus, J., Munz, M., Larsson, E. M., Schule, B., et al. (2007). Phenotypic variation in a large Swedish pedigree due to SNCA duplication and triplication. Neurology, 68(12), 916–922.

Fuchs, J., Tichopad, A., Golub, Y., Munz, M., Schweitzer, K. J., Wolf, B., et al. (2008). Genetic variability in the SNCA gene influences alpha-synuclein levels in the blood and brain. The FASEB Journal, 22(5), 1327–1334.

Funayama, M., Hasegawa, K., Kowa, H., Saito, M., Tsuji, S., & Obata, F. (2002). A new locus for Parkinson's disease (PARK8) maps to chromosome 12p11.2-q13.1. Annals of Neurology, 51(3), 296–301.

Fung, H. C., Scholz, S., Matarin, M., Simon-Sanchez, J., Hernandez, D., Britton, A., et al. (2006). Genome-wide genotyping in Parkinson's disease and neurologically normal controls: First stage analysis and public release of data. Lancet Neurology, 5(11), 911-916.

Gasser, T. (2008). Hunting for genes and mutations: It's worth remembering the basics. Neurology, 70(16 Pt 2), 1373-1374.

Gasser, T. (2009a). Mendelian forms of Parkinson's disease. Biochimica et Biophysica Acta, 1792(7), 587-596.

Gasser, T. (2009b). Molecular pathogenesis of Parkinson disease: Insights from genetic studies. Expert Reviews in Molecular Medicine, 11, e22.

Gilks, W. P., Abou-Sleiman, P. M., Gandhi, S., Jain, S., Singleton, A., Lees, A. J., et al. (2005). A common LRRK2 mutation in idiopathic Parkinson's disease. Lancet, 365(9457), 415-416.

Gloeckner, C. J., Kinkl, N., Schumacher, A., Braun, R. J., O'Neill, E., Meitinger, T., et al. (2006). The Parkinson disease causing LRRK2 mutation I2020T is associated with increased kinase activity. Human Molecular Genetics, 15(2), 223-232.

Goate, A., Chartier-Harlin, M. C., Mullan, M., Brown, J., Crawford, F., Fidani, L., et al. (1991). Segregation of a missense mutation in the amyloid precursor protein gene with familial Alzheimer's disease. Nature, 349(6311), 704-706

Goedert, M., Spillantini, M. G., & Davies, S. W. (1998). Filamentous nerve cell inclusions in neurodegenerative diseases. Current Opinion Neurobiology, 8(5), 619-632.

Goedert, M., Wischik, C. M., Crowther, R. A., Walker, J. E., & Klug, A. (1988). Cloning and sequencing of the cDNA encoding a core protein of the paired helical filament of Alzheimer disease: Identification as the microtubule-associated protein tau. Proceedings of the National Academy of Sciences of the United States of America, 85(11), 4051-4055.

Goker-Alpan, O., Giasson, B. I., Eblan, M. J., Nguyen, J., Hurtig, H. I., Lee, V. M., et al. (2006). Glucocerebrosidase mutations are an important risk factor for Lewy body disorders. Neurology, 67(5), 908-910.

Golbe, L. I., Di Iorio, G., Bonavita, V., Miller, D. C., & Duvoisin, R. C. (1990). A large kindred with autosomal dominant Parkinson's disease. Annals of Neurology, 27(3), 276-282.

Goldwurm, S., Di Fonzo, A., Simons, E. J., Rohe, C. F., Zini, M., Canesi, M., et al. (2005). The G6055A (G2019S) mutation in LRRK2 is frequent in both early and late onset Parkinson's disease and originates from a common ancestor. Journal of Medical Genetics, 42(11), e65.

Goris, A., Williams-Gray, C. H., Clark, G. R., Foltynie, T., Lewis, S. J., Brown, J., et al. (2007). Tau and alpha-synuclein in susceptibility to, and dementia in, Parkinson's disease. Annals of Neurology, 62(2), 145-153.

Grabowski, G. A. (2008). Phenotype, diagnosis, and treatment of Gaucher's disease. Lancet, 372(9645), 1263-1271.

Harbo, H. F., Finsterer, J., Baets, J., Van Broeckhoven, C., Di Donato, S., Fontaine, B., et al. (2009). EFNS guidelines on the molecular diagnosis of neurogenetic disorders: General issues, Huntington's disease, Parkinson's disease and dystonias. European Journal of Neurology, 16(7), 777-785.

Hatano, Y., Li, Y., Sato, K., Asakawa, S., Yamamura, Y., Tomiyama, H., et al. (2004). Novel PINK1 mutations in early-onset parkinsonism. Annals of Neurology, 56(3), 424–427.

Healy, D. G., Abou-Sleiman, P. M., Valente, E. M., Gilks, W. P., Bhatia, K., Quinn, N., et al. (2004). DJ-1 mutations in Parkinson's disease. Journal of Neurology, Neurosurgery, and Psychiatry, 75(1), 144–145.

Healy, D. G., Falchi, M., O'Sullivan, S. S., Bonifati, V., Durr, A., Bressman, S., et al. (2008). Phenotype, genotype, and worldwide genetic penetrance of LRRK2-associated Parkinson's disease: A case-control study. Lancet Neurology, 7(7), 583–590.

Hedrich, K., Djarmati, A., Schafer, N., Hering, R., Wellenbrock, C., Weiss, P. H., et al. (2004). DJ-1 (PARK7) mutations are less frequent than Parkin (PARK2) mutations in early-onset Parkinson disease. Neurology, 62(3), 389–394.

Hering, R., Strauss, K. M., Tao, X., Bauer, A., Woitalla, D., Mietz, E. M., et al. (2004). Novel homozygous p.E64D mutation in DJ1 in early onset Parkinson disease (PARK7). Human Mutation, 24(4), 321–329.

Hutton, M., Lendon, C. L., Rizzu, P., Baker, M., Froelich, S., Houlden, H., et al. (1998). Association of missense and 50splice-site mutations in tau with the inherited dementia FTDP-17. Nature, 393(6686), 702–705.

Ibanez, P., Lesage, S., Janin, S., Lohmann, E., Durif, F., Destee, A., et al. (2009). Alpha-synuclein gene rearrangements in dominantly inherited parkinsonism: Frequency, phenotype, and mechanisms. Archives of Neurology, 66(1), 102–108. International Human Genome Sequencing, C. (2004). Finishing the euchromatic sequence of the human genome. Nature, 431(7011), 931–945.

International Parkinson's Disease Genomic Consortium (2011). Imputations of sequence variants for identification of genetic risk for Parkinson's disease: a meta-analysis of genome-wide association studies. Lancet, 377 (9766): 641-9.

Ishikawa, A., & Tsuji, S. (1996). Clinical analysis of 17 patients in 12 Japanese families with autosomal-recessive type juvenile parkinsonism. Neurology, 47(1), 160–166.

Kachergus, J., Mata, I. F., Hulihan, M., Taylor, J. P., Lincoln, S., Aasly, J., et al. (2005). Identification of a Novel LRRK2 Mutation Linked to Autosomal Dominant Parkinsonism: Evidence of a Common Founder across European Populations. American Journal of Human Genetics, 76(4), 672–680.

Karpinar, D. P., Balija, M. B., Kugler, S., Opazo, F., Rezaei-Ghaleh, N., Wender, N., et al. (2009). Pre-fibrillar alphasynuclein variants with impaired beta-structure increase neurotoxicity in Parkinson's disease models. The EMBO Journal, 28(20), 3256–3268.

Kitada, T., Asakawa, S., Hattori, N., Matsumine, H., Yamamura, Y., Minoshima, S., et al. (1998). Mutations in the parkin gene cause autosomal recessive juvenile parkinsonism. Nature, 392, 605–608.

Klein, C., Schneider, S. A., & Lang, A. E. (2009). Hereditary parkinsonism: Parkinson disease look-alikes–an algorithm for clinicians to 'PARK' genes and beyond. Movement Disorders, 24(14), 2042–2058.

Krüger, R., Kuhn, W., Müller, T., Woitalla, D., Graeber, M., Ko¨ sel, S., et al. (1998). Ala30Pro mutation in the gene encoding a-synuclein in Parkinson's disease. Nature Genetics, 18, 106–108.

Kwok, J. B., Teber, E. T., Loy, C., Hallupp, M., Nicholson, G., Mellick, G. D., et al. (2004). Tau haplotypes regulate transcription and are associated with Parkinson's disease. Annals of Neurology, 55(3), 329–334.

Latourelle, J. C., Pankratz, N., Dumitriu, A., Wilk, J. B., Goldwurm, S., Pezzoli, G., et al. (2009). Genomewide association study for onset age in Parkinson disease. BMC Medical Genetics, 10, 98.

Lesage, S., Durr, A., Tazir, M., Lohmann, E., Leutenegger, A. L., Janin, S., et al. (2006). LRRK2 G2019S as a cause of Parkinson's disease in North African Arabs. The New England Journal of Medicine, 354(4), 422–423.

Levy, S., Sutton, G., Ng, P. C., Feuk, L., Halpern, A. L., Walenz, B. P., et al. (2007). The diploid genome sequence of an individual human. PLoS Biology, 5(10), e254.

Lu, C. S., Wu-Chou, Y. H., van Doeselaar, M., Simons, E. J., Chang, H. C., Breedveld, G. J., et al. (2008). The LRRK2 Arg1628Pro variant is a risk factor for Parkinson's disease in the Chinese population. Neurogenetics, 9(4), 271–276.

Lupski, J. R., Reid, J. G., Gonzaga-Jauregui, C., Rio Deiros, D., Chen, D. C., Nazareth, L., et al. (2010). Whole-Genome Sequencing in a Patient with Charcot-Marie-Tooth Neuropathy. The New England Journal of Medicine, 362(13), 1181- 1191.

Lücking, C. B., Dürr, A., Bonifati, V., Vaughan, J., De Michele, G., Gasser, T., et al. (2000). Association between Early-OnsetnParkinson's Disease and Mutations in the Parkin Gene. The New England Journal of Medicine, 342(21), 1560-1567.

Machaczka, M., Rucinska, M., Skotnicki, A. B., & Jurczak, W. (1999). Parkinson's syndrome preceding clinical manifestation of Gaucher's disease. American Journal of Hematology, 61(3), 216–217.

Maraganore, D. M., de Andrade, M., Elbaz, A., Farrer, M. J., Ioannidis, J. P., Kruger, R., et al. (2006). Collaborative analysis of alpha-synuclein gene promoter variability and Parkinson disease. JAMA, 296(6), 661–670.

Maraganore, D. M., de Andrade, M., Lesnick, T. G., Strain, K. J., Farrer, M. J., Rocca, W. A., et al. (2005). Highresolution whole-genome association study of Parkinson disease. American Journal of Human Genetics, 77(5), 685–693.

Martin, E. R., Scott, W. K., Nance, M. A., Watts, R. L., Hubble, J. P., Koller, W. C., et al. (2001). Association of Single Nucleotide Polymorphisms of the Tau Gene With Late-Onset Parkinson Disease. JAMA, 286(18), 2245–2250.

Mata, I. F., Samii, A., Schneer, S. H., Roberts, J. W., Griffith, A., Leis, B. C., et al. (2008). Glucocerebrosidase gene mutations: A risk factor for Lewy body disorders. Archives of Neurology, 65(3), 379–382.

Matsumine, H., Saito, M., Shimoda-Matsubayashi, S., Tanaka, H., Ishikawa, A., Nakagawa-Hattori, Y., et al. (1997). Localization of a gene for an autosomal recessive form of juvenile Parkinsonism to chromosome 6q25.2-27. American Journal of Human Genetics, 60(3), 588–596.

Metzker, M. L. (2009). Sequencing technologies - the next generation. Nature Reviews Genetics, 11(1), 31–46.

Mizuta, I., Satake, W., Nakabayashi, Y., Ito, C., Suzuki, S., Momose, Y., et al. (2006). Multiple candidate gene analysis identifies {alpha}-synuclein as a susceptibility gene for sporadic Parkinson's disease. Human Molecular Genetics, 15(7), 1151–1158.

Mueller, J. C., Fuchs, J., Hofer, A., Zimprich, A., Lichtner, P., Illig, T., et al. (2005). Multiple regions of alpha-synuclein are associated with Parkinson's disease. Annals of Neurology, 57 (4), 535–541.

Neumann, J., Bras, J., Deas, E., O'Sullivan, S. S., Parkkinen, L., Lachmann, R. H., et al. (2009). Glucocerebrosidase mutations in clinical and pathologically proven Parkinson's disease. Brain, 132(Pt 7), 1783–1794.

Ng, S.B., Buckingham, K.J., Lee, C., Bigham, A.W., Tabor, H.K., Dent, K.M., et al. (2010) Exome sequencing identifies the cause of a mendelian disorder. Nature Genetics, 42(1), 30–35.

Nichols, W. C., Pankratz, N., Hernandez, D., Paisan-Ruiz, C., Jain, S., Halter, C. A., et al. (2005). Genetic screening for a single common LRRK2 mutation in familial Parkinson's disease. Lancet, 365(9457), 410–412.

Ozelius, L. J., Senthil, G., Saunders-Pullman, R., Ohmann, E., Deligtisch, A., Tagliati, M., et al. (2006). LRRK2 G2019S as a cause of Parkinson's disease in Ashkenazi Jews. The New England Journal of Medicine, 354(4), 424–425.

Paisan-Ruiz, C., Jain, S., Evans, E. W., Gilks, W. P., Simon, J., van der Brug, M., et al. (2004). Cloning of the gene containing mutations that cause PARK8-linked Parkinson's disease. Neuron, 44(4), 595–600.

Pankratz, N., Wilk, J. B., Latourelle, J. C., DeStefano, A. L., Halter, C., Pugh, E. W., et al. (2009). Genomewide association study for susceptibility genes contributing to familial Parkinson disease. Human Genetics, 124(6), 593–605.

Pittman, A. M., Myers, A. J., Abou-Sleiman, P., Fung, H. C., Kaleem, M., Marlowe, L., et al. (2005). Linkage disequilibrium fine mapping and haplotype association analysis of the tau gene in progressive supranuclear palsy and corticobasal degeneration. Journal of Medical Genetics, 42(11), 837–846.

Polymeropoulos, M. H., Higgins, J. J., Golbe, L. I., Johnson, W. G., Ide, S. E., Di Iorio, G., et al. (1996). Mapping of a gene for Parkinson's disease to chromosome 4q21-q23. Science, 274, 1197–1199.

Polymeropoulos, M. H., Lavedan, C., Leroy, E., Ide, S. E., Dehejia, A., Dutra, A., et al. (1997). Mutation in the a-synuclein gene identified in families with Parkinson's disease. Science, 276, 2045–2047.

Rogaeva, E., Johnson, J., Lang, A. E., Gulick, C., Gwinn- Hardy, K., Kawarai, T., et al. (2004). Analysis of the PINK1 gene in a large cohort of cases with Parkinson disease. Archives of Neurology, 61(12), 1898–1904.

Rohe, C. F., Montagna, P., Breedveld, G., Cortelli, P., Oostra, B. A., & Bonifati, V. (2004). Homozygous PINK1 C-terminus mutation causing early-onset parkinsonism. Annals of Neurology, 56(3), 427–431.

Satake, W., Nakabayashi, Y., Mizuta, I., Hirota, Y., Ito, C.,Kubo, M., et al. (2009). Genome-wide association study identifies common variants at four loci as genetic risk factors for Parkinson's disease. Nature Genetics, 41(12), 1303–1307.

Scott, W. K., Nance, M. A., Watts, R. L., Hubble, J. P., Koller, W. C., Lyons, K., et al. (2001). Complete genomic screen in Parkinson disease: Evidence for multiple genes. JAMA, 286(18), 2239–2244.

Simon-Sanchez, J., Schulte, C., Bras, J. M., Sharma, M., Gibbs, J. R., Berg, D., et al. (2009). Genome-wide association study reveals genetic risk underlying Parkinson's disease. Nature Genetics, 41(12), 1308-1312.

Singleton, A. B., Farrer, M., Johnson, J., Singleton, A., Hague, S., Kachergus, J., et al. (2003). {alpha}-Synuclein locus triplication causes Parkinson's DISEASE. Science, 302(5646), 841.

Skipper, L., Wilkes, K., Toft, M., Baker, M., Lincoln, S., Hulihan, M., et al. (2004). Linkage disequilibrium and association of MAPT H1 in Parkinson disease. American Journal of Human Genetics, 75(4), 669-677.

Spillantini, M. G., Schmidt, M. L., Lee, V. M., Trojanowski, J. Q., Jakes, R., & Goedert, M. (1997). Alpha-synuclein in Lewy bodies. Nature, 388(6645), 839-840.

Spira, P. J., Sharpe, D. M., Halliday, G., Cavanagh, J., & Nicholson, G. A. (2001). Clinical and pathological features of a Parkinsonian syndrome in a family with an Ala53Thr alphasynuclein mutation. Annals of Neurology, 49(3), 313-319.

Tayebi, N., Callahan, M., Madike, V., Stubblefield, B. K., Orvisky, E., Krasnewich, D., et al. (2001). Gaucher disease and parkinsonism: A phenotypic and genotypic characterization. Molecular Genetics and Metabolism, 73(4), 313-321.

Tobin, J. E., Latourelle, J. C., Lew, M. F., Klein, C., Suchowersky, O., Shill, H. A., et al. (2008). Haplotypes and gene expression implicate the MAPT region for Parkinson disease: The GenePD Study. Neurology, 71(1), 28-34.

Valente, E. M., Abou-Sleiman, P. M., Caputo, V., Muqit, M. M., Harvey, K., Gispert, S., et al. (2004). Hereditary early-onset Parkinson's disease caused by mutations in PINK1. Science, 304(5674), 1158-1160.

Valente, E. M., Bentivoglio, A. R., Dixon, P. H., Ferraris, A., Ialongo, T., Frontali, M., et al. (2001). Localization of a novel locus for autosomal recessive early-onset parkinsonism, park6, on human chromosome 1p35-p36. American Journal of Human Genetics, 68(4), 895-900.

Valente, E. M., Salvi, S., Ialongo, T., Marongiu, R., Elia, A. E., Caputo, V., et al. (2004). PINK1 mutations are associated with sporadic early-onset parkinsonism. Annals of Neurology, 56(3), 336-341.

Wheeler, D. A., Srinivasan, M., Egholm, M., Shen, Y., Chen, L., McGuire, A., et al. (2008). The complete genome of an individual by massively parallel DNA sequencing. Nature, 452(7189), 872-876.

Williams, D. R. (2006). Tauopathies: Classification and clinical update on neurodegenerative diseases associated with microtubule-associated protein tau. Internal Medicine Journal, 36 (10), 652-660.

Winkler, S., Hagenah, J., Lincoln, S., Heckman, M., Haugarvoll, K., Lohmann-Hedrich, K., et al. (2007). Alpha-synuclein and Parkinson disease susceptibility. Neurology, 69(18), 1745-1750.

Zabetian, C. P., Hutter, C. M., Factor, S. A., Nutt, J. G., Higgins, D. S., Griffith, A., et al. (2007). Association analysis of MAPT H1 haplotype and subhaplotypes in Parkinson's disease. Annals of Neurology, 62(2), 137-144.

Zarranz, J. J., Alegre, J., Gomez-Esteban, J. C., Lezcano, E., Ros, R., Ampuero, I., et al. (2004). The new mutation, E46K, of alpha-synuclein causes Parkinson and Lewy body dementia. Annals of Neurology, 55(2), 164-173.

Zimprich, A., Biskup, S., Leitner, P., Lichtner, P., Farrer, M., Lincoln, S., et al. (2004). Mutations in LRRK2 cause autosomal-dominant parkinsonism with pleomorphic pathology. Neuron, 44(4), 601–607.

Zody, M. C., Jiang, Z., Fung, H. C., Antonacci, F., Hillier, L. W., Cardone, M. F., et al. (2008). Evolutionary toggling of the *MAPT* 17q21.31 inversion region. Nature Genetics, 40 (9), 1076–1083.

3

Parkin and Parkinson's Disease

Shiam-Peng Tay[1], Grace G.Y. Lim[1],
Calvin W.S. Yeo[1] and Kah-Leong Lim[1,2,3]
[1]*Department of Physiology, National University of Singapore,*
[2]*A*STAR Duke-NUS Neuroscience Research Partnership,*
[3]*National Neuroscience Institute*
Singapore

1. Introduction

Parkinson's disease (PD) is the most common neurodegenerative movement disorder affecting millions of predominantly elderly individuals worldwide. Originally described as "The Shaking Palsy" in 1817 by the British physician, James Parkinson, the disease is attended by a constellation of motoric deficits including bradykinesia (slowness in movements), postural instability, rigidity and tremor that ultimately result in near total immobility. Although pathological changes are distributed in the PD brain, the principal neuropathology that underlies the characteristic motor phenotype of PD patients is unequivocally the loss of midbrain dopaminergic (DA) neurons in the *substantia nigra pars compacta* (SNpc), which results in a severe depletion of striatal dopamine and thereby an impaired nigrostriatal system that otherwise allows an individual to execute proper, coordinated movements. This specific pattern of neurodegeneration in PD is often accompanied by the presence of eosinophilic intracytoplasmic inclusions known as Lewy bodies (LBs) in surviving neurons in the SN as well as in other affected brain regions such as the dorsal motor nucleus of the vagus, locus ceruleus (LC) and olfactory nuclei (Braak et al., 2003). In advanced stages of the disease, LB pathology can also be found in the limbic structures and neocortex (Braak et al., 2003). Non-motor features arising from these extra-nigral neuronal lesions, including autonomic, sensory and cognitive dysfunctions, present additional sources of considerable consternation and disability for affected individuals (Olanow et al., 2008). Thus, although SN pathology is often regarded as the most important hallmark of PD, the disease is increasingly being recognized as a multi-system disorder affecting not only dopaminergic, but also noradrenergic, cholinergic and serotonergic systems (Alexander, 2004).

Despite intensive research, the etiology of PD remains poorly understood and no current treatments can unequivocally slow or stop the degenerative process. Current therapies for PD are palliative at best and the mainstay is pharmacologic intervention via DA replacement (e.g. through L-DOPA administration). Major drawbacks with current therapies include the inevitable loss of effectiveness and increasing drug-induced side effects as the disease progresses. Invariably, the debilitating nature and morbidity of the disease present significant healthcare, socio-economic and emotional problems. As the world population rapidly ages, these problems undoubtedly would also increase. Notably, a recent study by Dorsey et al projected that the number of PD cases in Europe's five most

and the world's ten most populous countries would increase to 9 million in year 2030 (Dorsey et al., 2007). This is definitely a worrying trend, and one that aptly emphasizes the urgency to develop more effective treatment modalities for the PD patient.
In large part, the difficulty in identifying disease-modifying drugs for PD is due to: i) our current limited understanding of the molecular mechanism(s) that underlies the pathogenesis of PD (the illumination of which would allow the identification and therapeutic exploitation of key molecules involved in the pathogenic process), and ii) the lack of a truly representative mammalian model of PD that recapitulates accurately the progressive process as well as the nature and distribution of the human pathology. However, during the last decade or so, the identification and functional characterization of several genes whose mutations are causative of rare familial forms of PD have provided tremendous insights into the molecular events underlying neurodegeneration in PD. Alongside, several genetic models of PD have also been generated that replicate the disease phenotype to varying degrees of success. Collectively, these studies implicate aberrant mitochondrial and protein homeostasis as key contributors to the development of PD, with oxidative stress likely acting an important nexus between the two pathogenic events.

2. Parkin and Parkinson's disease

Mutations in *α-synuclein, parkin, DJ-1, PINK1,* and *LRRK2* are currently recognized to be unequivocally linked to familial parkinsonism (Table 1). Whereas *α-synuclein* and *LRRK2* mutations are causative of dominant parkinsonism, mutations in *parkin, DJ-1, PINK1* are associated with recessive parkinsonism (Thomas and Beal, 2007).

Locus	Chromosome	Gene	Inheritance	Function
PARK1 & 4	4q21-23	*α-synuclein (SNCA)*	Dominant	Unclear (presynaptic protein)
PARK2	6q25.2-27	*Parkin (PRKN)*	Recessive	Ubiquitin ligase
PARK3	2p13	*Unknown*	Dominant	-
PARK5	4p14	*UCHL1*	Dominant	Ubiquitin hydrolase
PARK6	1p35-36	*PINK1*	Recessive	Putative serine/threonine kinase
PARK7	1p36	*DJ-1*	Recessive	Redox sensor
PARK8	12p11.2-q13.1	*LRRK2/dardarin*	Dominant	Putative serine/threonine kinase
PARK9	1p36	*ATP13A2*	Recessive	Lysosomal P-type ATPase
PARK10	1p32	*Unknown*	Unknown	-
PARK11	2q37.1	*Unknown*	Dominant	-
PARK12	Xq21-q25	*Unknown*	Unknown	-
PARK13	2p12	*Omi/HtrA2*	Dominant	Mitochondrial serine protease
PARK14	22q13.1	*PLA2G6*	Recessive	Phospholipase
PARK15	22q12-q13	*FBXO7*	Recessive	Component of SCF E3 complex
PARK16	1q32	*Unknown*	Unknown	-

Table 1. PD-linked genes

Apart from these, mutations in *UCHL1*, *Omi/HtrA2* and *ATP13A2* have also been suggested to cause parkinsonism, but their relevance to PD is currently unclear because the purported disease-causing mutation is either extremely rare in occurrence (e.g. UCHL1 I93M) (Healy et al., 2004) or present in control population at similar frequencies (e.g. Omi/HtrA2 G399S) (Simon-Sanchez and Singleton, 2008) or otherwise results in a clinical phenotype that is rather divergent from classical PD (e.g. ATP13A2-linked parkinsonism that is characterized by mild parkinsonism and prominent cognitive defects) (Ramirez et al., 2006). More recently, two other genes, *PLA2G6* encoding a phospholipase and *FBXO7* encoding a component of the Skp-Cullin-Fbox (SCF) ubiquitin ligase complex, have also been identified to be associated with recessive parkinsonism (Di Fonzo et al., 2009; Paisan-Ruiz et al., 2009). The function of these various disease-associated genes, especially the unequivocal ones, has been extensively characterized. Interestingly, it turned out that these seemingly functionally disparate PD-linked proteins that have no clear relationship with each other at first glance may all influence either protein or mitochondrial homeostasis, with some, like parkin, being directly involved in both. Accordingly, in the absence of functional parkin, aberrations in both protein and mitochondrial quality control (QC) would ensue that may eventually trigger the demise of susceptible neurons. Indeed, the pivotal role parkin plays in maintaining DA neuronal survival is underscored by our current recognition that parkin dysfunction represents not only a predominant cause of familial parkinsonism but also a formal risk factor for the more common, sporadic form of PD. Here, we shall discuss the role of parkin in PD and why a better understanding of parkin function can help elucidate potential therapeutic strategies for the disease.

2.1 Parkin mutations and parkinsonism

Mutations in parkin were originally identified in Japan more than a decade ago to be causative of autosomal recessive juvenile parkinsonism (ARJP) (Kitada et al., 1998). Following this discovery, several ethnically diverse individuals with early-onset PD (age < 45 years) in other parts of the world were also found to carry parkin mutations, which occur at a frequency of about 10-20% and 50% in sporadic and familial early-onset cases respectively (Lucking et al., 2000; Mata et al., 2004; Periquet et al., 2003). Clinically, parkin-associated parkinsonism is often quite indistinguishable from idiopathic PD, with bradykinesia, rigidity and rest tremor being variably combined in both disorders. However, parkin-related patients tend to exhibit slower disease progression and better response to L-DOPA (and also a higher tendency to develop L-DOPA-induced dyskinesia) than those with parkinsonism of different etiologies. Additionally, other less typical features common to parkin cases include prominent dystonia, presence of hyperreflexia and more symmetrical presentation of symptoms, although none of these features are sufficiently specific to be diagnostic of parkin mutations. Limited post-mortem studies of known parkin cases conducted to date demonstrated neuronal loss predominantly in the SN and LC regions of the brain that is accompanied by gliosis. Importantly, the majority of parkin-related cases are devoid of classic LBs (Hayashi et al., 2000; Mori et al., 1998; Pramstaller et al., 2005), suggesting that parkin-associated parkinsonism is pathologically distinct from idiopathic PD, and as such may represent a phenocopy of the latter. However, this is debatable as LBs are found in at least two cases of parkin-related PD (Farrer et al., 2001; Pramstaller et al., 2005). An attractive corollary to this is that functional parkin may facilitate LB formation, which we favor as a working hypothesis (see section 2.2).

Structurally, the 465 amino acid-containing human parkin protein is comprised of a ubiquitin-like (UBL) domain at its N-terminus, a RING1-IBR-RING2 domain at its C-terminus and a unique middle segment that links the two domains (Fig. 1). Similar to other RING finger-containing proteins, parkin functions as an E3 ubiquitin ligase associated with the ubiquitin-proteasome system (UPS). To date, more than 100 different parkin mutations have been described with over 50 of these being missense/nonsense substitutions (Fig. 1). Although most of the missense mutations occur within the RING1-IBR-RING2 catalytic moiety, many of them are also found along the length of the protein outside this region. Further, exonic mutations are also frequently observed with deletion of exon 3 and/or 4 being the most common (Hedrich et al., 2004).

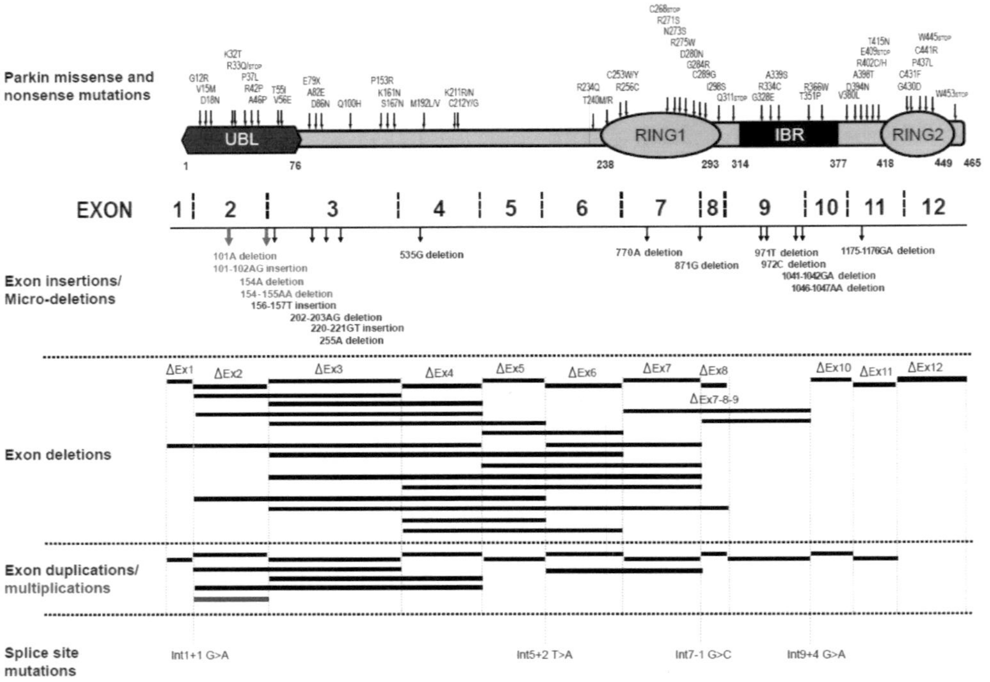

Fig. 1. Schematic depiction of parkin structure and associated disease-linked mutations including missense/nonsense substitutions, insertions, microdeletion as well as exonic multiplications and deletions.

Curiously, despite the heterogeneity, there is no discernable difference in the clinical manifestations among PD patients carrying different parkin mutations. This suggests that substitutions of amino acids resulting from missense mutations are as detrimental to parkin function as are truncation and deletion mutations. Another curious, albeit controversial feature of parkin-related cases is that a single allelic hit might be sufficient to cause disease, which contradicts the widely accepted notion that parkin mutations transmit in a classical autosomal recessive manner (Klein et al., 2007). Supporting this, Hilker and colleagues demonstrated via positron emission tomography that asymptomatic carriers of a single parkin mutation exhibit significantly reduced fluorodopa uptake in the striatal regions compared to control subjects, suggesting preclinical dopaminergic dysfunction (Hilker et al.,

2001). In concordance with this, a subsequent transcranial sonography-based study revealed SN hyperechogenicity in 5 out of 7 asymptomatic carriers of parkin mutations (Walter et al., 2004). Moreover, fMRI analysis of heterozygous parkin carriers demonstrated reorganization of striatocortical motor loops that possibly reflect a compensatory effort to overcome latent nigrostriatal dysfunction (Buhmann et al., 2005). Notwithstanding these evidences, the pathogenicity of single heterozygous parkin mutation is a subject of ongoing debate. An outstanding issue is whether heterozygous parkin mutations may have arisen incidentally. Several studies have sought to address this, but the findings have thus far been inconsistent, i.e. heterozygosity for parkin mutations was reported to be similar between patients and controls in some studies (Kay et al., 2007; Lincoln et al., 2003) but also found to be unique to PD cases in others (Clark et al., 2006b). Another issue is how mutations occurring on a recessive gene can contribute to disease pathogenesis. Given the neuroprotective role of parkin function (discussed in later section), one could envisage that parkin haploinsufficiency could increase the risk of heterozygous parkin mutation carriers for PD. Supporting this, a promoter variant of parkin associated with a lower expression of parkin was found to occur more commonly in PD cases than in controls (West et al., 2002). Alternatively, emerging evidence suggest that certain parkin mutations may also contribute to neurotoxicity directly. The role of single heterozygous parkin mutations thus remains unresolved.

Notwithstanding the controversy surrounding the role of heterozygous parkin mutations, how parkin mutations disrupt the function of the protein was a topic of intense research. Intuitively, one would posit that disease-associated mutations of parkin result in the loss of its enzymatic activity. Although this is true for mutations that occur on parkin's RING2 domain, several groups including ours have demonstrated that the majority of parkin missense mutants outside its RING2 domain retain their catalytic competency (Chung et al., 2001; Hampe et al., 2006; Matsuda et al., 2006; Sriram et al., 2005; Wang et al., 2005). Instead, misfolding of parkin triggered by these mutations appears to be the major mechanism underlying parkin inactivation. Notably, missense parkin mutations frequently alter the protein solubility and concomitantly promote its aggregation into inclusion bodies (Ardley et al., 2003; Cookson et al., 2003; Gu et al., 2003; Hampe et al., 2006; Muqit et al., 2004; Sriram et al., 2005; Wang et al., 2005b). Amongst the aggregation-producing parkin mutations is the R275W substitution, which frequently occurs in the heterozygous state. Alternatively, some mutations of parkin compromise its function by destabilizing the protein and accelerating its degradation via the proteasome (Schlehe et al., 2008).

2.2 Parkin-mediated ubiquitination and protein homeostasis

As mentioned earlier, parkin functions as an E3 ligase associated with the UPS, a major proteolytic machinery that normally identifies and degrades unwanted intracellular proteins. In this system, proteins that are destined for proteasome-mediated degradation are added a chain of ubiquitin via a reaction cascade that involves the ubiquitin-activating (E1), -conjugating (E2) and -ligating (E3) enzymes. Through the sequential and repetitive actions of these enzymes, successive isopeptide linkages are formed between the C-terminal glycine carboxyl group (G76) of the ubiquitin moiety being added and the ε-amino group of a free lysine (most commonly K48) on the ubiquitin that is attached to the protein. The (G76-K48) polyubiquitinated substrate is then recognized by the 26S proteasome as a target for degradation. It is important to highlight that the ubiquitin sequence contains seven lysine residues (at positions 6, 11, 27, 29, 33, 48 and 63) and that polyubiquitin chain assembly can occur at any of these lysine residues (Peng et al., 2003). In addition, proteins can also be monoubiquitinated. Notably, both K63-linked polyubiquitination and monoubiquitination of proteins are not typically associated with proteasome-mediated ubiquitination.

Shortly after the discovery of parkin as a PD-linked gene, three independent groups demonstrated that parkin-mediated ubiquitination is linked to protein degradation and that disease-associated parkin mutations compromise its role as an E3 enzyme (Imai et al., 2000; Shimura et al., 2000; Zhang et al., 2000). A logical and popular hypothesis that ensued is that loss of parkin function could lead to a toxic accumulation of one or several of its substrates, thereby leading to neurodegeneration. This had fuelled intense effort by many laboratories around the world to identify the culprit substrate(s) involved. To date, no less than 25 substrates (or putative substrates) of parkin has been reported since the identification of CDCrel1 as the first putative substrate for the ubiquitin ligase (Zhang et al., 2000) (Table 2). However, none of the parkin substrates identified thus far is exclusively expressed in DA neurons, which raises the question on why DA neurons in familial parkinsonism cases linked to parkin mutations are selectively vulnerable to deficient parkin function. Further, few from the laundry list fulfil an important criterion expected of an "authentic" parkin substrate: accumulation in the brains of ARJP patients and parkin-deficient models (Table 2). Although the pace of substrate identification has slowed down considerably in recent years, new parkin substrates continue to emerge periodically. Amongst the most recently isolated parkin substrates is the zinc finger-containing protein called PARIS (ZNF746) (Shin et al., 2011), a major transcriptional repressor of PGC-1α expression, which in turn regulates the transcription of many genes involved in cellular metabolism. Importantly, unlike most previously identified parkin substrates, PARIS accumulates in post-mortem brain tissues derived from ARJP and sporadic PD patients, as well as in the ventral midbrain region of mice that is conditionally ablated of parkin expression (Shin et al., 2011). Moreover, stereotactic injection of viral vector encoding PARIS into the SN of mice results in a selective loss of TH-positive DA neurons that can be rescued by either parkin or PGC-1α co-expression (Shin et al., 2011). Together, these results suggest that PARIS is an "authentic" parkin substrate and that its upregulation may underlie neurodegeneration due to parkin inactivation. Notwithstanding this and the fact that a few other substrates have similarly been reported to fulfil the criterion of a parkin substrate (Table 2), what constitutes an "authentic" substrate for parkin is really debatable, as discussed below.

Although protein ubiquitination is classically associated with proteasome-mediated degradation, the existence of non-classic ubiquitin modifications such as K63-linked polyubiquitination would caution against the fixation on the traditional view that substrates of a ubiquitin ligase must exhibit an accelerated, proteasome-dependent turnover in the presence of the enzyme. This is particularly relevant to parkin, which we and others have demonstrated to be a multifunctional enzyme capable of mediating alternative ubiquitin topologies such as monoubiquitination and K63-linked polyubiquitination - modifications that are typically uncoupled from the proteasome and often considered as "non-proteolytic" (Doss-Pepe et al., 2005; Hampe et al., 2006; Lim et al., 2005; Matsuda et al., 2006) (Fig. 2). Our results would argue that the catalytic function of parkin is not limited to targeting substrate for degradation by the proteasome. Thus, the lack of accumulation of an identified parkin substrate in the brains of ARJP patients and parkin-deficient models does not necessarily mean that it is less than an "authentic" substrate. For example, we have previously reported that parkin-mediated polyubiquitination of synphilin-1 (an interactor of α-synuclein) normally occurs via K63-linked chains, which does not appear to affect its steady-state turnover (Lim et al., 2005). Not surprisingly, the level of synphilin-1 is neither appreciably altered in ARJP brains nor in brain tissues derived from parkin null mice (Ko et al., 2005). A corollary to this is that proteasome-independent pathways may also be relevant to parkin-related neurodegeneration.

Substrates	Ub Type	Elevated in			Reference
		KO mice	ARJP Brain	PD brain	
CDCrel-1	-	Yes/No	Yes/No	-	(Ko et al., 2005)
CDCrel-2a	-	-	Yes	-	(Choi et al., 2003)
Synaptotagmin XI	-	Yes/No	-	-	(Periquet et al., 2005)
Synphilin-1	K63	No	No		(Chung et al., 2001; Ko et al., 2005; Lim et al., 2005)
P38/AIMP2	Multiple Mono	Yes	Yes	Yes	(Corti et al., 2003; Hampe et al., 2006; Ko et al., 2005; Periquet et al., 2005)
FBP1	-	Yes	Yes	Yes	(Ko et al., 2006)
PARIS (ZNF746)	K48	Yes	Yes	Yes	(Shin et al., 2011)
Cyclin E	-	No	Yes/No	Yes	(Ko et al., 2005; Staropoli et al., 2003)
PDCP2-1	-	-	Yes	Yes	(Fukae et al., 2009)
Pael-R	-	No	Yes/No	-	(Ko et al., 2005)
α/β tubulin	-	Yes/No	No	-	(Ko et al., 2005; Ren et al., 2003)
Hsp70	Multiple Mono	No	No	Yes	(Moore et al., 2008)
PICK1	Mono	No	-	-	(Joch et al., 2007)
VDAC1	K27, Mono	Yes	-	-	(Geisler et al., 2010; Narendra et al.; Periquet et al., 2005)
Ataxin-2	-	Yes	-	-	(Huynh et al., 2007)
O-glycosylated α-synuclein	-	-	Yes	-	(Shimura et al., 2001)
RanBP2	-	-	-	-	(Um et al., 2006)
Lim Kinase 1	-	-	-	-	(Lim et al., 2007)
Eps15	Mono	-	-	-	(Fallon et al., 2006)
DJ-1 L166P	K63	-	-	-	(Olzmann et al., 2007)
Bcl-2	Mono	-	-	-	(Chen et al., 2010)
Drp1	K48	-	-	-	(Wang et al., 2011)
Mitofusin	-	-	-	-	(Poole et al., 2010; Ziviani et al., 2010)
Dopamine Transporter	-	-	-	-	(Jiang et al., 2004)
Phospholipase Cγ1	-	Yes	-	-	(Dehvari et al., 2009)
Ataxin3 polyQ79	-	-	-	-	(Tsai et al., 2003)

Table 2. List of parkin substrates/putative substrates

By virtue of its apparent dissociation from the proteasome, we have originally proposed that parkin-mediated K63-linked ubiquitination may be involved in cargo diversion during proteasomal stress and accordingly, in the biogenesis of inclusion bodies associated with neurodegenerative diseases (Lim et al., 2006). Our proposal is consistent with the concept of aggresomes, which are juxtanuclear inclusion bodies formed in the presence of proteasomal stress and that have been suggested to act as staging grounds for the disposal of protein aggregates via the autophagic route (Kopito, 2000). Supporting our hypothesis, we found that parkin-mediated K63 polyubiquitination of synphilin-1 promotes its aggregation into aggresome-like inclusion bodies (Lim et al., 2005). Corroborating our findings, Olzmann et al demonstrated that parkin-mediated K63 polyubiquitination of misfolded DJ-1 couples the protein to the dynein motor complex via the histone deacetylase 6 (HDAC6) adaptor, thereby promoting its sequestration into aggresomes (Olzmann et al., 2007). Importantly, our recent work identified K63-linked polyubiquitin as a novel cargo selection signal for macroautophagy-mediated clearance of aggresomes (Tan et al., 2008a; Tan et al., 2008b). By being capable of mediating both proteasome-associated K48-polyubiquitination and macroautophagy-associated K63-linked polyubiquitination, parkin may potentially act as an important triage between the two major cellular degradation systems. This multi-functionality of parkin may in part help explain its apparent broad neuroprotective properties, as the flexibility of ubiquitin linkage usage presumably would allow the enzyme to adapt rapidly to changes in cellular environment.

2.3 Parkin-mediated ubiquitination and mitochondrial homeostasis

One of the first hints that parkin may play a role in mitochondrial homeostasis aside from its role as a regulator of protein turnover came from a study in fruit flies. Greene and colleagues analyzed adult *Drosophila parkin* null mutant and observed that the most prominent pathology is not in the brain but in the flight musculature of these mutant flies, which is plagued by muscle degeneration and pronounced mitochondrial lesions (Greene et al., 2003). Interestingly, *PINK1* null flies were subsequently found to phenocopy their *parkin*-deficient counterparts and importantly, *parkin* over expression in *PINK1-/-* flies is able to rescue all the mutant phenotypes tested, although the reverse, does not happen (Clark et al., 2006a; Park et al., 2006), suggesting that parkin acts in the same pathway but downstream of PINK1. We now know from several follow-up studies in flies and other model systems that the parkin/PINK1 pathway is a key regulator of mitochondrial dynamics, although it is currently controversial whether the pathway promotes mitochondrial fission or fusion [For a recent review, see (Burbulla et al., 2010)].

In an exciting development, Narendra and colleagues from Youle laboratory have recently demonstrated that parkin plays an essential role in removing damaged mitochondria from the cell via a specialized form of autophagy known as mitophagy (Narendra et al., 2008). This has fuelled widespread interest amongst many researchers directed at elucidating the mechanism underlying parkin-mediated mitophagy, which is reminiscent of the initial excitement shared by many to uncover novel parkin substrates. A model (Fig. 2) that has emerged from a flurry of follow-up studies proposed that a key initial event that occurs upon mitochondrial depolarization is the selective accumulation of PINK1 in the outer membrane of the damaged organelle (presumably after its segregation by fission). Notably, PINK1 accumulation in healthy mitochondria is prevented by a proteolytic event that rapidly cleaves the protein (Narendra et al., 2010; Vives-Bauza et al., 2010). Upon recruitment to depolarized mitochondria by PINK1, parkin then becomes activated

(Matsuda et al., 2010) and promotes the ubiquitination and subsequent p97 AAA-ATPase-regulated degradation of mitofusins (Poole et al., 2010; Ziviani et al., 2010), the elimination of which will prevent unintended fusion events involving damaged mitochondria and thereby their re-entry into undamaged mitochondrial network from occurring (Tanaka et al., 2010). The event is then followed by the induction of mitophagy, which is also parkin-dependent. Parkin-mediated K63 ubiquitination is apparently important here, as mitochondrial substrates that are modified by K63 polyubiquitin can presumably help in the recruitment of autophagy receptors such as HDAC6 and p62 to the damaged organelle. Notably, both HDAC6 and p62 are ubiquitin-binding proteins that preferentially recognize K63 ubiquitin chains (Lim and Lim, 2010; Olzmann et al., 2007; Tan et al., 2008a). The end result is the formation of "mito-aggresomes" and their subsequent clearance by lysosomes. The whole process thus resembles the formation and autophagic clearance of aggresomes.

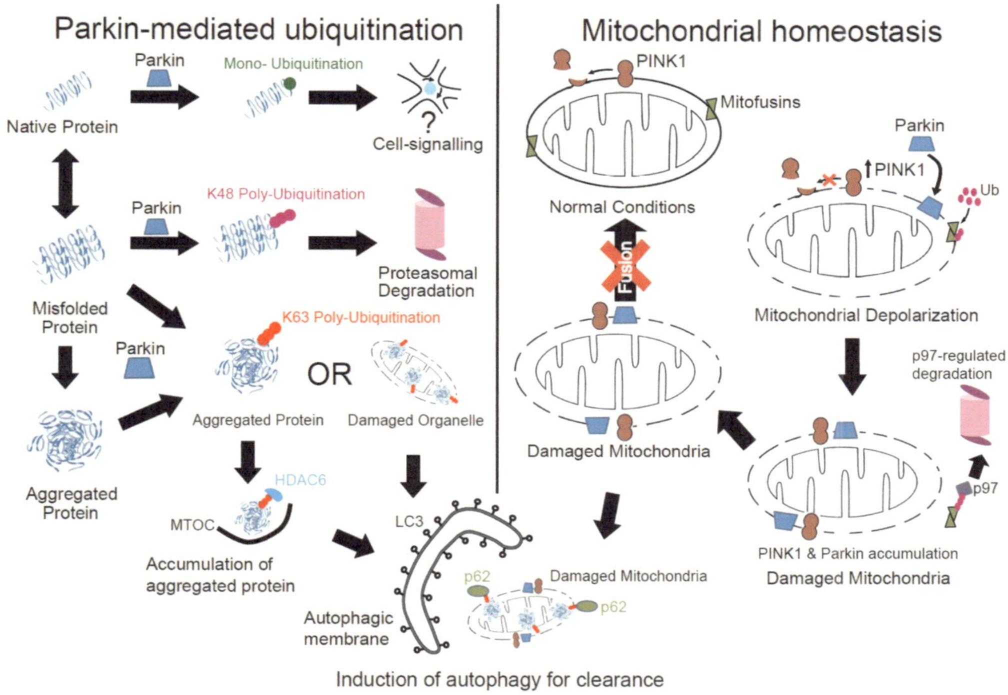

Fig. 2. Role of parkin in protein and mitochondrial QC. *(Left)* Parkin is a unique E3 enzyme capable of mediating various types of ubiquitin modification on its substrates that would result in different outcomes. *(Right)* A model of parkin/PINK1-mediated mitophagy.

Despite the logic and experimental support for the events surrounding parkin-mediated mitophagy as described above, the model is not without controversy. Because the majority of studies related to parkin-mediated mitophagy were carried out in cells grown in glucose-containing medium, a potential confounding factor is that these cells generate most of their ATP via glycolysis from glucose present in the medium, and not via oxidative phosphorylation. Notably, mitophagy is blocked in yeast that are made obligatorily dependent on mitochondrial metabolism, even under severe starvation conditions (Kanki and Klionsky, 2008). According to a recent study by Van Laar and colleagues, parkin-mediated mitophagy does not seem to take place appreciably in primary neurons treated with mitochondrial uncouplers such as CCCP (Van Laar et al., 2011). Unlike other cell types, neurons are strictly dependent on mitochondrial respiration. In HeLa cells (grown in glucose medium) where parkin-mediated mitophagy was originally observed, the phenomenon is similarly attenuated when these cells were forced into dependence on mitochondrial respiration (i.e. cultured in glucose-free medium) (Van Laar et al., 2011). Thus, parkin-mediated mitophagy appears to be dependent on the bioenergetic status of the cell. Presumably, additional mechanisms are involved in the regulation of mitophagy in neurons and other cell types that derive their energy from oxidative phosphorylation. Notwithstanding this, it is important to highlight that at least two groups have found that parkin accumulation on mitochondria does occur in primary neurons treated with CCCP (Narendra et al., 2008; Vives-Bauza et al., 2010). The reason for this discrepancy is presently unclear, but the conundrum obviously needs to be resolved as whether parkin-mediated mitophagy takes place appreciably in neurons has significant implications for its role in PD pathogenesis.

Interestingly, parkin is also involved in mitochondrial biogenesis. Kuroda and colleagues previously demonstrated that parkin over-expression enhances the transcription and replication of mitochondrial DNA by associating with mitochondrial transcription factor A (TFAM) and promoting TFAM-mediated transcription (Kuroda et al., 2006). Accordingly, the event is attenuated by parkin expression silencing with siRNA. However, an important caveat is that parkin-induced mitochondrial biogenesis only occurs in proliferating but not differentiated cells (Kuroda et al., 2006). Hence, its relevance to post-mitotic cells like neurons is unclear. From the recent work by Shin and colleagues, we now know that parkin can also potentially regulate mitochondrial biogenesis by regulating PGC-1α expression indirectly through its ability to down-regulate PARIS (which represses PGC-1α expression) (Shin et al., 2011). PGC-1α regulates a variety of genes that play important roles in mitochondrial biogenesis. Amongst these PGC-1α-regulated genes is nuclear respiratory factor-1 (NRF-1), whose activity contributes to the expression of respiratory subunits and mitochondrial transcription factors (Scarpulla, 2008). Notably, both PGC-1α and NRF-1 expression are reduced in the SN of PD brains (Shin et al., 2011), suggesting that impaired renewal of neuronal mitochondria may contribute to DA neurodegeneration in parkin-related cases. Based on these results, it is also logical to speculate that parkin might assist in the replenishment of exited mitochondria following extensive mitophagy. Thus, parkin appears to be involved in the entire spectrum of mitochondrial dynamics, i.e. from biogenesis to clearance.

2.4 Parkin is a potent neuroprotectant

Given the critical role of parkin in regulating protein and mitochondrial homeostasis, it is perhaps unsurprising to note that parkin is capable of protecting neurons against a wide variety of insults, including those mediated by α-synuclein or mutant LRRK2, as well as those generated by dopamine quinones, neurotoxins or metallic ions (Feany and Pallanck, 2003; Winklhofer, 2007). Yet, it remains rather amazing at the same time to note that a single ubiquitin ligase could do all that. Moreover, several studies have also demonstrated that parkin can afford protection against neurotoxicity elicited by agents that are not directly related to PD. For example, parkin is apparently capable of mitigating cytotoxicity induced by β-amyloid or by expanded polyglutamine-containing proteins through facilitating their elimination from the cell (Rosen et al., 2010; Tsai et al., 2003). While the removal of aberrant proteins or damaged mitochondria from cells undergoing various forms of stress may be common denominators underlying the broad neuroprotective capacity of parkin, recent studies also implicated a more direct role for parkin in neuroprotective signalling. Indeed, parkin-mediated ubiquitination is important for the activation of major cellular pro-survival pathways such as the NF-κB pathway (Henn et al., 2007). Henn and colleagues demonstrated in cells treated with kainate (an excitotoxin) or rotenone (a mitochondrial complex I inhibitor) that parkin-mediated protection against cell death is dependent on NF-κB activity (Henn et al., 2007). Interestingly, the authors further showed that the activation of NF-kB pathway by parkin is associated with its K63 polyubiquitination activity (Henn et al., 2007). Notably, several studies have also reported the ability of parkin to suppress stress-related mitogen-activated protein kinase (MAPK) signalling (e.g. JNK and p38) (Cha et al., 2005; Ren et al., 2009), although the effect may be an indirect consequence of reduced oxidative stress level in the presence of parkin.

Besides its catalytic role, parkin can also promote neuroprotection in an ubiquitination-independent manner. For example, Ren and colleagues have demonstrated that parkin does not require its ligase activity to stabilize microtubules and that this activity-independent function of parkin is important in the protection of DA neurons against microtubule-deploymerizing toxins (Ren et al., 2009). In a separate development, a provocative report suggested that parkin possesses ubiquitination-independent transcriptional activity, which in this case acts as a repressor of the tumor suppressor p53 expression. The repression of p53 expression by parkin ultimately leads to decreased Bax transcription, caspase 3 activity and apoptosis (da Costa et al., 2009). Although the subject of parkin's nuclear residency is currently still controversial, it is noteworthy that parkin localization to the nucleus has been independently observed by at least one other group (Kao, 2009a). Kao showed that parkin translocates to the nucleus following DNA damage (Kao, 2009a), apparently to assist in DNA repair (Kao, 2009b). Since parkin lacks a defined nucleus localization signal, precisely how the translocation of parkin occurs under different conditions remains to be elucidated. Notwithstanding the gaps in our current knowledge regarding the mechanisms underlying parkin-mediated protection, it is clear that parkin functions as a broad-spectrum neuroprotectant. Conceivably, parkin gene delivery could offer a novel avenue of PD therapy. Indeed, virus-mediated delivery of parkin has been shown to prevent DA neurodegeneration in rats either overexpressing α-synuclein (Lo Bianco et al., 2004; Yamada et al., 2005) or treated with parkinsonian neurotoxins (Paterna et al., 2007), or in a non-human primate model of α-synuclein overexpression (Yasuda et al., 2007). Another way to harness parkin's protective function is to look for molecules that can functionally compensate for loss of parkin function. Notably, Tain and colleagues have recently demonstrated that pharmacological activation of *4E-BP* (*Thor*) expression in parkin null flies by rapamycin can suppress all their pathologies (Tain et al., 2009), suggesting that rapamycin can somehow mimic parkin neuroprotection in the absence of the ubiquitin ligase.

2.5 Mammalian models of parkin-related parkinsonism

Given that parkin-related parkinsonism transmits in a largely recessive fashion and that parkin function is clearly important for neuronal homeostasis, one would intuitively be optimistic about generating a representative model of parkin-related parkinsonism through the ablation of endogenous parkin in animals. Although *Drosophila parkin* null mutants do exhibit prominent parkinsonian features (including DA neuronal loss and locomotive defects) that progress with age, germline-derived *parkin* knockout mice generally fail to exhibit robust signs of parkinsonism (Dawson et al., 2010; Perez and Palmiter, 2005). On the other hand, biochemical and proteomic analyses of brain samples prepared from these mice revealed deficits in dopamine handling, reduced mitochondrial respiration and antioxidant capacity, as well as increased ROS-mediated damage, all of which are consistent with the implicated cellular roles of parkin (Goldberg et al., 2003; Itier et al., 2003; Palacino et al., 2004). Conceivably, other proteins like PINK1 and DJ-1 that have overlapping functions with parkin may help to mitigate the overt manifestation of phenotypes in *parkin* null mice. However, it is noteworthy that even *parkin/PINK1/DJ-1* triple knockout mice do not exhibit any evidence of nigral degeneration or dramatic pathology, at as late as 24 months of age (Kitada et al., 2009).

Why conventional *parkin* knockout mice (and for that matter the majority of genetic mouse models of PD generated via traditional means) consistently failed to produce significant nigral cell loss and associated phenotypes remains a puzzle, although the controlled environment that these animals frequently lived in may deny them the entry of unknown disease-promoting factor(s) that might be present in the environment at large. Notably, even individuals with overt parkin mutations typically require a few decades for the disease to surface, suggesting pathogenic interaction between genetic mutations and age-associated or other factors. Alternatively, compensatory mechanisms that kicked in during development may influence the onset of disease symptoms in humans and mouse alike. Supporting this, virus-mediated delivery of PD-linked genes into the SN of adult rodents via stereotactic injections, which effectively bypass developmental compensation, usually results in marked DA neurodegeneration (Ulusoy et al., 2008). As mentioned earlier, such an approach was taken by Shin and colleagues, who generated a conditional *parkin* knockout mice by which exon 7 of the *parkin* gene flanked by loxP sites was removed from the SN of adult mice following stereotactic injection of a Cre recombinase-containing lentiviral vector (Shin et al., 2011). This elegant approach leads to a dramatic loss of parkin expression from the ventral midbrain of injected mice that is accompanied by an age-dependent loss of DA neurons, although the motor parameters of these mice were not reported. Thus, loss of parkin function in adult mice does promote DA neuronal loss, albeit in a conditional-dependent manner. At the same time, the study also provided indirect evidence supporting that the pathogenicity arising from the loss of parkin function can be developmentally compensated (at least in mice). Such compensatory mechanisms may conceivably operate in humans and may account for the age-dependency and the heterogeneity of age of onset of PD. At the least, we now have a model of parkin-linked recessive parkinsonism that exhibits substantial and progressive nigral cell loss.

A different approach was taken by Lu and colleagues in modelling parkin dysfunction in mice. In view of the possibility that single parkin mutations may also contribute to the disease, the group developed a BAC (bacterial artificial chromosome) transgenic mouse model expressing a C-terminal truncated human mutant parkin (Parkin-Q311X) in DA neurons under the direction of a dopamine transporter promoter (Lu et al., 2009). Expression of Parkin-Q311X, an aggregation-prone mutant, in mice produces age-dependent loss of SN DA neurons that is accompanied by progressive hypokinetic motor deficits. These results suggest that certain parkin mutants may exert direct neurotoxicity and support the role of heterozygous parkin mutations in disease pathogenesis. Notably, previous studies conducted in the *Drosophila* by the same group as well as by our group also arrived at the same suggestion (Sang et al., 2007; Wang et al., 2007). Indeed, transgenic flies expressing human parkin mutants such as R275W and Q311X display age-dependent, selective loss of DA neurons that is accompanied by progressive locomotion deficits (Sang et al., 2007; Wang et al., 2007).

2.6 Relevance of parkin to sporadic PD

That parkin mutations transmit in a recessive manner would suggest that the loss of parkin function predisposes DA neurons to degeneration. An important corollary to this is that any post-translational event that promotes the loss of parkin function could potentially mimic the effects brought about by overt mutations and be just as detrimental. Further, in view of the suggested contribution of parkin haploinsufficiency to disease risk, it is reasonable to assume that the down-regulation of normal parkin function mediated by such events need not result in the total abolition of its enzymatic activity to elicit a pathogenic effect.

We and others have found that a wide variety of PD-linked stressors, including those that produce oxidative and nitrosative stress, induce parkin solubility alterations and thereby its aggregation in a manner analogous to that brought about by several of its missense mutations (LaVoie et al., 2005; Wang et al., 2005; Winklhofer et al., 2003). Remarkably, dopamine also modifies parkin in a similar fashion (LaVoie et al., 2005; Wang et al., 2005). Furthermore, parkin appears to be uniquely susceptible to dopamine-induced modifications compared to several other related E3 members such as HHARI, Cbl and CHIP (LaVoie et al., 2007; LaVoie et al., 2005; Wong et al., 2007). Accordingly, detergent-insoluble parkin, but not HHARI, Cbl and CHIP, accumulates in the PD brain (LaVoie et al., 2005; Wang et al., 2005; Wong et al., 2007). As optimal level of soluble parkin is important for neuronal survival, the immobilization of the parkin within aggregates would not only deprive the protein of its function but also effectively reduce the pool of functional parkin available to the cell. Like haploinsufficiency, the biochemical depletion of soluble parkin levels is expected to increase the vulnerability of susceptible neurons to degeneration. Interestingly, normal parkin in the brain also becomes progressively more detergent-insoluble with aging (Pawlyk et al., 2003), which may provide an explanation to why age represents a risk factor for PD.

Besides stress-induced modifications, parkin phosphorylation is another post-translational modification that is linked to its inactivation. Notably, serine phosphorylation of parkin by casein kinase 1 (CK1) or cyclin-dependent kinase 5 (Cdk5) reportedly down-regulates its activity (Avraham et al., 2007; Yamamoto et al., 2005), and compound phosphorylation of parkin by both kinases further leads to its aggregation (Rubio de la Torre et al., 2009). While the physiological role of parkin phosphorylation remains unclear, it is conceivable that aberrant CK1 or Cdk5 activity can promote loss of parkin function and play a role in sporadic PD pathogenesis. Supporting this, parkin phosphorylation is elevated in distinct regions of sporadic PD brains and correlates with increased levels of p25, the activator of CDK5 (Rubio de la Torre et al., 2009). More recently, Ko and colleagues have demonstrated that tyrosine phosphorylation of parkin at residue 143 (Y143) by the src family kinase member, c-Abl, similarly inactivates its enzyme activity and compromises its protective function both *in vitro* and *in vivo* (Ko et al., 2010). They further showed that parkin is tyrosine-phosphorylated at Y143 in human post-mortem PD brains and that this modification of parkin is accompanied by the accumulation of parkin substrates such as

AIMP2. Together, the results by Ko and colleagues suggest a pathophysiologic regulation of parkin by c-Abl in sporadic PD (Ko et al., 2010).

Other than the above-mentioned post-translational modifications, a number of parkin interactors have also been demonstrated to be capable of inactivating its E3 ligase activity. For example, the bcl-2-associated athanogene 5 (BAG5) associates with and inhibits parkin activity (Kalia et al., 2004). Further, BAG5 promotes the sequestration of parkin within protein aggregates and compromises its neuroprotective function. Accordingly, targeted expression of BAG5 in the SNpc of mice enhances DA neurodegeneration following axotomy-induced DA neuronal injury or MPTP administration (Kalia et al., 2004). Although the authors suggested that BAG5 may serve as a useful therapeutic target for PD, the mechanism by which BAG5 inhibits parkin E3 activity remains unclear to this date. It is also curious why DA neuronal injury would induce BAG5 expression, an event that inhibits rather than stimulates the neuroprotective activity of parkin, which invariably will worsen the condition. Notably, besides BAG5, several other parkin interactors have also been identified as modulators of its catalytic activity. These include 14-3-3η, a chaperone-like protein, and Nrdp1, a RING-finger containing ubiquitin ligase (Sato et al., 2006; Zhong et al., 2005). Whereas 14-3-3η interacts with and reduces parkin activity directly (Sato et al., 2006), Nrdp1 promotes parkin degradation and depletes the availability of parkin to the cell (Zhong et al., 2005). Both events if unregulated would obviously be detrimental to parkin's protective function.

Taken together, it is apparent that loss of parkin function is not limited to those induced by disease-causing mutations, but also includes several biochemical and protein-protein modifications that can either alter the catalytic function of the E3 ligase directly, or indirectly through promoting its aggregation or degradation. Collectively, these mutation-independent modifications that inactivate parkin activity provide a mechanism for parkin dysfunction that is relevant to the pathogenesis of sporadic PD.

3. Conclusion

It is evident from the above discussion that parkin plays a key role in maintaining DA neuronal homeostasis and that its dysfunction is relevant to not just familial parkinsonism but also to sporadic PD. Parkin thus represents a neuroprotective PD-linked gene whose function can be and arguably should be exploited. Accordingly, a better understanding of parkin-mediated neuroprotective pathways would offer opportunities to uncover molecular targets that may be of therapeutic value to both familial and sporadic PD. The *Drosophila* model, with its powerful genetics as well as its amenability to drug screening, will be particularly useful here. Alternatively, given that the loss of parkin function can apparently be developmentally compensated (at least in mice), the identification and validation of components of the compensatory network will represent another approach to elucidate rational therapeutic strategies. Indeed, from a therapeutics point of view, it may be equally (if not more) beneficial to understand how parkin-related cases as well as PD in general are kept in check for decades before disease onset than to map the precise pathogenic events that occur after disease onset.

4. Acknowledgment

This work was supported by grants from A*STAR Biomedical Research Council, Khoo's Discovery Award, Singapore Millennium Foundation and the National University of

Singapore (LKL). C.Y. and G.L. are supported by graduate scholarships from the Singapore Millennium Foundation. We thank Xiao-Hui Ng for illustrations.

5. References

Alexander, G. E. (2004). Biology of Parkinson's disease: pathogenesis and pathophysiology of a multisystem neurodegenerative disorder. *Dialogues in Clinical Neuroscience*, Vol.6, pp. 259-280.

Ardley, H. C., Scott, G. B., Rose, S. A., Tan, N. G., Markham, A. F. & Robinson, P. A. (2003). Inhibition of proteasomal activity causes inclusion formation in neuronal and non-neuronal cells overexpressing Parkin. *Mol Biol Cell*, Vol.14, No.11, pp. 4541-4556.

Avraham, E., Rott, R., Liani, E., Szargel, R. & Engelender, S. (2007). Phosphorylation of Parkin by the cyclin-dependent kinase 5 at the linker region modulates its ubiquitin-ligase activity and aggregation. *J Biol Chem*, Vol.282, No.17, pp. 12842-12850.

Braak, H., Del Tredici, K., Rub, U., de Vos, R. A., Jansen Steur, E. N. & Braak, E. (2003). Staging of brain pathology related to sporadic Parkinson's disease. *Neurobiol Aging*, Vol.24, No.2, pp. 197-211.

Buhmann, C., Binkofski, F., Klein, C., Buchel, C., van Eimeren, T., Erdmann, C., Hedrich, K., Kasten, M., Hagenah, J., Deuschl, G., Pramstaller, P. P. & Siebner, H. R. (2005). Motor reorganization in asymptomatic carriers of a single mutant Parkin allele: a human model for presymptomatic parkinsonism. *Brain*, Vol.128, No.Pt 10, pp. 2281-2290.

Burbulla, L. F., Krebiehl, G. & Kruger, R. (2010). Balance is the challenge--the impact of mitochondrial dynamics in Parkinson's disease. *Eur J Clin Invest*, Vol.40, No.11, pp. 1048-1060.

Cha, G. H., Kim, S., Park, J., Lee, E., Kim, M., Lee, S. B., Kim, J. M., Chung, J. & Cho, K. S. (2005). Parkin negatively regulates JNK pathway in the dopaminergic neurons of Drosophila. *Proc Natl Acad Sci U S A*, Vol.102, No.29, pp. 10345-10350.

Chen, D., Gao, F., Li, B., Wang, H., Xu, Y., Zhu, C. & Wang, G. (2010). Parkin Mono-ubiquitinates Bcl-2 and Regulates Autophagy. *Journal of Biological Chemistry*, Vol.285, No.49, pp. 38214-38223.

Choi, P., Snyder, H., Petrucelli, L., Theisler, C., Chong, M., Zhang, Y., Lim, K., Chung, K. K. K., Kehoe, K., D'Adamio, L., Lee, J. M., Cochran, E., Bowser, R., Dawson, T. M. & Wolozin, B. (2003). SEPT5_v2 is a parkin-binding protein. *Molecular Brain Research*, Vol.117, No.2, pp. 179-189.

Chung, K. K., Zhang, Y., Lim, K. L., Tanaka, Y., Huang, H., Gao, J., Ross, C. A., Dawson, V. L. & Dawson, T. M. (2001). Parkin ubiquitinates the alpha-synuclein-interacting protein, synphilin-1: implications for Lewy-body formation in Parkinson disease. *Nat Med*, Vol.7, No.10, pp. 1144-1150.

Clark, I. E., Dodson, M. W., Jiang, C., Cao, J. H., Huh, J. R., Seol, J. H., Yoo, S. J., Hay, B. A. & Guo, M. (2006a). Drosophila pink1 is required for mitochondrial function and interacts genetically with parkin. *Nature*, Vol.441, No.7097, pp. 1162-1166.

Clark, L. N., Afridi, S., Karlins, E., Wang, Y., Mejia-Santana, H., Harris, J., Louis, E. D., Cote, L. J., Andrews, H., Fahn, S., Waters, C., Ford, B., Frucht, S., Ottman, R. & Marder, K. (2006b). Case-control study of the parkin gene in early-onset Parkinson disease. *Arch Neurol*, Vol.63, No.4, pp. 548-552.

Cookson, M. R., Lockhart, P. J., McLendon, C., O'Farrell, C., Schlossmacher, M. & Farrer, M. J. (2003). RING finger 1 mutations in Parkin produce altered localization of the protein. *Hum Mol Genet*, Vol.12, No.22, pp. 2957-2965.

Corti, O., Hampe, C., Koutnikova, H., Darios, F., Jacquier, S., Prigent, A., Robinson, J. C., Pradier, L., Ruberg, M., Mirande, M., Hirsch, E., Rooney, T., Fournier, A. & Brice, A. (2003). The p38 subunit of the aminoacyl-tRNA synthetase complex is a Parkin substrate: linking protein biosynthesis and neurodegeneration. *Hum Mol Genet*, Vol.12, No.12, pp. 1427-1437.

da Costa, C. A., Sunyach, C., Giaime, E., West, A., Corti, O., Brice, A., Safe, S., Abou-Sleiman, P. M., Wood, N. W., Takahashi, H., Goldberg, M. S., Shen, J. & Checler, F. (2009). Transcriptional repression of p53 by parkin and impairment by mutations associated with autosomal recessive juvenile Parkinson's disease. *Nat Cell Biol*, Vol.11, No.11, pp. 1370-1375.

Dawson, T. M., Ko, H. S. & Dawson, V. L. (2010). Genetic animal models of Parkinson's disease. *Neuron*, Vol.66, No.5, pp. 646-661.

Dehvari, N., Sandebring, A., Flores-Morales, A., Mateos, L., Chuan, Y.-C., Goldberg, M. S., Cookson, M. R., Cowburn, R. F. & Cedazo-Mínguez, A. (2009). Parkin-mediated ubiquitination regulates phospholipase C-γ1. *Journal of Cellular and Molecular Medicine*, Vol.13, No.9b, pp. 3061-3068.

Di Fonzo, A., Dekker, M. C., Montagna, P., Baruzzi, A., Yonova, E. H., Correia Guedes, L., Szczerbinska, A., Zhao, T., Dubbel-Hulsman, L. O., Wouters, C. H., de Graaff, E., Oyen, W. J., Simons, E. J., Breedveld, G. J., Oostra, B. A., Horstink, M. W. & Bonifati, V. (2009). FBXO7 mutations cause autosomal recessive, early-onset parkinsonian-pyramidal syndrome. *Neurology*, Vol.72, No.3, pp. 240-245.

Dorsey, E. R., Constantinescu, R., Thompson, J. P., Biglan, K. M., Holloway, R. G., Kieburtz, K., Marshall, F. J., Ravina, B. M., Schifitto, G., Siderowf, A. & Tanner, C. M. (2007). Projected number of people with Parkinson disease in the most populous nations, 2005 through 2030. *Neurology*, Vol.68, No.5, pp. 384-386.

Doss-Pepe, E. W., Chen, L. & Madura, K. (2005). Alpha-synuclein and parkin contribute to the assembly of ubiquitin lysine 63-linked multiubiquitin chains. *J Biol Chem*, Vol.280, No.17, pp. 16619-16624.

Fallon, L., Belanger, C. M. L., Corera, A. T., Kontogiannea, M., Regan-Klapisz, E., Moreau, F., Voortman, J., Haber, M., Rouleau, G., Thorarinsdottir, T., Brice, A., van Bergen en Henegouwen, P. M. P. & Fon, E. A. (2006). A regulated interaction with the UIM protein Eps15 implicates parkin in EGF receptor trafficking and PI(3)K-Akt signalling. *Nat Cell Biol*, Vol.8, No.8, pp. 834-842.

Farrer, M., Chan, P., Chen, R., Tan, L., Lincoln, S., Hernandez, D., Forno, L., Gwinn-Hardy, K., Petrucelli, L., Hussey, J., Singleton, A., Tanner, C., Hardy, J. & Langston, J. W. (2001). Lewy bodies and parkinsonism in families with parkin mutations. *Ann Neurol*, Vol.50, No.3, pp. 293-300.

Feany, M. B. & Pallanck, L. J. (2003). Parkin: a multipurpose neuroprotective agent? *Neuron*, Vol.38, No.1, pp. 13-16.

Fukae, J., Sato, S., Shiba, K., Sato, K.-i., Mori, H., Sharp, P. A., Mizuno, Y. & Hattori, N. (2009). Programmed cell death-2 isoform1 is ubiquitinated by parkin and increased in the substantia nigra of patients with autosomal recessive Parkinson's disease. *FEBS Letters*, Vol.583, No.3, pp. 521-525.

Geisler, S., Holmstrom, K. M., Skujat, D., Fiesel, F. C., Rothfuss, O. C., Kahle, P. J. & Springer, W. (2010). PINK1/Parkin-mediated mitophagy is dependent on VDAC1 and p62/SQSTM1. *Nat Cell Biol*, Vol.12, No.2, pp. 119-131.

Goldberg, M. S., Fleming, S. M., Palacino, J. J., Cepeda, C., Lam, H. A., Bhatnagar, A., Meloni, E. G., Wu, N., Ackerson, L. C., Klapstein, G. J., Gajendiran, M., Roth, B. L., Chesselet, M. F., Maidment, N. T., Levine, M. S. & Shen, J. (2003). Parkin-deficient mice exhibit nigrostriatal deficits but not loss of dopaminergic neurons. *J Biol Chem*, Vol.278, No.44, pp. 43628-43635.

Greene, J. C., Whitworth, A. J., Kuo, I., Andrews, L. A., Feany, M. B. & Pallanck, L. J. (2003). Mitochondrial pathology and apoptotic muscle degeneration in Drosophila parkin mutants. *Proc Natl Acad Sci U S A*, Vol.100, No.7, pp. 4078-4083.

Gu, W. J., Corti, O., Araujo, F., Hampe, C., Jacquier, S., Lucking, C. B., Abbas, N., Duyckaerts, C., Rooney, T., Pradier, L., Ruberg, M. & Brice, A. (2003). The C289G and C418R missense mutations cause rapid sequestration of human Parkin into insoluble aggregates. *Neurobiol Dis*, Vol.14, No.3, pp. 357-364.

Hampe, C., Ardila-Osorio, H., Fournier, M., Brice, A. & Corti, O. (2006). Biochemical analysis of Parkinson's disease-causing variants of Parkin, an E3 ubiquitin-protein ligase with monoubiquitylation capacity. *Hum Mol Genet*, Vol.15, No.13, pp. 2059-2075.

Hayashi, S., Wakabayashi, K., Ishikawa, A., Nagai, H., Saito, M., Maruyama, M., Takahashi, T., Ozawa, T., Tsuji, S. & Takahashi, H. (2000). An autopsy case of autosomal-recessive juvenile parkinsonism with a homozygous exon 4 deletion in the parkin gene. *Mov Disord*, Vol.15, No.5, pp. 884-888.

Healy, D. G., Abou-Sleiman, P. M. & Wood, N. W. (2004). Genetic causes of Parkinson's disease: UCHL-1. *Cell Tissue Res*, Vol.318, No.1, pp. 189-194.

Hedrich, K., Eskelson, C., Wilmot, B., Marder, K., Harris, J., Garrels, J., Meija-Santana, H., Vieregge, P., Jacobs, H., Bressman, S. B., Lang, A. E., Kann, M., Abbruzzese, G., Martinelli, P., Schwinger, E., Ozelius, L. J., Pramstaller, P. P., Klein, C. & Kramer, P. (2004). Distribution, type, and origin of Parkin mutations: review and case studies. *Mov Disord*, Vol.19, No.10, pp. 1146-1157.

Henn, I. H., Bouman, L., Schlehe, J. S., Schlierf, A., Schramm, J. E., Wegener, E., Nakaso, K., Culmsee, C., Berninger, B., Krappmann, D., Tatzelt, J. & Winklhofer, K. F. (2007). Parkin mediates neuroprotection through activation of IkappaB kinase/nuclear factor-kappaB signaling. *J Neurosci*, Vol.27, No.8, pp. 1868-1878.

Hilker, R., Klein, C., Ghaemi, M., Kis, B., Strotmann, T., Ozelius, L. J., Lenz, O., Vieregge, P., Herholz, K., Heiss, W. D. & Pramstaller, P. P. (2001). Positron emission tomographic analysis of the nigrostriatal dopaminergic system in familial parkinsonism associated with mutations in the parkin gene. *Ann Neurol*, Vol.49, No.3, pp. 367-376.

Huynh, D. P., Nguyen, D. T., Pulst-Korenberg, J. B., Brice, A. & Pulst, S. M. (2007). Parkin is an E3 ubiquitin-ligase for normal and mutant ataxin-2 and prevents ataxin-2-induced cell death. *Experimental Neurology*, Vol.203, No.2, pp. 531-541.

Imai, Y., Soda, M. & Takahashi, R. (2000). Parkin suppresses unfolded protein stress-induced cell death through its E3 ubiquitin-protein ligase activity. *J Biol Chem*, Vol.275, No.46, pp. 35661-35664.

Itier, J. M., Ibanez, P., Mena, M. A., Abbas, N., Cohen-Salmon, C., Bohme, G. A., Laville, M., Pratt, J., Corti, O., Pradier, L., Ret, G., Joubert, C., Periquet, M., Araujo, F., Negroni, J., Casarejos, M. J., Canals, S., Solano, R., Serrano, A., Gallego, E., Sanchez, M., Denefle, P., Benavides, J., Tremp, G., Rooney, T. A., Brice, A. & Garcia de Yebenes, J. (2003). Parkin gene inactivation alters behaviour and dopamine neurotransmission in the mouse. *Hum Mol Genet*, Vol.12, No.18, pp. 2277-2291.

Jiang, H., Jiang, Q. & Feng, J. (2004). Parkin Increases Dopamine Uptake by Enhancing the Cell Surface Expression of Dopamine Transporter. *Journal of Biological Chemistry*, Vol.279, No.52, pp. 54380-54386.

Joch, M., Ase, A. R., Chen, C. X. Q., MacDonald, P. A., Kontogiannea, M., Corera, A. T., Brice, A., Seguela, P. & Fon, E. A. (2007). Parkin-mediated Monoubiquitination of the PDZ Protein PICK1 Regulates the Activity of Acid-sensing Ion Channels. *Mol. Biol. Cell*, Vol.18, No.8, pp. 3105-3118.

Kalia, S. K., Lee, S., Smith, P. D., Liu, L., Crocker, S. J., Thorarinsdottir, T. E., Glover, J. R., Fon, E. A., Park, D. S. & Lozano, A. M. (2004). BAG5 inhibits parkin and enhances dopaminergic neuron degeneration. *Neuron*, Vol.44, No.6, pp. 931-945.

Kanki, T. & Klionsky, D. J. (2008). Mitophagy in yeast occurs through a selective mechanism. *J Biol Chem*, Vol.283, No.47, pp. 32386-32393.

Kao, S. Y. (2009a). DNA damage induces nuclear translocation of parkin. *J Biomed Sci*, Vol.16, pp. 67.

Kao, S. Y. (2009b). Regulation of DNA repair by parkin. *Biochem Biophys Res Commun*, Vol.382, No.2, pp. 321-325.

Kay, D. M., Moran, D., Moses, L., Poorkaj, P., Zabetian, C. P., Nutt, J., Factor, S. A., Yu, C. E., Montimurro, J. S., Keefe, R. G., Schellenberg, G. D. & Payami, H. (2007). Heterozygous parkin point mutations are as common in control subjects as in Parkinson's patients. *Ann Neurol*, Vol.61, No.1, pp. 47-54.

Kitada, T., Asakawa, S., Hattori, N., Matsumine, H., Yamamura, Y., Minoshima, S., Yokochi, M., Mizuno, Y. & Shimizu, N. (1998). Mutations in the parkin gene cause autosomal recessive juvenile parkinsonism. *Nature*, Vol.392, No.6676, pp. 605-608.

Kitada, T., Tong, Y., Gautier, C. A. & Shen, J. (2009). Absence of nigral degeneration in aged parkin/DJ-1/PINK1 triple knockout mice. *J Neurochem*, Vol.111, No.3, pp. 696-702.

Klein, C., Lohmann-Hedrich, K., Rogaeva, E., Schlossmacher, M. G. & Lang, A. E. (2007). Deciphering the role of heterozygous mutations in genes associated with parkinsonism. *Lancet Neurol*, Vol.6, No.7, pp. 652-662.

Ko, H. S., Kim, S. W., Sriram, S. R., Dawson, V. L. & Dawson, T. M. (2006). Identification of Far Upstream Element-binding Protein-1 as an Authentic Parkin Substrate. *J. Biol. Chem.*, Vol.281, No.24, pp. 16193-16196.

Ko, H. S., Lee, Y., Shin, J. H., Karuppagounder, S. S., Gadad, B. S., Koleske, A. J., Pletnikova, O., Troncoso, J. C., Dawson, V. L. & Dawson, T. M. (2010). Phosphorylation by the c-Abl protein tyrosine kinase inhibits parkin's ubiquitination and protective function. *Proc Natl Acad Sci U S A*, Vol.107, No.38, pp. 16691-16696.

Ko, H. S., von Coelln, R., Sriram, S. R., Kim, S. W., Chung, K. K., Pletnikova, O., Troncoso, J., Johnson, B., Saffary, R., Goh, E. L., Song, H., Park, B. J., Kim, M. J., Kim, S., Dawson, V. L. & Dawson, T. M. (2005). Accumulation of the authentic parkin substrate aminoacyl-tRNA synthetase cofactor, p38/JTV-1, leads to catecholaminergic cell death. *J Neurosci*, Vol.25, No.35, pp. 7968-7978.

Kopito, R. R. (2000). Aggresomes, inclusion bodies and protein aggregation. *Trends Cell Biol*, Vol.10, No.12, pp. 524-530.

Kuroda, Y., Mitsui, T., Kunishige, M., Shono, M., Akaike, M., Azuma, H. & Matsumoto, T. (2006). Parkin enhances mitochondrial biogenesis in proliferating cells. *Hum Mol Genet*, Vol.15, No.6, pp. 883-895.

LaVoie, M. J., Cortese, G. P., Ostaszewski, B. L. & Schlossmacher, M. G. (2007). The effects of oxidative stress on parkin and other E3 ligases. *J Neurochem*, Vol.103, No.6, pp. 2354-2368.

LaVoie, M. J., Ostaszewski, B. L., Weihofen, A., Schlossmacher, M. G. & Selkoe, D. J. (2005). Dopamine covalently modifies and functionally inactivates parkin. *Nat Med*, Vol.11, No.11, pp. 1214-1221.

Lim, K. L., Chew, K. C., Tan, J. M., Wang, C., Chung, K. K., Zhang, Y., Tanaka, Y., Smith, W., Engelender, S., Ross, C. A., Dawson, V. L. & Dawson, T. M. (2005). Parkin mediates nonclassical, proteasomal-independent ubiquitination of synphilin-1: implications for Lewy body formation. *J Neurosci*, Vol.25, No.8, pp. 2002-2009.

Lim, K. L., Dawson, V. L. & Dawson, T. M. (2006). Parkin-mediated lysine 63-linked polyubiquitination: a link to protein inclusions formation in Parkinson's and other conformational diseases? *Neurobiol Aging*, Vol.27, No.4, pp. 524-529.

Lim, K. L. & Lim, G. G. (2011). K63-linked ubiquitination and neurodegeneration. *Neurobiol Dis*, 43, 9-16.

Lim, M. K., Kawamura, T., Ohsawa, Y., Ohtsubo, M., Asakawa, S., Takayanagi, A. & Shimizu, N. (2007). Parkin interacts with LIM Kinase 1 and reduces its cofilin-phosphorylation activity via ubiquitination. *Experimental cell research*, Vol.313, No.13, pp. 2858-2874.

Lincoln, S. J., Maraganore, D. M., Lesnick, T. G., Bounds, R., de Andrade, M., Bower, J. H., Hardy, J. A. & Farrer, M. J. (2003). Parkin variants in North American Parkinson's disease: cases and controls. *Mov Disord*, Vol.18, No.11, pp. 1306-1311.

Lo Bianco, C., Schneider, B. L., Bauer, M., Sajadi, A., Brice, A., Iwatsubo, T. & Aebischer, P. (2004). Lentiviral vector delivery of parkin prevents dopaminergic degeneration in an alpha-synuclein rat model of Parkinson's disease. *Proc Natl Acad Sci U S A*, Vol.101, No.50, pp. 17510-17515.

Lu, X. H., Fleming, S. M., Meurers, B., Ackerson, L. C., Mortazavi, F., Lo, V., Hernandez, D., Sulzer, D., Jackson, G. R., Maidment, N. T., Chesselet, M. F. & Yang, X. W. (2009). Bacterial artificial chromosome transgenic mice expressing a truncated mutant parkin exhibit age-dependent hypokinetic motor deficits, dopaminergic neuron degeneration, and accumulation of proteinase K-resistant alpha-synuclein. *J Neurosci*, Vol.29, No.7, pp. 1962-1976.

Lucking, C. B., Durr, A., Bonifati, V., Vaughan, J., De Michele, G., Gasser, T., Harhangi, B. S., Meco, G., Denefle, P., Wood, N. W., Agid, Y. & Brice, A. (2000). Association between early-onset Parkinson's disease and mutations in the parkin gene. French Parkinson's Disease Genetics Study Group. *N Engl J Med*, Vol.342, No.21, pp. 1560-1567.

Mata, I. F., Lockhart, P. J. & Farrer, M. J. (2004). Parkin genetics: one model for Parkinson's disease. *Hum Mol Genet*, Vol.13 Spec No 1, pp. R127-133.

Matsuda, N., Kitami, T., Suzuki, T., Mizuno, Y., Hattori, N. & Tanaka, K. (2006). Diverse effects of pathogenic mutations of Parkin that catalyze multiple monoubiquitylation in vitro. *J Biol Chem*, Vol.281, No.6, pp. 3204-3209.

Matsuda, N., Sato, S., Shiba, K., Okatsu, K., Saisho, K., Gautier, C. A., Sou, Y. S., Saiki, S., Kawajiri, S., Sato, F., Kimura, M., Komatsu, M., Hattori, N. & Tanaka, K. (2010). PINK1 stabilized by mitochondrial depolarization recruits Parkin to damaged mitochondria and activates latent Parkin for mitophagy. *J Cell Biol*, Vol.189, No.2, pp. 211-221.

Moore, D. J., West, A. B., Dikeman, D. A., Dawson, V. L. & Dawson, T. M. (2008). Parkin mediates the degradation-independent ubiquitination of Hsp70. *J Neurochem*, Vol.105, No.5, pp. 1806-1819.

Mori, H., Kondo, T., Yokochi, M., Matsumine, H., Nakagawa-Hattori, Y., Miyake, T., Suda, K. & Mizuno, Y. (1998). Pathologic and biochemical studies of juvenile parkinsonism linked to chromosome 6q. *Neurology*, Vol.51, No.3, pp. 890-892.

Muqit, M. M., Davidson, S. M., Payne Smith, M. D., MacCormac, L. P., Kahns, S., Jensen, P. H., Wood, N. W. & Latchman, D. S. (2004). Parkin is recruited into aggresomes in a stress-specific manner: over-expression of parkin reduces aggresome formation but can be dissociated from parkin's effect on neuronal survival. *Hum Mol Genet*, Vol.13, No.1, pp. 117-135.

Narendra, D., Tanaka, A., Suen, D. F. & Youle, R. J. (2008). Parkin is recruited selectively to impaired mitochondria and promotes their autophagy. *J Cell Biol*, Vol.183, No.5, pp. 795-803.

Narendra, D. P., Jin, S. M., Tanaka, A., Suen, D. F., Gautier, C. A., Shen, J., Cookson, M. R. & Youle, R. J. (2010). PINK1 is selectively stabilized on impaired mitochondria to activate Parkin. *PLoS Biol*, Vol.8, No.1, pp. e1000298.

Narendra, D. P., Kane, L. A., Hauser, D. N., Fearnley, I. M. & Youle, R. J. p62/SQSTM1 is required for Parkin-induced mitochondrial clustering but not mitophagy; VDAC1 is dispensable for both. *Autophagy*, Vol.6, No.8.

Olanow, C. W., Hauser, R. A., Jankovic, J., Langston, W., Lang, A., Poewe, W., Tolosa, E., Stocchi, F., Melamed, E., Eyal, E. & Rascol, O. (2008). A randomized, double-blind, placebo-controlled, delayed start study to assess rasagiline as a disease modifying therapy in Parkinson's disease (the ADAGIO study): rationale, design, and baseline characteristics. *Mov Disord*, Vol.23, No.15, pp. 2194-2201.

Olzmann, J. A., Li, L., Chudaev, M. V., Chen, J., Perez, F. A., Palmiter, R. D. & Chin, L. S. (2007). Parkin-mediated K63-linked polyubiquitination targets misfolded DJ-1 to aggresomes via binding to HDAC6. *J Cell Biol*, Vol.178, No.6, pp. 1025-1038.

Paisan-Ruiz, C., Bhatia, K. P., Li, A., Hernandez, D., Davis, M., Wood, N. W., Hardy, J., Houlden, H., Singleton, A. & Schneider, S. A. (2009). Characterization of PLA2G6 as a locus for dystonia-parkinsonism. *Ann Neurol*, Vol.65, No.1, pp. 19-23.

Palacino, J. J., Sagi, D., Goldberg, M. S., Krauss, S., Motz, C., Wacker, M., Klose, J. & Shen, J. (2004). Mitochondrial dysfunction and oxidative damage in parkin-deficient mice. *J Biol Chem*, Vol.279, No.18, pp. 18614-18622.

Park, J., Lee, S. B., Lee, S., Kim, Y., Song, S., Kim, S., Bae, E., Kim, J., Shong, M., Kim, J. M. & Chung, J. (2006). Mitochondrial dysfunction in Drosophila PINK1 mutants is complemented by parkin. *Nature*, Vol.441, No.7097, pp. 1157-1161.

Paterna, J. C., Leng, A., Weber, E., Feldon, J. & Bueler, H. (2007). DJ-1 and Parkin Modulate Dopamine-dependent Behavior and Inhibit MPTP-induced Nigral Dopamine Neuron Loss in Mice. *Mol Ther.*

Pawlyk, A. C., Giasson, B. I., Sampathu, D. M., Perez, F. A., Lim, K. L., Dawson, V. L., Dawson, T. M., Palmiter, R. D., Trojanowski, J. Q. & Lee, V. M. (2003). Novel monoclonal antibodies demonstrate biochemical variation of brain parkin with age. *J Biol Chem*, Vol.278, No.48, pp. 48120-48128.

Peng, J., Schwartz, D., Elias, J. E., Thoreen, C. C., Cheng, D., Marsischky, G., Roelofs, J., Finley, D. & Gygi, S. P. (2003). A proteomics approach to understanding protein ubiquitination. *Nat Biotechnol*, Vol.21, No.8, pp. 921-926.

Perez, F. A. & Palmiter, R. D. (2005). Parkin-deficient mice are not a robust model of parkinsonism. *Proc Natl Acad Sci U S A*, Vol.102, No.6, pp. 2174-2179.

Periquet, M., Corti, O., Jacquier, S. & Brice, A. (2005). Proteomic analysis of parkin knockout mice: alterations in energy metabolism, protein handling and synaptic function. *Journal of Neurochemistry*, Vol.95, No.5, pp. 1259-1276.

Periquet, M., Latouche, M., Lohmann, E., Rawal, N., De Michele, G., Ricard, S., Teive, H., Fraix, V., Vidailhet, M., Nicholl, D., Barone, P., Wood, N. W., Raskin, S., Deleuze, J. F., Agid, Y., Durr, A. & Brice, A. (2003). Parkin mutations are frequent in patients with isolated early-onset parkinsonism. *Brain*, Vol.126, No.Pt 6, pp. 1271-1278.

Poole, A. C., Thomas, R. E., Yu, S., Vincow, E. S. & Pallanck, L. (2010). The mitochondrial fusion-promoting factor mitofusin is a substrate of the PINK1/parkin pathway. *PLoS One*, Vol.5, No.4, pp. e10054.

Pramstaller, P. P., Schlossmacher, M. G., Jacques, T. S., Scaravilli, F., Eskelson, C., Pepivani, I., Hedrich, K., Adel, S., Gonzales-McNeal, M., Hilker, R., Kramer, P. L. & Klein, C. (2005). Lewy body Parkinson's disease in a large pedigree with 77 Parkin mutation carriers. *Ann Neurol*, Vol.58, No.3, pp. 411-422.

Ramirez, A., Heimbach, A., Grundemann, J., Stiller, B., Hampshire, D., Cid, L. P., Goebel, I., Mubaidin, A. F., Wriekat, A. L., Roeper, J., Al-Din, A., Hillmer, A. M., Karsak, M., Liss, B., Woods, C. G., Behrens, M. I. & Kubisch, C. (2006). Hereditary parkinsonism with dementia is caused by mutations in ATP13A2, encoding a lysosomal type 5 P-type ATPase. *Nat Genet*, Vol.38, No.10, pp. 1184-1191.

Ren, Y., Jiang, H., Yang, F., Nakaso, K. & Feng, J. (2009). Parkin protects dopaminergic neurons against microtubule-depolymerizing toxins by attenuating microtubule-associated protein kinase activation. *J Biol Chem*, Vol.284, No.6, pp. 4009-4017.

Ren, Y., Zhao, J. & Feng, J. (2003). Parkin binds to alpha/beta tubulin and increases their ubiquitination and degradation. *J Neurosci*, Vol.23, No.8, pp. 3316-3324.

Rosen, K. M., Moussa, C. E., Lee, H. K., Kumar, P., Kitada, T., Qin, G., Fu, Q. & Querfurth, H. W. (2010). Parkin reverses intracellular beta-amyloid accumulation and its negative effects on proteasome function. *J Neurosci Res*, Vol.88, No.1, pp. 167-178.

Rubio de la Torre, E., Luzon-Toro, B., Forte-Lago, I., Minguez-Castellanos, A., Ferrer, I. & Hilfiker, S. (2009). Combined kinase inhibition modulates parkin inactivation. *Hum Mol Genet*, Vol.18, No.5, pp. 809-823.

Sang, T. K., Chang, H. Y., Lawless, G. M., Ratnaparkhi, A., Mee, L., Ackerson, L. C., Maidment, N. T., Krantz, D. E. & Jackson, G. R. (2007). A Drosophila model of mutant human parkin-induced toxicity demonstrates selective loss of dopaminergic neurons and dependence on cellular dopamine. *J Neurosci*, Vol.27, No.5, pp. 981-992.

Sato, S., Chiba, T., Sakata, E., Kato, K., Mizuno, Y., Hattori, N. & Tanaka, K. (2006). 14-3-3eta is a novel regulator of parkin ubiquitin ligase. *EMBO J*, Vol.25, No.1, pp. 211-221.

Scarpulla, R. C. (2008). Nuclear control of respiratory chain expression by nuclear respiratory factors and PGC-1-related coactivator. *Ann N Y Acad Sci*, Vol.1147, pp. 321-334.

Schlehe, J. S., Lutz, A. K., Pilsl, A., Lammermann, K., Grgur, K., Henn, I. H., Tatzelt, J. & Winklhofer, K. F. (2008). Aberrant folding of pathogenic Parkin mutants: aggregation versus degradation. *J Biol Chem*, Vol.283, No.20, pp. 13771-13779.

Shimura, H., Hattori, N., Kubo, S., Mizuno, Y., Asakawa, S., Minoshima, S., Shimizu, N., Iwai, K., Chiba, T., Tanaka, K. & Suzuki, T. (2000). Familial Parkinson disease gene product, parkin, is a ubiquitin-protein ligase. *Nat Genet*, Vol.25, No.3, pp. 302-305.

Shimura, H., Schlossmacher, M. G., Hattori, N., Frosch, M. P., Trockenbacher, A., Schneider, R., Mizuno, Y., Kosik, K. S. & Selkoe, D. J. (2001). Ubiquitination of a New Form of alpha -Synuclein by Parkin from Human Brain: Implications for Parkinson's Disease. *Science*, Vol.293, No.5528, pp. 263-269.

Shin, J. H., Ko, H. S., Kang, H., Lee, Y., Lee, Y. I., Pletinkova, O., Troconso, J. C., Dawson, V. L. & Dawson, T. M. (2011). PARIS (ZNF746) Repression of PGC-1alpha Contributes to Neurodegeneration in Parkinson's Disease. *Cell*, Vol.144, No.5, pp. 689-702.

Simon-Sanchez, J. & Singleton, A. B. (2008). Sequencing analysis of OMI/HTRA2 shows previously reported pathogenic mutations in neurologically normal controls. *Hum Mol Genet*, Vol.17, No.13, pp. 1988-1993.

Sriram, S. R., Li, X., Ko, H. S., Chung, K. K., Wong, E., Lim, K. L., Dawson, V. L. & Dawson, T. M. (2005). Familial-associated mutations differentially disrupt the solubility, localization, binding and ubiquitination properties of parkin. *Hum Mol Genet*, Vol.14, No.17, pp. 2571-2586.

Staropoli, J. F., McDermott, C., Martinat, C., Schulman, B., Demireva, E. & Abeliovich, A. (2003). Parkin Is a Component of an SCF-like Ubiquitin Ligase Complex and Protects Postmitotic Neurons from Kainate Excitotoxicity. *Neuron*, Vol.37, No.5, pp. 735-749.

Tain, L. S., Mortiboys, H., Tao, R. N., Ziviani, E., Bandmann, O. & Whitworth, A. J. (2009). Rapamycin activation of 4E-BP prevents parkinsonian dopaminergic neuron loss. *Nat Neurosci*, Vol.12, No.9, pp. 1129-1135.

Tan, J. M., Wong, E. S., Dawson, V. L., Dawson, T. M. & Lim, K. L. (2008a). Lysine 63-linked polyubiquitin potentially partners with p62 to promote the clearance of protein inclusions by autophagy. *Autophagy*, Vol.4, No.2, pp. 251-253.

Tan, J. M., Wong, E. S., Kirkpatrick, D. S., Pletnikova, O., Ko, H. S., Tay, S. P., Ho, M. W., Troncoso, J., Gygi, S. P., Lee, M. K., Dawson, V. L., Dawson, T. M. & Lim, K. L. (2008b). Lysine 63-linked ubiquitination promotes the formation and autophagic clearance of protein inclusions associated with neurodegenerative diseases. *Hum Mol Genet*, Vol.17, No.3, pp. 431-439.

Tanaka, A., Cleland, M. M., Xu, S., Narendra, D. P., Suen, D. F., Karbowski, M. & Youle, R. J. (2010). Proteasome and p97 mediate mitophagy and degradation of mitofusins induced by Parkin. *J Cell Biol*, Vol.191, No.7, pp. 1367-1380.

Thomas, B. & Beal, M. F. (2007). Parkinson's disease. *Hum Mol Genet*, Vol.16 Spec No. 2, pp. R183-194.

Tsai, Y. C., Fishman, P. S., Thakor, N. V. & Oyler, G. A. (2003). Parkin facilitates the elimination of expanded polyglutamine proteins and leads to preservation of proteasome function. *J Biol Chem*, Vol.278, No.24, pp. 22044-22055.

Ulusoy, A., Bjorklund, T., Hermening, S. & Kirik, D. (2008). In vivo gene delivery for development of mammalian models for Parkinson's disease. *Exp Neurol*, Vol.209, No.1, pp. 89-100.

Um, J. W., Min, D. S., Rhim, H., Kim, J., Paik, S. R. & Chung, K. C. (2006). Parkin Ubiquitinates and Promotes the Degradation of RanBP2. *J. Biol. Chem.*, Vol.281, No.6, pp. 3595-3603.

Van Laar, V. S., Arnold, B., Cassady, S. J., Chu, C. T., Burton, E. A. & Berman, S. B. (2011). Bioenergetics of neurons inhibit the translocation response of Parkin following rapid mitochondrial depolarization. *Hum Mol Genet*, Vol.20, No.5, pp. 927-940.

Vives-Bauza, C., Zhou, C., Huang, Y., Cui, M., de Vries, R. L., Kim, J., May, J., Tocilescu, M. A., Liu, W., Ko, H. S., Magrane, J., Moore, D. J., Dawson, V. L., Grailhe, R., Dawson, T. M., Li, C., Tieu, K. & Przedborski, S. (2010). PINK1-dependent recruitment of Parkin to mitochondria in mitophagy. *Proc Natl Acad Sci U S A*, Vol.107, No.1, pp. 378-383.

Walter, U., Klein, C., Hilker, R., Benecke, R., Pramstaller, P. P. & Dressler, D. (2004). Brain parenchyma sonography detects preclinical parkinsonism. *Mov Disord*, Vol.19, No.12, pp. 1445-1449.

Wang, C., Ko, H. S., Thomas, B., Tsang, F., Chew, K. C., Tay, S. P., Ho, M. W., Lim, T. M., Soong, T. W., Pletnikova, O., Troncoso, J., Dawson, V. L., Dawson, T. M. & Lim, K. L. (2005). Stress-induced alterations in parkin solubility promote parkin aggregation and compromise parkin's protective function. *Hum Mol Genet*, Vol.14, No.24, pp. 3885-3897.

Wang, C., Lu, R., Ouyang, X., Ho, M. W., Chia, W., Yu, F. & Lim, K. L. (2007). Drosophila overexpressing parkin R275W mutant exhibits dopaminergic neuron degeneration and mitochondrial abnormalities. *J Neurosci*, Vol.27, No.32, pp. 8563-8570.

Wang, C., Tan, J. M., Ho, M. W., Zaiden, N., Wong, S. H., Chew, C. L., Eng, P. W., Lim, T. M., Dawson, T. M. & Lim, K. L. (2005b). Alterations in the solubility and intracellular localization of parkin by several familial Parkinson's disease-linked point mutations. *J Neurochem*, Vol.93, No.2, pp. 422-431.

Wang, H., Song, P., Du, L., Tian, W., Yue, W., Liu, M., Li, D., Wang, B., Zhu, Y., Cao, C., Zhou, J. & Chen, Q. (2011). Parkin ubiquitinates Drp1 for proteasome-dependent degradation: implication of dysregulated mitochondrial dynamics in Parkinson's disease. *J Biol Chem*.

West, A. B., Maraganore, D., Crook, J., Lesnick, T., Lockhart, P. J., Wilkes, K. M., Kapatos, G., Hardy, J. A. & Farrer, M. J. (2002). Functional association of the parkin gene promoter with idiopathic Parkinson's disease. *Hum Mol Genet*, Vol.11, No.22, pp. 2787-2792.

Winklhofer, K. F. (2007). The parkin protein as a therapeutic target in Parkinson's disease. *Expert Opin Ther Targets*, Vol.11, No.12, pp. 1543-1552.

Winklhofer, K. F., Henn, I. H., Kay-Jackson, P. C., Heller, U. & Tatzelt, J. (2003). Inactivation of parkin by oxidative stress and C-terminal truncations: a protective role of molecular chaperones. *J Biol Chem*, Vol.278, No.47, pp. 47199-47208.

Wong, E. S., Tan, J. M., Wang, C., Zhang, Z., Tay, S. P., Zaiden, N., Ko, H. S., Dawson, V. L., Dawson, T. M. & Lim, K. L. (2007). Relative sensitivity of parkin and other cysteine-containing enzymes to stress-induced solubility alterations. *J Biol Chem*, Vol.282, No.16, pp. 12310-12318.

Yamada, M., Mizuno, Y. & Mochizuki, H. (2005). Parkin gene therapy for alpha-synucleinopathy: a rat model of Parkinson's disease. *Hum Gene Ther*, Vol.16, No.2, pp. 262-270.

Yamamoto, A., Friedlein, A., Imai, Y., Takahashi, R., Kahle, P. J. & Haass, C. (2005). Parkin phosphorylation and modulation of its E3 ubiquitin ligase activity. *J Biol Chem*, Vol.280, No.5, pp. 3390-3399.

Yasuda, T., Miyachi, S., Kitagawa, R., Wada, K., Nihira, T., Ren, Y. R., Hirai, Y., Ageyama, N., Terao, K., Shimada, T., Takada, M., Mizuno, Y. & Mochizuki, H. (2007). Neuronal specificity of alpha-synuclein toxicity and effect of Parkin co-expression in primates. *Neuroscience*, Vol.144, No.2, pp. 743-753.

Zhang, Y., Gao, J., Chung, K. K., Huang, H., Dawson, V. L. & Dawson, T. M. (2000). Parkin functions as an E2-dependent ubiquitin- protein ligase and promotes the degradation of the synaptic vesicle-associated protein, CDCrel-1. *Proc Natl Acad Sci U S A*, Vol.97, No.24, pp. 13354-13359.

Zhong, L., Tan, Y., Zhou, A., Yu, Q. & Zhou, J. (2005). RING finger ubiquitin-protein isopeptide ligase Nrdp1/FLRF regulates parkin stability and activity. *J Biol Chem*, Vol.280, No.10, pp. 9425-9430.

Ziviani, E., Tao, R. N. & Whitworth, A. J. (2010). Drosophila parkin requires PINK1 for mitochondrial translocation and ubiquitinates mitofusin. *Proc Natl Acad Sci U S A*, Vol.107, No.11, pp. 5018-5023.

4

Modeling LRRK2 Parkinsonism

Kelly Hinkle and Heather Melrose
Dept. Of Neuroscience, Mayo Clinic Jacksonville, USA

1. Introduction

Mutations in the LRRK2 gene were first described in 2004 and have now emerged as the most important genetic finding in Parkinson's Disease (PD) (Paisan-Ruiz et al., 2004, Zimprich et al., 2004). Incredibly, they account for up to 40% of familial parkinsonism in certain ethnic populations (Ishihara et al., 2007; Kachergus et al., 2005; Ozelius et al., 2006). Moreover LRRK2 mutations also are responsible for about 2 % of PD in sporadic (idiopathic) patients and two risk factors increase the risk for sporadic PD in Asian populations by two-fold (Di Fonzo et al., 2006; Farrer et al., 2007; Ross et al., 2008; Tan, 2006). While the precise functional role of LRRK2 protein is still emerging, it has attracted intense pharmaceutical interest as a highly "druggable" target. This, and other unique properties including variable penetrance and pathologies that overlap with other neurodegenerative disorders, have fueled theories that a LRRK2 therapeutic will benefit not just familial parkinsonism, but also sporadic parkinsonism and perhaps even neurodegeneration in general. Development of LRRK2 agents relies on the availability of animal models, which provide not only information of physiological and pathological functions but also a means for testing and phenotypic reversal. In this chapter we summarize the progress to date for both invertebrate and vertebrate models of LRRK2 parkinsonism and briefly discuss opportunities for therapeutic development.

2. Background

2.1 LRRK2 mutations

There are five LRRK2 mutations (R1441C, R1441G; Y1699C; G2019S; I2020T) proven to segregate with disease and cause pathogenicity (Paisan-Ruiz et al., 2004; Zimprich et al., 2004) and two variants that are considered risk factors (LRRK2 G2385R and R1628P) (Farrer et al., 2007; Ross et al., 2008; Tan, 2006). While all leading to the same disease, the substitutions are not all found in the same functional domain. LRRK2 R1441C and G substitutions affect the Roc domain, a 'Ras-like' part of the protein (Mata et al., 2005). The LRRK2 Y1699C substitution and the R1628P risk factor are found in the COR domain and LRRK2 G2019S and I2020T are encoded within exon 41 at the 'activation hinge' of the MAPKKK domain (Mata et al., 2005). To date, the only substitution affecting risk of disease in the WD40 domain is the G2385R risk factor. The most common substitution, *LRRK2* G2019S, originates from a common founder and presents with variable, age-dependent penetrance (Healy et al., 2008; Hulihan et al., 2008; Kachergus et al., 2005).

2.2 Clinical and neuropathological features of LRRK2 parkinsonism

The overall clinical profile in individuals with LRRK2 mutations is similar to that of typical late-onset PD (Aasly et al., 2005; Djaldetti et al., 2008; Healy et al., 2008). In agreement with observations in idiopathic PD, individuals with LRRK2-parkinsonism are generally responsive to levodopa treatment. While tremor, bradykinesia, and rigidity occurs in individuals with idiopathic PD, tremor is more frequently observed in individuals with LRRK2 G2019S (Djaldetti et al., 2008; Healy et al., 2008; Hulihan et al., 2008).

Disease duration, severity and response to treatment do not differ between G2019S carriers, regardless of zygosity (Ishihara et al., 2007, (Djaldetti et al., 2008) Individuals harboring LRRK2 G2019S present with similar non-motor features to idiopathic PD with the exception of a lower rate of cognitive impairment and hyposmia (Healy et al., 2008; Hulihan et al., 2008). Remarkably, there are aged G2019S carriers that escape disease (Carmine Belin et al., 2006; Kay et al., 2005). The LRRK2 G2019S mutation is primarily associated with transitional or brainstem Lewy body pathology, reminiscent of typical, late-onset idiopathic PD (Ross et al., 2006). LRRK2 mutation carriers presenting with tauopathy or ubiquitin-positive inclusions, with nigral neuronal loss and gliosis, have also been described (Wszolek et al., 2004; Dachsel et al., 2007; Rajput et al., 2006) Neuropathologic studies of affected individuals from other PARK8-linked kindreds, including Family A (Y1699C), Family D (R1441C), and the Sagamihara family (I2020T) have presented with pleomorphic pathology, including neuronal loss without co-existing pathology or with α-synuclein, ubiquitin-positive inclusions or tau pathology (Taylor et al., 2006).

2.2.1 LRRK2 expression

LRRK2 mRNA is highly expressed in the lungs, kidney, spleen and leucocytes; (Biskup et al., 2006; Li et al., 2007; Westerlund et al., 2008; White et al., 2007; Zimprich et al., 2004) however, its expression profile suggests that LRRK2 is unlikely to be an essential developmental protein (Biskup et al., 2007). In adult rodent brain, LRRK2 mRNA is somewhat restricted, with highest levels found in dopamine receptive areas but surprisingly low levels in the dopamine synthesizing areas (Biskup et al., 2006; Galter et al., 2006; Melrose et al., 2006; Simon-Sanchez et al., 2006; Taymans et al., 2006). LRRK2 protein levels do not entirely correlate with mRNA levels, suggesting transport following synthesis. LRRK2 protein is highly expressed in the spiny neurons in the striatum and in the dopamine neurons of the substantia nigra, (Biskup et al., 2006; Melrose et al., 2007) but robust expression is also found in many non-dopaminergic areas throughout the brain, for example the hippocampus and cerebellum (Biskup et al., 2006; Greggio et al., 2006; Higashi et al., 2007a; Higashi et al., 2007b; Melrose et al., 2007; Miklossy et al., 2006).

2.3 Predicted function

LRRK2 protein contains a GTPase domain as well as a kinase domain containing homologous sequence to tyrosine-like kinase (TLK), including mixed-lineage kinases (MLKs) and receptor-interacting kinases (RIPKs) (Mata et al., 2006). Given the size of the protein monomer (286kDa), its protein-protein interaction domains (ANK, LRR, WD40) and its propensity to dimerize, (Greggio et al., 2008) it is reasonable to postulate LRRK2 is part of a larger scaffolding complex. While *in silico* modeling suggests that LRRK2 mutations may have increased kinase activity and

act through a dominant "gain-of-function", data on kinase activity across the different mutations has been controversial, with only the G2019S mutation consistently reported to enhance kinase activity compared to wild-type activity (Adams et al., 2005; Jaleel et al., 2007; Luzon-Toro et al., 2007; MacLeod et al., 2006; Smith et al., 2006; West et al., 2005).
LRRK2 has been characterized extensively in vitro. Although it is beyond the scope of this review to discuss these studies detail, several lines of evidence several lines of evidence point to a role in synaptic function (possibly by regulation of vesicle synthesis or transport and/or regulation of membranous structure) and as a regulator of neuronal outgrowth and guidance.

3. Invertebrate models

3.1 LRRK2 worm models

LRK-1, the paralogue of LRRK2 in *Caenorhabditis elegans,* shares ~35% identity and 57% similarity with the enzymatic GTPase and kinase domains (Samann et al., 2009) and is expressed ubiquitously, including in muscle, intestine and importantly in neurons (Sakaguchi-Nakashima et al., 2007; Samann et al., 2009). Experimental approaches to study LRRK2 in worms have included loss of LRK-1 function, over-expression of LRK-1 and transgenic insertion of human wild type and mutant LRRK2.

3.1.1 LRK-1 loss of function worm models

Sakaguchi-Nakashima et al first described loss-of-function LRK-1 mutants, the km17 line, which has a deletion in the kinase and WD40 domains, and km41 line that has the GTPase and kinase domain deleted (Sakaguchi-Nakashima et al., 2007). A third deletion strain, tm1898 (also lacking the GTPAse and kinase domain) was later described (Saha et al., 2009). All three deletion mutants result in mislocalization of synaptobrevin to dendrites, suggesting that normally LRK-1 plays a role in sorting and/or localization of synaptic vesicle proteins (Sakaguchi-Nakashima et al., 2007; Samann et al., 2009) possibly by excluding them from dendrite-specific transport machinery in the Golgi (Sakaguchi-Nakashima et al., 2007). Loss-of-function LRK-1 (km17 and km41) worms also exhibited defects in movement and chemotaxis (Sakaguchi-Nakashima et al., 2007). Both the km41 and tm1898 mutants were reported to have increased sensitivity to endoplasmic reticiulum stress, following tunicamycin exposure but were resistant to mitochondrial stress via paraquat (Samann et al., 2009). Conversely, Saha reported that RNAi knockdown of LRK-1, while not affecting baseline viability, did sensitize nemotodes to mictochrondrial dysfunction via rotenone treatment, a response that was confirmed in the km17 deletion line (Saha et al., 2009). Interestingly, loss of LRK-1 has been found to suppress the neurite outgrowth defects, mitochondrial abnormalities and increased paraquat sensitivity in PINK-1 loss-of-function mutants. Additionally, the increased sensitivity of LRK-1 loss-of-function worms to tunicamycin was reduced in PINK-1 loss-of-function mutants, suggesting an antagonistic role of PINK-1 and LRK-1 (Samann et al., 2009). Curiously, loss of LRK-1 also attenuates transgenic LRRK2-induced DA neurodegeneration and basal slowing behavioral phenotype (Yao et al., 2010)

3.1.2 Transgenic worm models

Transgenic worms have been created by either overexpressing wild-type (WT) LRK-1 and/or comparable mutant LRK-1 or by overexpressing human WT or mutant LRRK2 with fluorescent tags (Sakaguchi-Nakashima et al., 2007; Samann et al., 2009) driven by tissue-specific promoters whereas others have over-expressed human LRRK2 WT and pathogenic mutants via the dopamine neuron-specific DAT promoters (Saha et al., 2009; Wolozin et al., 2008; Yao et al., 2010).

Over-expression of endogenous WT and mutant LRK-1 in neurons resulted in axon guidance defects and embryonic lethality (Samann et al., 2009). Surprisingly, worms expressing human LRRK2 had increased longevity and reduced vulnerability to mitochondrial toxicity, with human WT LRRK2 offering more protection than mutant G2019S, R1441C or R1441C kinase dead LRRK2 (Saha et al., 2009; Wolozin et al., 2008). Despite this protection, transgenic LRRK2 WT and G2019S worms exhibited DA neuron degeneration and decreased dopamine levels, with G2019S mutants exhibiting more severe phenotypes (Saha et al., 2009). These findings were confirmed by Yao et al, who also demonstrated that G2019S and R1441C mutant worms displayed progressive behavioral and locomotor dysfunction, which could be rescued by exogenous dopamine (Yao et al., 2010).

Taken together, the data from worm models of LRRK2 suggests that WT LRK/LRRK2 may work in a gain-of-function manner which is antagonistic to DA neuronal survival. While it does seem likely that LRK-1 is linked to mitochondrial pathways in some manner, the contrasting data makes any inferences difficult.

3.2 Fruit fly models

The Drosophila melanogster paralogue of human LRRK2, dLRRK (CG5483) has similar GTPase and kinase domains among others, with 46% and 44% homology respectively. Expression of LRRK is ubiquitous in the adult fly brain, which suggests that *Drosophila* is a good model for *LRRK2* (Imai et al., 2008). As with the worm models, fly modelers have employed a number of similar experimental approaches including deletion and manipulation of dLRRK and overexpression of WT and mutant human LRRK2.

3.2.1 dLRRK loss of function

Several groups have used the loss of function e03680 line which has a piggyback transposon that results in kinase-null dLRRK2 (Imai et al., 2008; Kanao et al., 2010; Lee et al., 2010b; Lee et al., 2007; Lin et al., 2010; Tain et al., 2009; Wang et al., 2008) or a chromosomally deficient line $dLRRK^{df}$ (Imai et al., 2008; Lee et al., 2007). Additionally, loss of dLRRK activity has been achieved by RNAi knock-down (Gehrke et al., 2010; Imai et al., 2008) and by 3KD kinase-dead mutation (Imai et al., 2008; Kanao et al., 2010; Lee et al., 2010b). Results have been contrasting, even between groups using the same line. For example, the e03680 line was reported to have no loss of dopaminergic neurons (Wang et al., 2008, Imai et al , 2008), however locomotive impairment (Lee et al., 2007; Tain et al., 2009), degenerative changes in DA neurons (Lee et al., 2007), irregular nerve terminal morphology/overgrowth and changes in neurotransmission (Lee et al., 2010b) were also reported in this line. Interestingly, Imai and colleagues did report increased levels of dopamine in the e03680 line, supporting neurotransmission or storage changes (Imai et al., 2008). Additionally, heterozygous e03680 flies expressing toxic Tau-GFP had longer dendrites and branching and decreased Tau inclusions (Lin et al., 2010).

Data on second hit response has also been contradictory, with the e03680 flies exhibiting increased (Wang et al., 2008) and decreased sensitivity (Imai et al., 2008) although both groups reported resistance of this line to paraquat. Chromosomally deficient line $dLRRK^{df}$

was also resistant to hydrogen peroxide, and RNAi knockdown of LRRK2 decreased sensitivity to both hydrogen peroxide and paraquat (Imai et al., 2008).

3.2.2 Transgenic fly models

Many transgenic models of *Drosophila* employ the bipartite GAL4/UAS system (Brand and Perrimon, 1993) giving rise to tissue-specific gene expression. Some groups have used dLRRK WT and comparable mutant ectopic expressors utilizing GAL4 drivers directed to pan neuronal- and dopaminergic neuronal-specific expression among others (Gehrke et al., 2010; Imai et al., 2008; Kanao et al., 2010; Lee et al., 2010b; Lee et al., 2007; Lin et al., 2010). Some studies showed no deleterious effects, such as with locomotion or DA neuronal changes (Lee et al., 2007), whereas others showed that dLRRK mutants and/or WT overexpressors had decrease in dopamine and DA neurons (Imai et al., 2008) decreased dendrite arborization (Lee et al., 2010b; Lin et al., 2010) and neuromuscular junction (NMJ) bouton loss (Lee et al., 2010b). Other groups have utilized transgenic human LRRK2 GAL4-driven *Drosophila* models (Gehrke et al., 2010; Kanao et al., 2010; Lee et al., 2010b; Lin et al., 2010; Liu et al., 2008; Ng et al., 2009; Venderova et al., 2009). Significant retinal degeneration and other eye abnormalities were observed in eye-specific hLRRK2 WT- and mutant-expressing cells (Liu et al., 2008; Venderova et al., 2009) whereas others did not observe this effect (Kanao et al., 2010; Ng et al., 2009).

Flies with ectopic neuronal expression of mutant and/or WT transgenes exhibited locomotive impairment and DA neuron loss (Lin et al., 2010; Liu et al., 2008; Ng et al., 2009; Venderova et al., 2009) and decreased boutons, NMJ length and arborization (Lee et al., 2010b). Endogenous dLRRK (Imai et al., 2008) and transgenic WT hLRRK2 (Ng et al., 2009) protein appeared punctate and localized to the cytoplasm and exogenous dLRRK colocalized to endosomal structures that partially overlapped with synaptic markers (Imai et al., 2008). Interestingly, transgenic mutant LRRK2 tended to form intracellular aggregates (Ng et al., 2009). Lin et al expressed hLRRK2 WT and mutants in *Drosophila* with GAL4 drivers specific for DA neuron dendrites and showed their degeneration (Lin et al., 2010). The hLRRK2 G2019S fly showed the most severe defect, including aberrant localization of axonal proteins, including microtubule-associated protein tau, to dendrites. Dendrite degeneration was exacerbated by overexpression of tau and conversely rescued by knock-down of tau in the transgenic mutant flies, this toxic effect being attributed to increased tau phosphorylation phosphorylation through Sgg (GSK3b homologue) (Lin et al., 2010). Both dLRRK mutants and/or WT overexpressors were significantly sensitive to oxidative stressors paraquat and hydrogen peroxide (Imai et al., 2008). Additionally, transgenic hLRRK WT (Venderova et al., 2009) and mutant (Ng et al., 2009) flies had increased sensitivity to mitochondria Complex I toxin rotenone and WT hLRRK2 flies had a decrease in the number of mitochondria at presynaptic nerve terminals (Lee et al., 2010b).

Taken together, dLRRK2 appears to have some role in the maintenance of dopaminergic neurons and the over-expression of LRRK2 results in locomotive impairment, DA neuron loss, decreased dendrite arborization, protein sorting or trafficking defects and increased sensitivity to oxidative stress. Although mortality rates differed among the studies, most groups saw that the hLRRK2 pathogenic mutants tended to have a more severe phenotype, providing evidence for the gain-of-function hypothesis. Like the worm models, the second hit data, while somewhat contrasting, do go some way to support LRRK2 involvement in stress response and mitochondrial pathways.

3.2.3 Fly interactor studies

Studies have been performed utilizing double transgenic hLRRK2 flies concomitantly expressing human PINK1, DJ-1 or Parkin. These fly models exhibited various eye abnormalities and some had decreased DA neuron survival (Venderova et al., 2009) whereas coexpression of Parkin with mutant LRRK2 provided significant protection against DA neuron degeneration that occurs with age or in response to rotenone (Ng et al., 2009) Also, loss-of-function dLRRK suppressed Parkin and PINK1 pathology in flies (Tain et al., 2009). Thus, this data further supports the observations that wild-type *d*LRRK negatively regulates DA neuron survival and provides evidence that there is some sort of relationship between LRRK2 and these other PD-associated genes.

Drosophila models have been utilized for the search and characterization of LRRK2 substrates and/or interacting proteins (Imai et al., 2008; Lee et al., 2010b; Tain et al., 2009; Venderova et al., 2009). Imai and colleagues showed that both *Drosophila* and human LRRK2 phosphorylate 4E-BP (a negative regulator of translation and mediator of stress response), and that pathogenic mutations caused hyper-phosphorylation of 4E-BP, which led to reduced resistance to oxidative stress and increased dopaminergic neurodegeneration in flies (Imai et al., 2008). Likewise, loss-of-function e03680 flies had a decrease in the amount of phosphorylated 4E-BP (Tain et al., 2009). This association was confirmed in a study that not only showed that LRRK2 interacted with 4E-BP at the postsynaptic compartment, but also found that hLRRK2 phosphorylated Futsch (MAP1b homolog) and possibly interacted with Tubulin (Lee et al., 2010b). Another study found that dLRRK/hLRRK2 phosphorylated FoxO (a transcription factor involved in cell metabolism and oxidative stress which regulates 4E-BP), which subsequently activated downstream cell death regulators and resulted in neurodegeneration (such as eye defects and DA neuron loss) in dFoxO overexpressing flies (Kanao et al., 2010). However, it has been found that LRRK2 phosphorylates itself and other substrates more strongly than 4E-BP in mammals (Kumar et al., 2010), so the negative effects may be *Drosophila* specific. Another study recently reported that dLRRK/hLRRK2 targeted microRNA pathways and that pathogenic LRRK2 antagonized these miRNAs, which negatively affected cell cycle and DA neuron survival (Gehrke et al., 2010). Additionally, the group found that LRRK2 associated with and negatively regulated Argonaute (dAgo1/hAgo2) RISC proteins and LRRK2 mutants promoted the association of phospho-4E-BP1 with hAgo2. Thus, it appears that WT LRRK2 can regulate protein expression by targeting microRNA silencing pathways, and mutations in LRRK2 can upset a delicate balance.

4. Rodent LRRK2 models

While invertebrate LRRK2 models have been and will continue to be highly informative, it is important to remember that the LRRK genes are not true orthologues of LRRK2 (Marin, 2008). In addition, physiological limitations include not only the lack of basal ganglia but also their short lifespan, leaving the effects of aging impossible to determine. Given that age is the biggest risk factor for development of LRRK2 parkinsonism, the development of mammalian LRRK2 models is key for understanding pathophysiology and for drug screening.

To date a number of rodent models have been published in the literature, with experimental approaches Including knock-out of LRRK2, over-expression of human wild-type and mutant LRRK2, over-expression of mouse wild-type and mutant LRRK2 and targeted knock-in of human mutations into the murine genome.

4.1 Murine LRRK2 knockouts

Several groups have reported LRRK2 knockout mice in varying detail. In 2009, Andreas-Mateo et al reported that mice with partial knockout of exon 39 and complete knockout of exon 40 are viable, grossly normal and have completely intact dopaminergic system in terms of dopamine levels and neuronal number up to 2 years of age and show no altered sensitivity to 1-methyl-4-phenyl-1,2,3,6-tetrahydropyridine (MPTP) (Andres-Mateos et al., 2009). Around the same time Lin et al also reported that no pathological or behavioral abnormalities were observed in their knockout mice that lack LRRK2 exon 2 (Lin et al., 2010). Interestingly, when they crossed the LRRK2 knockout to conditional A53T mice, a complete amelioration of α-synuclein mediated neuropathological abnormalities was observed. The third report which described two lines of knockout mice (one with ablation of exon 1, the other ablation of exons 29/30) also reported a lack of any dopaminergic phenotypes or brain neuropathology (Tong et al., 2010). Surprisingly, a major renal phenotype was found in these mice which included dramatic morphological changes and shrinkage, accumulation of alpha-synuclein and pSer 129 alpha-synuclein, impaired ubiquitin degradation, impaired autophagy, apoptosis and inflammation. Interestingly, in a different exon 1 knockout model, yet to be fully described, decreased phospho-tau levels and concurrent increased soluble tubulin levels were reported, implying a role for LRRK2 in regulation microtubule dynamics (Gillardon, 2009).

Our group has also created LRRK2 KO mice, which are in the final stages of characterization. Microdialysis in these mice has revealed that while the dopamine release following KCl stimulated is not different in magnitude to the wild-type controls, it appears to be slightly delayed. Starting from about 4 months we have also seen progressive darkening of the kidneys and histopathological analysis reveals severe inflammation.

4.2 Over-expression of LRRK2

The first rodent over-expression models were described by McLeod et al in 2006 (MacLeod et al., 2006), whose group investigated both embryonic cDNA electroporation and adult adeno-associated viral expression of WT and mutant LRRK2 kinase domain constructs in rats. A reduction in neurite outgrowth and branching was observed in the embryos expressing mutant G2019S and Y1699C in periventricular layer neural progenitors. In adult rats, viral expression of WT and G2019S in the nigra resulted apotosis in nigral neurons and striatal abnormalities including phospho-tau increases.

Three years later, Chenjian Li's group published the first bacterial artificial chromosome (BAC) mouse models, using human WT and ROC domain mutant R1441G BACs (Li et al., 2009). The mice showed an expression pattern of transgenic LRRK2 that mirrored endogenous expression patterns at levels around 5-fold on an FVB/N background. Striking phenotypes were reported including progressive levodopa-responsive slowness of movement associated with ~33% decreased dopamine release following nomifensine treatment and axonal pathology of nigrostriatal dopaminergic projection. While nigral neuronal loss was absent, the R1441G mice displayed a marked reduction in the number of tyrosine hydroxylase-positive nigral dendrites and accumulation of microtubule associated protein tau pathology in the striatum. Extensive characterization of their expression matched human WT BAC model model was not presented, however no overt phenotypes were noted.

Two groups have since published data on BAC models expressing the kinase domain mutant G2019S. Li et al expressed a murine wild type and mutant G2019S BAC on a C57BL/6 background, with expression levels around 6 fold over endogenous LRRK2 (Li et al., 2010). Total dopamine content in the striatum was normal in WT BAC mice and G2019S mice at 6 months but declined by 25% in G2019S BAC mice by 12 months, suggesting an age related decline. Despite normal striatal dopamine levels, voltammetry in brain slices derived from 12 month old wild-type BAC transgenic mice showed a 25% increase in evoked dopamine release following a single pulse, whereas the decline in DA release following repeated stimulation was comparable to non-transgenic controls, as was their dopamine transporter (DAT)-mediated uptake. Conversely, the G2019S BAC mice displayed a 35% decrease in dopamine release by voltammetry, poorly sustained evoked dopamine release after repeated stimulation and a lower rate of dopamine uptake, presumably as a compensatory mechanism. No dopamine neuronal loss was seen in either model. Behaviorally the wild-type transgenic mice displayed enhanced ability on the beam test and increase spontaneous activity, whereas the G2019S BAC mice did not display any abnormalites. While no overt pathological lesions were reported, the authors did reveal that phospho- tau was decreased in the WT transgenic mice.

Our group (Melrose et al., 2010) also reported WT and mutant G2019S BAC mice, utilizing a human LRRK2 BAC rather than a murine BAC. Using *in vivo* microdialysis we demonstrated that basal extracellular dopamine levels were reduced by ~33% in G2019S BAC mice at ~8 months and an enhanced response to amphetamine challenge was noted. Total striatal dopamine, dopamine neuronal number, DAT levels and D1 and D2 receptor density were all unchanged up to 22 months. Behaviorally, the G2019S mice displayed some abnormal open field behavior but no motor deficits. Surprisingly, and in contrast to Li et al, we found that our human WT BAC mice also displayed reduced basal dopamine levels, even more pronounced (~66% versus 33%) than in our G2019S BAC mice. While this is likely attributed to differential expression levels in the two lines (WT BAC mice around 3.5 fold overexpression in half brain extracts and 2.5 fold in G2019S mice) it nevertheless supports a gain of function mechanism. Interestingly, D1 receptors were slightly upregulated in aged human WT BAC mice, although no changes were found in D2 receptors or DAT levels. Pathologically we did not detect any alpha-synuclein pathology in either line, but we did see changes in the phosphorylation of tau. Modest phosphorylation changes, detected by immunohistochemistry, were restricted to the hippocampus in the human WT BAC mice (the area of highest expression). In the G2019S mice however, tau alterations were much more pronounced and widespread. Biochemical analysis of tau revealed enhanced phosphorylation at several phospho-epitopes and upon de-phosphorylation the tau species distribution was still different from the non-transgenic controls, suggesting that other post-translational modifications may be altered in G2019S mice and we hypothesize that these processing changes may increase the likelihood of abberant phosphorylation. One final observation worth noting is that we recently showed that neurogenesis is altered in our G2019S mice (Winner et al., 2011). Proliferation and migration of new neurons was impaired in the subventricular zone/rostral migratory stream and in the subgranular zone of the hippocampus. Furthermore, new neurons in the hippocampus had impaired outgrowth and a diminished number of spines. Curiously, exercise was found to partially recover the neuroblast deficit in the hippocampus, which may suggest that exercise induced signaling can at least partially compensate abberant LRRK2 activity caused by the G2019S mutation.

In a different transgenic approach Lin et al generated hemagglutinin tagged conditional human WT and G2019S using cDNA fragments inserted into the mouse prion protein expression vector controlled by the tetracycline-responsive promoter (tetP) (Lin et al., 2009). Expression levels were between 8-16 fold for the human WT and G2019S lines and mice were on a C57BL/6 background. Human WT mice were behaviorally normal, but G2019S mice were found to gain less weight than controls and had increased ambulatory and rearing activities. One month old human WT and G2019S and mice were also reported to have perturbed microtubule dynamics, evidenced by a dramatic shift of β-tubulin from soluble to insoluble fractions prepared from brain lysates. Finally, ubiquitin staining increased in cortical neurons of 6 month old human WT and G2019S mice and by 20 months this increase became more pronounced and was clustered with LRRK2 staining, which the authors suggest may hint to inhibition of ubiquitin-proteasome activities. Interestingly, both the human WT and G2019S mice enhanced α-synuclein pathology when crossed with inducible A53T mutant mice. Curiously, double A53T/ kinase dead G2019S mice also exhibited similar enhanced phenotype, suggesting that kinase activity was not involved in α-synuclein mediating toxicity. The authors instead attributed the synergistic effects to impairment of golgi function, microtubule transport and the ubiquitin-proteasomal pathway, which occurred when LRRK2 was co-expressed, regardless of the transgene type or expression level.

Two recently described viral models are the only LRRK2 models to date that document dopamine neuronal loss. Lee et al (Lee et al., 2010a) developed herpes simplex virus (HSV) amplicon-based mouse models expressing either human WT, G2019S and G2019S-D1994A (kinase dead) LRRK2, in which up to 75% of nigral neurons were infected after injection. HSV amplicon-mediated delivery of LRRK2 G2019S induced significant loss (~50%) of tyrosine hydroxylase-positive neurons 3 weeks after stereotaxic injection into the ipsilateral striatum of mice compared to control viruses expressing WT LRRK2 and eGFP and G2019S-D1994A. This model is the first model that directly implicates kinase activity being responsible for toxicity *in vivo* in a mammalian model, supported by the lack of effect in the kinase dead model, as well as attenuation of the neuronal loss by kinase inhibitors GW5074 and indirubin-3'-monooxime. The second viral model, the only published rat model to date, used a second generation adeno-viral serotype 5 vector, with transgene expression driven by the neuronal-specific human synapsin-1 promoter to express human WT and G2019S LRRK2 in rat brain (Dusonchet et al., 2011). Injections were delivered to the striatum and retrograde expression in the nigra was around 2 fold expression level overall, although with only 30% of all neurons transduced, this suggested very high levels in individual neurons. G2019S, but not WT mice exhibited a progressive neuronal loss that reached ~20% by 42 days as well as a 10% decrease in tyrosine hydroxylase fiber density. No alpha- synuclein pathology was observed but the authors noted some transient abnormal phosphorylation of tau for both WT and G2019S which did not correlate with neuronal cell death in G2019S.

4.3 Targeted knockin of LRRK2

For large proteins such as LRRK2, the over-expression approach is not without caveat and within the field there has been much concern about over-expression artifacts. To circumvent this, targeting the models' own genome, known as "knockin" is an alternative and potentially more physiological approach, since gene expression is recapitulated in the correct temporal, anatomical and quantitative manner and under the endogenous transcriptional and translational controls. Nevertheless, many would still argue, justifiably, that over-expression models and their phenotypes, even if exaggerated, often give vital clues to normal and pathological functions. Equally, the risk with the knockin approach is that the relatively low mutant expression levels, within a species that doesn't normally develop the disease, may yield no or very subtle phenotypes.

To date only one knockin model has been published, by Tong et al, who created a ROC domain R1441C mutant (Tong et al., 2009). Whilst the homozygous knockin mice were grossly normal and did not exhibit dopamine neuronal loss, amperometric recordings in chromaffin cells derived from the R1441C, stimulated with high KCl, revealed significant reductions in the total catecholamine release per cell, quantal size and the frequency of release events. Slice recordings from dopaminergic neurons in the nigra of R1441C mice also exhibited smaller amplitude and duration of hyperpolarization after dopamine application, as well as slower recover times, and reduced responses to amphetamine and the D2 agonist quinpirole, compared with WT controls. Locomotor testing in the open field also revealed the knockin mice had a reduced behavioral response to amphetamine and quinpirole, providing *in vivo* evidence that dopamine release and D2 autoceptor feedback mechanisms may be impaired. No neuropathology was noted in these mice.

4.4 What do the models tell us about LRRK2?

At first glance, the success of the LRRK2 models appears to be nominal, with not a single model recapturing all the key features desired for a PD model - dopamine cell loss, motor impairment and alpha-synculein pathology. However, independent of the approach, a unifying theme is emerging from both invertebrate and vertebrate LRRK2 models, suggesting an important role for LRRK2 in dopaminergic neurotransmission, even in the absence of dopamine neuronal loss. Several other genetic PD mouse models also have abnormalities in dopamine transmission without neuronal loss including PINK1, parkin, DJ-1 and SNCA knockouts and SNCA WT over-expression mice (Abeliovich et al., 2000; Goldberg et al., 2003; Goldberg et al., 2005; Kitada et al., 2009; Nemani et al., 2010). Imaging studies have long established that in asymptomatic PD, the earliest detectable changes occur in the dopamine transporter and the same holds true for asymptomatic LRRK2 (Nandhagopal et al., 2008; Sossi et al., 2010) and SNCA patients (Bostantjopoulou et al., 2008; Perani et al., 2006; Samii et al., 1999). Thus, the data evolving from LRRK2 models (and other PD genetic models) may be recapturing early preclinical events. In reality this may make the models more valuable because the onset of motor symptoms in PD is only after 50-70% of the dopamine neurons are lost, by which point neuro-protective therapy would be futile. Understanding these early events in disease is key to allow us identify biomarkers to detect at risk patients and design neuro-protective therapies.

Aside from the effects on dopamine neurotransmission, the other consistent theme arising from LRRK2 *in vivo* data appears to be the impairment of cytoskeletal function, evidenced by the alterations observed in tau phosphorylation and perturbed microtubule dynamics. Although tau pathology is rare in LRRK2 brains, there is mounting evidence of the involvement of tau in PD in general, with over 15 genetic studies in small populations implicating variability in the tau gene with Parkinson's disease and a recent study of a large number of European PD samples unequivocally showing that tau gene (MAPT) variability is a major risk factor for PD, along with the alpha-synculein gene (SNCA) (Simon-Sanchez et al., 2009). Even though it has been proven already that there is no direct interaction between tau and LRRK2 protein, there appears to be an indirect link that warrants further investigation. If LRRK2 regulates tau physiology, this could have important implication for LRRK2 therapies in Alzheimer's disease.

Less consistent/investigated *in vivo*, but nevertheless still compelling are the changes in the inflammatory, autophagy/lysosomal, apoptotic, mitochondrial and proteosomal pathways observed in some models. These pathways may be particularly important in unraveling how LRRK2 leads to α-synuclein pathology in humans. While studies in invertebrates are suggestive of a potential role for LRRK2, more mammalian studies are needed into the role of LRRK2 in mitochrondrial/stress pathways. As it stands, there is no evidence for a direct interaction between LRRK2 and α-synuclein and the only instance of *in vivo* α-synuclein pathology in a LRRK2 model is in the kidneys, but not brain, of the LRRK2 knockout model (Tong et al., 2010). Notably, accumulation was accompanied by autophagic, proteasomal and inflammatory changes. Furthermore in double LRRK2 and α-synuclein A53T mice, enhancement of α-synuclein pathology was attributed to impairments in microtubule dynamic, golgi organization, mitochondrial toxicity and ubiquitin-proteasomal pathway (Lin et al., 2009). What is difficult to resolve though, is that double LRRK2 KO/ A53T mice have ameliorated α-synuclein brain pathology (Lin et al., 2009). These complex findings reiterate the notion that LRRK2 is likely a multi-faceted protein, which may have distinct cellular specific roles.

4.5 The future for LRRK2 therapeutics

Intense pharmaceutical interest has surrounded LRRK2 since its discovery and many companies are developing inhibitors of LRRK2 and screening is already underway in many of the models described above. It is still not clear exactly what function of LRRK2 mediates its toxicity and data attributing it to enzymatic kinase activity is conflicting. Although the general consensus appears to be that LRRK2 pathogenicity is a toxic gain of function, the kidney phenotype in LRRK2 KO mice suggests that peripheral effects may be an important loss-of-function consideration. A highly selective LRRK2 inhibitor (LRRK2-IN1) was recently developed by Nathaniel Gray and colleagues (Deng et al., 2011) which abolished Ser910 and Ser935 phosphorylation of LRRK2 in the kidney of mice after 1 hour. No changes were observed in brain because the compound is unable to cross the blood brain barrier. Once CNS drug delivery issues are overcome, it will be interesting to see the effects of LRRK-IN1in in vivo LRRK2 models.

5. References

Aasly, J. O., et al., 2005. Clinical features of LRRK2-associated Parkinson's disease in central Norway. Ann Neurol. 57, 762-5.

Abeliovich, A., et al., 2000. Mice lacking alpha-synuclein display functional deficits in the nigrostriatal dopamine system. Neuron. 25, 239-52.

Adams, J. R., et al., 2005. PET in LRRK2 mutations: comparison to sporadic Parkinson's disease and evidence for presymptomatic compensation. Brain. 128, 2777-85.

Andres-Mateos, E., et al., 2009. Unexpected lack of hypersensitivity in LRRK2 knock-out mice to MPTP (1-methyl-4-phenyl-1,2,3,6-tetrahydropyridine). J Neurosci. 29, 15846-50.

Biskup, S., et al., 2006. Localization of LRRK2 to membranous and vesicular structures in mammalian brain. Ann Neurol. 60, 557-69.

Biskup, S., et al., 2007. Dynamic and redundant regulation of LRRK2 and LRRK1 expression. BMC Neurosci. 8, 102.

Bostantjopoulou, S., et al., 2008. (123)I-FP-CIT SPET striatal uptake in parkinsonian patients with the alpha-synuclein (G209A) mutation A. Hell J Nucl Med. 11, 157-9.

Brand, A. H., Perrimon, N., 1993. Targeted gene expression as a means of altering cell fates and generating dominant phenotypes. Development. 118, 401-15.

Carmine Belin, A., et al., 2006. Leucine-rich repeat kinase 2 (LRRK2) mutations in a Swedish Parkinson cohort and a healthy nonagenarian. Mov Disord. 21, 1731-4.

Dachsel, J. C., et al., 2007. Lrrk2 G2019S substitution in frontotemporal lobar degeneration with ubiquitin-immunoreactive neuronal inclusions. Acta Neuropathol. 113, 601-6.

Deng, X., et al., 2011. Characterization of a selective inhibitor of the Parkinson's disease kinase LRRK2. Nat Chem Biol. 7, 203-5.

Di Fonzo, A., et al., 2006. Comprehensive analysis of the LRRK2 gene in sixty families with Parkinson's disease. Eur J Hum Genet. 14, 322-31.

Djaldetti, R., et al., 2008. Clinical characteristics of Parkinson's disease among Jewish Ethnic groups in Israel. J Neural Transm. 115, 1279-84.

Dusonchet, J., et al., 2011. A rat model of progressive nigral neurodegeneration induced by the Parkinson's disease-associated G2019S mutation in LRRK2. J Neurosci. 31, 907-12.

Farrer, M. J., et al., 2007. Lrrk2 G2385R is an ancestral risk factor for Parkinson's disease in Asia. Parkinsonism Relat Disord. 13, 89-92.

Galter, D., et al., 2006. LRRK2 expression linked to dopamine-innervated areas. Ann Neurol. 59, 714-9.

Gehrke, S., et al., 2010. Pathogenic LRRK2 negatively regulates microRNA-mediated translational repression. Nature. 466, 637-41.

Gillardon, F., 2009. Leucine-rich repeat kinase 2 phosphorylates brain tubulin-beta isoforms and modulates microtubule stability--a point of convergence in parkinsonian neurodegeneration? J Neurochem. 110, 1514-22.

Goldberg, M. S., et al., 2003. Parkin-deficient mice exhibit nigrostriatal deficits but not loss of dopaminergic neurons. J Biol Chem. 278, 43628-35.

Goldberg, M. S., et al., 2005. Nigrostriatal dopaminergic deficits and hypokinesia caused by inactivation of the familial Parkinsonism-linked gene DJ-1. Neuron. 45, 489-96.

Greggio, E., et al., 2006. Kinase activity is required for the toxic effects of mutant LRRK2/dardarin. Neurobiol Dis. 23, 329-41.

Greggio, E., et al., 2008. The Parkinson disease-associated leucine-rich repeat kinase 2 (LRRK2) is a dimer that undergoes intramolecular autophosphorylation. J Biol Chem. 283, 16906-14.

Healy, D. G., et al., 2008. Phenotype, genotype, and worldwide genetic penetrance of LRRK2-associated Parkinson's disease: a case-control study. Lancet Neurol. 7, 583-90.

Higashi, S., et al., 2007a. Localization of Parkinson's disease-associated LRRK2 in normal and pathological human brain. Brain Res. 1155, 208-19.

Higashi, S., et al., 2007b. Expression and localization of Parkinson's disease-associated leucine-rich repeat kinase 2 in the mouse brain. J Neurochem. 100, 368-81.

Hulihan, M. M., et al., 2008. LRRK2 Gly2019Ser penetrance in Arab-Berber patients from Tunisia: a case-control genetic study. Lancet Neurol. 7, 591-4.

Imai, Y., et al., 2008. Phosphorylation of 4E-BP by LRRK2 affects the maintenance of dopaminergic neurons in Drosophila. EMBO J. 27, 2432-43.

Ishihara, L., et al., 2007. Screening for Lrrk2 G2019S and clinical comparison of Tunisian and North American Caucasian Parkinson's disease families. Mov Disord. 22, 55-61.

Jaleel, M., et al., 2007. LRRK2 phosphorylates moesin at threonine-558: characterization of how Parkinson's disease mutants affect kinase activity. Biochem J. 405, 307-17.

Kachergus, J., et al., 2005. Identification of a novel LRRK2 mutation linked to autosomal dominant parkinsonism: evidence of a common founder across European populations. Am J Hum Genet. 76, 672-80.

Kanao, T., et al., 2010. Activation of FoxO by LRRK2 induces expression of proapoptotic proteins and alters survival of postmitotic dopaminergic neuron in Drosophila. Hum Mol Genet. 19, 3747-58.

Kay, D. M., et al., 2005. Escaping Parkinson's disease: a neurologically healthy octogenarian with the LRRK2 G2019S mutation. Mov Disord. 20, 1077-8.

Kitada, T., et al., 2009. Impaired dopamine release and synaptic plasticity in the striatum of parkin-/- mice. J Neurochem. 110, 613-21.

Kumar, A., et al., 2010. The Parkinson's disease associated LRRK2 exhibits weaker in vitro phosphorylation of 4E-BP compared to autophosphorylation. PLoS One. 5, e8730.

Lee, B. D., et al., 2010a. Inhibitors of leucine-rich repeat kinase-2 protect against models of Parkinson's disease. Nat Med. 16, 998-1000.

Lee, S., et al., 2010b. LRRK2 kinase regulates synaptic morphology through distinct substrates at the presynaptic and postsynaptic compartments of the Drosophila neuromuscular junction. J Neurosci. 30, 16959-69.

Lee, S. B., et al., 2007. Loss of LRRK2/PARK8 induces degeneration of dopaminergic neurons in Drosophila. Biochem Biophys Res Commun. 358, 534-9.

Li, X., et al., 2007. Leucine-rich repeat kinase 2 (LRRK2)/PARK8 possesses GTPase activity that is altered in familial Parkinson's disease R1441C/G mutants. J Neurochem. 103, 238-47.

Li, Y., et al., 2009. Mutant LRRK2(R1441G) BAC transgenic mice recapitulate cardinal features of Parkinson's disease. Nat Neurosci. 12, 826-8.

Lin, C. H., et al., 2010. LRRK2 G2019S mutation induces dendrite degeneration through mislocalization and phosphorylation of tau by recruiting autoactivated GSK3ss. J Neurosci. 30, 13138-49.

Lin, X., et al., 2009. Leucine-rich repeat kinase 2 regulates the progression of neuropathology induced by Parkinson's-disease-related mutant alpha-synuclein. Neuron. 64, 807-27.

Liu, Z., et al., 2008. A Drosophila model for LRRK2-linked parkinsonism. Proc Natl Acad Sci U S A. 105, 2693-8.

Luzon-Toro, B., et al., 2007. Mechanistic insight into the dominant mode of the Parkinson's disease-associated G2019S LRRK2 mutation. Hum Mol Genet. 16, 2031-9.

MacLeod, D., et al., 2006. The familial Parkinsonism gene LRRK2 regulates neurite process morphology. Neuron. 52, 587-93.

Marin, I., 2008. Ancient origin of the Parkinson disease gene LRRK2. J Mol Evol. 67, 41-50.

Mata, I. F., et al., 2005. Lrrk2 pathogenic substitutions in Parkinson's disease. Neurogenetics. 6, 171-7.

Mata, I. F., et al., 2006. LRRK2 mutations are a common cause of Parkinson's disease in Spain. Eur J Neurol. 13, 391-4.

Melrose, H., et al., 2006. Anatomical localization of leucine-rich repeat kinase 2 in mouse brain. Neuroscience. 139, 791-4.

Melrose, H. L., et al., 2010. Impaired dopaminergic neurotransmission and microtubule-associated protein tau alterations in human LRRK2 transgenic mice. Neurobiol Dis. 40, 503-17.

Melrose, H. L., et al., 2007. A comparative analysis of leucine-rich repeat kinase 2 (Lrrk2) expression in mouse brain and Lewy body disease. Neuroscience. 147, 1047-58.

Miklossy, J., et al., 2006. LRRK2 expression in normal and pathologic human brain and in human cell lines. J Neuropathol Exp Neurol. 65, 953-63.

Nandhagopal, R., et al., 2008. Progression of dopaminergic dysfunction in a LRRK2 kindred: a multitracer PET study. Neurology. 71, 1790-5.

Nemani, V. M., et al., 2010. Increased expression of alpha-synuclein reduces neurotransmitter release by inhibiting synaptic vesicle reclustering after endocytosis. Neuron. 65, 66-79.

Ng, C. H., et al., 2009. Parkin protects against LRRK2 G2019S mutant-induced dopaminergic neurodegeneration in Drosophila. J Neurosci. 29, 11257-62.

Ozelius, L. J., et al., 2006. LRRK2 G2019S as a cause of Parkinson's disease in Ashkenazi Jews. N Engl J Med. 354, 424-5.

Paisan-Ruiz, C., et al., 2004. Cloning of the gene containing mutations that cause PARK8-linked Parkinson's disease. Neuron. 44, 595-600.

Perani, D., et al., 2006. Positron emission tomography changes in PARK1 mutation. Mov Disord. 21, 127-30.

Rajput, A., et al., 2006. Parkinsonism, Lrrk2 G2019S, and tau neuropathology. Neurology. 67, 1506-8.

Ross, O. A., et al., 2006. Lrrk2 and Lewy body disease. Ann Neurol. 59, 388-93.

Ross, O. A., et al., 2008. Analysis of Lrrk2 R1628P as a risk factor for Parkinson's disease. Ann Neurol. 64, 88-92.

Saha, S., et al., 2009. LRRK2 modulates vulnerability to mitochondrial dysfunction in Caenorhabditis elegans. J Neurosci. 29, 9210-8.

Sakaguchi-Nakashima, A., et al., 2007. LRK-1, a C. elegans PARK8-related kinase, regulates axonal-dendritic polarity of SV proteins. Curr Biol. 17, 592-8.

Samann, J., et al., 2009. Caenorhabditits elegans LRK-1 and PINK-1 act antagonistically in stress response and neurite outgrowth. J Biol Chem. 284, 16482-91.

Samii, A., et al., 1999. PET studies of parkinsonism associated with mutation in the alpha-synuclein gene. Neurology. 53, 2097-102.

Simon-Sanchez, J., et al., 2006. LRRK2 is expressed in areas affected by Parkinson's disease in the adult mouse brain. Eur J Neurosci. 23, 659-66.

Simon-Sanchez, J., et al., 2009. Genome-wide association study reveals genetic risk underlying Parkinson's disease. Nat Genet. 41, 1308-12.

Smith, W. W., et al., 2006. Kinase activity of mutant LRRK2 mediates neuronal toxicity. Nat Neurosci. 9, 1231-3.

Sossi, V., et al., 2010. Dopamine turnover increases in asymptomatic LRRK2 mutations carriers. Mov Disord. 25, 2717-23.

Tain, L. S., et al., 2009. Rapamycin activation of 4E-BP prevents parkinsonian dopaminergic neuron loss. Nat Neurosci. 12, 1129-35.

Tan, E. K., 2006. Identification of a common genetic risk variant (LRRK2 Gly2385Arg) in Parkinson's disease. Ann Acad Med Singapore. 35, 840-2.

Taylor, J. P., et al., 2006. LRRK2: a common pathway for parkinsonism, pathogenesis and prevention? Trends Mol Med. 12, 76-82.

Taymans, J. M., et al., 2006. Distribution of PINK1 and LRRK2 in rat and mouse brain. J Neurochem. 98, 951-61.

Tong, Y., et al., 2009. R1441C mutation in LRRK2 impairs dopaminergic neurotransmission in mice. Proc Natl Acad Sci U S A. 106, 14622-7.

Tong, Y., et al., 2010. Loss of leucine-rich repeat kinase 2 causes impairment of protein degradation pathways, accumulation of alpha-synuclein, and apoptotic cell death in aged mice. Proc Natl Acad Sci U S A. 107, 9879-84.

Venderova, K., et al., 2009. Leucine-Rich Repeat Kinase 2 interacts with Parkin, DJ-1 and PINK-1 in a Drosophila melanogaster model of Parkinson's disease. Hum Mol Genet. 18, 4390-404.

Wang, D., et al., 2008. Dispensable role of Drosophila ortholog of LRRK2 kinase activity in survival of dopaminergic neurons. Mol Neurodegener. 3, 3.

West, A. B., et al., 2005. Parkinson's disease-associated mutations in leucine-rich repeat kinase 2 augment kinase activity. Proc Natl Acad Sci U S A. 102, 16842-7.

Westerlund, M., et al., 2008. Developmental regulation of leucine-rich repeat kinase 1 and 2 expression in the brain and other rodent and human organs: Implications for Parkinson's disease. Neuroscience. 152, 429-36.

White, L. R., et al., 2007. MAPK-pathway activity, Lrrk2 G2019S, and Parkinson's disease. J Neurosci Res. 85, 1288-94.

Winner, B., et al., 2011. Adult neurogenesis and neurite outgrowth are impaired in LRRK2 G2019S mice. Neurobiol Dis. 41, 706-16.

Wolozin, B., et al., 2008. Investigating convergent actions of genes linked to familial Parkinson's disease. Neurodegener Dis. 5, 182-5.

Wszolek, ZK et al., 2004. Autosomal dominant parkinsonism associated with variable synuclein and tau pathology. Neurology. 62(9):1619-22.

Yao, C., et al., 2010. LRRK2-mediated neurodegeneration and dysfunction of dopaminergic neurons in a Caenorhabditis elegans model of Parkinson's disease. Neurobiol Dis. 40, 73-81.

Zimprich, A., et al., 2004. Mutations in LRRK2 cause autosomal-dominant parkinsonism with pleomorphic pathology. Neuron. 44, 601-7.

5

Alpha-Synuclein Interactions with Membranes

Katja Pirc[1] and Nataša Poklar Ulrih[1,2]
[1]*University of Ljubljana, Biotechnical faculty*
[2]*Centre of excellence CIPKeBiP*
Slovenia

1. Introduction

Synucleinopathies are a group of neurodegenerative disorders that share common pathological intracellular deposits that contain aggregates of the protein α-synuclein. Substantial evidence suggests that fibril formation by α-synuclein is a critical step in the development of Parkinson's disease (PD). Indeed, *in vitro*, α-synuclein forms fibrils with morphologies and staining characteristics similar to those extracted from disease-affected brains. Also, three single-point mutations and duplication or triplication of the α-synuclein locus correlate with early onset of PD.

However, the function of α-synuclein remains unknown. A significant portion of α-synuclein is localized within membrane fractions, and especially synaptic vesicles associated with vesicular transport processes. These observations suggest that α-synuclein has a role in vesicular trafficking. Although α-synuclein belongs to a group of natively unfolded proteins, there is strong evidence that the membrane affinity of the protein induces an α-helical conformation. A large number of studies have investigated α-synuclein–lipid interactions in the search for a physiological function, as well as to understand this potential membrane involvement in the pathogenesis of α-synuclein. In this review, we will predominantly focus on current opinion about the native wild-type α-synuclein–lipid interactions and the structure of α-synuclein that is established at the membrane surface. However, it should be noted that membranes have been reported to both accelerate and inhibit the fibril formation of α-synuclein, although this will not be the focus of the present review.

2. Intrinsically disordered proteins

A significant number of proteins involved in protein deposition diseases have been seen to be intrinsically disordered proteins. Well-known examples include amyloid β-protein and tau protein in Alzheimer's disease, prion protein (PrP) in prion diseases, exon 1 region of huntingtin in Huntington's disease, and α-synuclein in PD (Fink, 2005).

It has been estimated that more than 30% of eukaryotic proteins have disordered regions that are greater than 50 consecutive residues (Dunker et al., 2001). This term "disordered protein" refers to proteins that in their purified state at neutral pH, have been either shown experimentally or predicted to lack an ordered structure; such proteins are also known as natively unfolded, or intrinsically unstructured. Disordered proteins, or disordered regions of a protein, lack specific tertiary structure and can be composed of an ensemble of conformations (Fink, 2005). Intrinsically unstructured proteins are frequently involved in important regulatory functions in the cell, and the lack of intrinsic structure is in many cases removed when the protein binds to its target molecule. Some functional advantages of these proteins might be an ability to bind to several different targets, the precise control of their binding thermodynamics, and their involvement in cell-cycle control and both transcriptional and translational regulation (Wright & Dyson, 1999). Gunasekaran et al. proposed that disordered proteins provide a simple solution to the need for large intermolecular interfaces while maintaining smaller proteins, and hence a smaller genome and a smaller cell size. For monomeric proteins with extensive intermolecular interfaces, such proteins would need to be 2-3-fold larger, and this would either increase intracellular crowding or enlarge the size of the cell by some 15% to 30%, owing to the increase in the sequence length (Gunasekaran et al., 2003).

3. Synucleinopathies

Protein-conformation-dependent toxicity is an emerging theme in neurodegenerative disorders, including the synucleinopathies (Ulrih et al., 2008). The group of synucleinopathies comprises many neurodegenerative diseases, among which the best known and most common is PD, but it also includes Lewy body dementia, multiple system atrophy, neurodegeneration with brain iron accumulation type I, diffuse Lewy body disease, and Lewy body variant of Alzheimer's disease (Arawaka et al., 1998; Gai et al., 1998; Spillantini et al., 1997; Wakabayashi et al., 1997). These are all brain amyloidoses with the common characteristic of pathological intracellular inclusions of aggregates that have α-synuclein as the key component (Spillantini et al., 1997; Wakabayashi et al., 1997).

PD is characterized by the death of neurons that produce dopamine and are located in the *substantia nigra pars compacta* brain region (see below). This is accompanied by the appearance of Lewy bodies and Lewy neurites (Galvin et al., 1999). Lewy bodies are spherical protein inclusions that are found in the cytoplasm of surviving *substantia nigra* neurons, and they consist of a dense core surrounded by a halo of radiating fibrils of α-synuclein; they also contain a variety of other proteins. The fibrils seen in PD are structurally similar to those in the amyloid diseases, and they appear as linear rods of 5 nm to 10 nm diameter (Fink, 2006). PD affects more than 1% of the population over 65 years of age (Goedert, 2001), and typical symptoms include tremor, slow movements, fine motor difficulties, and loss of postural reflexes (Jankovic, 2008). The cause of PD remains unknown, but considerable evidence suggests a multifactorial etiology that involves genetic susceptibility and environmental factors (Fink, 2006). However, substantial evidence indicates that aggregation of α-synuclein is a critical step in the etiology of PD (Trojanowski & Lee, 2003).

Most cases of PD are of the late onset idiopathic type (Beyer, 2007). Evidence for an important role for α-synuclein in triggering PD also emerged when certain mutations were discovered that are associated with rare inherited autosomal dominant cases of PD. While, as indicated, familial early onset PD is caused by overexpression of α-synuclein due to duplication (Chartier-Harlin et al., 2004) or triplication (Singleton et al., 2003) of the α-synuclein gene locus, three specific point mutations have also been identified: A53T in a large kindred of Italian and Greek origin (Polymeropoulos et al., 1997); A30P in a German family (Kruger et al., 1998); and E46K in a Spanish family (Zarranz et al., 2004).

4. Alpha-synuclein

In brain homogenates, α-synuclein represents 0.5% to 1% of the total protein (Iwai et al., 1995). Northern blotting and *in-situ* hybridization in human and mice have show relatively high expression of α-synuclein in a restricted number of brain regions, one of which is the *substantia nigra* (Abeliovich et al., 2000; Lavedan, 1998). Here, α-synuclein is localized in the presynaptic terminals (George et al., 1995; Iwai et al., 1995), with about 15% found in the membrane fraction (Lee et al., 2002); after synaptosomal lysis, α-synuclein is in the soluble fraction (Iwai et al., 1995).

Although the normal physiological function of α-synuclein remains unknown, it appears to be involved in maintenance of the synaptic vesicle reserve pool of the brain (Davidson et al., 1998; Fortin et al., 2004; Iwai et al., 1995; Nuscher et al., 2004). However, other roles for α-synuclein have been considered: roles in lipid metabolism and transport (Scherzer et al., 2003; Sharon et al., 2001; Willingham et al., 2003), vesicle docking at the membrane (Larsen et al., 2006), exocytosis (Srivastava et al., 2007), lipid organisation (Madine et al., 2006) and prevention of oxidation of unsaturated lipids (Zhu et al., 2006). To date, no conclusive evidence showing the precise role of α-synuclein in cell physiology has been provided.

4.1 Primary sequence

Alpha-synuclein is a small (140 amino acid; 14 kDa) highly acidic protein (Figure 1), and it is intrinsically disordered under physiological conditions *in vitro* (Bisaglia et al., 2009; Fink, 2006). The first 89 residues are composed almost entirely of seven 11-amino-acid imperfect repeats, with a consensus sequence of KTKEGV (George et al., 1995). This strongly resembles sequence motifs found in exchangeable apolipoproteins, which are believed to constitute amphipathic helical lipid-binding domains (Segrest et al., 1992). This 11-residue periodicity is broken in one point by the insertion of four uncharged amino acids, separating units 4 and 5. There are no Cys or Trp residues in the α-synuclein sequence (George et al., 1995).

The structure of α-synuclein can be divided into three regions (Figure 1). The N-terminal domain (residues 1-60) is positively charged and contains five of the imperfect repeats (Fink, 2006; George et al., 1995). The sequence 61-95 is the most hydrophobic portion of the protein, and this was originally described as the "non-amyloid-beta component" (NAC) of Alzheimer´s disease plaques (Takeda et al., 1998). Several studies have defined this region as responsible for α-synuclein aggregation and β-sheet formation (Bodles et al., 2001; Giasson et al., 2001). The homologous β-synuclein, which is distinct from α-synuclein by the absence of the central hydrophobic sequence, is much less prone to self-aggregation. The interaction between β-synuclein and α-synuclein has been argued to inhibit aggregation (Park & Lansbury, 2003). The highly acidic C-terminal domain of α-synuclein is rich in Pro and acidic residues, with a predominance of Glu residues over Asp (George et al., 1995). This domain contains three of the four Tyr residues, at positions 125, 133 and 136; the fourth Tyr residue is at position 39. It has been shown that monomeric α-synuclein has a more compact structure than expected for a completely unfolded polypeptide, and this compactness has been linked to its inhibition of fibril formation due to burial of the hydrophobic NAC domain (Bertoncini et al., 2005; Dedmon et al., 2005). In addition, it has been shown that the 1–102 and 1–110 C-terminal-truncated α-synuclein fragments, but not that of 1–120, are efficient in the promotion of α-synuclein aggregation. The negatively charged 104, 105, 114 and 115 residues in the C-terminus have been suggested to be responsible for reduced α-synuclein aggregation and a lack of seeding of wild-type α-synuclein (Murray et al., 2003).

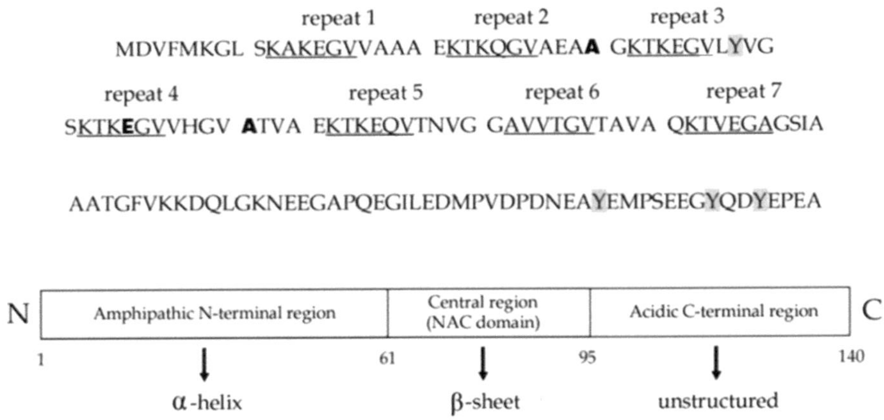

Fig. 1. Top: Amino-acid sequence of human α-synuclein. The imperfect 11-mer repeats are as indicated, with the predominant KTKEGV consensus sequences underlined. The locations of the three point mutations that have been linked to early-onset PD (A30T, E46K, A53T) are shown in bold type, and the four Tyr residues are shaded. Bottom: The α-synuclein sequence can be divided into three regions: the N-terminus adopts an α-helix upon binding to lipids, the hydrophobic NAC domain can form β-sheet structure, and the negatively charged C-terminus is unstructured.

4.2 Alpha-synuclein structure under physiological conditions

Weinreb et al. were the first to attempt to define the secondary structure of α-synuclein. Sedimentation of α-synuclein under physiological conditions is slower than for globular proteins of a similar molecular weight, suggesting an elongated structure of the native protein. Circular dichroism has demonstrated the lack of α-synuclein secondary structure in solution: 68% as random coils and less than 2% as helical content. The reminder of the protein is β-sheet, although it is difficult to quantify the β-sheet structure by circular dichroism. Fourier-transform infrared spectroscopy has confirmed that native α-synuclein is unstructured. The conformational properties of α-synuclein were not changed by heat denaturation and were independent of α-synuclein concentration, salt concentration, chemical denaturants and pH. These features prompted the conclusion that under physiological conditions, α-synuclein exists as a mixture of rapidly equilibrating extended conformers, and that it is representative of a class of natively unfolded proteins (Weinreb et al., 1996). With a slightly different isolation protocol, circular dichroism showed 9% α-helix, 35% β-sheet, and 56% random coil structure in solution (Narayanan & Scarlata, 2001).
Dedmon et al. (2005) used paramagnetic relaxation enhancement and nuclear magnetic resonance (NMR) to show interactions between different parts of the α-synuclein molecule. Some α-synuclein mutants were prepared, with the insertion of nitroxide-labeled cysteine residues, which allowed the observation of short-life-time interactions. Partial condensation of α-synuclein is driven by long-range contacts between residues 30-100 in the center of the molecule, and residues 120-140 in the C-terminal tail. It appears that this interaction can shield the NAC region (residues 61-95) from aggregation, which is the most hydrophobic part of α-synuclein (Dedmon et al., 2005). Bertoncini et al. used a similar methodology to show that the most important interaction is a hydrophobic cluster that comprises the C-terminal part of the NAC region (residues 85-95) and the C-terminus (residues 110-130),

which is probably mediated by Met^{116}, Val^{118}, Tyr^{125} and Met^{127}. Within the C-terminal domain, residues 120-130 contact residues 105-115, and the region around residue 120 also interacts with the N-terminus around residue 20. These long-range interactions that stabilize the monomeric conformations of α-synuclein also inhibit its oligomerization and aggregation. The autoinhibitory conformations fluctuate in the range of nanoseconds to microseconds (Bertoncini et al., 2005). Consistent with this, small-angle X-ray scattering analysis has shown that the radius of gyration, which is used to describe the dimensions of polypeptide chain, is ~40 Å with native α-synuclein, which is much larger than that predicted for a folded globular protein of 140 residues (15 Å), although it is significantly smaller than that of a fully unfolded random coil (52 Å) (Uversky et al., 2001).

Using an atomic-force-microscopy-based single-molecule mechanical unfolding methodology, Sandal et al. (2008) studied the α-synuclein conformation equilibrium under various conditions. Their method allowed the measuring of the force required for unfolding a single protein molecule. It was thus possible to detect conformers with a lifetime that was longer than 10^{-3} s, which due to their longevity, might be the most biologically relevant structures. In 10 mM TRIS/HCl buffer solution at pH 7.5, the α-synuclein secondary structure contains a random coil (38.2%) and β-structure (7.3%) (Sandal et al., 2008).

5. Fibril formation

In-vitro studies of recombinant α-synuclein have demonstrated that purified α-synuclein forms fibril aggregates that resemble those found in Lewy bodies (Serpell et al., 2000). In contrast to its helical secondary structure in the presence of lipids, α-synuclein monomers form soluble oligomers (sometimes referred to as protofibrils) that can undergo a conformational change from disordered to predominantly beta secondary structure. These oligomers can assemble and form insoluble fibrils, which are found in inclusion bodies, together with other proteins (Conway et al., 2000; Fink, 2006; Wood et al., 1999).

Extensive data suggest that the first step of fibrillogenesis is the formation of a partially folded intermediate that promotes self-association of α-synuclein and formation of various oligomeric species (Uversky et al., 2001). Factors that increase the concentrations of these intermediates will favor aggregation (Fink, 2006). Protein aggregation and the kinetics of fibril formation typically appear sigmoidal, and they are usually attributed to a nucleated polymerization process in which the initial lag phase corresponds to the requirement for the formation of critical nuclei; the subsequent exponential growth phase corresponds to fibril elongation, and the final plateau is ascribed to the exhaustion of the soluble monomers and intermediates (Ulrih et al., 2008).

All three of the above-mentioned PD-related point mutations have been shown to accelerate α-synuclein aggregation *in vitro* (Uversky, 2007). The A53T and A30P point mutations both accelerate oligomer formation, although only A53T readily forms large amyloid fibrils (Conway et al., 2000). E46K appears to be even more effective in the promotion of aggregate formation in cultured cells than these other two mutations (Pandey et al., 2006).

As fibril formation of native α-synuclein occurs in most cases of synucleinopathies, most studies have deal with the mechanisms that trigger this process. Both physical and chemical factors have been demonstrated to affect this aggregation process (Lundvig et al., 2008).

As mentioned above, it is believed that interactions between the C-terminus and the central portion of α-synuclein can prevent or minimize its aggregation/fibril formation. As the majority of hydrophobic interactions in the C-terminal of α-synuclein arise through its three

Tyr, we created Tyr to Ala mutants to examine the importance of these Tyr residues in fibril formation of α-synuclein *in vitro*. This was completely inhibited in the timescale over which measurements were made (70 hours) when the three C-terminal Tyr were replaced with Ala. In addition, substitution of Tyr^{133} by Ala also inhibitted fibril formation, whereas the individual Y125A and Y136A mutants showed limited inhibition. Replacement of Tyr^{39} by Ala also resulted in substantial inhibition of fibril formation. Structural analysis showed that the Y133A α-synuclein mutant has a substantially different conformation, as it is rich in α-helical secondary structure, as compared with wild-type α-synuclein and its other mutants. However, no formation of any tertiary structure was seen, as judged from the near-UV circular-dichroism spectra. These observations suggest that the long-range intramolecular interactions between the N-terminal and C-terminal of α-synuclein are crucial for the process of fibril formation (Ulrih et al., 2008).

6. Alpha-synuclein and membranes

6.1 Lipid-binding domains

A characteristic feature of the α-synuclein amino-acid sequence is the set of seven degenerate 11-residue repeating motifs. These are reminescent of the amphipathic α-helical domains of the exchangeable apolipoproteins, which mediate a variety of lipid and protein interactions (Davidson et al., 1998, George et al., 1995). Amphipathicity corresponds to the segregation of polar and nonpolar residues to the two opposite faces of the α-helix, a distribution that is well suited for membrane binding (Drin & Antonny, 2009).

Depending upon the distribution of residues to the polar and nonpolar faces of the helices, Segrest et al. divided the apolipoprotein α-helices into different classes: class A helices bind lipids and are characterized by a clustering of basic residues at the polar/nonpolar interface and acidic residues at the center of the polar face, while class G helices are implicated in protein interactions and are characterized by a random radial distribution of charged residues to the polar face of the helix (Segrest et al., 1992). Davidson et al. subjected the entire α-synuclein sequence to helical wheel analysis and identified five potential amphipathic α-helices that encompass all of the 11-mer repeats and some of the adjacent amino acids. The first four of these five theoretical helices share the defining properties of class A_2 lipid-binding helices, and they are distinguished by clustered basic residues at the polar-apolar interface and positioned ±100° from the center of the nonpolar face, with a preponderence of Lys over Arg, and the presence of Glu residues on the polar face. The α-helix on the fifth 11-mer repeat resembles a class G helix, and it is thus a candidate for protein-protein interactions (Davidson et al., 1998).

There is a notable feature that can be used to distinguish between putative amphipathic α-synuclein helices and those in the exchangeable apolipoproteins: the Thr residues at the center of the nonpolar faces of helices 2-4 (Davidson et al., 1998). Although polar, these can reside on the nonpolar face of the helix due to its relatively long aliphatic side chain (Segrest et al., 1992). Thr are conserved among the α-synuclein sequences from canary, human and rat, suggesting that they indeed have an important function. Another unique aspect of the α-synuclein 11-mer repeat sequences is the absence of Pro, which in exchangeable apolipoproteins introduces helix-breaking hairpin turns. In contrast, α-synuclein helices 1-4 appear to be punctuated by nonpolar residues that are predicted to disrupt the amphipathicity of a helix (Davidson et al., 1998).

6.2 Lipid and membrane selectivity

Data that have documented the tendency of α-synuclein to colocalize with synaptic vesicles *in vivo* (Maroteaux et al., 1988) and the presence of the 11-residue repeated domains in a pattern similar to that found in the apolipoproteins (George et al., 1995) sparked a series of studies to determine the α-synuclein lipid-binding ability. Alpha-synuclein interactions with membranes have been found to be one of the most contentious areas regarding this protein (Fink, 2006), as there have been numerous reports on sometimes completely contradicting results, and as there might be major differences between the situation *in vivo* and *in vitro*. Also, membranes have been reported to both accelerate (Lee et al., 2002) and inhibit (Narayanan & Scarlata, 2001; Zhu & Fink, 2003) α-synuclein fibril formation, so this probably reflects the varying conditions used in the different studies (Zhu & Fink, 2003).

All three of these α-synuclein mutations occur within the N-terminus, which is responsible for its membrane binding, hence suggesting an effect on membrane interactions (Fortin et al., 2010). The A30P α-synuclein mutation, and to a lesser extent that of A53T, disrupts the helical structure of α-synuclein (Bussell & Eliezer, 2001), although it does not significantly affect the structure of membrane-associated α-synuclein (Bussell & Eliezer, 2004). The E46K α-synuclein mutant binds to negatively charged vesicles with a higher protein/lipid ratio than does wild-type α-synuclein (Choi et al., 2004), while A30P affects the localization, and presumably the membrane binding, of α-synuclein *in vivo* (Fortin et al., 2010).

6.2.1 Membrane interactions *in vitro*

It is generally accepted that α-synuclein preferentially interacts with small unilamellar vesicles (SUVs) containing negatively charged head groups (Davidson et al., 1998; Jo et al., 2000) or interfacial packing defects (Kamp & Beyer, 2006; Nuscher et al., 2004), and that upon SUV binding, α-synuclein undergoes a conformational transition from an intrinsically disordered state to an α-helical structure (Davidson et al., 1998; Jo et al., 2000; Nuscher et al., 2004). Various combinations of charged and uncharged lipids have been used in these studies. These negatively charged acidic phospholipids include phosphatidylglycerol (PG), phosphatidic acid (PA), phosphatidylserine (PS) and phosphatidylinositol (PI), while the uncharged, neutral lipids commonly used include phosphatidylcholine (PC) and phosphatidylethanolamine (PE) (Valenzuela, 2007).

The interactions of α-synuclein with membranes have been shown to affect the properties of both the protein and the membranes, and both electrostatic and hydrophobic interactions are important in the protein-bilayer association (Zhu et al., 2003). There are several factors that are believed to have central roles in modulation of the binding equilibrium of α-synuclein to membranes, including chemical properties of the membranes (Davidson et al., 1998; Jo et al., 2000), ionic strength of the solution (Davidson et al., 1998; Zhu et al., 2003), vesicle size, or more precisely, the curvature of the phospholipid surface (Davidson et al., 1998; Narayanan & Scarlata, 2001; Rhoades et al., 2006), and mass ratio of α-synuclein to the lipids (Zhu & Fink, 2003). Here, an overview of some of the more important findings regarding the lipid specificities of α-synuclein are given.

Davidson et al. were the first to demonstrate that α-synuclein binds only to acidic phospholipids and preferentially to vesicles with smaller diameters. Circular dichroism spectroscopy was used to determine the effects of this lipid binding on the secondary structure of α-synuclein. In buffer solution, α-synuclein is mainly unstructured, with less than 3% of the structure as α-helix. Incubation of α-synuclein with vesicles made of a mixture of acidic and neutral phospholipids is accompanied by a large increase in its α-helical content. Alpha-synuclein does not bind to SUVs or multilamellar vesicles composed of PC only, or of a mixture of PC and PE. Here, α-synuclein binds to SUVs containing at least 30% to 50% acidic lipids, per vesicle weight. Comparisons of the ability of α-synuclein to bind to vesicles of different sizes, as SUVs with 20 nm to 25 nm diameters and large unilamellar vesicles (LUV) with 125 ±30 nm diameter, have shown that α-synuclein does not bind to vesicles that contained neutral 1-palmitoyl 2-oleoyl PC (POPC) alone. Also, binding to LUVs composed of POPC/1-palmitoyl 2-oleoyl PA (POPA) was less than to SUVs of the same composition (Davidson et al., 1998).

Binding to negatively charged SUVs was confirmed in another study where they incubated α-synuclein together with vesicles and then fractionated the solution with gel filtration chromatography. Alpha-synuclein eluted together with the SUV fraction when incubated with either POPC/POPA or POPC/1-palmitoyl 2-oleoyl PS (POPS) phospholipids, while its binding to vesicles composed of POPC alone was not detected (Perrin et al., 2000). Althought in nervous tissue PA comprises approximately 1% to 3% of the total phospholipids, while PS is more abundant (12% to 22% of the total phospholipids) (Sastry et al., 1985), it is difficult to relate these values directly to the local composition of specific membranes inside the cell, since these lipids are not distributed evenly in the cell and are generated and metabolized rapidly (Perrin et al., 2000).

Using thin-layer chromatography overlay, it has been shown that α-synuclein binds to the brain or commercially available lipids PE, PI and lyso-PE. These interactions were much weaker with POPS and brain PS, and absent with POPC, POPA, sphingomyelin and cholesterol (Jo et al., 2000). Surprisingly, in contrast with a previous report (Davidson et al., 1998), α-synuclein does not bind to PA, which was attributed to the properties of the thin-layer chromatography overlay method. Replacing PC with PE in acidic lipid vesicles greatly increased the binding of α-synuclein (Jo et al., 2000). Althought both PE and PC are neutral phospholipids that have similar electrostatic properties, they differ in their head-group orientation, lipid bilayer packing, and hydrogen-bonding capacity (Hauser et al., 1981, as cited in Jo et al., 2000). When the neutral head-groups are tightly packed, PE forms a lipid monolayer with high negative curvature (Bazzi et al., 1992). It is believed that α-synuclein can relieve this negative curvature strain, and hence stabilize the PE/acidic lipid vesicles. This study also showed that both SUVs and multilamellar vesicles composed of POPC/POPS induce α-helical secondary structures, which suggests that the vesicle size does not impact on the α-synuclein secondary structure. With the neutral charged PE in the presence of acidic phospholipids (PA and PI), this significant increases the α-synuclein α-helicity. However, it should be emphasized that the changes in α-synuclein secondary structure are much lower in the presence of neutral PC in combination with negatively charged lipids (Jo et al., 2000).

In contrast to previous studies that used prolonged incubation times and mechanical separation of the products, and which found that α-synuclein only bound to SUVs composed of acidic phospholipids (Davidson et al., 1998; Jo et al., 2000; Perrin et al., 2000), in another study, the association between α-synuclein and lipids was viewed immediately after the addition of lipids to α-synuclein. Data were then obtained either by monitoring the change in intrinsic fluorescence emanating from four α-synuclein Tyr residues, or by adding the Laurdan fluorescent probe to the vesicles. Surprisingly, α-synuclein bound with similar affinities to LUVs composed of the negatively charged POPS and the electrically neutral

POPC. This initial binding did not induce changes in the secondary structure of α-synuclein. This study also supported the role of the α-synuclein C-terminus in membrane binding, by showing that lowering the pH of folded α-synuclein, which reduces the negative charge of α-synuclein, greatly increases the binding affinity without altering the secondary structure (Narayanan & Scarlata, 2001).

Fluorescence correlation spectroscopy was used as a tool for rapid and quantitative analysis of the lipid binding of α-synuclein. Some studies have confirmed the importance of the negatively charged lipids (PA and PS) for α-synuclein binding to LUVs with 120 nm diameter, when no pre-incubation of α-synuclein and the vesicles was used. Alpha-synuclein has a significantly higher affinity for vesicles that contain some POPA, over those that contain an equivalent amount of POPS. The reason for this could be the polar POPA head-group, which is smaller in size compared to that of POPS and might therefore be able to pack more closely together in a lipid bilayer, producing a higher charge density. Alpha-synuclein shows slightly higher binding affinity to POPE compared to POPC (Rhoades et al., 2006). Combined with other data in the literature (Davidson et al., 1998; Jo et al., 2000; Nuscher et al., 2004), these suggest that each molecule of α-synuclein can bind to a lipid bilayer patch composed of ≤85 acidic lipid molecules, corresponding in the case of POPS to a weight ratio of bound protein to total lipid of approximately 1:5. Interestingly, at higher α-synuclein concentrations, the amount of bound α-synuclein decreases, suggesting a destabilization of the membrane. This study also confirmed the importance of electrostatic interactions for the binding between α-synuclein and the lipids (Rhoades et al., 2006).

The binding of α-synuclein to SUVs has been monitored by measuring the changes in intrinsic fluorescence emanating from the four Tyr residues in α-synuclein. These data have suggested that α-synuclein binds to both negatively charged and electrically neutral SUVs, although slightly weaker for the latter. This binding to electrically neutral vesicles is presumably due to electrostatic interactions between the negatively charged C-terminal region of α-synuclein and the positively charged choline. Binding to different types of vesicles was also detected in high ionic strength solutions. These data indicate that for α-synuclein binding to lipids, not only are electrostatic interactions important, but also hydrophobic interactions. The influence of α-synuclein binding to the membrane has also been examined. Due to the differences in the excitation spectra and polarisation of the Laurdan dye after incubation of dipalmitoyl PA (DPPA)/dipalmitoyl PC (DPPC) and dipalmitoyl PG (DPPG)/DPPC SUVs with α-synuclein, this study concluded that α-synuclein is inserted deep into the membrane and does not remain bound only on the surface. A lack of significant penetration of α-synuclein into the DPPC vesicle bilayer was observed. Random coil–helix structure transition was most notable when SUVs composed of DPPG or dipalmitoyl PS (DPPS) or their mixtures with DPPC or dipalmitoyl PE (DPPE) were used. The amount of helix induced was smaller for DPPA/DPPC. SUVs made of DPPC only do not trigger the formation of the α-synuclein α-helix structure; presumably α-synuclein binds to the surface of these vesicles due to electrostatic interactions, but does not induce the helical structure (Zhu et al., 2003).

The small diameter of the SUVs leads to curvature stress in the bilayer, which results in a rather broad phase transition that is centered at ~4-5 °C below the chain-melting phase-transition temperature (T_m), and thus vesicles made of DPPC undergo melting transition at 36 °C rather than at 41 °C (Gaber & Sheridan, 1982). Using isothermal titration calorimetry, differential scanning calorimetry (Nuscher et al., 2004), spin label electron paramagnetic resonance (EPR), and fluorescence spectroscopy (Kamp & Beyer, 2006), it has been shown that α-synuclein affects the lipid packing in neutral SUVs. Here α-synuclein induces chain ordering below the T_m, but not in the liquid crystalline state of zwitterionic vesicle membranes. Binding of α-synuclein leads to an increase in the temperature and cooperitivity of the phase transition, which was attributed to defect healing in the curved vesicle membranes. Binding to the vesicles also induces coil-helix transitions of α-synuclein (Kamp & Beyer, 2006; Nuscher et al., 2004). SUVs made of POPC/POPG at a molar ratio of 1:1 and 2:1 cause α-helix formation in the structure of α-synuclein, and this is more pronounced at the 1:1 ratio. A helix structure is not observed in LUVs of the same composition. This again hightlights the importance of the negative charge and size of lipid vesicles for α-synuclein α-helix formation. A more important finding is the formation of the helical structure by binding to SUVs of neutrally charged DPPC under the T_m and not above that temperature (Nuscher et al., 2004).

Recently, Bartels et al. used circular dichroism spectroscopy and isotermal titration calorimetry to investigate peptide fragments from different domains of the full-length α-synuclein protein. They showed that membrane recognition of the N-terminus is essential for the cooperative formation of helical domains in the protein. This suggests that the membrane-induced helical folding of the first 25 residues of α-synuclein might be driven simultaneously by electrostatic attraction and by changes in lipid ordering (Bartels et al., 2010).

6.2.2 Membrane interactions *in vivo*

Compared with the α-synuclein–lipid interaction *in vitro*, the interaction of α-synuclein with membranes in cells is less well understood. Cole et al. investigated α-synuclein interactions with intracellular lipid stores in cultured cells treated with high concentrations of fatty acids. Here, α-synuclein accumulated on phospholipid monolayers surrounding triglyceride-rich lipid droplets and protected the stored triglycerides from hydrolysis. Chemical cross-linking experiments led to the suggestion that dimers or trimers of α-synuclein were associated with the droplet surface (Cole et al., 2002).

Alpha-synuclein can be imported into cells (Sung et al., 2001) and can be secreted from cells, althought it lacks a conventional signal sequence for secretion (Lee et al., 2005). Lee et al. reported that a portion of α-synuclein is stored in the lumen of vesicles in the cytoplasm, and that the α-synuclein in vesicles might be secreted through an unconventional exocytosis pathway. This study also demonstrated that intravesicular α-synuclein is more prone to aggregation than cytosolic α-synuclein, and that aggregated forms of α-synuclein are also secreted from cells (Lee et al., 2005). They thus used a series of deletion mutants and recombinant peptides to determine the amino-acid sequence motifs of α-synuclein that were required for its membrane translocation. The N-terminal region and the NAC peptide were shown to be necessary for translocation, althought the NAC was less effective than the N-terminal region. This thus suggested that the 11-amino acid repeat sequences bind to the lipid bilayer and that this binding interaction is crucial for α-synuclein translocation. Cellular uptake of α-synuclein was not significantlly affected by treatment with inhibitors of endocytosis, suggesting that this occurs via a mechanism distinct from normal endocytosis (Ahn et al., 2006).

Sharon et al. showed that free fatty acids have specific roles in the formation and maintenance of the soluble α-synuclein oligomers, and they suggested that α-synuclein might be a fatty-acid-binding protein (Sharon et al., 2001). In contrast, a later NMR study excluded high-affinity binding of fatty-acid molecules to specific α-synuclein sites (Lucke et al., 2006). Exposure of living mesencephalic neurons to polyunsaturated fatty acids (PUFAs) increased the α-synuclein oligomer levels, whereas saturated fatty acids decreased these. Here, α-synuclein interacts with the free PUFAs to form the first soluble oligomers, which then aggregate into insoluble high-molecular-weight complexes (Sharon et al., 2003a). Indeed, elevated PUFA levels have been detected in the soluble fractions of PD and Lewy bodies dementia brains. The levels of saturated and monounsaturated fatty acids did not change in these PD brains or in cells overexpressing α-synuclein, which indicated that α-synuclein is involved specifically in the maintenance of PUFA levels (Sharon et al., 2003b).

Using binding assays, it has been demonstrated that α-synuclein binds saturably and with high affinity to detergent-resistant membranes, to lipid rafts, in permeabilized HeLa cells, and in the presence of synaptosomal membranes from transgenic mice expressing human α-synuclein. The A53T α-synuclein mutation has no detectable effects on this binding, while the A30P mutation disrupts the association, which supports the specificity of the interaction (Fortin et al., 2004). It should also be mentioned that both of these mutations do not generally affect the interactions of α-synuclein with artificial membranes (Perrin et al., 2000), probably because these membranes fail to reproduce the full characteristics of lipid rafts (Fortin et al., 2004). In contrast, the A30P mutation distrupts α-synuclein association with native membranes, such as those of axonal transport vesicles, lipid droplets produced in HeLa cells by the administration of oleic acid, and yeast (Cole et al., 2002; Jensen et al., 1998; Outeiro et al., 2003). Alterations in the electrophoretic mobility of α-synuclein upon membrane binding have confirmed its binding to lipid rafts, with this interaction resistant to digestion of the rafts with proteinase K, which suggests that the lipids, rather than proteins, are required. This assumption is also supported by high affinity binding of α-synuclein to artificial membranes that do indeed mimic lipid rafts. Cholesterol does not appear to be required for the binding, but rather for maintenance of raft integrity; sphingolipid also appears not to be crucial for these interactions (Kubo et al., 2005).

Similar to previous reports (Davidson et al., 1998; Perrin et al., 2000), Kubo et al. reported that α-synuclein binding requires acidic phospholipids, with a preference for PS. Synthetic PS with defined acyl chains did not support this binding when used individually, with the combination of 18:1 PS and PS with polyunsaturated acyl chains required both to bind to and to shift the electrophoretic mobility of α-synuclein. The addition of 18:1 PC to 20:4 PS, or conversely, the addition of 20:4 PC to 18:1 PS, also promoted α-synuclein binding. The requirement for both monounsaturated and polyunsaturated acyl chains suggests that the interaction of α-synuclein requires membranes with two distinct phases: lipid rafts in a liquid-ordered phase, and the rest of the cell membrane in a liquid-disordered phase. Alpha-synuclein binds with higher affinity to artificial membranes with the PS head-group on the polyunsaturated fatty acyl chain rather than on the oleoyl side chain, apparently reflecting an interaction of α-synuclein with both the acyl chain and the head-group (Kubo et al., 2005).

In contrast to artificial membranes, the interactions of α-synuclein with biological membranes are highly dynamic and they show rapid dissociation. Thus, rather than electrostatic interactions, Kim et al. suggested the involment of hydrophobic interactions. Furthermore, the interactions of α-synuclein with cellular membranes occured only in the presence of nonprotein and nonlipid cytosolic components, which distinguished it from the spontanous interaction with artificial membranes. Here, addition of a cytosolic preparation to the artificial membranes resulted in similar binding of α-synuclein as for biological membranes (Kim et al., 2006).

Lipid rafts contain a lot of the ganglioside GM1, and it has been suggested that the gangliosides mediate or facilitate the association of α-synuclein with neuronal membranes (Martinez et al., 2007). However, recently Di Pasquale et al. identifed a ganglioside-binding domain in α-synuclein that showed a marked preference for interactions with GM3, which is a minor brain ganglioside for which the expression increases with age; the Lys^{34} and Tyr^{39} residues were shown to have critical roles in the GM3 recognition by α-synuclein (Di Pasquale et al., 2010).

7. Structural properties of membrane-bound α-synuclein

High resolution structural and dynamics information of α-synuclein in its lipid-bound state appear to be sufficient for the development of a better understanding of the physiological role of α-synuclein, as well as to identify the structural features that appear to be relevant to α-synuclein misfolding (Ulmer et al., 2005). However, despite the abundance of structural information for soluble proteins, relatively little is known about the structures of membrane-associated proteins in the physiologically important lipid bilayer environment (Jao et al., 2008). Consistent with this, the conformation of membrane-bound α-synuclein still remains unclear and somewhat contradictory.

Several biophysical methods have provided valuable insights into the structural features of the disordered and folded α-synuclein, including circular dichroism spectroscopy (Davidson et al., 1998; Chandra et al., 2003; Perrin et al., 2000), fluorescence spectroscopy (Rhoades et al., 2006), NMR (Bisaglia et al., 2005; Bussel & Eliezer, 2001, 2003; Bussel et al., 2005; Chandra et al., 2003; Dedmon et al., 2005; Eliezer et al., 2001; Ulmer et al., 2005), and EPR (Bortolus et al., 2008; Drescher et al., 2008; Georgieva et al., 2008; Jao et al., 2004, 2008). Binding of α-synuclein to anionic membranes induces folding of its N-terminal part into an amphipathic helix, whereas the C-terminus (residues ~98-140) remains unstructured (Bisaglia et al., 2005; Bussel & Eliezer, 2003; Chandra et al., 2003; Davidson et al., 1998; Eliezer et al., 2001; Ulmer et al., 2005). The helical content of α-synuclein is much lower in buffer and in the presence of zwitterionic membranes (Davidson et al., 1998; Zhu & Fink; 2003).

It has generally been proposed that the natural binding target of α-synuclein *in vivo* is the synaptic vesicles, the surface topology of which is most closely approximated *in vitro* by synthetic lipid vesicles (Bisaglia et al., 2005; Bussel & Eliezer, 2003; Bussell et al., 2005; Chandra et al., 2003; Jao et al., 2004; Ulmer et al., 2005). The slow tumbling rate of intact phospholipid vesicles has hindered direct studies of the vesicle-bound conformation of α-synuclein using solution NMR methods (Georgieva et al., 2008). Consequently, most of the structural information available concerns studies where detergent micelles were used as membrane-mimetic environments, because their small size facilitates high-resolution structural analysis by NMR. The conformation of micelle-bound α-synuclein has thus been thoroughly investigated, and there is a general consensus on the presence of two curved helices, with a break in the α-synuclein 38−44 region (Bisaglia et al., 2005; Bussell & Eliezer, 2003; Chandra et al., 2003; Ulmer et al., 2005). On the contrary, the structure of α-synuclein bound to lipid vesicles, which would be more relevant physiologically, remains a matter of debate. EPR analyses of α-synuclein derivatives bound to SUVs have provided evidence for an elongated helical structure that is devoid of any significant tertiary packing (Jao et al., 2004), or they have suggested a broken helical structure (Bortolus et al., 2008; Drescher et al., 2008). A number of recent studies have highlighted the ongoing debate regarding the physiologically relevant form, as the bent or extended membrane-bound helix (Figure 2).

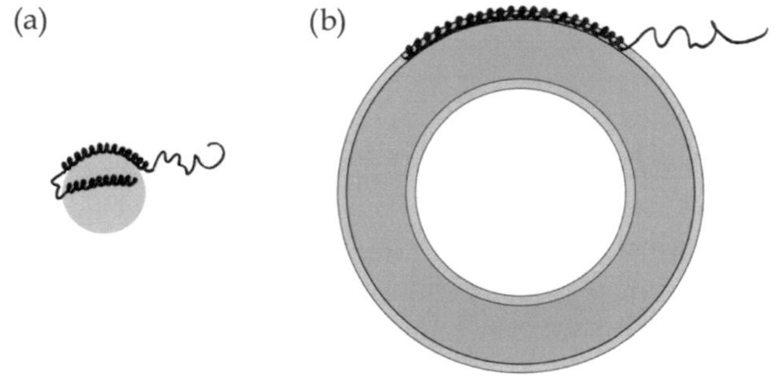

Fig. 2. Illustrations of the generally proposed α-synuclein structures on (a) micelles (bent helix model) and (b) SUVs (elongated helix model) (Jao et al., 2008; Trexler & Rhoades, 2009).

7.1 Helix periodicity

Several studies have raised the question of the periodicity of the helix that is formed upon binding of α-synuclein to membranes. As indicated above, the N-terminus of α-synuclein contains seven imperfect 11-residue repeats. Using site-directed spin-labeling, it has been shown that repeats 5–7 of α-synuclein are bound to SUVs with an 11/3 periodicity (11 residues to complete three full turns) (Jao et al., 2004). Sodium dodecyl sulphate (SDS) micelle-bound α-synuclein shows the same periodicity, as opposed to the 18/5 periodicity of an ideal α-helix (Bussell et al., 2005). In this ideal 18/5 periodicity, there are 3.6 residues per turn and the rotation per residue is 100°. In the α-synuclein 11/3 periodicity, the number of residues per turn is 3.67 and the rotation per residue is 98.18°. Using theoretical methods, it has indeed been concluded that the periodicity of α-synuclein is 11/3, and that through the positioning of the charged residues, this has implications for α-synuclein membrane binding. These calculations show that the energy penalty for a change in periodicity from the 18/5 to 11/3 on anionic membranes is overcome by the favorable solvation energy (Mihajlovic & Lazaridis, 2008).

7.2 Analysis of α-synuclein structure by nuclear magnetic resonance

Eliezer et al. were the first to use NMR spectroscopy to characterize the conformational properties of α-synuclein when bound to lipid vesicles and lipid-mimetic detergent micelles. They demonstrated that only the first 100 residues of the N-terminal region of α-synuclein bind to both SDS micelles and PA/PC vesicles and fold into an amphipathic helix, while the acidic C-terminal region of α-synuclein remains unstructured (Eliezer et al., 2001).
Ulmer et al. have described the structure and dynamics of α-synuclein in the micelle-bound form according to solution NMR spectroscopy. In binding to SDS micelles or SDS micelles with dodecylPC (DPC), α-synuclein forms two curved α-helices (Figure 3), helix-N (Val^{3}-Val^{37}) and helix-C (Lys^{45}-Thr^{92}). These helices are connected by a well-ordered, extended linker in an unexpected anti-parallel arrangement, which is followed by another short extended region (Gly^{93}-Lys^{97}) that overlaps with a chaperone-mediated autophagy recognition motif and a predominantly unstructured highly mobile tail (Asp^{98}-Ala^{140}) (Ulmer et al., 2005).

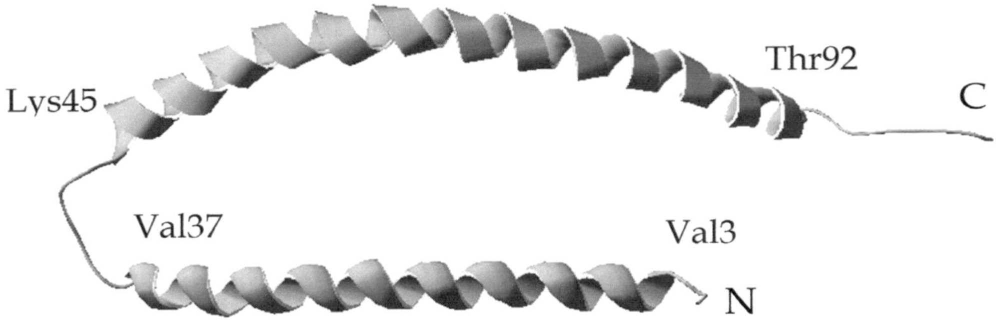

Fig. 3. Structure of α-synuclein bound to SDS micelles. Picture represents the two curved α-helices (Val^{3}-Val^{37} and Lys^{45}-Thr^{92}), connected by extended linker. The disordered C-terminus has been partially omitted. The image was generated from the PDB (accession number 1XQ8).

Although the presence of the helix break in the micelle-bound state of α-synuclein has been suggested to be a consequence of the small size of the micelle (Jao et al., 2004), the well-ordered conformation of the helix-helix connector indicates a defined interaction of α-synuclein with the lipid surfaces, suggesting that when it is bound to larger diameter synaptic vesicles, this can act as a switch between this broken helix structure and the uninterrupted helix structure (Ulmer et al., 2005). Therefore, the presence or absence of the helical break in α-synuclein appears to be the more controversial structural feature of α-synuclein when bound to lipids (Bisaglia et al., 2009). Other studies have also shown that there are two helical regions in the N-terminal sequence of α-synuclein that are interrupted by a single helix break around residue 42 (Bisaglia et al., 2005; Bussel & Eliezer, 2003; Chandra et. al., 2003). Data from Bisaglia et al. show that the region of residues 61-95 (the NAC region) is partially embedded in the micelle (Bisaglia et al., 2005)

Analysis of the dynamic processes of the α-synuclein backbone on a fast timescale (picoseconds to nanoseconds) revealed the presence of three distinct helical regions that have greater mobility with respect to the other helical fragments: Ala^{30}-Val^{37}, Asn^{65}-Val^{70}, and Glu^{83}-Ala^{89} (Ulmer et al., 2005). All three of these regions have two Gly residues in close sequential proximity, which might serve to mitigate a possible effect of α-synuclein binding on membrane fluidity. The helix curvature is significantly less than predicted based on the native globular micelle shape, which indicates a deformation of the micelle by α-synuclein. Ulmer et al. suggested that the interactions of the positively charged Lys side chains, which emanate sidewards from the helices, with the negatively charged headgroups of SDS can lead to the deformation of the globular micelle along the helix axes, to form a prolate, ellipsoid particle (Ulmer et al., 2005).

As indicated above, there are four Tyr residues in α-synuclein. One of these, Tyr^{39}, is located in the break region. Bisaglia et al. (2005) suggested that this Tyr^{39} is buried in the SDS micelle and proposed that this insertion might protect α-synuclein from aggregation (Zhou & Freed, 2004; Ulrih et al., 2008), as well as to protect Tyr^{39} from phosphorylation by $p72^{syk}$ tyrosine kinase (Negro et al., 2002, as cited in Bisaglia et al., 2005). This is in contrast with other models that have predicted that this Tyr^{39} is located either on the hydrophilic side of the helix or at the membrane-water interface (Bussell & Eliezer, 2003; Chandra et al., 2003; Jao et al., 2004; Mihajlovic & Lazaridis, 2008).

7.3 Analysis of α-synuclein structure by electron paramagnetic resonance

EPR analysis of 47 singly labeled α-synuclein mutants has shown that the membrane interactions are mediated by major conformational changes within seven of the N-terminal 11-amino-acid repeats: these reorganize from highly dynamic structures into an elongated helical structure. The equivalent positions within each of these different repeats are located in structurally comparable positions with respect to the membrane proximity, which suggests a curved membrane-dependent α-helical structure of α-synuclein, wherein each of these 11-aminoacid repeats takes up three helical turns (Jao et al., 2004). The α-synuclein helix is over 90 amino acids in length and it extends parallel to the curved membrane in a manner that allows the conserved Lys and Glu residues to interact with the zwitterionic headgroups, while the uncharged residues penetrate into the acyl-chain region (Jao et al., 2008). This structural arrangement is significantly different from that of α-synuclein in the presence of the commonly used membrane-mimetic detergent, SDS (Bisaglia et al., 2005, Ulmer et al., 2005). Thus these structural analyses also show that it is important to consider the lipid composition of any given bilayer, as this can have pronounced effects on the protein and bilayer structures (Jao et al., 2008).

Several other independent studies have appeared, with contradictory results. In one such study (Bortolus et al., 2008), the 35-43 region of α-synuclein bound to SUVs and to SDS micelles was investigated using site-directed spin labeling and EPR spectroscopy. The distance distributions were compatible with the presence of conformational disorder in this region, rather than for the formation of a continuous helical structure. These data showed that α-synuclein shows very similar behavior in micelles and in SUVs, and they ruled out an unbroken helical structure of the region around residue 40. This propensity for helix breaking was confirmed by their molecular dynamics simulations of the 31-52 fragment interacting with a lipid bilayer (Bortolus et al., 2008).

In a study by Drescher et al. (2008), four α-synuclein mutants were prepared by inserting Cys residues labeled with the spin-label reagent (*S*-(2,2,5,5-tetramethyl-2,5-dihydro-1H-pyrrol-3-yl)methyl methanesulfonothioate) (MTSL), with each containing one label in the proposed helix 1, and a second label in helix 2. Between the labeled Cys residues within the molecule the distance resulting from their binding to the membrane was measured using dual-frequency pulsing EPR (double electron-electron resonance). Consistent with a previous report (Bortolus et al., 2008), these data showed that α-synuclein even adopts a two-helix, antiparallel arrangement on vesicles that are large enough to accommodate an extended helix, which suggests that this bent structure is also the preferred conformation of α-synuclein on larger vesicles (Drescher et al., 2008).

Also using pulsed dipolar EPR, Georgieva et al. came to somewhat different conclusions. Here the distances measured between the pairs of nitroxide spin labels introduced were close to those expected for a single continuous helix. To circumvent problems associated with SUVs and rodlike SDS micelles, here they used lipid bicelles (providing a lipid-bilayer structure, yet having a particle size nearly as small as that of micelles), which produced very similar results to liposomes while offering a major improvement in experimentally accessible distance ranges and resolution. According to these data, they suggested that when α-synuclein is bound to SUVs, it forms a single α-helix, without the intermediate region of the interruption. The idea that α-synuclein can interconvert between these broken and extended helical forms was also suggested, and it thus remains possible that *in vivo* α-synuclein occupies one or the other form depending on conditions (Georgieva et al., 2008).

7.4 Analysis of α-synuclein structure with other methods

Contradictory to these current models of membrane-bound α-synuclein that have been deduced mostly from NMR studies, limited proteolysis experiments have indicated that the C-terminal part of membrane-bound α-synuclein has a more rigid structure. The negatively charged C-terminus appears to bind Ca^{2+} in the presence of SDS micelles, and in doing so it becomes sufficiently rigid and structured to resist extensive proteolysis (de Laureto et al., 2006). In another study based on site-directed fluorescence labeling, they also examined the effects of Ca^{2+} on the acidic tail conformation of lipid-bound α-synuclein (Tamamizu-Kato et al., 2006). Here, they suggested that the Ca^{2+} either bridges α-synuclein to the membrane, possibly by coordinating with the negative charge on the α-synuclein acidic tail and the acidic head-groups in the phospholipid bilayer, or it facilitates the traversing of the membrane bilayer by this segment of α-synuclein (Tamamizu-Kato et al., 2006).

Another study highlighted the role of the physical parameters of the membrane mimetic in determining the α-synuclein conformation (Trexler & Rhoades, 2009). Single molecule Förster resonance energy transfer was used to probe the helical structure of α-synuclein bound to SDS micelles and LUVs. Single and double Cys α-synuclein mutants were engineered to allow for site-specific labeling with maleimide fluorophores. When bound to highly curved detergent micelles, α-synuclein formed a bent-helix, whereas the structure of the elongated helix was adopted when bound to the more physiological 100-nm-diameter lipid vesicles (Trexler & Rhoades, 2009).

Single-molecule Förster resonance energy transfer was also used to provide evidence for the structural interplay between the broken and extended α-helix structures of α-synuclein, as induced by the binding of α-synuclein to SDS and phospholipid SUVs (Ferreon et al., 2009). The switch between a broken and an extended helical structure can be triggered by changing the concentrations of the binding partners or by varying the curvature of the binding surfaces presented by the micelles or bilayers composed of SDS. The use of lipid vesicles of various compositions showed that a low fraction of the negatively charged lipids, as similar to that found in biological membranes, was sufficient to drive α-synuclein binding and folding that resulted in the induction of the extended helical structure (Ferreon et al., 2009).

The structure of the N-terminal domain of α-synuclein has also been determined using theoretical methods (Mihajlovic & Lazaridis, 2008). This computional study of the binding of truncated α-synuclein (residues 1-95) to planar bilayers showed that α-synuclein forms a bent helix, with the largest bend around residue 47. This bending of the helix was not due to the protein sequence or membrane-protein interactions, but to the collective motions of the long helix (Mihajlovic & Lazaridis, 2008).

8. Conclusions

In this chapter, we have presented the state-of-the-art for the field of α-synuclein structure, and for its fibril formation and interactions with membranes. There are still many unanswered questions regarding the correlation between α-synuclein membrane affinity, and its function and its role in synucleinopathies. As the disruption of membranes by α-synuclein correlates with the binding affinity of α-synuclein for particular membrane compositions and with the induced helical conformation of α-synuclein, this suggests that inappropriate membrane permeabilization is the cause of cell dysfunction, and even cell death, in amyloid diseases. Protofibrillar or fibrillar α-synuclein results in a much more rapid destruction of membranes than soluble monomeric α-synuclein, which indicates that protofibrils or fibrils are likely to be significantly neurotoxic. Further studies of α-synuclein interactions with membranes are still very important to provide us with a fuller undertanding of the molecular mechanisms of its implications in Parkinson's disease.

9. References

Abeliovich, A., Schmitz, Y., Farinas, I., Choi-Lundberg, D., Ho, W.H., Castillo, P.E., Shinsky, N., Verdugo, J.M.G., Armanini, M., Ryan, A., Hynes, M., Phillips, H., Sulzer, D. & Rosenthal, A. (2000). Mice lacking alpha-synuclein display functional deficits in the nigrostriatal dopamine system. *Neuron*, Vol.25, No.1, (January 2000), pp. 239-252, ISSN 0896-6273

Ahn, K.J., Paik, S.R., Chung, K.C. & Kim, J. (2006). Amino acid sequence motifs and mechanistic features of the membrane translocation of alpha-synuclein. *Journal of Neurochemistry*, Vol.97, No.1, (April 2006), pp. 265-279, ISSN 0022-3042

Arawaka, S., Saito, Y., Murayama, S. & Mori, H. (1998). Lewy body in neurodegeneration with brain iron accumulation type 1 is immunoreactive for alpha-synuclein. *Neurology*, Vol.51, No.3, (September 1998), pp. 887-889, ISSN 0028-3878

Bartels, T., Ahlstrom, L.S., Leftin, A., Kamp, F., Haass, C., Brown, M.F. & Beyer K. (2010). The N-terminus of the intrinsically disordered protein alpha-synuclein triggers membrane binding and helix folding. *Biophysical Journal*, Vol.99, No.7, (October 2010), pp. 2116-2124, ISSN 0006-3495

Bazzi, M.D., Youakim, A. & Nelsestuen, G.L. (1992). Importance of phosphatidylethanolamine for association of proteine kinase-c and other cytoplasmic proteins with membranes. *Biochemistry*, Vol.31, No.4, (February 1992), pp. 1125-1134, ISSN 0006-2960

Bertoncini, C.W., Jung, Y.S., Fernandez, C.O., Hoyer, W., Griesinger, C., Jovin, T.M. & Zweckstetter, M. (2005). Release of long-range tertiary interactions potentiates aggregation of natively unstructured alpha-synuclein. *Proceedings of the National Academy of Sciences of the United States of America*, Vol.102, No.5, (February 2005), pp. 1430-1435, ISSN 0027-8424

Beyer, K. (2007). Mechanistic aspects of Parkinson's disease: alpha-synuclein and the biomembrane. *Cell Biochemistry and Biophysics*, Vol.47, No.2, (April 2007), pp. 285-299, ISSN 1085-9195

Bisaglia, M., Tessari, I., Pinato, L., Bellanda, M., Giraudo, S., Fasano, M., Bergantino, E., Bubacco, L. & Mammi, S. (2005). A topological model of the interaction between α-synuclein and sodium dodecyl sulfate micelles. *Biochemistry*, Vol.44, No.1, (January 2005), pp. 329-339, ISSN 0006-2960

Bisaglia, M., Mammi, S. & Bubacco, L. (2009). Structural insights on physiological functions and pathological effects of alpha-synuclein. *Faseb Journal*, Vol.23, No.2, (February 2009), pp. 329-340, ISSN 0892-6638

Bodles, A.M., Guthrie, D.J., Greer, B. & Irvine, G B. (2001). Identification of the region of non-A beta component (NAC) of Alzheimer's disease amyloid responsible for its aggregation and toxicity. *Journal of Neurochemistry*, Vol.78, No.2, (July 2001), pp. 384-395, ISSN 0022-3042

Bortolus, M., Tombolato, F., Tessari, I., Bisaglia, M., Mammi, S., Bubacco, L., Ferrarini, A. & Maniero, A.L. (2008). Broken helix in vesicle and micelle-bound alpha-synuclein: Insights from site-directed spin labeling-EPR experiments and MD simulations. *Journal of the American Chemical Society*, Vol.130, No.21, (May 2008), pp. 6690-6691, ISSN 0002-7863

Bussell, R. & Eliezer, D. (2001). Residual structure and dynamics in Parkinson's disease-associated mutants of alpha-synuclein. *Journal of Biological Chemistry*, Vol.276, No.49, (December 2001), pp. 45996-46003, ISSN 0021-9258

Bussell, R. & Eliezer, D. (2003). A structural and functional role for 11-mer repeats in alpha-synuclein and other exchangeable lipid binding proteins. *Journal of Molecular Biology*, Vol.329, No.4, (June 2003), pp. 763-778, ISSN 0022-2836

Bussell, R. & Eliezer, D. (2004). Effects of Parkinson's disease-linked mutations on the structure of lipid-associated alpha-synuclein. *Biochemistry*, Vol.43, No.16, (April 2004), pp. 4810-4818, ISSN 0006-2960

Bussell, R., Ramlall, T.F. & Eliezer, D. (2005). Helix periodicity, topology, and dynamics of membrane-associated alpha-Synuclein. *Protein Science*, Vol.14, No.4, (April 2005), pp. 862-872, ISSN 0961-8368

Chandra, S., Chen, X.C., Rizo, J., Jahn, R. & Sudhof, T.C. (2003). A broken alpha-helix in folded alpha-synuclein. *Journal of Biological Chemistry*, Vol.278, No.17, (April 2003), pp. 15313-15318, ISSN 0021-9258

Chartier-Harlin, M.C., Kachergus, J., Roumier, C., Mouroux, V., Douay, X., Lincoln, S., Levecque, C., Larvor, L., Andrieux, J., Hulihan, M., Waucquier, N., Defebvre, L., Amouyel, P., Farrer, M. & Destee, A. (2004). Alpha-synuclein locus duplication as a cause of familial Parkinson's disease. *Lancet*, Vol.364, No.9440, (September 2004), pp. 1167-1169, ISSN 0140-6736

Choi, W., Zibaee, S., Jakes, R., Serpell, L.C., Davletov, B., Crowther, R.A. & Goedert, M. (2004). Mutation E46K increases phospholipid binding and assembly into filaments of human alpha-synuclein. *Febs Letters*, Vol.576, No.3, (October 2004), pp. 363-368, ISSN 0014-5793

Cole, N.B., Murphy, D.D., Grider, T., Rueter, S., Brasaemle, D. & Nussbaum, R.L. (2002). Lipid droplet binding and oligomerization properties of the Parkinson's disease protein alpha-synuclein. *Journal of Biological Chemistry*, Vol.277, No.8, (February 2002), pp. 6344-6352, ISSN 0021-9258

Conway, K A., Lee, S.J., Rochet, J.C., Ding, T.T., Williamson, R.E. & Lansbury, P T. (2000). Acceleration of oligomerization, not fibrillization, is a shared property of both alpha-synuclein mutations linked to early-onset Parkinson's disease: Implications for pathogenesis and therapy. *Proceedings of the National Academy of Sciences of the United States of America*, Vol.97, No.2, (January 2000), pp. 571-576, ISSN 0027-8424

Davidson, W.S., Jonas, A., Clayton, D.F. & George, J.M. (1998). Stabilization of alpha-synuclein secondary structure upon binding to synthetic membranes. *Journal of Biological Chemistry*, Vol.273, No.16, (April 1998), pp. 9443-9449, ISSN 0021-9258

de Laureto, P.P., Tosatto, L., Frare, E., Marin, O., Uversky, V.N. & Fontana, A. (2006). Conformational properties of the SDS-bound state of R-synuclein probed by limited proteolysis: Unexpected rigidity of the acidic C-terminal tail. *Biochemistry*, Vol.45, No.38, (September 2006), pp. 11523-11531, ISSN 0006-2960

Dedmon, M.M., Lindorff-Larsen, K., Christodoulou, J., Vendruscolo, M. &. Dobson, C.M. (2005). Mapping long-range interactions in alpha-synuclein using spin-label NMR and ensemble molecular dynamics simulations. *Journal of the American Chemical Society*, Vol.127, No.2, (January 2005), pp. 476-477, ISSN 0002-7863

Di Pasquale, E., Fantini, J., Chahinian, H., Maresca, M., Taieb, N. & Yahi, N. (2010). Altered ion channel formation by the Parkinson's-disease-linked E46K mutant of alpha-synuclein is corrected by GM3 but not by GM1 gangliosides. *Journal of Molecular Biology*, Vol.397, No.1, (March 2010), pp. 202-218, ISSN 0022-2836

Drescher, M., Veldhuis, G., van Rooijen, B.D., Milikisyants, S., Subramaniam, V. & Huber, M. (2008). Antiparallel arrangement of the helices of vesicle-bound alpha-synuclein. *Journal of the American Chemical Society*, Vol.130, No.25, (June 2008), pp. 7796-7797, ISSN 0002-7863

Drin, G. & Antonny, B. (2010). Amphipathic helices and membrane curvature. *Febs Letters*, Vol.584, No.9, (May 2010), pp. 1840-1847, ISSN 0014-5793

Dunker, A.K., Lawson, J.D., Brown, C.J., Williams, R.M., Romero, P., Oh, J.S., Oldfield, C.J., Campen, A.M., Ratliff, C.R., Hipps, K.W., Ausio, J., Nissen, M.S., Reeves, R., Kang, C.H., Kissinger, C.R., Bailey, R.W., Griswold, M.D., Chiu, M., Garner, E.C. & Obradovic, Z. (2001). Intrinsically disordered protein. *Journal of Molecular Graphics & Modelling*, Vol.19, No.1, pp. 26-59, ISSN 1093-3263

Eliezer, D., Kutluay, E., Bussell, R. & Browne, G. (2001). Conformational properties of alpha-synuclein in its free and lipid-associated states. *Journal of Molecular Biology*, Vol.307, No.4, (April 2001), pp. 1061-1073, ISSN 0022-2836

Ferreon, A.C.M., Gambin, Y., Lemke, E.A. & Deniz, A.A. (2009). Interplay of alpha-synuclein binding and conformational switching probed by single-molecule fluorescence. *Proceedings of the National Academy of Sciences of the United States of America*, Vol.106, No.14, (April 2009), pp. 5645-5650, ISSN 0027-8424

Fink, A.L. (2005). Natively unfolded proteins. *Current Opinion in Structural Biology*, Vol.15, No.1, (February 2005), pp. 35-41, ISSN 0959-440X

Fink, A.L. (2006). The aggregation and fibrillation of alpha-synuclein. *Accounts of Chemical Research*, Vol.39, No.9, (September 2006), pp. 628-634, ISSN 0001-4842

Fortin, D.L., Nemani, V.M., Nakamura, K. & Edwards, R.H. (2010). The behavior of alpha-synuclein in neurons. *Movement Disorders*, Vol.25, No.3, (July 2009), pp. S21-S26, ISSN 0885-3185

Fortin D.L., Troyer M.D., Nakamura K., Kubo S., Anthony M.D. & Edwards R.H. (2004). Lipid rafts mediate the synaptic localization of α-synuclein. *Journal of Neuroscience*, Vol.24, No.30, (July 2004), pp. 6715-6723, ISSN 0270-6474

Gaber, B.P. & Sheridan, J.P. (1982). Kinetic and thermodynamic studies of the fusion of small unilamellar phospholipid-vesicles. *Biochimica Et Biophysica Acta*, Vol.685, No.1, pp. 87-93, ISSN 0006-3002

Gai, W.P., Power, J.H., Blumbergs, P.C. & Blessing, W.W. (1998). Multiple-system atrophy: a new alpha-synuclein disease? *Lancet*, Vol.352, No.9127, (August 1998), pp. 547-548, ISSN 0140-6736

Galvin, J.E., Uryu, K., Lee, V.M.J. & Trojanowski, J.Q. (1999). Axon pathology in Parkinson's disease and Lewy body dementia hippocampus contains alpha-, beta-, and gamma-synuclein. *Proceedings of the National Academy of Sciences of the United States of America*, Vol.96, No.23, (November 1999), pp. 13450-13455, ISSN 0027-8424

George, J.M., Jin, H., Woods, W.S. & Clayton, D.F. (1995). Characterization of a novel protein regulated during the critical period for song learning in the zebra finch. *Neuron*, Vol.15, No.2, (August 1995), pp. 361-372, ISSN 0896-6273

Georgieva, E.R., Ramlall, T.F., Borbat, P.P, Freed, J.H. & Eliezer, D. (2008). Membrane-bound alpha-synuclein forms an extended helix: Long-distance pulsed ESR measurements using vesicles, bicelles, and rodlike micelles. *Journal of the American Chemical Society*, Vol.130, No.39, (October 2008), pp. 12856-12857, ISSN 0002-7863

Giasson, B.I., Murray, I.V., Trojanowski, J.Q. & Lee, V.M. (2001). A hydrophobic stretch of 12 amino acid residues in the middle of alpha-synuclein is essential for filament assembly. *Journal of Biological Chemistry*, Vol.276, No.4, (January 2001), pp. 2380-2386, ISSN 0021-9258

Goedert, M. (2001). Alpha-synuclein and neurodegenerative diseases. *Nature Reviews Neuroscience*, Vol.2, No.7, (July 2001), pp. 492-501, ISSN 1471-0048

Gunasekaran, K., Tsai, C.J., Kumar, S., Zunay, D. & Nussinov, R. (2003). Extended disordered proteins: targeting function with less scaffold. *Trends in Biochemical Sciences*, Vol.28, No.2, (February 2003), pp. 81-85, ISSN 0968-0004

Iwai, A., Masliah, E., Yoshimoto, M., Ge, N., Flanagan, L., de Silva, H.A., Kittel, A. & Saitoh, T. (1995). The precursor protein of non-A β component of Alzheimer's disease amyloid is a presynaptic protein of the central nervous system. *Neuron*, Vol.14, No.2, (February 1995), pp. 467-475, ISSN 0896-6273

Jankovic, J. (2008). Parkinson's disease: clinical features and diagnosis. *Journal of Neurology Neurosurgery and Psychiatry*, Vol.79, No.4, (April 2008), pp. 368-376, ISSN 0022-3050

Jao, C.C., Der-Sarkissian, A. & Langen, R. (2004). Structure of membrane-bound alpha-synuclein studied by site-directed spin labeling. *Proceedings of the National Academy of Sciences of the United States of America*, Vol.101, No.22, (June 2004), pp. 8331-8336, ISSN 0027-8424

Jao, C.C., Hegde, B.G., Chen, J., Haworth, I.S. & Langen, R. (2008). Structure of membrane-bound alpha-synuclein from site-directed spin labeling and computational refinement. *Proceedings of the National Academy of Sciences of the United States of America*, Vol.105, No.50, (December 2008), pp. 19666-19671, ISSN 0027-8424

Jensen, P.H., Nielsen, M.S., Jakes, R., Dotti, G. & Goedert, M. (1998). Binding of alpha-synuclein to brain vesicles is abolished by familial Parkinson's disease mutation. *Journal of Biological Chemistry*, Vol.273, No.41, (October 1998), pp. 26292-26294, ISSN 0021-9258

Jo, E., McLaurin, J., Yip, C.M., George-Hyslop, P., Fraser, P.E. (2000). Alpha-synuclein membrane interactions and lipid specificity. *Journal of Biological Chemistry*, Vol.275, No.44, (November 2000), pp. 34328-34334, ISSN 0021-9258

Kamp, F. & Beyer, K. (2006). Binding of alpha-synuclein affects the lipid packing in bilayers of small vesicles. *Journal of Biological Chemistry*, Vol.281, No.14, (April 2006), pp. 9251-9259, ISSN 0021-9258

Kim, Y.S., Laurine, E., Woods, W. & Lee, S.J. (2006). A novel mechanism of interaction between alpha-synuclein and biological membranes. *Journal of Molecular Biology*, Vol.360, No.2, (July 2006), pp. 386-397, ISSN 0022-2836

Kruger, R., Kuhn, W., Muller, T., Woitalla, D., Graeber, M., Kosel, S., Przuntek, H., Epplen, J.T., Schols, L. & Riess, O. (1998). Ala30Pro mutation in the gene encoding alpha-synuclein in Parkinson's disease. *Nature Genetics*, Vol.18, No.2, (February 1998), pp. 106-108, ISSN 1061-4036

Kubo, S., Nemani, V.M., Chalkley, R.J., Anthony, M.D., Hattori, N., Mizuno, Y., Edwards, R.H. & Fortin, D.L. (2005). A combinatorial code for the interaction of alpha-synuclein with membranes. *Journal of Biological Chemistry*, Vol.280, No.36, (September 2005), pp. 31664-31672, ISSN 0021-9258

Larsen, K.E., Schmitz, Y., Troyer, M.D., Mosharov, E., Dietrich, P., Quazi, A.Z., Savalle, M., Nemani, V., Chaudry, F.A., Edwards, R.H., Stefanis, L., Sulzer., D. (2006). Alpha-synuclein overexpression in PC12 and chromaffin cells impairs catecholamine release by interfering with a late step in exocytosis. *Journal of Neuroscience*, Vol.26, No.46, (November 2006), pp. 11915-11922, ISSN 0270-6474

Lavedan, C. (1998). The synuclein family. *Genome Research*, Vol.8, No.9, (September 1998), pp. 871-880, ISSN 1054-9803

Lee, H.J., Choi, C. & Lee, S.J. (2002). Membrane-bound alpha-synuclein has a high aggregation propensity and the ability to seed the aggregation of the cytosolic form. *Journal of Biological Chemistry*, Vol.277, No.1, (January 2002), pp. 671-678, ISSN 0021-9258

Lee, H.J., Patel, S., Lee, S.J. (2005). Intravesicular localization and exocytosis of alpha-synuclein and its aggregates. *Journal of Neuroscience*, Vol.25, No.25, (June 2005), pp. 6016-6024, ISSN 0270-6474

Lucke, C., Gantz, D.L., Klimtchuk, E. & Hamilton, J.A. (2006). Interactions between fatty acids and alpha-synuclein. *Journal of Lipid Research*, Vol.47, No.8, (August 2006), pp. 1714-1724, ISSN 0022-2275

Lundvig, D., Lindersson, E. & Jensen, P.H. (2005). Pathogenic effects of alpha-synuclein aggregation. *Molecular Brain Research*, Vol.134, No.1, (March 2005), pp. 3-17, ISSN 0169-328X

Madine, J., Doig, A.J. & Middleton, D.A. (2006). A study of the regional effects of alpha-synuclein on the organization and stability of phospholipid bilayers. *Biochemistry*, Vol.45, No.18, (May 2006), pp. 5783-5792, ISSN 0006-2960

Maroteaux, L., Campanelli, J.T. & Scheller, R.H. (1988). Synuclein - a neuron-specific protein localized to the nucleous and presynaptic nerve-terminal. *Journal of Neuroscience*, Vol.8, No.8, (August 1988), pp. 2804-2815, ISSN 0270-6474

Martinez, Z., Zhu, M., Han, S.B. & Fink, A.L. (2007). GM1 specifically interacts with alpha-synuclein and inhibits fibrillation. *Biochemistry*, Vol.46, No.7, (February 2007), pp. 1868-1877, ISSN 0006-2960

Mihajlovic, M. & Lazaridis, T. (2008). Membrane-bound structure and energetics of alpha-synuclein. *Proteins-Structure Function and Bioinformatics*, Vol.70, No.3, (February 2008), pp. 761-778, ISSN 0887-3585

Murray, I.V., Giasson, B.I., Quinn, S.M., Koppaka, V., Axelsen, P.H., Ischiropoulos, H., Trojanowski, J. Q. & Lee, V.M. (2003). Role of alpha-synuclein carboxy-terminus on fibril formation in vitro. *Biochemistry*, Vol.42, No.28, (July 2003), pp. 8530-8540, ISSN 0006-2960

Narayanan, V. & Scarlata, S. (2001). Membrane binding and self-association of alpha-synucleins. *Biochemistry*, Vol.40, No.33, (August 2001), pp. 9927-9934, ISSN 0006-2960

Nuscher, B., Kamp, F., Mehnert, T., Odoy, S., Haass, C., Kahle, P.J. & Beyer, K. (2004). Alpha-synuclein has a high affinity for packing defects in a bilayer membrane - A thermodynamics study. *Journal of Biological Chemistry*, Vol.279, No.21, (May 2004), pp. 21966-21975, ISSN 0021-9258

Outeiro, T.F. & Lindquist, S. (2003). Yeast cells provide insight into alpha-synuclein biology and pathobiology. *Science*, Vol.302, No.5651, (December 2003), pp. 1772-1775, ISSN 0036-8075

Pandey, N., Schmidt, R.E. & Galvin, J.E. (2006). The alpha-synuclein mutation E46K promotes aggregation in cultured cells. *Experimental Neurology*, Vol.197, No.2, (February 2006), pp. 515-520, ISSN 0014-4886

Park, J.Y. & Lansbury, P.T. (2003). Beta-synuclein inhibits formation of alpha-synuclein protofibrils: A possible therapeutic strategy against Parkinson's disease. *Biochemistry*, Vol.42, No.13, (April 2003), pp. 3696-3700, ISSN 0006-2960

Perrin, R.J., Woods, W.S., Clayton, D.F. & George, J.M. (2000). Interaction of human alpha-synuclein and Parkinson's disease variants with phospholipids - Structural analysis using site-directed mutagenesis. *Journal of Biological Chemistry*, Vol.275, No.44, (November 2000), pp. 34393-34398, ISSN 0021-9258

Polymeropoulos, M.H., Lavedan, C., Leroy, E., Ide, S.E., Dehejia, A., Dutra, A., Pike, B., Root, H., Rubenstein, J., Boyer, R., Stenroos, E.S., Chandrasekharappa, S., Athanassiadou, A., Papapetropoulos, T., Johnson, W.G., Lazzarini, A.M., Duvoisin, R.C., DiIorio, G., Golbe, L.I. & Nussbaum, R.L. (1997). Mutation in the alpha-synuclein gene identified in families with Parkinson's disease. *Science*, Vol.276, No.5321, (June 1997), pp. 2045-2047, ISSN 0036-8075

Rhoades, E., Ramlall, T.F., Webb, W.W. & Eliezer, D. (2006). Quantification of alpha-synuclein binding to lipid vesicles using fluorescence correlation spectroscopy. *Biophysical Journal*, Vol.90, No.12, (June 2006), pp. 4692-4700, ISSN 0006-3495

Sandal, M., Valle, F., Tessari, I., Mammi, S., Bergantino, E., Musiani, F., Brucale, M., Bubacco, L. & Samori, B. (2008). Conformational equilibria in monomeric alpha-synuclein at the single-molecule level. *Plos Biology*, Vol.6, No.1, (January 2008), pp. 99-108, ISSN 1544-9173

Sastry, P.S. (1985). Lipids of nervous-tissue – composition and metabolism. *Progress in Lipid Research*, Vol.24, No.2, pp. 69-176, ISSN 0163-7827

Scherzer, C.R., Jensen, R.V., Gullans, S.R. & Feany, M.B. (2003). Gene expression changes presage neurodegeneration in a Drosophila model of Parkinson's disease. *Human Molecular Genetics*, Vol.12, No.19, (October 2003), pp. 2457-2466, ISSN 0964-6906

Segrest, J.P., Jones, M.K., Deloof, H., Brouillette, C.G., Venkatachalapathi, Y.V. & Anantharamaiah, G.M. (1992). The amphiphathic helix in the exchangeable apolipoproteins – a review of secondary structure and function. *Journal of Lipid Research*, Vol.33, No.2, (February 1992), pp. 141-166, ISSN 0022-2275

Serpell, L.C., Berriman, J., Jakes, R., Goedert, M. & Crowther, R.A. (2000), Fiber diffraction of synthetic alpha-synuclein filaments shows amyloid-like cross-beta conformation. *Proceedings of the National Academy of Sciences of the United States of America*, Vol.97, No.9, (April 2000), pp. 4897-4902, ISSN 0027-8424

Sharon, R., Goldberg, M.S., Bar-Joseph, I., Betensky, R.A., Shen, J. & Selkoe, D.J. (2001). Alpha-synuclein occurs in lipid-rich high molecular weight complexes, binds fatty acids, and shows homology to the fatty acid-binding proteins. *Proceedings of the*

National Academy of Sciences of the United States of America, Vol.98, No.16, (July 2001), pp. 9110-9115, ISSN 0027-8424

Sharon, R., Bar-Joseph, I., Frosch, M.P., Walsh, D.M., Hamilton, J.A. & Selkoe, D.J. (2003a). The formation of highly soluble oligomers of alpha-synuclein is regulated by fatty acids and enhanced in Parkinson's disease. *Neuron*, Vol.37, No.4, (February 2003), pp. 583-595, ISSN 0896-6273

Sharon, R., Bar-Joseph, I., Mirick, G.E., Serhan, C.N. & Selkoe, D.J. (2003b). Altered fatty acid composition of dopaminergic neurons expressing alpha-synuclein and human brains with alpha-synucleinopathies. *Journal of Biological Chemistry*, Vol.278, No.50, (December 2003), pp. 49874-49881, ISSN 0021-9258

Singleton, A.B., Farrer, M., Johnson, J., Singleton, A., Hague, S., Kachergus, J., Hulihan, M., Peuralinna, T., Dutra, A., Nussbaum, R., Lincoln, S., Crawley, A., Hanson, M., Maraganore, D., Adler, C., Cookson, M.R., Muenter, M., Baptista, M., Miller, D., Blancato, J., Hardy, J. & Gwinn-Hardy, K. (2003). Alpha-synuclein locus triplication causes Parkinson's disease. *Science*, Vol.302, No.5646, (October 2003), pp. 841-841, ISSN 0036-8075

Spillantini, M.G., Schmidt, M.L., Lee, V.M.Y., Trojanowski, J.Q., Jakes, R. & Goedert, M. (1997). Alpha-synuclein in Lewy bodies. *Nature*, Vol.388, No.6645, (August 1997), pp. 839-840, ISSN 0028-0836

Srivastava, K., Lee, M. & Morrell, C. (2007). Mechanism of alpha-synuclein inhibition of platelet granule exocytosis. *Circulation*, Vol.116, No.16, (October 2007), pp. 76-76, ISSN 0009-7322

Sung, J.Y., Kim, J., Paik, S.R,, Park, J.H., Ahn, Y.S. & Chung, K.C. (2001). Induction of neuronal cell death by Rab5A-dependent endocytosis of alpha-synuclein. *Journal of Biological Chemistry*, Vol.276, No.29, (July 2001), pp. 27441-27448, ISSN 0021-9258

Takeda, A., Hashimoto, M., Mallory, M., Sundsumo, M., Hansen, L., Sisk, A., & Masliah, E. (1998). Abnormal distribution of the non-A beta component of Alzheimer's disease amyloid precursor/alpha-synuclein in Lewy body disease as revealed by Proteinase K and formic acid pretreatment. *Laboratory Investigation*, Vol.78, No.9, (September 1998), pp. 1169-1177, ISSN 0023-6837

Tamamizu-Kato, S., Kosaraju, M.G., Kato, H., Raussens, V., Ruysschaert, J.M. & Narayanaswami, V. (2006). Calcium-triggered membrane interaction of the alpha-synuclein acidic tail. *Biochemistry*, Vol.45, No.36, (September 2006), pp. 10947-10956, ISSN 0006-2960

Trexler, A.J. & Rhoades, E. (2009). Alpha-synuclein binds large unilamellar vesicles as an extended Helix. *Biochemistry*, Vol.48, No.11, (March 2009), pp. 2304-2306, ISSN 0006-2960

Trojanowski, J. Q. & Lee, V. M. Y. (2003). Parkinson's disease and related alpha-synucleinopathies are brain amyloidoses. In: *Parkinson's Disease: the Life Cycle of the Dopamine Neuron*, Federoff, H. J.;Burke, R. E., *et al* (Ed.), 107-110, Annals of the New York Academy of Sciences, ISBN 0077-8923 1-57331-448-X.

Ulmer, T.S., Bax, S., Cole, N.B. & Nussbaum, R.L. (2005). Structure and dynamics of micelle-bound human alpha-synuclein. *Journal of Biological Chemistry*, Vol.280, No.10, (March 2005), pp. 9595-9603, ISSN 0021-9258

Ulrih, N.P., Barry, C.H. & Fink, A.L. (2008). Impact of Tyr to Ala mutations on alpha-synuclein fibrillation and structural properties. *Biochimica Et Biophysica Acta-*

Molecular Basis of Disease, Vol.1782, No.10, (October 2008), pp. 581-585, ISSN 0925-4439

Uversky, V.N., Li, J. & Fink, A.L. (2001). Evidence for a partially folded intermediate in alpha-synuclein fibril formation. *Journal of Biological Chemistry*, Vol.276, No.14, (April 2001), pp. 10737-10744, ISSN 0021-9258

Uversky, V.N. (2007). Neuropathology, biochemistry, and biophysics of alpha-synuclein aggregation. *Journal of Neurochemistry*, Vol.103, No.1, (October 2007), pp. 17-37, ISSN 0022-3042

Valenzuela, S. M. (2007). Liposome Techniques for Synthesis of Biomimetic Lipid Membranes. In: *Nanobiotechnology of Biomimetic Membranes*, Martin, D. K. (Ed.), Springer US, 75-87, ISBN 978-0-387-37740-7, Sydney, Australia.

Wakabayashi, K., Matsumoto, K., Takayama, K., Yoshimoto, M. & Takahashi, H. (1997). NACP, a presynaptic protein, immunoreactivity in Lewy bodies in Parkinson's disease. *Neuroscience Letters*, Vol.239, No.1, (December 1997), pp. 45-48, ISSN 0304-3940

Weinreb, P.H., Zhen, W.G., Poon, A.W., Conway, K.A. & Lansbury, P.T. (1996). NACP, a protein implicated in Alzheimer's disease and learning, is natively unfolded. *Biochemistry*, Vol.35, No.43, (October 1996), pp. 13709-13715, ISSN 0006-2960

Willingham, S., Outeiro, T.F., DeVit, M.J., Lindquist, S.L. & Muchowski, P.J. (2003). Yeast genes that enhance the toxicity of a mutant huntingtin fragment or alpha-synuclein. *Science*, Vol.302, No.5651, (December 2003), pp. 1769-1772, ISSN 0036-8075

Wood S.J., Wypych J., Steavenson S., Louis J.C., Citron M. & Biere A.L. (1999). Alpha-synuclein fibrillogenesis is nucleation-dependent - Implications for the pathogenesis of Parkinson's disease. *Journal of Biological Chemistry*, Vol.274, No.28, (July 1999), pp. 19509-19512, ISSN 0021-9258

Wright, P.E. & Dyson, H.J. (1999). Intrinsically unstructured proteins: Re-assessing the protein structure-function paradigm. *Journal of Molecular Biology*, Vol.293, No.2, (October 1999), pp. 321-331, ISSN 0022-2836

Zarranz, J.J., Alegre, J., Gomez-Esteban, J.C., Lezcano, E., Ros, R., Ampuero, I., Vidal, L., Hoenicka, J., Rodriguez, O., Atares, B., Llorens, V., Tortosa, E.G., del Ser, T., Munoz, D.G. & de Yebenes, J.G. (2004). The new mutation, E46K, of alpha-synuclein causes Parkinson and Lewy body dementia. *Annals of Neurology*, Vol.55, No.2, (February 2004), pp. 164-173, ISSN 0364-5134

Zhou, W.B. & Freed, C.R. (2004). Tyrosine-to-cysteine modification of human alpha-synuclein enhances protein aggregation and cellular toxicity. *Journal of Biological Chemistry*, Vol.279, No.11, (March 2004), pp. 10128-10135, ISSN 0021-9258

Zhu, M. & Fink, A.L. (2003). Lipid binding inhibits alpha-synuclein fibril formation. *Journal of Biological Chemistry*, Vol.278, No.19, (May 2003), pp. 16873-16877, ISSN 0021-9258

Zhu, M., Li, J. & Fink, A.L. (2003). The association of alpha-synuclein with membranes affects bilayer structure, stability, and fibril formation. *Journal of Biological Chemistry*, Vol.278, No.41, (October 2003), pp. 40186-40197, ISSN 0021-9258

Zhu, M., Qin, Z.J., Hu, D., Munishkina, L.A. & Fink, A.L. (2006). Alpha-synuclein can function as an antioxidant preventing oxidation of unsaturated lipid in vesicles. *Biochemistry*, Vol.45, No.26, (July 2006), pp. 8135-8142, ISSN 0006-2960

6

Alpha-Synuclein, Oxidative Stress and Autophagy Failure: Dangerous Liaisons in Dopaminergic Neurodegeneration

Giovanni Stefanoni[1,2], Gessica Sala[1], Lucio Tremolizzo[1,2], Laura Brighina[1,2] and Carlo Ferrarese[1,2]
[1]*Department of Neuroscience and Biomedical Technologies, University of Milano-Bicocca*
[2]*Department of Neurology, San Gerardo Hospital, Monza.*
Italy

1. Introduction

The molecular mechanisms of neurodegeneration in Parkinson's disease and the cause of the selective dopaminergic neuronal loss are mostly unknown. Many pathogenetic factors have been found to play a role but the relationships among these factors, together with the reasons of the high vulnerability of dopaminergic neurons to them, have not been completely defined. Only a small fraction of Parkinson's disease cases have a defined etiology: this fraction include the monogenic hereditary variants of the disease and the sporadic cases determined by prolonged exposition to toxic agents inhibiting mitochondrial complex I, such as 1,1'-dimethyl-4,4'-5 bipyridinium (paraquat), rotenone and 1-methyl-4-phenyl-1,2,3,6-tetrahydropyridine (MPTP). Parkinson's disease-related toxins and pathogenetic mutations have been indispensable to create cell and animal models with the aim to clarify the molecular physiopathology of the disease. Little is known about the primitive causes of idiopathic Parkinson's disease, that probably represents a multi-factorial disease influenced by various genetic and environmental factors, all characterized by high incidence in general population. The different risk factors together would contribute to initiate the complex pathogenetic sequence of events leading to the death of dopaminergic neurons.

Recently, Parkinson's disease has been placed in the large category of neurodegenerative diseases caused by protein misfolding. In particular, alpha-synuclein has been proposed as the central and most specific factor implied in the pathogenesis of this syndrome, which, as a consequence, has been classified among synucleinopathies, together with dementia with Lewy bodies and multiple system atrophy, other neurodegenerative diseases having alpha-synuclein pathology as a major feature.

Aim of this chapter is to provide an organic revision of evidences for the involvement of alpha-synuclein in the pathogenesis of Parkinson's disease. We will define the mechanisms responsible for the toxic gain of function of α-synuclein and the processes triggered by aberrant alpha-synuclein and mediating its neurotoxic effect. Particular attention will be paid to establish the links that correlate the deleterious action of alpha-synuclein with oxidative stress and with the efficiency of the processes involved in the clearance of aberrant proteins; these last include the ubiquitin-proteasome system and the autophagic-lysosomal pathways. Both oxidative stress and impairment of protein degradation machinery exert a neurotoxic effect contributing to the pathogenesis of Parkinson's disease and partially mediated, in dopaminergic neurons, by qualitative and quantitative alterations in alpha-synuclein. This protein in turn is able to boost the processes responsible for its toxic gain of function. Therefore, a physiopathologic circuit emerges constituted by a complex interaction among different pathogenetic mechanisms, everyone able to support the others; the death of dopaminergic neurons represents the ultimate and irreversible outcome of all these events. This chapter aims at clarifying this complex dynamics responsible for the neurodegenerative process, with particular regard to mechanisms both determining and mediating the deleterious effect of alpha-synuclein. Furthermore, we will report data on the development of biochemical tests helpful for diagnosis and prognosis and useful as objective criteria to determine the neuroprotective effectiveness of drugs in clinical trials: in this regard, levels and modifications of α-synuclein, as well as parameters of oxidative stress and autophagy, could represent suitable peripheral biomarkers of disease risk and progression. Finally, we will discuss about the opportunity of interfering with all the reported pathogenetic mechanisms as putative neuroprotective pharmacologic strategy.

2. Alpha-synuclein toxicity

Alpha-synuclein is a 144aa protein encoded by the gene SNCA, localized at 4q chromosome. Three different SNCA transcripts can be detected in neurons. The physiological functions of alpha-synuclein is still not fully understood. It is abundantly expressed in nervous tissues and it localizes in the cytoplasm or associated with lipid membranes. In particular, this protein is mainly localized in the pre-synaptic compartment, where it seems to have a role in regulating neurotransmitter release, vesicle turnover, membrane stability and neuronal plasticity.

The hypothesis of an active involvement of alpha-synuclein in the pathogenesis of Parkinson's disease was proposed when this protein was identified as the main component of Lewy bodies, intraneuronal aggregates constituting a constant report in the neuropathology of Parkinson's disease (Spillantini et al 1997). Beside alpha-synuclein, Lewy bodies also contain components of proteasome machinery, chaperone proteins, alpha-tubulin, synphilin-1, glyceraldehyde 3-phosphate dehydrogenase and several other proteins known to be involved in nigral neurodegeneration. Residues 71 to 82 of alpha-synuclein are essential for the assembly of Lewy bodies. The exact role of these inclusions in the disease physiopathology was unknown for several years.

The key function of alpha-synuclein protein in the pathogenesis of Parkinson's disease was first elucidated by genetic studies: the finding of familial cases of Parkinson's disease genetically linked to missense mutations in the SNCA gene and to genomic triplication of the wild type gene gave evidence of the potential neurotoxic effect of this protein. The first causal mutation of hereditary Parkinson's disease was identified in a large Italian family ("Contursi kindred", from the name of the town): it was the missense mutation Ala53Thr in the SNCA gene (Polymeropoulos et al 1997). Only two other pathogenetic missense mutations have been identified in SNCA: Ala30Pro and Glu46Lys. All these variants are located in the N-terminus of the protein and are linked to autosomal dominant forms of Parkinson's disease. Anyway, the missense mutation frequency in SNCA in different populations is very low, whereas SNCA multiplications are a bit more frequent. The

Ala53Thr alpha-synuclein mutant is responsible for the greater in vivo neurotoxicity in transgenic animal models.

The deleterious effects of these genetic alterations on dopaminergic neurons have been demonstrated in cellular and animal models, confirming the hypothesis that both qualitative and quantitative alterations of alpha-synuclein are able to trigger its toxic effect: mutant alpha-synuclein protein exerts a selective toxicity in dopaminergic neurons when expressed in rats; at the same time, the mutant protein causes aggregation and formation of Lewy bodies in dopaminergic neurons of mouse models.

The toxicity of both mutant and wild type alpha-synuclein seems to require the acquisition of a misfolded conformation which prevents alpha-synuclein degradation and favors its fibrillization, firstly into protofibrillar oligomeric species and then to fibrillar aggregates. Recently, it has become clear that insoluble aggregates probably do not have an intrinsic toxic function, as suggested by the finding that Lewy bodies–positive dopaminergic neurons are less vulnerable to degeneration. Furthermore, the increased size of Lewy bodies and the decreased levels of soluble alpha-synuclein correlate with a higher resistance to cytotoxic agents. Therefore, formation of Lewy bodies could represent a protective phenomenon favoring the removal of soluble oligomers. Different mechanisms can explain the negative effects exerted by alpha-synuclein oligomers, which seem to be directly responsible for the neurotoxic effect of the protein (Vekrellis et al 2004):

- Binding to microtubules and dysregulation of cytoskeleton functions.
- Damaging of mitochondrial and other cellular membranes.
- Interaction with other proteins and modulation of their activity.

Alpha-synuclein oligomers directly interfere with proteasome subunits. Furthermore, alpha-synuclein impairs microtubule stability through binding to alpha-tubulin and to the microtubule associated protein TAU. Alpha synuclein induces the aggregation of TAU, which in turn favors alpha-synuclein fibrillization; interestingly, polymorphisms in the TAU gene have proved to modify the risk of developing Parkinson's disease.

In monogenic forms of Parkinson's disease the direct neurotoxic effect of mutant alpha-synuclein may depend on specific conformational modifications, modulating the propensity of the protein to aggregate, to interact with other proteins and to be processed by clearance mechanisms. Pathogenetic mutations of alpha-synuclein protein are known to confer a tendency to acquire abnormal conformation substantially easier than the wild type protein, which accounts for the development of Parkinson's disease in patients having these mutations.

The fact that over-expressed wild type alpha-synuclein is responsible for neurotoxicity suggests that even simple protein accumulation is able to trigger the misfolded conformation and to promote protein aggregation.

As well as in familial cases, even in sporadic Parkinson's disease the toxic gain of function of alpha-synuclein could derive from the intraneuronal accumulation of the protein or from biochemical modifications enhancing the propensity of the protein to aggregate. Anyway, the ubiquitous expression and the high levels of alpha-synuclein in the brain suggests that its simple presence in dopaminergic neurons is not sufficient to explain the selective degeneration of these cells, which must have specific characteristics able to induce or to accelerate alpha-synuclein misfolding, oligomerization and aggregation. Oxidative stress and production of highly reactive aldehydes, both depending on high levels of dopamine, can modify alpha-synuclein, partially explaining the high tendency of this protein to acquire a misfolded conformation in dopaminergic neurons. Indeed, dopamine promotes alpha-synuclein protofibrils formation. Oxidative stress, which is known to be one of the main pathogenetic factors leading to the death of dopaminergic neurons in Parkinson's disease, has been identified as a major responsible for alpha-synuclein post-translational modifications, consisting in oxidation and nitration of specific aminoacid residues; these alterations in alpha-synuclein have been detected in nigral neurons of brain samples from patients with Parkinson's disease (Giasson et al 2000) and from animal models of disease (Gao et al 2008).

An increase in alpha-synuclein levels, correlated with the degree of nigrostriatal dopamine depletion, has been demonstrated in the substantia nigra of patients with sporadic Parkinson's disease (Chu et al 2007). It is conceivable to suppose that this accumulation of the toxic protein might derive from an increase in transcription and translation of the SNCA gene or from a decrease in the protein degradation.

The variability in codifying and non-codifying SNCA gene sequences has demonstrated to modify the risk of developing sporadic Parkinson's disease, probably through a mild modulatory effect on transcription activity and, as a consequence, on intraneuronal levels of alpha-synuclein. SNCA duplication was found in sporadic cases of Parkinson's disease. Increasing length in the dinucleotide repeat sequence (REP1) of the SNCA gene promoter has been demonstrated to be correlated with an increased risk of developing sporadic Parkinson's disease (Maraganore et al 2006; Brighina et al 2008). Furthermore, single nucleotide polymorphisms at the promoter region and at the 3' end of SNCA gene have been found to modify the risk of disease.

Anyway, aging remains the most evident risk factor for sporadic Parkinson's disease. An interesting hypothesis suggests that senescence of dopaminergic neurons could promote the accumulation of misfolded alpha-synuclein through two main mechanisms: slowing alpha-synuclein turnover through the impairment of clearance machinery; impairing the function of mitochondria and antioxidant systems, with consequent increase in oxidative stress.

Great efforts have been done in order to identify genetic and environmental factors able to modulate the aging process. Caloric restriction represents the only environmental condition which has demonstrated to delay aging in a wide range of organisms. This evidence suggests that caloric restriction might guarantee protection from developing Parkinson's disease and could delay the disease progression. As it was supposed, caloric restriction has shown a protective effect in MPTP-induced animal models of Parkinson's disease, even if an epidemiologic correlation between diet and incidence of Parkinson's disease has not been demonstrated. The molecular basis of the protective role of caloric restriction in animal models has been elucidated in yeast, where a family of NAD^+-dependent protein deacetylases, called sirtuins (SIRTs), have been identified as mediators of the changes induced by starvation in cells; many sirtuins analogs have been discovered in mammals. These proteins regulate cell homeostasis partially through an epigenetic mechanism: they modulate histones acetylation and chromatin condensation. SIRT1 is a major responsible for protective cell modifications during starvation, whereas other SIRTs seem to exert a specific deleterious effect on dopaminergic neurons. In particular, SIRT2, an alpha-tubulin deacetylase, promotes formation of alpha-tubulin oligomers, which destabilize microtubules and form toxic complexes with alpha-synuclein oligomers. The interaction of alpha-synuclein oligomers with alpha-tubulin plays an important role in mediating alpha-synuclein toxicity. The NAD^+ concentration-dependency of SIRT2 activity suggests a possible modulation of alpha-synuclein misfolding and aggregation by energy metabolism.

3. Oxidative stress, mitochondrial dysfunction and excitotoxicity

An impairment in multiple steps of the mitochondrial respiratory chain has been demonstrated in Parkinson's disease (Schapira et al 1998). The importance of this pathogenetic mechanism mainly depends on its role of main source of reactive oxygen species. At the same time, the loss of mitochondrial function and the consequent energetic deficit interfere with glutamate uptake and increase neuronal vulnerability to glutamate excitotoxicity.

3.1 Mitochondrial dysfunction

Several epidemiologic and experimental data confirm the importance of mitochondrial derangement in the pathogenesis of Parkinson's disease. First of all, electron transport complex I represents the main molecular target of paraquat, rotenone and MPTP, the exogenous substances known to determine degeneration of human dopaminergic neurons. The selective toxicity of MPTP on dopaminergic neurons derives from its transformation to the metabolite 1-methyl-4-phenyl-pyridium (MPP^+), which is concentrated within dopaminergic neurons by dopamine transporters. Even paraquat, which is structurally similar to MPP^+, is carried into dopaminergic cells by the same transporter. In contrast to MPTP and paraquat, rotenone is not concentrated in nigral neurons, nevertheless it produces selective death of these cells. The development of parkinsonism after exposure to rotenone represents a further proof of the high susceptibility of dopaminergic neurons to mitochondrial impairment. Toxic derangement in complex I induces alpha-synuclein aggregation and formation of Lewy body-like inclusions (Betarbet et al 2000).

A reduced activity of the mitochondrial complexes I and IV has been observed in the substantia nigra of patients with Parkinson's disease and in animal models of disease (Palacino et al 2004). Decreased levels of coenzyme Q10 together with a higher ratio of oxidized vs. reduced Coenzyme Q10 have been observed in patients. An increase of cerebral lactate levels, suggesting an alteration in aerobic metabolism as a consequence of derangement of mitochondrial respiratory chain, has been detected by brain magnetic resonance spectroscopy in patients with Parkinson's disease (Henchcliffe et al 2008). Experiments performed on cytoplasmic hybrid cell lines from patients with Parkinson's disease suggest that the complex I deficit associated to the disease might be genetically determined by defects in mitochondrial DNA. A single nucleotide polymorphism within the gene encoding NADH dehydrogenase 3 of complex I has been associated to a decrease in the risk of sporadic Parkinson's disease, providing genetic evidence of the pathogenetic relevance of complex I activity (van der Walt et al 2003).

An endogenous substance able to impair mitochondrial function is salsolinol, which is synthesized from dopamine and acetaldehyde by salsolinol synthase. This molecule has been found in various regions of the brain, including striatum and substantia nigra. Salsolinol inhibits mitochondrial complex II and this effect may explain the fact that high levels of this molecule are able to induce degeneration of dopaminergic neurons (Storch et al 2000).

Alpha-synuclein contains a mitochondrial targeting sequence. Over-expression of this protein favors its translocation to the mitochondria. The damage of these organelles seems to be one of the mechanisms mediating the toxic effects of alpha-synuclein oligomers.
An additional confirmation of the importance of mitochondrial function for the homeostasis of dopaminergic neurons is the finding that some proteins linked to hereditary forms of Parkinson's disease exert their function within mitochondria; furthermore, pathogenetic mutations of the genes encoding for some of these proteins are associated with the impairment of mitochondrial function, which might be the main neurotoxic action exerted by these mutations:

- PTEN induced putative kinase 1 (PINK1/PARK6) is a kinase that localizes in the mitochondrial membrane. Its loss of function is associated with a decrease in complex I activity determining an increase in oxidative stress. Mutations of PINK1 gene are responsible for recessive forms of Parkinson's disease.
- DJ-1 (PARK7) is a protein found to be mutated in recessive forms of Parkinson's disease. It plays a role in cell protection during oxidative stress, which induces the translocation of the protein to the mitochondrial matrix and the intermembrane space. The loss of DJ1 has been associated to depolarization and fragmentation of mitochondria.
- Leucine-rich repeat kinase 2 (LRRK2/PARK8) is a kinase linked to dominant forms of Parkinson's disease. It is mainly localized in the cytosol but a fraction can be found in the outer mitochondrial membrane. Pathogenetic mutations determine an increase in the kinase activity of the protein.
- High temperature requirement proteinA2 (HTRA2/Omi/PARK13) is a mitochondrial protease which has been associated with recessive forms of Parkinson's disease. Its loss of function has revealed to produce mitochondrial damage.

3.2 Oxidative stress

Free radicals include reactive oxygen species and reactive nitrogen species. During cell metabolism some of these substances are normally produced: superoxide anion, hydrogen peroxide, nitric oxide, peroxynitrite, nitroxyl and hydroxy radical. These products can be responsible for the damage of protein, DNA and lipid.
The brain contains a high amount of substances, such as phospholipids and free fatty acids, which are vulnerable to oxidative modifications and, as a consequence, are responsible for the high vulnerability of the central nervous system to the deleterious action of free radicals. Lipid peroxidation represents a key mechanism mediating the toxicity of free radicals on a wide range of cell organelles and functions. Free radicals initiate peroxidation of the membrane lipids making them lose a hydrogen atom from a methylene group, with formation of a diene; this product mediates the formation of a peroxy radical through reaction with oxygen; the peroxy radical abstracts a hydrogen atom from another lipid to form hydroperoxides, which mediates the propagation of lipid peroxidation.
In physiologic conditions free radicals are rapidly converted into non toxic molecules by antioxidants, which prevent oxidation of other molecules, thus protecting cell from oxidative stress. The cell antioxidant system include four main molecules:

- Catalase is a heme-protein localized in peroxisomes, which catalyzes the decomposition of hydrogen peroxide to water and oxygen.

- Superoxide dismutase is a cytosolic, mithocondrial and extracellular metallo-protein which catalyzes the transformation of superoxide into O_2 and H_2O_2.
- Reduced glutathione is a tripeptide which exerts an important reducing activity of reactive oxygen species through its conversion to glutathione disulfide.
- Glutathione peroxidase is an enzyme which catalyzes the reduction of H_2O_2 to water and O_2 by reduced glutathione.

A large amount of studies have demonstrated that oxidative damage plays a major pathogenetic role in Parkinson's disease and represents a key contributor to the loss of dopaminergic neurons (Jenner & Olanow 1998). The high concentration of dopamine is presumed to be essential to determine the high vulnerability of dopaminergic cells to oxidative stress. Dopamine itself does not seem to exert direct toxic effects at physiologic concentrations, but toxic intermediates derive from its catabolism:

- Auto-oxidation of dopamine leads to the production of semiquinones, which have an intrinsic toxic effect and generate reactive oxygen species.
- The enzymatic metabolism of dopamine, mediated by monoamine oxidase B, leads to the generation of $H_2 0_2$; therefore, the inhibition of monoamine oxidase B by selective drugs may protect against production of some toxins and free radicals deriving from dopamine oxidation.

The experimental stimulation of dopamine catabolism by monoamine oxidase B leads to an increase in oxidative stress levels, thus confirming the deleterious role of dopamine derivatives on neuronal oxidoreductive equilibrium.

Extensive studies performed on postmortem brain samples have provided evidence supporting the involvement of oxidative stress in the pathogenesis of Parkinson's disease. Elevated levels of reactive oxygen species have been detected by assessment of lipid peroxidation, protein oxidation and DNA damage in nigrostriatal regions of patients with Parkinson's disease and in animal models:

- Malondialdehyde, 4-hydroxy-2,3-nonenal and thiobarbituric acid reactive substances (TBARS) are markers of lipid peroxidation which are elevated in the substantia nigra and striatum of diseased patients (Yoritaka et al 1996).
- Markers of oxidative damage to proteins, such as carbonyl modifications of aminoacid residues, are increased in substantia nigra of patients with Parkinson's disease (Alam et al 1997).
- An increase in oxidative alterations of nucleic acids was detected in midbrain of diseased patients (Zhang et al 1999).

On the other hand, a dysregulation of multiple antioxidant systems has been demonstrated in Parkinson's disease:

- An increase in superoxide dismutase and catalase levels has been detected in striatum and midbrain of animal models (Keeney et al 2006). This feature probably represents a compensatory reaction of cell control systems, aimed at neutralizing the increasing levels of reactive oxygen species.
- A decrease of reduced glutathione levels was detected in the substantia nigra and corpus striatum of patients with Parkinson's disease and in animal models (Pearce et al 1997). Glutathione deficiency could be a consequence of the high levels of free radicals, which rapidly oxidize glutathione to glutathione disulfide, or, alternatively, it might represent an early pathogenetic feature which contributes to the high vulnerability of dopaminergic neurons to oxidative stress.

The iron-catalyzed conversion of H_20_2 into hydroxyl radicals is supposed to contribute to oxidative stress and neurodegeneration in Parkinson's disease; this remark is based on the finding of increased iron content in postmortem brain samples from diseased patients.
Various proteins linked to recessive hereditary forms of Parkinson's disease play an important role in cell response to oxidative stress. In particular, an increase in protein and lipid peroxidation has been demonstrated in parkin defective animal models, suggesting that a defect in the ubiquitin-proteasome pathway or in formation of Lewy bodies can favor the generation of free radicals.
The mechanisms mediating the neurotoxic effects of oxidative species in dopaminergic neurons are complex and only partially understood, but a central role seems to be played by the alterations that free radicals produce on alpha-synuclein conformational status and degradation. Indeed, it has been demonstrated that oxidative stress induces intraneuronal accumulation and aggregation of alpha-synuclein and formation of Lewy bodies-like inclusions. This effect might be produced through a double mechanism:

- Reactive oxygen species directly generate post-translational modifications in alpha-synuclein residues, enhancing the tendency of the protein to aggregate.
- High levels of free radicals determine a down-regulation of both the ubiquitin-proteasome system and the autophagy-lysosomal pathway, thus impairing the entire degradative machinery of alpha-synuclein.

The deleterious effect of oxidative stress on the function of clearance systems might partially depend on direct alteration of proteins regulating and mediating these pathways; at the same time, oxidative stress produces ATP depletion through damage of mitochondrial membranes, thus interfering with all energy-dependent processes, such as the clearance of proteins and organelles.

3.3 Excitotoxicity

Several lines of experimental evidence indicate that a toxic effect exerted by high levels of glutamate in the synaptic cleft contributes to the neurodegeneration of dopaminergic neurons in Parkinson's disease. Excitotoxicity is a pathogenetic mechanism that has demonstrated a role in the neuronal death in different neurologic diseases, both acute and chronic (Ferrarese & Beal 2004).
The molecular processes that mediate glutamate effects on neuronal survival consist on a complex cascade of events that ultimately results in neuronal death. Overactivation of the N-methyl-D-aspartate (NMDA) receptors seem to mediate a great part of this neurotoxic effect through generation of a calcium overload. Indeed, NMDA receptors are permeable to calcium ions, so that their activation results in an increase in the cytoplasmatic concentration of this element; high intracellular levels of calcium are responsible for the activation of several pro-apoptotic pathways and for induction of oxidative stress through activation of oxygenases and perturbation of mitochondrial homeostasis.
Oxidative and nitrosative stress represent important processes both favoring and mediating excitotoxic damage. An increase in the production of free radicals has been demonstrated in neurons exposed to excitotoxic insults. Nitric oxide is produced in response to NMDA receptors activation thanks to the interaction of nitric oxide synthase with these receptors; nitric oxide contributes to the generation of free radicals and is involved in the activation of the pro-apoptotic cascade. These data suggest that oxidative stress gives an important contribution to the excitotoxic process downstream of glutamate receptor activation.

Furthermore, reactive oxygen species have been identified as agents able to induce the increased release of glutamate during pathologic conditions. In fact, lipid peroxidation of presynaptic membrane seems to impair the function of transporters involved in the maintenance of calcium homeostasis, resulting in sustained elevation of this ion in the presynaptic terminal, which is depolarized and so releases glutamate into the synaptic cleft; moreover, oxidative stress directly impairs glutamate transporter function in astrocytes and neurons, leading to an increase in concentrations of extracellular glutamate, which can bind postsynaptic receptors and mediate excitotoxicity.

Glutamate transport is an energy-dependent process, which explains, together with oxidative stress, the fact that mitochondrial dysfunction determine a decrease in the reuptake of glutamate and, as a consequence, an increase in neuron vulnerability to excitotoxicity.

Based on this strong relationship among oxidative stress, mitochondrial dysfunction and excitotoxicity, it is easy to imagine an involvement of glutamate toxicity in the pathogenesis of Parkinson's disease, where free radicals and mitochondrial impairment are known to play a major role. In animal models of disease modifications in the abundance and phosphorylation status of the different NMDA receptor subunits have been detected (Dunah et al 2000). Anyway, the importance of excitotoxicity in the degeneration of nigral dopaminergic neurons might be increased by the complex set of changes that nigrostriatal dopamine depletion triggers in functional anatomy of basal ganglia circuitry. In particular, the reduction of the nigrostriatal dopaminergic transmission produces a strong increase in the glutammatergic activity of the subthalamic projection, normally inhibited by nigral neurons. This hyperactivity critically contributes to the onset of parkinsonian motor symptoms, as confirmed by the evidence that electric suppression of subthalamic nucleus through deep brain stimulation improves motor functions. Furthermore, these functional alterations in basal ganglia circuitry might have pathogenetic implications: overactivation of subthalamic glutammatergic transmission to substantia nigra could promote the excitotoxic damage of dopaminergic neurons, favoring neuronal death and accelerating disease progression; this concept has been confirmed by the beneficial effects obtained by blockade of subthalamic activity in animal models of Parkinson's disease (Blandini et al 2001).

Therefore, excitotoxicity appears to be an important contributor to neuronal death in the substantia nigra of patients with Parkinson's disease; this mechanism correlates with oxidative stress and is amplified by subthalamic overactivation.

4. Role of clearance mechanisms

Emerging data support the view that dysregulation of alpha-synuclein clearance machinery might represent the key feature leading to the intraneuronal accumulation of this protein. These mechanisms include the ubiquitin-proteasome system and the autophagic-lysosomal pathways; the autophagic pathways involved in the degradation of alpha-synuclein are chaperone-mediated autophagy and macroautophagy (Webb et al 2000). Anyway, the accumulation of alpha-synuclein does not represent the only negative consequence of clearence systems failure.

4.1 Impairment of the ubiquitin-proteasomal system

Increasing evidences indicate that the ubiquitin–proteasome pathway is defective in Parkinson's disease. The finding that Lewy bodies are ubiquitin-positive aggregates has suggested that a dysfunction in proteasome might contribute to the accumulation and aggregation of alpha-synuclein and other neurotoxic proteins. The first confirmation of this hypothesis has derived from the identification of hereditary forms of Parkinson's disease linked to two genes within the ubiquitin-proteasome system: parkin and UCHL1.

Parkin (PARK2) is an ubiquitin E3 ligase, an enzyme that catalyzes the addition of ubiquitin chains to substrate proteins which must be degraded by the proteasome. Mutations in parkin gene are responsible for almost half of autosomal recessive cases of hereditary Parkinson's disease (Kitada et al 1998); most of the pathogenetic mutations are associated with a defect in the E3 ubiquitin ligase activity of the protein. Furthermore, parkin is responsible for K63 ubiquitination of alpha-synuclein; this function is not involved in the degradation of substrate proteins through proteasome but favors protein aggregation and generation of insoluble inclusions. Mutations in the parkin gene prevent the formation of Lewy bodies in the substantia nigra, thus suggesting that the K63 ubiquitin ligase function of parkin is essential for the fibrillization of alpha-synuclein and formation of insoluble inclusions; the degeneration of dopaminergic neurons deriving from parkin loss of function supports the hypothesis that Lewy bodies might contrast the toxic effects of the protofibrillar protein.

Ubiquitin C-terminal hydrolase L1 (UCHL1/PARK5) is an enzyme that cleaves peptide-ubiquitin bonds and recycles ubiquitin monomers. Variants of UCHL1 gene have been associated to familial forms of Parkinson's disease. The I93M mutation was identified in a family with probable autosomal dominant Parkinson's disease; in vitro studies have demonstrated that this mutation results in partial loss of UCHL1 hydrolytic activity. In addition to the hydrolase activity, UCHL1 exerts a dimerization-dependent ubiquitin ligase activity that promotes alpha-synuclein aggregation. The single nucleotide polymorphism S18Y, which has been found to decrease the susceptibility to sporadic disease, seems to be associated with reduced ligase activity.

A direct proof of proteasome dysfunction in Parkinson's disease has been the finding of structural and functional alterations in the 20S proteasome subunit in the substantia nigra of patients with sporadic disease. The pathogenetic relevance of proteasome impairment has been reinforced by the observation that administration of proteasomal inhibitors to animals can produce the neuropathological and motor manifestations of Parkinson's disease, including selective nigral cell loss, Lewy-bodies-like inclusions and typical clinical signs.

Two mechanisms are known to be responsible for a dysfunction in the ubiquitin-proteasome system: aging is associated with a physiologic decrease of proteasome efficiency and ubiquitination activity; oxidative species and alpha-synuclein protofibrils exert a deleterious effects on proteasome subunits.

Alpha-synuclein oligomers have demonstrated to inhibit proteasome function through direct interaction with 20S subunit; this effect might favor further accumulation of alpha-synuclein, which in turn may worsen proteasome impairment.

The mechanisms behind proteasome inhibition by oligomeric alpha-synuclein require further investigation in order to be clarified. Synphilin-1 has been associated to the pathogenesis of Parkinson's disease since its identification as an alpha-synuclein-interacting protein, a component of Lewy bodies and a substrate of the E3 ligase parkin. This protein has been found to interact with the protein S6 ATPase, which exerts a regulatory function on proteasome. Furthermore, recent studies indicate that synphilin-1 exerts an inhibitory effect on proteasome activity partially due to the interaction with alpha-synuclein (Alvarez-Castelao et al 2010); mutations in synphilin-1 gene have been detected in patients with sporadic Parkinson's disease.

Chronic oxidative stress alters the subunits of proteasome, so that even reactive oxygen species might be responsible for proteasome impairment in Parkinson's disease.

4.2 Autophagy dysfunction

Autophagy is a finely regulated intracellular process that mediates lysosomal degradation of proteins and organelles. Its function allows the clearance of substrates characterized by alterations limiting their physiologic function or responsible for a cytotoxic effect. This degradative process exerts a cytoprotective role that is probably dependent on the clearance of toxic intracellular structures and the catabolism of substrates in order to obtain energy during starvation. Anyway, in particular situations autophagy seems to mediate a specific pathway of programmed cell death; this function requires a strong activation of autophagy and until now, in vivo, has been identified only during involutional physiologic processes in embryonic tissues (Nixon et al 2006).

In mammalian cells autophagy encompasses three main processes: microautophagy, macroautophagy and chaperone-mediated autophagy. Microautophagy is a constitutive, non selective process consisting on endocytosis of small amounts of cytoplasm into lysosomes through invagination of lysosomal membrane. Macroautophagy and chaperone-mediated autophagy are inducible processes: the first one allows lysosomal degradation of organelles and proteins after their sequestration within a double-membrane-limited vacuole called autophagosome; the second one is a selective device for degradation of aberrant proteins, which are directly transported into the lysosomal lumen by a translocation system constituted by specific carrier proteins.

Recent research has revealed the existence of a dysfunction in autophagy pathways in the cerebral regions involved in neurodegenerative processes. A decrease in the activity of both autophagic-lysosomal pathway and the ubiquitin-proteasome system has been reported during aging in every tissue, included neurons (Martinez-Vicente et al 2005). This deficit might be a major responsible for the intracellular accumulation of misfolding proteins and aberrant mitochondria, representing factors leading to oxidative stress and neuronal damage. Therefore, autophagy impairment might be a primum movens of the neurodegenerative processes and, at the same time, a limiting factor that is necessary for preventing early onset of massive neuronal loss.

In the last years the pathogenetic role of altered clearance machinery has become a central subject of research in Parkinson's disease: indeed, the impairment of chaperone-mediated autophagy and macroautophagy, together with the dysfunction of ubiquitin-proteasome system, seems to give a major contribute to the development and progression of nigral degeneration. The loss of function of these degradative pathways might produce a deleterious effect through induction of the pathogenetic processes more directly responsible for neuronal death, such as the accumulation and oligomerization of alpha-synuclein, the persistence of damaged mitochondria and the consequent production of reactive oxygen species. In turn, these key mediators of dopaminergic neurodegeneration can further worsen the impairment of clearance machinery and, in particular, of autophagic pathways (Cuervo et al 2010).

4.2.1 Impairment of chaperone-mediated autophagy

Chaperone mediated autophagy mediates the translocation of proteins containing a Lys-Phe-Glu-Arg-Gln (KFERQ) motif into lysosomes. This process requires the presence of three main proteins: cytosolic heat shock protein 70 (hsc70), lysosomal hsc70, lysosomal-associated membrane protein 2A (lamp2A). Cytosolic hsc70 binds the KFERQ sequence of substrate proteins and carries them to the lysosomal membrane, where lamp2A, after interaction with cytosolic hsc70, multimerizes and forms a translocation complex with lysosomal hsc70, thus mediating the transport of the substrate protein into the lysosomal lumen. Several proteins with neuropathologic relevance, such as alpha-synuclein, amyloid precursor protein β and huntingtin, contain a KFERQ motif.

The binding of the substrate protein to lamp2A represents the limiting step of chaperone mediated autophagy. Oxidative stress, accumulation of substrates and the lack of nutrients and growth factors are all conditions determining a compensatory and cytoprotective activation of chaperone mediated autophagy through an increase of lamp2A levels on lysosomal membrane.

The hypothesis that a dysfunction of chaperone mediated autophagy might be involved in the pathogenesis of Parkinson's disease was proposed when this process was demonstrated to be the main degradative pathway for alpha-synuclein; indeed, this protein accumulates when chaperone-mediated autophagy is suppressed by down-regulation of lamp2A expression. Therefore, the efficiency of this clearance pathway appears to be crucial in regulating the intraneuronal levels of alpha-synuclein. The evidence of a strong correlation between the functional state of chaperone mediated autophagy and the deleterious action of alpha-synuclein has been reinforced by demonstration that both pathogenetic mutations and overexpression of α-synuclein inhibit this process (Cuervo et al 2004, Xilouri et al 2009). Experiments performed on animal models over-expressing alpha-synuclein have revealed that down-regulation of chaperone mediated autophagy is responsible for part of the alpha-synuclein toxicity in dopaminergic neurons. A reduced turnover of proteins directly involved in the neuronal survival and in the apoptotic machinery may mediate the deleterious effect of alpha-synuclein-mediated inhibition of this clearance pathway.

Therefore, it is conceivable to assume that other substrates of chaperone mediated autophagy contribute to neuronal death through their accumulation. For example, glyceraldehyde-3-phosphate dehydrogenase (GAPDH) (Tatton 2000) and myocyte enhancer factor 2D (MEF2D) (Yang et al 2009) are substrates of this degradative pathway and, at the same time, are specifically involved in the molecular physiopathology of Parkinson's disease; these factors could represent key mediators of the neuronal death when chaperone mediated autophagy is impaired.

Besides mutations and multiplications of alpha-synuclein gene, other mutations linked to hereditary Parkinson's disease are responsible for the impairment of chaperone mediated autophagy. Pathogenetic mutation I93M of PARK5 gene has been demonstrated to determine the inhibition of chaperone mediated autophagy and the accumulation of alpha-synuclein (Kabuta et al 2008).

The finding of low levels of lamp2A and total hsc70 in post-mortem substantia nigra of patients with sporadic disease indicates that a reduced activity of chaperone mediated autophagy is likely to be a pathogenetic mechanism even in idiopathic Parkinson's disease (Alvarez-Erviti 2010).

In conclusion, the failure of chaperone mediated autophagy seems to be a pathogenetic mechanism favoring the death of dopaminergic neurons and, as a consequence, contributing to the development and progression of Parkinson's disease.

4.2.2 Macroautophagy failure

Macroautophagy starts with sequestration of a region of cytoplasm containing proteins and organelles designed for degradation within a double-membrane vacuole called autophagosome. Once formed, the autophagic vacuole undergoes a process of maturation, which is essential for the subsequent fusion with lysosome and the degradation of substrates. The proper function of macroautophagy allows the removal of misfolded proteins and aberrant organelles, which are unsuitable for degradation through other pathways.

Macroautophagy is regulated by the mammalian target of rapamycin (mTOR), a serine/threonine kinase on which two main signal transduction pathways converge:

- The AKT pathway, modulated by neurotrophic growth factors.
- The AMPK pathway, modulated by intracellular levels of aminoacids and ATP.

Macroautophagy is suppressed by mTOR in presence of high levels of nutrients or when growth factors stimulate the cell.

Several exogenous molecules are known to activate macroautophagy independently of mTOR activity. These include drugs actually used in the treatment of neurologic and non neurologic diseases, such as calcium antagonists, lithium and valproate.

Macroautophagy proceeds through various steps, each requiring the presence of specific autophagy related genes (Atg). Four main phases can be distinguished:

1. Nucleation of the autophagosome.
2. Sequestration of a region of cytoplasm containing substrates to be degraded.
3. Maturation of the autophagosome.
4. Fusion with lysosome and degradation of substrates.

Therefore, regulation and biological function of macroautophagy appear to be characterized by a remarkable complexity. Since different variants of this process exist, each one characterized by specific activators, regulatory pathways and biological effects.

Although macroautophagy, chaperone mediated autophagy and ubiquitin-proteasome system are responsible for the degradation of different preferential substrates, a functional correlation among them have been demonstrated. In particular, macroautophagy is able to modulate its own activity depending on the efficiency of the other two pathways. Both proteasome and chaperone mediated autophagy inhibition determine a cytoprotective activation of macroautophagy.

Macroautophagy has been implied in the pathogenesis of several neurodegenerative diseases, such as Parkinson's disease, Alzheimer's disease, Huntington's disease and frontotemporal dementia, as well as acute injuries. A role of macroautophagy in the development of these pathologies was proposed when intraneuronal accumulation of autophagic vacuoles was detected in postmortem brains of diseased patients; increasing experimental data indicate that this feature is likely to mirror a dysfunction in maturation and lysosomal clearance of autophagosomes.

Macroautophagy seems to play a relevant role in the clearance of alpha-synuclein. Both pathogenetic mutations and over-expression of alpha-synuclein determine an induction of macroautophagy, which is dependent on the inhibition of chaperone mediated autophagy (Xilouri et al 2009).

Anyway, the impairment of alpha synuclein degradation seems not to have a major role in mediating the deleterious effect of macroautophagy impairment: the accumulation of other substrates might be more decisive. In this regard, it is important to remind that macroautophagy represents the only mechanism able to mediate the clearance of damaged mitochondria through a process named mitophagy. The intraneuronal accumulation of aberrant mitochondria determines neurotoxic effects linked to the generation of reactive oxygen species and the release of pro-apoptotic mediators. Increasing evidence from transgenic models of disease suggests that a defect in the mitophagy pathway might exert an key pathogenetic role in Parkinson's disease. In fact, genes responsible for hereditary disease are essential components of mitophagy machinery: PINK1 and parkin, two genes linked to recessive forms of Parkinson's disease, encode proteins that work synergistically to ensure the sequestration of aberrant mitochondria within the autophagic vacuole Narendra et al 2010).

Even DJ1, a gene linked to autosomal recessive Parkinson's disease, encodes for a protein that activates macroautophagy and favors mitochondrial turnover (Krebiehl et al 2010).

Loss of function of PINK1, parkin or DJ1 causes hereditary Parkinson's disease and the death of dopaminergic neurons in cell and animal models: the decreased efficiency of macroautophagy and mitophagy might be responsible for part of this neurotoxic effect.

Based on these assumptions, the efficacy of mitochondria turnover should be evaluated as a putative defective step linked to macroautophagy dysfunction even in idiopathic Parkinson's disease.

4.2.3 Loss of lysosomal function

The hypothesis that macroautophagy might be impaired in Parkinson's disease only apparently contrasts with the accumulation of autophagosomes and the increase of LC3II levels that have been demonstrated in postmortem substantia nigra of diseased patients. As previously reported, recent data suggest that a defect in maturation of autophagosome and in its fusion with lysosome could be the major responsible for the accumulation of autophagic vacuoles. Indeed, a depletion of the intraneuronal lysosomal pool and decreased levels of lysosome associated proteins, such as LAMP1, cathepsin D and heat shock protein 73, have been detected in nigral neurons of patients with sporadic Parkinson's disease. Furthermore, lysosomal depletion has been found in dopaminergic neurons of a MPTP mouse model (Dehay et al 2010); in this study the loss of lysosomes has been identified as an early alteration preceding the accumulation of autophagosomes and the neuronal degeneration. Oxidative injury has been found to favor lipid peroxidation of lysosomal membrane and, at last, to reduce the pool of lysosomes. Therefore, a strong and synergistic correlation seems to exist between oxidative stress and the dysfunction of autophagic-lysosomal pathway.

An additional proof of the protective role of lysosomal function in dopaminergic neurons has derived from the finding that mutations of genes encoding lysosomal proteins can modify the risk of developing Parkinson's disease. ATP13A2 (PARK9) is a lysosomal transmembrane cation transporting ATPase that is necessary to maintain acidity in the lysosomal lumen; low pH is indispensable for the function of lysosomal hydrolases and, as a consequence, for degradation of autophagy substrates. Homozygous mutations of ATP13A2 gene causes Kufor-Rakeb syndrome, characterized by early-onset parkinsonism with pyramidal degeneration and dementia. In vitro experiments have demonstrated that loss of ATP13A2 impairs lysosomal degradation of alpha-synuclein and cause intraneuronal accumulation of this protein (Gitler et al 2009).

Glucocerebrosidase (GBA) is a lysosomal enzyme that catalyzes the hydrolysis of the lipid glucosylceramide into glucose and ceramide. Homozygous mutations of GBA gene are responsible for Gaucher syndrome, a multisystem lysosomal storage disease characterized by neurodegenerative manifestations. Recently, carriers of GBA pathogenetic mutations have been identified at higher risk of sporadic Parkinson's disease (Sidransky et al 2009). This confirms the great importance of lysosomal function for the survival of dopaminergic neurons.

5. Neuropathologic outcome of molecular physiopathology: More than nigral degeneration

In the previous paragraphs we have reported evidences regarding the occurrence of specific deleterious processes in degeneration of dopaminergic neurons; furthermore, we have highlighted the functional correlations that have been demonstrated among these processes. A wide body of data confirms that each of these mechanisms can be responsible for degeneration of dopaminergic neurons and involutional modifications of the substantia nigra. These modifications are responsible for the motor symptoms that represent the major criteria for diagnosis of Parkinson's disease. The reasons of the selective damage of nigral neurons is not currently known; particular biological conditions might favor the onset of pathogenetic mechanisms in these neurons or could be responsible for an extreme vulnerability to systemic biochemical alterations.
However, the selectiveness of nigral involvement in Parkinson's disease is not absolute. In fact, the cardinal symptoms of Parkinson's disease are often preceded by a series of early manifestations, such as depression, sleep disturbances, eye movement disorders, hyposmia, constipation and loss of cardiac and vasomotor reflexes, which can start several years before the motor disturbances. The neuropathologic substrate of these aspecific manifestations does not seem to be ascribable to the degeneration of substantia nigra, rather they would derive from the involvement of other monoaminergic neurons in central and peripheral nervous system. Postmortem studies in patients with Parkinson's disease have provided evidence of a typical temporal pattern of pathology progression from peripheral neurons, spinal cord and brainstem to basal ganglia and cortical regions. These studies have revealed the precocious degeneration of autonomic ganglia of mesenteric plexus, dorsal motor nucleus of vagus, rafe nuclei, locus ceruleus and ventral tegmental area; the involvement of these centers is consistent with the clinical symptoms preceding parkinsonian signs. Based on these premises, the degeneration of substantia nigra appears as a late manifestation of the neuropathologic process; moreover, the onset of the characteristic motor manifestations is usually insidious and can be appreciated only when about 50% to 60% of dopaminergic neurons have been lost. These remarks indicate that the diagnosis of Parkinson's disease is always made when the underlying neuropathologic process has already reached an advanced phase; this limits the benefits that can be expected from putative neuroprotective therapies. Hence, it would be desirable to be endowed of diagnostic tools useful to make diagnosis of Parkinson's disease during early or even pre-clinical stages. This assumption has promoted the pre-clinical and clinical research aimed at identifying biomarkers of disease.

5.1 Peripheral biomarkers

Different rationales justify the use of biomarkers for Parkinson's disease:

- To study disease mechanisms.
- To identify individuals with an increased risk of disease.
- To diagnose patients before or at the threshold of motor symptoms.
- To monitor disease progression throughout its course.
- To establish drug mechanisms, assess drug dosing and secondary outcomes in clinical studies.

Neuroimaging biomarkers include detection of dopamine transporter (DAT) levels in basal ganglia with radiolabeled tracers; 123I-FP-CIT SPECT, commonly known as DATscan, is actually used in clinical practice to assist in the differential diagnosis of movement disorders. Anyway, DAT depletion follows the death of nigral neurons; furthermore, the exposure to radiations and the high costs limit the use of this test in screening and follow up.

Peripheral biochemical markers would offer the advantage of being easily accessible for repeated measurements, feature that makes them particularly useful not only for diagnosis but even for monitoring the course of the disease. Various peripheral cell types share with neurons the molecular machinery for several biochemical processes; this provides the chance of testing peripheral ex-vivo models to seek for disease-specific biochemical alterations. The ideal biomarker should reflect a pathogenetic mechanism operative at central level (core biomarker) and playing a major role in the patophysiology of Parkinson's disease, such as alpha-synuclein aggregation, mitochondrial dysfunction, oxidative stress and impairment of the clearance machinery. Therefore, it is essential to identify peripheral models reproducing the molecular alterations detected in the affected neurons. Up to now, a wide range of putative peripheral models of disease have been proposed: platelets, peripheral blood mononuclear cells and fibroblasts represent ex vivo tissues which are actually under investigation with the aim of disclosing differences in biochemical parameters between patients with Parkinson's disease and controls; even plasma is currently studied with the same purpose. The accessibility of peripheral tissues represent the clearest advantage of their use, significantly compensating the fact that they are not the main target of the disease.

Cerebrospinal fluid (CSF) cannot be considered a peripheral sample, because it is not easily accessible; anyway, CSF represents a more direct window on central nervous system than blood, so that it can be analysed in pilot studies to determine biochemical alterations which could be more extensively assessed in peripheral models.

The development of therapies demonstrating a pre-clinical neuroprotective effect has raised the need of peripheral biomarkers more and more pressing. In fact, new drugs tested to delay the progression of Parkinson's disease are targeted to specific biochemical alterations occurring in the central nervous system; in this context, a great help would derive from the availability of reliable biochemical parameters linked to the targeted pathway, useful to monitor therapies in clinical studies. Biomarkers expected to predict the effect of a therapeutic intervention and assessed as substitutes for a clinically relevant endpoint are named surrogate markers; their use would allow to overcome some difficulties that often occur in clinical trials of neuroprotective therapies: a biomarker could give short-term information on drug biochemical efficacy, whereas clinical outcome can be evaluated only after years of treatment; a biomarker would not be influenced by a symptomatic effect that could complicate the demonstration of the neuroprotective effect of the drug.

Actually, among the putative peripheral biochemical markers which have been investigated, no one has a reliability which could justify its use in clinical practice.

Alpha-synuclein levels in peripheral blood cells from patients with Parkinson's disease do not seem to differ from controls (Brighina et al 2010), even if an increased expression of the alpha-synuclein gene has been detected in fibroblasts from patients (Hoepken et al 2008). Data on total plasma level of the protein in patients compared to controls are contrasting but new alpha-synuclein assays able to detect oligomeric protein have demonstrated changes in plasma and cerebrospinal fluid from diseased patients. Recently, the concentration of alpha-synuclein oligomers and the ratio of oligomers on total alpha-synuclein have been found significantly increased in cerebrospinal fluid from diseased patients compared to controls (Tokuda et al 2010). The oligomeric soluble fraction of alpha-synuclein has been reported to be increased in plasma samples obtained from patients.

A reduction of glutamate uptake has been observed in platelets from patients and the decrease has showed a positive correlation with clinical severity of the disease (Ferrarese et al. 1999, 2001). This finding indicates that a systemic defect in glutamate transport occurs in patients with Parkinson's disease.

Some studies have reported a decrease in proteasome function in lymphocytes from diseased patients (Blandini et al 2006), but this finding has not been confirmed by subsequent experiments (Brighina et al 2010).

Oxidative stress is induced in lymphocytes from patients with Parkinson's disease and inversely correlates with L-dopa daily doses (Prigione et al 2006, 2009). Increased nitrotyrosine modifications of alpha-synuclein have been found in peripheral blood mononuclear cells obtained from individuals with idiopathic Parkinson's disease compared to controls; moreover, the amount of nitrotyrosine-modified alpha-synuclein has been demonstrated to positively correlate with intracellular levels of reactive oxygen species; in the same ex vivo model a significant increase in LC3II level have been demonstrated in diseased patients (Prigione et al 2010). Therefore, in patients with sporadic Parkinson's disease, a systemic dysregulation of autophagy and oxidative stress seem to exist and correlate with alpha-synuclein post-translational modifications. This confirms the chance of identifying peripheral biomarkers able to mirror the activation of pathogenetic processes in the central nervous system: biochemical parameters of autophagy and oxidative stress, together with qualitative and quantitative alterations of alpha-synuclein, could be useful for diagnostic or prognostic purposes and to monitor the biochemical effects of putative neuroprotective therapies. Moreover, the physiopathologic correlation among these mechanisms could offer the possibility of a combined use of these parameters to increase the accuracy of single biomarkers. In particular, the specificity of autophagy dysregulation in peripheral models, not confirmed in other neurodegenerative diseases, qualifies autophagy machinery as a new and promising target of research in the field of peripheral biochemical markers of disease.

It is conceivable that neuroprotective drugs would have more chance of success if they are administered during early stages of disease, when the molecular pathogenetic processes occurring in dopaminergic neurons could be more easily blocked; therefore, the availability of tools useful to make early diagnosis would increase the potential neuroprotective effects of old and new putative therapies. Therefore, development of disease biomarkers is strongly related to the identification of drugs able to delay the progression of Parkinson's disease or even to prevent its onset if diagnosis is made in preclinical stages.

5.2 Therapeutic perspectives

Several pharmacological approaches have been tested in order to prevent dopaminergic neurodegeneration. It is obvious that the most promising targets of neuroprotective strategy for Parkinson's disease are represented by the molecular pathogenetic mechanisms known to contribute to nigral degeneration.

An ideal therapeutic approach would consist in preventing alpha-synuclein misfolding, accumulation and aggregation in dopaminergic neurons. Means to achieve this aim include the suppression of alpha-synuclein expression through siRNA technology, the development of agents able to rescue the formation of toxic oligomeric intermediates, the induction of the neuronal pathways involved in alpha-synuclein degradation. The first two strategies will be tested in the near future, whereas the stimulation of clearance pathways is actually subjected to intense research.

Different drugs have been successfully used to induce macroautophagy in cell and animal models of disease. Anyway, the use of these interventions to prevent neurodegeneration is limited by the lack of specificity; indeed, most of the tested drugs affect major intracellular pathways, thus explaining a series of undesired side effects. Molecules that activate the transcriptional factor EB, responsible for the induction of lysosomal biogenesis, have proved a neuroprotective effect in cell and animal models of disease (Dehay et al 2010). In particular, rapamycin and trehalose, two largely used macroautophagy inducers, have demonstrated to rescue neurons from the toxicity of various stimuli related to Parkinson's disease. The effectiveness of these two molecules seems to derive from their property to modulate the two most critical steps of macroautophagy: they induce the formation of autophagosomes through an mTOR-dependent (rapamycin) or mTOR-independent (trehalose) mechanism; furthermore, they activate the transcription factor EB, determining an increase of lysosomal biogenesis, so that the increased sequestration of cargoes within the autophagosomes is balanced by an increase of lysosomal function, thus preventing the intracellular accumulation of autophagic vacuoles. This might represent a reasonable model to develop therapeutic tools aimed at activating macroautophagy. Ongoing screenings to identify novel specific macroautophagy enhancers should provide, in coming years, novel agents useful to modulate macroautophagy for therapeutic purposes.

No effective strategies are available to activate the ubiquitin-proteasome system; pharmacologic research has focused on increasing the proteolytic activity of proteasome subunits, but ubiquitin targeting and substrate deubiquitinization are all possible target of future therapies which could be tested.

The importance of chaperone mediated autophagy in the degradation of alpha-synuclein makes it a priority to identify compounds able to stimulate this pathway. In this regard, the pharmacologic increase of lamp2a levels on lysosomal membrane appears as the most reasonable approach. Genetic overexpression of lamp2A has been demonstrated to upregulate chaperone mediated autophagy in animal models but pharmacologic tools able to obtain the same effect are currently not available; cholesterol-depleting agents has shown to enhance the activity of chaperone mediated autophagy through disruption of lysosome membrane lipid microdomains, where inactive lamp2A is stored.

As previously reported, sirtuins have been identified as mediators of modifications induced by starvation in dopaminergic neurons of animals; in particular, SIRT2 seems to enhance the toxic effect of alpha-synuclein, whereas SIRT1 has demonstrated to exert a protective role in dopaminergic neurons. These discoveries have led to the search for potential therapeutic targets among SIRTs. Promising pharmacologic approaches include stimulation of SIRT1, which imitates the protective effects produced by caloric restriction in animals, and inhibition of SIRT2.

Stimulation of mitochondrial function might represent another target of putative neuroprotective drugs for Parkinson's disease. Resveratrol is a molecule that has been demonstrated to induce genes involved in mitochondrial biogenesis and aerobic metabolism; this drug rescues dopaminergic neurons in MPTP mouse models.

Several studies have evaluated the putative neuroprotective role of treatments aimed at reducing oxidative stress. An evidence of the potential benefit of antioxidant treatment in Parkinson's disease has been the finding that induction of glutathione peroxidase expression determines a protective effect against 6-hydroxydopa toxicity in dopaminergic neurons of mice. Similarly, overexpression of glutathione peroxidase, as well as Cu, Zn-superoxide dismutase, protects murine brain against paraquat-induced neurodegeneration.

Several foods and natural molecules are supposed to exert a neuroprotective effect thanks to their antioxidant properties. Soy component genistein increases cellular reduced glutathione. Green tea contains polyphenols and flavonoids that prevent lipid peroxidation; another substance contained in green tea, epigallocatechin 3-gallate, has been demonstrated to stimulate nigrostriatal transmission and prevent dopaminergic neuronal loss through suppression of nitric oxide levels in a MPTP mouse model; this finding has qualified nitrosative stress as a putative target of neuroprotective therapies: 7-nitroindazole, a synthetic inhibitor of nitric oxide synthase, has been shown to prevent neurodegeneration in MPTP animal models. Administration of supplements of coenzyme Q10, an endogenous antioxidant that acts as an electron transporter for mitochondrial complexes I and II, has been found to increase the activity of mitochondrial complex I in patients with Parkinson's disease and to prevent dopaminergic neuronal degeneration in a mouse model of disease.

Different plant extracts have antioxidant properties and produce positive effects on experimental models of Parkinson's disease. Withania somnifera belongs to the solanaceae family, extensively used in Indian Ayurvedic medicine. This plant contains various alkaloids which might mediate its putative therapeutic effects. Recent studies have shown that administration of extract from w. somnifera increases the levels of antioxidant molecules in the midbrain and corpus striatum of mouse models of Parkinson's disease; furthermore, this treatment has produced an improvement in dopaminergic transmission and motor function in the same models (Rajasankar et al 2009).

Use of non-steroidal anti-inflammatory medications seems to reduce the risk of Parkinson's disease, probably as a consequence of a decreased generation of free radicals and nitric oxide in dopaminergic neurons.

Antioxidant therapies have demonstrated to be effective at preventing alpha-synuclein aggregation and neuronal death in many cellular and animal models of PD but clinical studies have failed to demonstrate any significant effect on disease progression in patients. Propalgylamines (selegiline and rasagiline) are drugs actually used in clinical practice for the treatment of Parkinson's disease. These molecules seem to positively modify the natural history of the disease thanks to their antioxidant effect, partially related to the inhibition of MAO-B-mediated dopamine catabolism (Magyar et al 2010). The neuroprotective effect of propalgylamines has been demonstrated in various models of disease but it has not been definitely proved in patients. In fact, MAO-B inhibition is also responsible for an improvement in motor symptoms, based on the increase of dopaminergic nigrostriatal transmission, so that it is difficult to distinguish symptomatic from neuroprotective effect. this confirms the need of a peripheral, pathology-related biomarker, useful as a surrogate endpoint in clinical trials of neuroprotective drugs. Anyway, molecular mechanisms different from MAO-B inhibition are supposed to contribute to the putative neuroprotective effect of selegiline and rasagiline: propargylamines have demonstrated to prevent mitochondrial permeabilization, cytochrome c release, caspase activation and nuclear translocation of glyceraldehyde 3-phosphate dehydrogenase; moreover, rasagiline induces the expression of anti-apoptotic proteins, such as Bcl-2 and glial cell-line derived neurotrophic factor (GDNF).

Drugs interfering with excitotoxic insult, such as the NMDA antagonist amantadine, produce little improvement in motor parkinsonian symptoms and significantly reduce motor side effects of L-dopa treatment. Although NMDA antagonists have been found to prevent nigral degeneration in animal models of Parkinson's disease (Blandini et al 2001), no neuroprotective effect has been demonstrated in patients.

Dopaminergic drugs, such as L-dopa and dopamine agonists, as well as deep brain stimulation, might determine neuroprotective effects based on the hypothesis that an increase of dopaminergic transmission should inhibit the glutammatergic projection from subthalamus to the substantia nigra.

6. Conclusions

Molecular physiopathology of Parkinson's disease represents an intricate cascade of events that researchers have only begun to clarify (Fig. 1). The association that has been established between nigral degeneration and alpha-synuclein modifications has found its confirmation in a growing body of experimental evidences. Anyway, the primitive conditions that are responsible for the toxic gain of function of this protein, as well as the molecular properties of aberrant alpha-synuclein that are responsible for its deleterious effect on neuronal homeostasis, are mostly unknown and must be further explored. The precise assessment of the sequence of events leading to alpha-synuclein oligomerization and to neuronal death is undoubtedly an essential step in the research of neuroprotective tools; an ideal goal would consist in the identification of critical nodes in the molecular physiopathology of Parkinson's disease, which may provide novel promising targets of therapies aimed at blocking the degenerative process.

Mitochondrial impairment and oxidative stress seem to be early features responsible for alpha-synuclein modifications favoring protein misfolding and aggregation, but the same mechanisms can be induced by the same alpha-synuclein oligomers that they contribute to produce, so that a linear sequence of events cannot be established. Glutammatergic overstimulation of nigral neurons seems to exert a major role in the genesis of motor symptoms, whereas excitotoxicity probably plays a secondary role that only accelerates the death of neurons when these are exposed to energetic defects, oxidative stress and other toxic features. Therefore, it is possible to argue that a significant neuroprotective effect is unlikely to be obtained through pharmacologic interference with only one of these mechanisms, as it is confirmed by the failure of multiple selective strategies aimed at stimulating mitochondrial function or at contrasting oxidative stress or excitotoxicity.

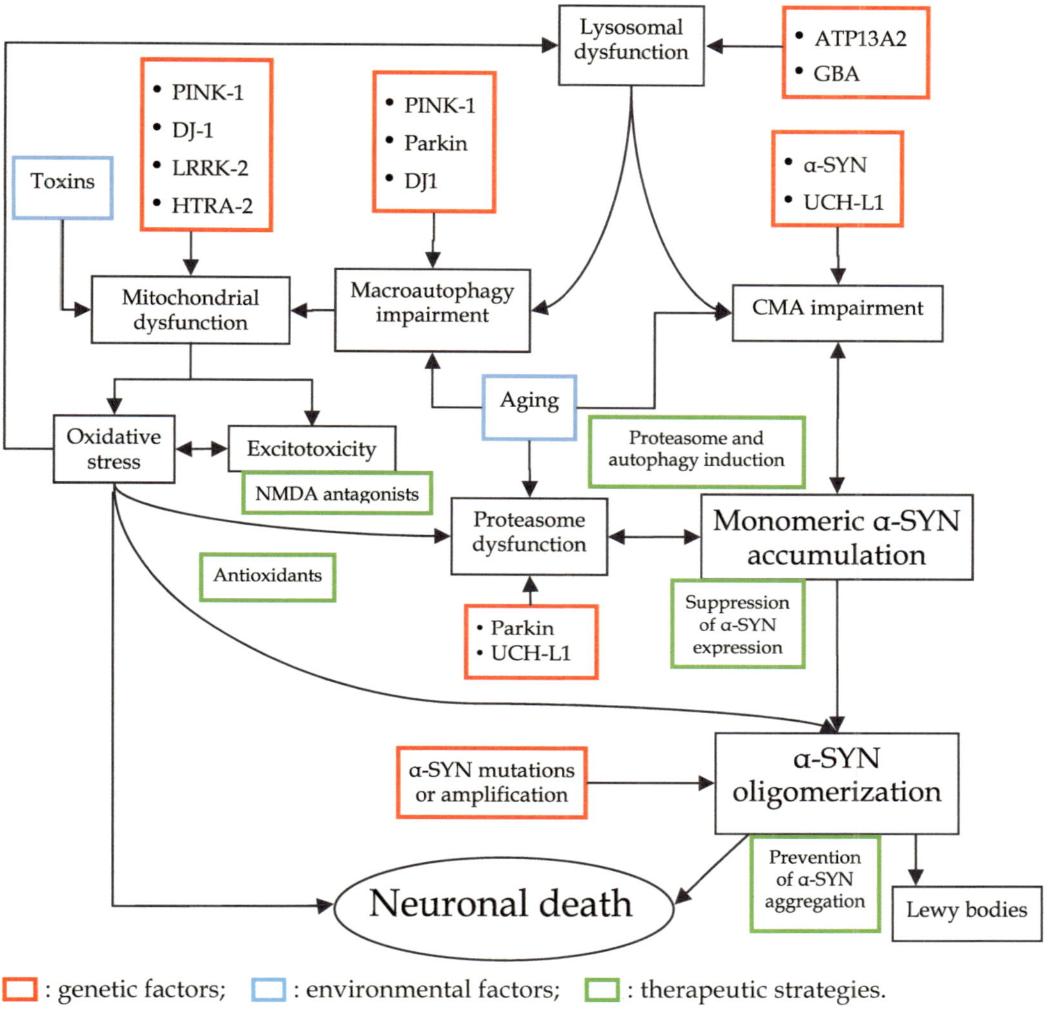

Fig. 1. Scheme illustrating genetic and enviromental factors involved in alpha-synuclein (α-SYN) toxicity and possible therapeutic targets. CMA: chaperone mediated autophagy

Therapeutic tools able to remove alpha-synuclein oligomers or to favor the protein refolding are not currently available. Anyway, several data support a critical role for the efficiency of the intracellular clearance machinery in the maintenance of neuronal integrity; in fact, strong links have been established between abnormal functioning of surveillance pathways and the pathogenesis of Parkinson's disease. Ubiquitin-proteasome system represents the first degradative pathway which has been investigated, however its importance has been downsized by the finding of its secondary role in the degradation of alpha-synuclein, which remains the most disease-specific pathogenetic factor. In this context, the scientific attention has switched to autophagy. Alpha-synuclein, UCH-L1, ATP13A2, DJ1 and PINK1 have all been demonstrated to regulate the clearance of proteins and mitochondria through autophagic-lysosomal pathway. Furthermore, the loss of a single allele of the glucocerebrosidase gene seems to be sufficient to increase the risk of developing the disease.

Pathogenetic mutations of genes responsible for recessive forms of Parkinson's disease, such as DJ1, PINK1 and ATP13A2, inhibit autophagy or lysosomal function through a loss of function of the encoded protein, whereas mutations of genes linked to dominant forms of the disease, such as alpha-synuclein and UCH-L1, impair autophagy through a gain of an aberrant function. Therefore, a correspondence exists between the type of transmission of the hereditary disease and the mechanism through which muted proteins impair autophagy. Furthermore, several studies performed on postmortem brains and on cell and animal models of disease have confirmed that a failure of the autophagic-lysosomal pathway is likely to be a key feature of the disease physiopathology. This defect can trigger all the well-known pathogenetic mechanisms involved in Parkinson's disease, which in turn can worsen the efficiency of autophagy. Together, these evidences sustain the hypothesis of a central involvement of autophagic and lysosomal dysfunction in the pathogenesis of Parkinson's disease.

The fact that the intraneuronal surveillance machinery has been demonstrated to contrast the onset of most pathogenetic mechanisms of Parkinson's disease makes the recovery and the improvement of this cell quality-control a priority in the development of new therapeutic strategies. Pharmacologic approaches aimed at promoting the removal of aberrant proteins and organelles could reveal as the most rationale and global solution applicable to delay the progression of Parkinson's disease and other neurodegenerative disease related to protein misfolding.

In conclusion, restoring the normal function of autophagic-lysosomal pathway, together with reducing oxidative stress and favouring alpha-synuclein refolding, represent promising strategies of neuroprotective therapies. Anyway, all these approaches still face some limitations that need to be overcome; the identification of early diagnostic biomarkers remains an absolute priority that could allow to overcome part of these limitations.

An accurate knowledge of the wide range of mechanisms involved in the physiopathology of Parkinson's disease and, firstly, the definition of the complex interactions connecting these mechanisms represent basic requirements to develop diagnostic instruments and therapeutic tools able to modify the natural course of this disease.

7. References

Alam ZI, Daniel SE, Lees AJ, Marsden DC, Jenner P & Halliwell B. (1997). A generalised increase in protein carbonyls in the brain in Parkinson's but not incidental Lewy body disease. *Journal of Neurochemistry*. Vol.69, No.3, (September 1997), pp. 1326-9, ISSN 0022-3042

Alvarez-Castelao B & Castaño JG. (2010). Synphilin-1 inhibits alpha-synuclein degradation by the proteasome. *Cellular and Molecular Life Sciences*, (November 2010). ISSN 1420-9071

Alvarez-Erviti L Rodriguez-Oroz MC, Cooper JM, Caballero C, Ferrer I, Obeso JA & Schapira AH. (2010). Chaperone-Mediated Autophagy Markers in Parkinson Disease Brains. *Archives of Neurology*,(August 2010), ISSN 1538-3687

Betarbet R, Sherer TB, MacKenzie G, Garcia-Osuna M, Panov AV & Greenamyre JT. (2000). Chronic systemic pesticide exposure reproduces features of Parkinson's disease. *Nature Neuroscience*, Vol.3, No.12, (December 2000), pp. 1301-6, ISSN 1097-6256

Blandini F, Nappi G & Greenamyre JT. (2001). Subthalamic infusion of an NMDA antagonist prevents basal ganglia metabolic changes and nigral degeneration in a rodent model of Parkinson's disease. *Annals of Neurology*, Vol.49, No.4, (April 2001), pp. 525-9, ISSN 1097-6256

Blandini F, Sinforiani E, Pacchetti C, Samuele A, Bazzini E, Zangaglia R, Nappi G & Martignoni E. (2006). Peripheral proteasome and caspase activity in Parkinson disease and Alzheimer disease. *Neurology*, Vol.66, No.4, (February 2006), pp. 529-34, ISSN 0028-3878

Brighina L, Frigerio R, Schneider NK, Lesnick TG, de Andrade M, Cunningham JM, Farrer MJ, Lincoln SJ, Checkoway H, Rocca WA & Maraganore DM. (2008). Alpha-synuclein, pesticides, and Parkinson disease: a case-control study. *Neurology*, ol.70, No.16, (April 2008), pp. 1461-9, ISSN 0028-3878

Brighina L, Prigione A, Begni B, Galbussera A, Andreoni S, Piolti R & Ferrarese C. (2010). Lymphomonocyte alpha-synuclein levels in aging and in Parkinson disease. *Neurobiology of Aging*, Vol.31, No.5, (May 2010), pp. 884-5, ISSN 0197-4580

Chu Y & Kordower JH. (2007). Age-associated increases of alpha-synuclein in monkeys and humans are associated with nigrostriatal dopamine depletion: Is this the target for Parkinson's disease? *Neurobiology of Disease*, Vol.25, No.1, (January 2007), pp. 134-49, ISSN 0969-9961

Cuervo AM, Wong ES & Martinez-Vicente M. (2010). Protein degradation, aggregation, and misfolding. *Movement Disorders*, Vol.25, Suppl.1, (2010), pp. S49-54, ISSN 0885-3185.

Cuervo AM, Stefanis L, Fredenburg R, Lansbury PT & Sulzer D. (2004). Impaired degradation of mutant alpha-synuclein by chaperone-mediated autophagy. *Science*, Vol.305, No.5688, (August 2004), pp. 1292-5, ISSN 0193-4511

Dehay B, Bové J, Rodríguez-Muela N, Perier C, Recasens A, Boya P & Vila M. (2010). Pathogenic lysosomal depletion in Parkinson's disease. *The Journal of Neuroscience*, Vol.30, No.37, (September 2010), pp. 12535-44, ISSN 0270-6474

Dunah AW, Wang Y, Yasuda RP, Kameyama K, Huganir RL, Wolfe BB & Standaert DG. (2000). Alterations in subunit expression, composition, and phosphorylation of striatal N-methyl-D-aspartate glutamate receptors in a rat 6-hydroxydopamine model of Parkinson's disease. *Molecular Pharmacology*, Vol.57, No.2, (February 2000), pp. 342-52, ISSN 0026-895X

Ferrarese C, Zoia C, Pecora N, Piolti R, Frigo M, Bianchi G, Sala G, Begni B, Riva R & Frattola L. (1999). Reduced platelet glutamate uptake in Parkinson's disease. *Journal of Neural Transmission*, Vol.106, No.7-8, (1999), pp. 685-92, ISSN 0300-9564

Ferrarese C, Tremolizzo L, Rigoldi M, Sala G, Begni B, Brighina L, Ricci G, Albizzati MG, Piolti R, Crosti F, Dalprà L & Frattola L. (2001). Decreased platelet glutamate uptake and genetic risk factors in patients with Parkinson's disease. *Neurological Sciences*, Vol.22, No.1, (February 2001), pp. 65-6, ISSN 1590-1874

Ferrarese C & Beal MF (Eds.). (2004). *Excitotoxicity in neurological diseases. New therapeutic challenge.* Kluwer Academic Publisher, ISBN 1-4020-7680-0, Norwell, Massachusetts, USA

Gao HM, Kotzbauer PT, Uryu K, Leight S, Trojanowski JQ & Lee VM. (2008). Neuroinflammation and oxidation/nitration of alpha-synuclein linked to dopaminergic neurodegeneration. *The Journal of Neuroscience*, Vol.28, No.30, (July 2008), pp. 7687-98, ISSN 0270-6474

Giasson BI, Duda JE, Murray IV, Chen Q, Souza JM, Hurtig HI, Ischiropoulos H, Trojanowski JQ & Lee VM. (2000). Oxidative damage linked to neurodegeneration by selective alpha-synuclein nitration in synucleinopathy lesions. *Science, Vol.290, No.5493, (November* 2000), pp. 985-9, ISSN 0193-4511

Gitler AD, Chesi A, Geddie ML, Strathearn KE, Hamamichi S, Hill KJ, Caldwell KA, Caldwell GA, Cooper AA, Rochet JC & Lindquist S. (2009). Alpha-synuclein is part of a diverse and highly conserved interaction network that includes PARK9 and manganese toxicity. *Nature Genetics,* Vol.41, No.3, (March 2009), pp. 308-15, ISSN 1061-4036

Henchcliffe C, Shungu DC, Mao X, Huang C, Nirenberg MJ, Jenkins BG & Beal MF. (2008). Multinuclear magnetic resonance spectroscopy for in vivo assessment of mitochondrial dysfunction in Parkinson's disease. *Annals of the New York Academy of Sciences,* No. 1147, (December 2008), pp. 206-20, ISSN 0077-8923

Hoepken HH, Gispert S, Azizov M, Klinkenberg M, Ricciardi F, Kurz A, Morales-Gordo B, Bonin M, Riess O, Gasser T, Kögel D, Steinmetz H & Auburger G. (2008). Parkinson patient fibroblasts show increased alpha-synuclein expression. *Experimental Neurology,* Vol.212, No.2, (August 2008), pp. 307-13, ISSN 0014-4886

Jenner P & Olanow CW. (1998). Understanding cell death in Parkinson's disease. *Annals of Neurology,* Vol.44, No.3 Suppl.1, (September 1998), pp. S72-84, ISSN 0364-5134

Kabuta T, Furuta A, Aoki S, Furuta K & Wada K. (2008). Aberrant interaction between Parkinson disease-associated mutant UCH-L1 and the lysosomal receptor for chaperone-mediated autophagy. *The Journal of Biological Chemistry,* Vol.283, No.35, (August 2008), pp. 23731-8, ISSN 0021-9258

Keeney PM, Xie J, Capaldi RA & Bennett JP Jr. (2006). Parkinson's disease brain mitochondrial complex I has oxidatively damaged subunits and is functionally impaired and misassembled. *The Journal of Neuroscience,* Vol.26, No.19, (May 2006), pp. 5256-64, ISSN 0270-6474

Kitada T, Asakawa S, Hattori N, Matsumine H, Yamamura Y, Minoshima S, Yokochi M, Mizuno Y & Shimizu N. (1998). Mutations in the parkin gene cause autosomal recessive juvenile parkinsonism. *Nature,* Vol.392, No.6676, (April 1998), pp. 605-8, ISSN 0028-0836

Krebiehl G, Ruckerbauer S, Burbulla LF, Kieper N, Maurer B, Waak J, Wolburg H, Gizatullina Z, Gellerich FN, Woitalla D, Riess O, Kahle PJ, Proikas-Cezanne T & Krüger R. (2010). Reduced basal autophagy and impaired mitochondrial dynamics due to loss of Parkinson's disease-associated protein DJ-1. *PLoS One,* Vol.5, No.2, (February 2010), pp. e9367, ISSN 1932-6203

Magyar K, Szende B, Jenei V, Tábi T, Pálfi M & Szökő E. (2010). R-Deprenyl: Pharmacological Spectrum of its Activity. *Neurochemistry Research,* Vol.35, No.12, (August 2010), pp1922-32, ISSN 0364-3190

Maraganore DM, de Andrade M, Elbaz A, Farrer MJ, Ioannidis JP, Krüger R, Rocca WA, Schneider NK, Lesnick TG, Lincoln SJ, Hulihan MM, Aasly JO, Ashizawa T, Chartier-Harlin MC, Checkoway H, Ferrarese C, Hadjigeorgiou G, Hattori N, Kawakami H, Lambert JC, Lynch T, Mellick GD, Papapetropoulos S, Parsian A, Quattrone A, Riess O, Tan EK & Van Broeckhoven C; Genetic Epidemiology of Parkinson's Disease (GEO-PD) Consortium. (2006). Collaborative analysis of alpha-synuclein gene promoter variability and Parkinson disease. *JAMA,* Vol. 296, No. 6, (August 2006), pp. 661-70, ISSN 0098-7484

Narendra DP, Jin SM, Tanaka A, Suen DF, Gautier CA, Shen J, Cookson MR & Youle RJ. (2010). PINK1 is selectively stabilized on impaired mitochondria to activate Parkin. *PLoS Biology*, Vol.8, No.1, (January 2010), pp. e1000298, ISSN 1544-9173

Nixon RA (2006). Autophagy in neurodegenerative disease: friend, foe or turncoat? *Trends in Neurosciences*, Vol.29, No.9, (September 2006), pp. 528-35, ISSN 0166-2236

Palacino JJ, Sagi D, Goldberg MS, Krauss S, Motz C, Wacker M, Klose J & Shen J. (2004). Mitochondrial dysfunction and oxidative damage in parkin-deficient mice. *The Journal of Biological Chemistry*, Vol. 279, No.18, (April 2004), pp. 18614-22, ISSN 0021-9258

Pearce RK, Owen A, Daniel S, Jenner P & Marsden CD. (1997). Alterations in the distribution of glutathione in the substantia nigra in Parkinson's disease. *Journal of Neural Transmission*, Vol.104, No.6-7, pp. 661-77, ISSN 0300-9564

Polymeropoulos MH, Lavedan C, Leroy E, Ide SE, Dehejia A, Dutra A, Pike B, Root H, Rubenstein J, Boyer R, Stenroos ES, Chandrasekharappa S, Athanassiadou A, Papapetropoulos T, Johnson WG, Lazzarini AM, Duvoisin RC, Di Iorio G, Golbe LI & Nussbaum RL. (1997). Mutation in the alpha-synuclein gene identified in families with Parkinson's disease. *Science*, Vol. 276, No.5321, (June 1997), pp. 2045-7, ISSN 0193-4511

Prigione A, Begni B, Galbussera A, Beretta S, Brighina L, Garofalo R, Andreoni S, Piolti R & Ferrarese C. (2006). Oxidative stress in peripheral blood mononuclear cells from patients with Parkinson's disease: negative correlation with levodopa dosage. *Neurobiology of Disease*. Vol.23, No.1, (July 2006), pp. 36-43, ISSN 0969-9961

Prigione A, Isaias IU, Galbussera A, Brighina L, Begni B, Andreoni S, Pezzoli G, Antonini A & Ferrarese C. (2009). Increased oxidative stress in lymphocytes from untreated Parkinson's disease patients. *Parkinsonism & Related Disorders*, Vol.15, No.4, (May 2009), pp. 327-8, ISSN 1353-8020

Prigione A, Piazza F, Brighina L, Begni B, Galbussera A, Difrancesco JC, Andreoni S, Piolti R & Ferrarese C. (2010). Alpha-synuclein nitration and autophagy response are induced in peripheral blood cells from patients with Parkinson disease. *Neuroscience Letters*, Vol.477, No.1, (June 2010), pp. 6-10, ISSN 0304-3940

Rajasankar S, Manivasagam T & Surendran S. (2009). Ashwagandha leaf extract: a potential agent in treating oxidative damage and physiological abnormalities seen in a mouse model of Parkinson's disease. *Neuroscience Letters*, Vol.454, No.1, (April 2009), pp. 11-5, ISSN 0304-3940

Schapira AH, Gu M, Taanman JW, Tabrizi SJ, Seaton T, Cleeter M & Cooper JM. (1998). Mitochondria in the etiology and pathogenesis of Parkinson's disease. *Annals of Neurology*, Vol.44, No.3 Suppl1, (September 1998), pp. S89-98, ISSN 0364-5134

Sidransky E, Nalls MA, Aasly JO et al. (2009). Multicenter analysis of glucocerebrosidase mutations in Parkinson's disease. *N Engl J Med*, Vol.361, No.17, (October 2009), pp. 1651-61, ISSN 0028-4793

Spillantini MG, Schmidt ML, Lee VM, Trojanowski JQ, Jakes R & Goedert M. (1997). Alpha-synuclein in Lewy bodies. *Nature*, Vol.388, No.6645, (August 1997), pp. 839-40, ISSN 0028-0836

Storch A, Kaftan A, Burkhardt K & Schwarz J. (2000). 1-Methyl-6,7-dihydroxy-1,2,3,4-tetrahydroisoquinoline (salsolinol) is toxic to dopaminergic neuroblastoma SH-

SY5Y cells via impairment of cellular energy metabolism. *Brain Research*, Vol.855, No.1, (February 2000), pp. 67-75, ISSN 0006-8993

Tatton NA. (2000). Increased caspase 3 and Bax immunoreactivity accompany nuclear GAPDH translocation and neuronal apoptosis in Parkinson's disease. *Experimental Neurology*, Vol. 166, No.1, (November 2000), pp. 29-43, ISSN 0014-4886

Tokuda T, Qureshi MM, Ardah MT, Varghese S, Shehab SA, Kasai T, Ishigami N, Tamaoka A, Nakagawa M & El-Agnaf OM. (2010). Detection of elevated levels of α-synuclein oligomers in CSF from patients with Parkinson disease. *Neurology*, Vol.75, No.20, (November 2010), pp. 1766-72, ISSN 0028-3878

Van der Walt JM, Martin ER, Scott WK et al. (2003). Genetic polymorphisms of the N-acetyltransferase genes and risk of Parkinson's disease. *Neurology*, Vol.60, No.7, (April 2003), pp. 1189-91, ISSN 0028-3878

Vekrellis K, Rideout HJ & Stefanis L. Neurobiology of alpha-synuclein. *Molecular Neurobiology*,Vol.30, No.1, (August 2004), pp. 1-21, ISSN 0893-7648

Webb JL, Ravikumar B, Atkins J, Skepper JN & Rubinsztein DC. (2003). Alpha-Synuclein is degraded by both autophagy and the proteasome. *The Journal of Biological Chemistry*, Vol.278, No.27, (July 2003), pp. 25009-13, ISSN 0021-9258

Xilouri M, Vogiatzi T, Vekrellis K, Park D & Stefanis L. (2009). Aberrant alpha-synuclein confers toxicity to neurons in part through inhibition of chaperone-mediated autophagy. *PLoS One,* Vol.4, No.5, (May 2009), pp. e5515, ISSN 1932-6203

Yang Q, She H, Gearing M, Colla E, Lee M, Shacka JJ & Mao Z. (2009). Regulation of neuronal survival factor MEF2D by chaperone-mediated autophagy. *Science,* Vol.323, No.5910, (January 2009), pp. 124-7, ISSN 0193-4511

Yoritaka A, Hattori N, Uchida K, Tanaka M, Stadtman ER & Mizuno Y. (1996). Immunohistochemical detection of 4-hydroxynonenal protein adducts in Parkinson disease. *Proceedings of the National Academy of Sciences of the United States of America,* Vol.93, No.7, (April 1996), pp. 2696-701, ISSN 0027-8424

Zhang J, Perry G, Smith MA, Robertson D, Olson SJ, Graham DG & Montine TJ. (1999). Parkinson's disease is associated with oxidative damage to cytoplasmic DNA and RNA in substantia nigra neurons. *The American Journal of Pathology,* Vol.154, No.5, (May 1999), pp. 1423-9, ISSN 0002-9440

7

Targeting α-Synuclein-Related Synaptic Pathology: Novel Clues for Parkinson's Disease Therapy

Arianna Bellucci[1] and PierFranco Spano[1,2]

[1]*Division of Pharmacology, Department of Biomedical Sciences and Biotechnologies and National Institute of Neuroscience –Italy, School of Medicine, University of Brescia, Brescia (BS),*

[2]*IRCCS San Camillo Hospital, Venice, Italy*

1. Introduction

Parkinson's disease (PD) is the most diffuse movement disorder, affecting approximately 6 milion individuals worldwide and presenting tremor, rigidity and bradykinesia as the main clinical features. The onset of PD typically occur in patients over the age of 50 years and its incidence slowly progresses with increasing age. Neuropathologically, it is characterized by loss of striatal-projecting dopaminergic neurons of the substantia nigra pars compacta, and by the presence of Lewy bodies (LB) and Lewy neurites (LN) (Forno, 1996). To date, LB and LN are the characteristic neuropathological alterations of another neurodegenerative disease: Dementia with Lewy bodies (DLB), a form of late-life dementia which eventually overlaps with Alzheimer's disease.

It is noteworthy that, despite the staggering impact of PD on society, the available therapeutic armamentarium for this disease is still limited. Indeed, the gold-standard treatment for PD from the 60'- the dopamine precursor L-DOPA - induces severe motor side effects and its efficacy declines with the progression of the disease. The rest of the pharmacological treatments for PD mainly include drugs that are usually employed in association with L-DOPA such as dopamine agonists, which however fail to match L-DOPA's efficacy. Best results are currently achieved with invasive strategies via subcutaneous or intraduodenal delivery of apomorphine or L-DOPA, or deep brain stimulation of the subthalamic nucleus. Nonetheless, usually after 15 years of pharmacological and therapeutical interventions, most of the patients start to present several motor complications, thus requesting multiple adjuvant strategies such as physiotherapy, hospitalization or social assistance.

For these reasons, in recent years, much effort has been made in order to outline novel therapeutical approaches to cure PD. In particular, interventions such as stem-cell based approaches have been tested as potential treatments for PD. Although results indicate that patients may gain a long-term clinical benefit from the intrastriatal transplantation of human embryonic mesencephalic tissue (Piccini et al., 1999), part of the graft-derived dopaminergic cells develop LB after 11-16 years (Li et al., 2008;Kordower et al., 2008a;Kordower et al., 2008b), probably because α-synuclein can be transmitted from cell to cell (Desplats et al., 2009), and what's more, the availability of human mesencephalic tissue is limited. Thus, it became clear that lentiviral vectors are ideal candidates to design novel gene-based disease modifying strategies for neurodegenerative diseases such as PD. Indeed, surgical infusion is currently required for viral vector delivery into the brain and PD is the only neurodegenerative disorder routinely treated with neurosurgery (Bjorklund et al., 2009;Bjorklund and Kirik, 2009;Kaplitt, 2010). Furthermore, several animal models of PD are available to test new therapies. Actually, promising preclinical gene therapy studies focusing on the correction of dopamine deficiency are currently in progress (Azzouz et al., 2002;Jarraya et al., 2009). However, a limitation with this level of analysis is that it sidesteps the main goal that a current therapeutical approach for PD should afford: to block and/or counteract dopamine neuron derangement. Indeed, a disease modifying gene therapy approach is missing, as the mechanisms underlying dopamine neuron derangement in PD are not yet completely clear. For these reasons, unravelling the molecular mechanisms underlying PD onset is essential to discover new therapeutic targets to cure the disease.

In recent years, the idea that α-synuclein is a causative agent of PD has spread upon the scientific community, the link being that α-synuclein is deposited in the pathological hallmark of PD, the LB and that α-synuclein mutations are responsible for the onset of familial form of PD (Cookson and van der, 2008;Cookson, 2005). These considerations leave us with the simplest possible sketch of the pathogenesis of PD: α-synuclein is an initiator of damage and the final outputs, after many years, are cell loss and LB formation. However, it has to be taken into account that the majority of PD cases are idiopatic, thus: what are the causes underlying the pathological accumulation of α-synuclein? Many epidemiological studies have been conducted to verify whether environmental or genetic factors may predispose to the development of PD (Elbaz and Moisan, 2008). From these latter, it became evident that a correlation exists between pesticide or chemicals exposure and PD onset. Furthermore, besides α-synuclein, 12 other gene mutations, some of which with unknown function (Belin and Westerlund, 2008) have been found to be responsible for the development of early onset PD. Some of these genes encode mitochondrial associated proteins or members of the ubiquitin-proteasome system. Remarkably, mitochondrial and proteasomal dysfunctions have been linked to the onset of PD (Tritschler et al., 1994). Thus, the overall conclusions of epidemiological studies indicate that PD is a complex, multifactoriated disorder and that α-synuclein aggregation, mitochondrial and proteasomal dysfunctions play central pathogenic roles. Noteworthy, the observation that both mitochondrial and proteasomal inhibitors induce α-synuclein accumulation as well as dysfunction and degeneration of nigrostriatal dopaminergic neurons "in vivo" (Xiong et al., 2009;Xie et al., 2010) remind to the hypothesis that α-synuclein deposition is a central step event during the pathogenesis of PD. This notion has been reinforced by findings showing that the area that degenerate in PD (substantia nigra, striatum and ventral tegmental area) express low levels of α-synuclein in physiological conditions (Wersinger et al., 2004), and that α-synuclein levels in the substantia nigra decrease with age (Mak et al., 2009) supporting the hypothesis that these regions may be more vulnerable to a pathological increase of α-synuclein levels, especially during the aging process. At present, the neuropathological diagnosis of PD and DLB is based on the detection and quantification of LB (Beach et al., 2009b;Beach et al., 2009a;McKeith et al., 1996;McKeith et al., 2005;McKeith, 2006). Indeed, the spreading of LB pathology correlates with the progression of the disease In PD, LB are mainly found at predilection sites of neuronal loss such as the substantia nigra

(Braak et al., 2003;Jellinger, 2009;Halliday and McCann, 2010), thus indicating that LB may be somehow related to nerve cell loss. Later on, it was shown that the number of LB in patients with mild to moderate loss of neurons in the substantia nigra is higher than in patients with severe neuronal depletion, thus indicating that LB-containing neurons may be the dying neurons (Wakabayashi et al., 2007). Furthermore, it seems that the presence of LB is not always related to nerve cell degeneration as every dying nerve cell does not necessarely form LB. Indeed, LB-containing neurons of the substantia nigra don't undergo apoptotic cell death to a greater degree than the general population and most neurons that undergo cell death do not contain LB (Schulz-Schaeffer, 2010;Tompkins and Hill, 1997). Finally, substantia nigra neurons, whether they contain LB or not, are similarly affected by morphological dendritic abnormalities or biochemical changes, thus indicating that the neurons in general are involved in the disease process (Bergeron et al., 1996;Hill, 1996;Javoy-Agid et al., 1990;Patt et al., 1991;Kramer et al., 2008;Schulz-Schaeffer, 2010).

In addition, recent findings indicate that in DLB 90% or even more α-synuclein aggregates are located at presynapses in the form of very small deposits, pointing out that not cell death but rather α-synuclein aggregate-related synaptic dysfunctions may cause the neurodegeneration (Schulz-Schaeffer, 2010;Kramer et al., 2008). It may thus be feasible that PD may be characterized by dying back mechanisms that begin at the synapse and lead to axonal degeneration in the striatum as a consequence of the pathological accumulation of α-synuclein at the synapse. These events may lately drive dopaminergic cells of the substantia nigra toward neurodegeneration. Therefore, α-synuclein is central to the pathogenesis of PD. This view opens the way to a novel question: is it the α-synuclein deposition-associated synaptic pathology which may affect the function and resilience of dopaminergic neurons?

Alpha-synuclein is a 140 amino acids protein, a fragment of which has been identified as a non A-β component (NAC) in amyloid preparations of Alzheimer's disease (Ueda et al., 1993). It was firstly described as a brain specific protein (Nakajo et al., 1993;George et al., 1995) and since the initial findings indicated that the protein localizes at presynaptic site and portions of the nucleus in brain neuronal cells (Jakes et al., 1994;Iwai et al., 1995) it was denominated with the acronym "synuclein". Recombinant α-synuclein does not assume a uniform consistent secondary structure in aqueous solution, thus the protein is said to be natively unfolded (Weinreb et al., 1996). Several observations have shown that α-synuclein is implicated in the control of synaptic membrane processes and biogenesis (Jenco et al., 1998;Davidson et al., 1998). From these studies, it was hypothesized that α-synuclein could play a key role in the modulation of synaptic activity. Consequently, it has been demonstrated that α-synuclein interacts with- and modulates the expression, subcellular distribution and activity of numerous synaptic proteins as well as cytoskeletal components (Engelender et al., 1999;Bonini and Giasson, 2005;Chandra et al., 2005;Sousa et al., 2009;Scott et al., 2010;Garcia-Reitbock et al., 2010;Darios et al., 2010;Burre et al., 2010). Alpha-synuclein also shares numerous biochemical and functional similarities with synaptic proteins such as synapsins. Furthermore, it has been found to be implicated in the control of neurotransmitter release (Abeliovich et al., 2000;Gureviciene et al., 2007;Nemani et al., 2010) and since the protein is specifically upregulated in a discrete population of presynaptic terminals of the songbird during a period of song acquisition (George et al., 1995), it has been hypothesized that it may be implicated in synaptic plasticity. Thus, it emerges that α-synuclein has a critical role in the control of synaptic activity in specific neuronal populations, rendering it possible to outline a whole new scenario to single out novel therapeutical targets among the α-synuclein synaptic partners. Modulation of these proteins may open new ways toward the development of disease modifying strategies to cure PD-related synaptic dysfunctions.

By performing a critical review of the PD-related α-synuclein proteome, this article will outline the most relevant findings defining the specific modulatory effects exerted by α-synuclein in the control of synaptic functions in physiological and pathological conditions. The overall conclusions of these studies will spot novel potential therapeutic targets for the development of pharmacological and gene-based strategies aimed at straightening α-synuclein-related synaptic dysfunctions as new clues to cure PD.

2. Alpha-synuclein: Biophysical characteristics

Alpha-synuclein was first described in Torpedo californica (Maroteaux et al., 1988). It belongs to the synuclein family, which includes β- and γ-synucleins. These proteins have a common amino-terminal sequence containing a different number of repeat regions while they differ in the carboxy-terminal part (Tofaris and Spillantini, 2005). Alpha-synuclein from different organisms possesses an high degree of sequence conservation (Clayton and George, 1998). Three α-synuclein isoforms are produced by alternative splicing (Bayer et al., 1999) in humans. The best known isoform is 140 amino acids in length and constitutes the whole and major transcript of the protein. Two other isoforms, of 126 and 112 amino acids in length, derive from the selective deletion of exon 3 and 5, respectively.

The full length α-synuclein transcript (Figure 1) can be divided into three regions: 1) The N-terminal region, residues 1-60, includes the sites of three familial PD mutations and contains four 11-amino acid imperfect repeats with a highly conserved hexameric motif (KTKEGV). This region is involved in the formation of amphipatic α-helices, similar to the lipid-binding domain of apolipoproteins (George et al., 1995;Clayton and George, 1998); 2) The central region, containing residues 61-95, comprises the NAC highly aggregation-prone sequence (Ueda et al., 1993;Han et al., 1995); 3) The C-terminal region, from residue 96 to 140, is highly enriched in proline acidic residues, and contains three highly conserved tyrosine residues, which are considered a signature of the α- and β-synuclein family.

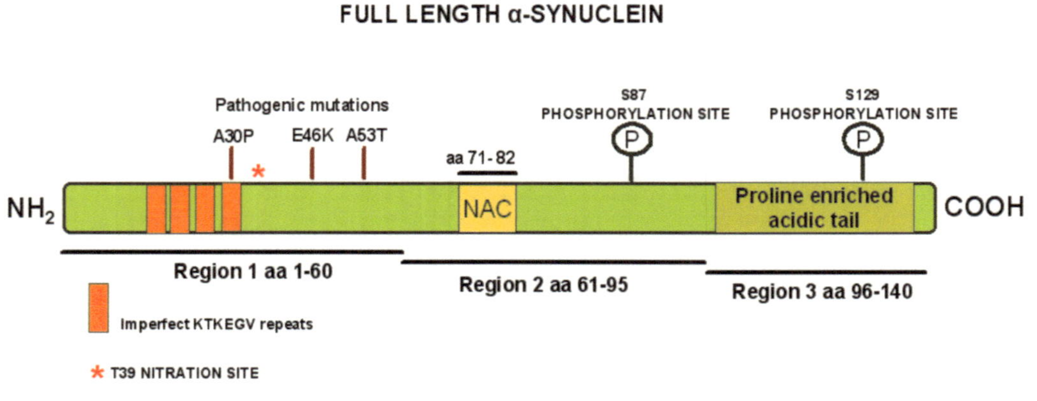

Fig. 1. Schematic representation of the full length 140 amino acid α-synuclein transcript. Pathogenic mutations as well as phosphorylation and nitration sites are indicated.

The amino acid sequence and subcellular localization of α-synuclein indicate that it can interact with lipid membranes. Indeed, the repeat region, mediates reversible binding to acidic phospholipids by making up a conserved apolipoprotein-like class-A2 helix which is associated with a large shift in protein secondary structure from around 3% to about 80% α-helical (Davidson et al., 1998). Consistently, it has been observed that α-synuclein can inhibit a protein which is localized to plasma membrane and submembraneous vesicles: phospholipase D2, whose activity produces phosphatidic acid, which is implicated in vesicle budding (Jenco et al., 1998). Membrane-bound α-synuclein has an high aggregation propensity and seeds the aggregation of the cytosolic form (Lee and Lee, 2002). Lipids can facilitate the incorporation of α-synuclein into membranes and influence α-synuclein fibril elongation (Gai et al., 2000) suggesting that α-synuclein may be strongly implicated in synaptic membrane biogenesis. Furthermore, the key role of α-synuclein in membrane-associated processes is supported by findings indicating that α-synuclein knock-out mice have enhanced dopamine release at nigrostriatal terminals in response to electrical stimulation, indicating that α-synuclein is an activity-dependent negative regulator of dopaminergic transmission (Abeliovich et al., 2000). On this line, it has been shown that depletion of α-synuclein results in a decrease in the distal pool of presynaptic vesicles in cultured hippocampal neurons (Murphy et al., 2000). Furthermore, its overexpression reduces neurotransmitter release by inhibiting synaptic vesicle reclustering after endocytosis (Nemani et al., 2010). Cytosolic proteins regulate α-synuclein membrane interactions, thus suggesting that cytosolic cofactors may be implicated in disease pathogenesis (Wislet-Gendebien et al., 2006;Wislet-Gendebien et al., 2008). In particular, protein-protein interactions may affect α-synuclein ability to bind to synaptic membranes, thus affecting its biochemical properties and modulating its tendency toward aggregation, suggesting that, in the α-synuclein synaptic proteome, it could be possible to modulate α-synuclein aggregation by selectively regulating the expression of some o its protein partners.

The relevance of the formation of protein complexes in the modulation of α-synuclein function is supported by several findings which suggest that the protein likely behave like a molecular chaperone. Indeed, some studies have shown that α-synuclein shares functional and physical homologies with a family of ubiquitous cytoplasmic chaperones: the 14-3-3 proteins (Ostrerova et al., 1999). Alpha-synuclein can bind 14-3-3 proteins as well as other protein members of its family proteome such as protein kinase C. Thus, it was hypothesized that an increase of α-synuclein levels could be harmful for the cells as it could affect signal transduction pathways involved in cell differentiation and survival. On this line, in 2001, Iwata and colleagues showed that α-synuclein inhibited mitogen-activated protein (MAP) kinase signaling and accelerated cell death following serum reduction in neuro2a cells. However, results from later studies indicated that overexpression of wild type α-synuclein can protect neuronal cells from apoptotic stimuli and delay cell death induced by serum withdrawal (Alves da Costa et al., 2000;Lee et al., 2001b), thus leading to controversial conclusions. Indeed, it has also been reported that α-synuclein protects against oxidative stress by inactivating c-jun-N-terminal kinase, which is strongly implicated in stress responses (Hashimoto et al., 2002). However, it is likely that the neuroprotective/toxic effects of α-synuclein may be ascribed to a different sensitivity of cells to α-synuclein levels. Indeed, it has been shown that at a nanomolar scale TAT-α-synuclein is neuroprotective against oxidative stress, while at a micromolar scale it is able to aggregate and trigger neurotoxic mechanisms (Albani et al., 2004;Batelli et al., 2008).

Finally, recent evidence showed that cells from transgenic mice expressing the truncated form of α-synuclein are more susceptible to environmental conditions and that overexpression of the wild type from of the protein in neuronal progenitor cells affect their fate of differentiation, thus supporting the notion that full length α-synuclein is involved in dopaminergic cell differentiation and survival (Michell et al., 2007;Schneider et al., 2007).

3. Alpha-synuclein pathology in PD and α-synucleinopathies

The term α-synucleinopathies is usually employed to define a group of neurodegenerative disorders that show common pathologic proteinaceous accumulation of α-synuclein aggregates. In these diseases, α-synuclein aggregates are deposited in selective vulnerable populations of neuronal and glial cells (Goedert, 1999;Spillantini and Goedert, 2000;Galvin et al., 2001;Trojanowski and Lee, 2003). From a clinical point of view, α-synucleinopathies include symptomatically heterogeneous disorders, among them LB-associated diseased such as PD, DLB, multiple system atrophy (MSA) LB dysphagia as well as neurodegeneration with brain iron accumulation type I, pure autonomic failure, and the LB variant of Alzheimer's disease (Uversky, 2007).

However, since α-synuclein has been found to be the main component of LB and LN in the PD brain (Spillantini et al., 1997), and it has been described that mutations in the gene encoding α-synuclein (SNCA gene) are responsible for the onset of familiar forms of PD (Polymeropoulos et al., 1997), in the last decade, much effort has been devoted to the characterization of the molecular basis of α-synuclein-related neuronal degeneration in PD and DLB.

Missense mutations in the gene encoding α-synuclein, as well as duplication and triplication of the locus containing the SNCA gene, have been identified in familial forms of PD (Tofaris and Spillantini, 2007;Lee and Trojanowski, 2006). However, familial forms of PD linked to missense mutations are extremely rare and have different clinical and histopathological features, although they may provide insights into pathogenic mechanisms leading to LB formation. Fibril formation is accelerated by the A53T mutated α-synuclein with respect to A30P-mutated or wild type form of the protein. However, in fibril-producing conditions, the A30P monomer is consumed more rapidly than the wild type monomer, although less rapidly than the A53T monomer, thus indicating that both mutations trigger the accelerated formation of pre-fibrillar α-synuclein oligomers (Conway et al., 2000). A30P-mutated α-synuclein display a reduced binding to vesicles, thus increasing the neuropathology and the bioavailability of the protein for aberrant interactions (Choi et al., 2004). The E46K mutation significantly increases the binding of α-synuclein to negatively charged liposomes and enhances the rate of filament assembly comparably to the A53T mutation (Greenbaum et al., 2005). The deleterious effects of point mutations and the effect of high expression levels have been investigated "in vivo" in transgenic and viral infected animals. Transgenic mice where the expression of A53T α-synuclein has been driven by the mouse prion protein promoter (mPrP) showed accumulation of α-synuclein in cell bodies and dystrophic neuritis as well as motor impaiment (Neumann et al., 2002). However, these transgenic mice showed an extensive α-synuclein pathology in motor neurons and axons which may account for their behavioural phenotype. Other studies showed that transgenic overexpression of the wild type form of α-synuclein under the guidance of the mPrP was not associated to protein accumulation or behavioural deficits. Conversely, transgenic mice overexpressing the A30P mutant α-synuclein under the guidance of the Thy1 promoter developed age dependent LB-like changes such as proteinase K-resistant protein aggregates, neuritic pathology and formation of some argyrophilic and thioflavin S-positive α-synuclein inclusions. Remarkably, although mPrP but not Thy1 promoter drives high expression of the transgene in the substantia nigra neurons, the tyrosine hydroxylase (TH)–positive neurons of this area in the mPrP-driven transgenic mice were devoid of α-synclein aggregates, and didn't show loss of striatal dopamine or DAT (Giasson et al., 2002;Lee et al., 2002). In line with these findings another study showed that TH-driven expression of wt or mutant α-synuclein didn't result in the formation of intracellular α-synuclein aggregates.

From these studies, it became evident that adeno- or lentiviral-mediated expression of α-synuclein may represent a powerful tool to induce the selective expression of the protein in dopaminergic neurons of the substantia nigra of adult rodents (Kirik et al., 2002;Klein et al., 2002;Lo et al., 2002). Indeed, overexpression of either wild type or mutant form of the protein led to cellular and axonal pathology associated with loss of nigral neurons, reduction in striatal dopamine levels and motor deficits without the formation of fibrillary inclusions (Lo et al., 2002), thus contradicting evidences from studies on transgenic animals. These observations suggest that dopaminergic neurons are vulnerable to high levels of human α-synuclein and that wild type or mutant form of the protein are both toxic. Nonetheless, it may be taken into account that these discrepancies may be related to the high rate of transgene expression that can be achieved by either technology or by the high toxicity which is induced by gene transfection in viral models. To date, neither transgenic nor viral-mediated rodent models expressing wild type or mutated α-synuclein show fibrillary inclusions. Thus the mechanisms by which wild type human α-synuclein assembles in LB in the substantia nigra of PD patients hasn't been clarified by using these models. Nonetheless, filamentous α-synuclein inclusions have been observed in a *Drosophila* model in association with loss of dopaminergic cells and locomotor defects (Feany and Bender, 2000).

Although studies of genetic mutations in α-synuclein helped in the understanding some of the function and pathogenic properties of α-synuclein, they only account for a very small proportion of PD cases. Indeed, more than 90% of PD cases are sporadic, thus characterized by the accumulation of insoluble fibrils of WT α-synuclein (Spillantini et al., 1997;Spillantini et al., 1998). Therefore, much effort has been made in order to understand what are the alterations which convert wild type α-synuclein to a toxic species. It has been shown that wild type α-synuclein aggregates form fibrils identical to those isolated from disease brains, even though the rate of fibril formation is slower than that of the mutant form (Serpell et al., 2000;Conway et al., 1998). To date, several post-translational modifications of α-synuclein can alter its biophysical properties. Thus, it has been hypothesized that these modifications are implicated in the induction of the fibrillation process (Oueslati et al., 2010). These studies indicate that α-synuclein has numerous potential sites for post-translational modifications such as phosphorylation, tyrosine nitration or protein cleavage. In transfected cells, it is constitutively phosphorylated at serine residues 87 and 129, with the latter being the predominant site (Okochi et al., 2000). Residue 129 in α-synuclein lies a consensus sequence for casein kinase 1, which is also present in β- and γ-synuclein, and casein kinase 1 and 2 have been found to phosphorylate this site. Alpha-synuclein can be phosphorylated also by several G-protein-coupled receptor kinases, events which reduce the ability of the protein to interact with phospholipids and PLD2 (Pronin et al., 2000). Tyrosine kinase 72syk can phosphorylate the tyrosine residues in the carboxy-terminus of the protein both *in vitro* and in CHO cells (Negro et al., 2002). The specific phosphorylation of serine 129 in the C-terminal region can decrease the ability of this portion to prevent fibril formation (Fujiwara et al., 2002). Other post translational modifications, such as tyrosine nitration of α-synuclein, which have been reported in LB, seem to promote fibril formation (Giasson et al., 2000;Hodara et al., 2004). Indeed, it has been shown that the specific nitration of the tyrosine at position 39 in the N-terminal region of α-synuclein decreases its ability to bind to lipid vesicles and shows the efficiency of both the proteasome and calpain I to degrade the protein, thus fostering its accumulation. Thus, collectively it seems that modifications of specific regions of α-synuclein may differentially affect its tendency toward aggregation. In particular, modifications in the C-terminal part of α-synuclein are likely. This is confirmed by the fact that modifications in this region, such as oxidation, nitration and phosphorylation, may influence the propensity of α-synuclein to aggregate "in vivo" in a similar way to truncation (Giasson et al., 2000;Fujiwara et al., 2002;Hashimoto et al., 1999). Similarly, polyamines, dopamine or other positively charged molecules can interact with the C-terminal portion of α-synuclein and promote its aggregation (Antony et al., 2003;Fernandez et al., 2004;Goers et al., 2003;Norris et al., 2005).

Remarkably, it has been reported that LB are rich of C-terminally-truncated α-synuclein (Campbell et al., 2001;Baba et al., 1998) which derives from proteolitic cleavage operated by calpain I (Mishizen-Eberz et al., 2005;Dufty et al., 2007). Several studies demonstrated that C-terminally truncated α-synuclein has an high tendency towards aggregation both "in vitro" and "in vivo" (Crowther et al., 1998;Tofaris et al., 2003;Tofaris et al., 2006;Bellucci et al., 2011) thus indicating that these α-synuclein species could play a role in inducing LB formation. On this line, other findings (Murray et al., 2003) indicate that, while the middle region of α-synuclein forms the core of filaments, the negative charges in the carboxy-terminal part of α-synuclein counteract its aggregation, thus implying that a lack or biochemical modifications of this region may increase the propensity of the protein to aggregate.

It is noteworthy that abnormal protein degradation is another process which has been involved in the formation of LB. Indeed, accumulation of misfolded proteins can overwhelm the ubiquitin-proteasome system, leading to aberrant degradation (Bence et al., 2001;Venkatraman et al., 2004) and binding of α-synuclein filaments and soluble oligomers to the proteasome results in marked inhibition of chymotrypsin-like hydrolytic activity (Lindersson et al., 2004). Monomeric WT α-synuclein can be directly degraded by the 20S proteasome in a ubiquitin-independent manner (Tofaris et al., 2003) a process that is slowed down by nitrosylation of monomeric α-synuclein (Hodara et al., 2004) and that can lead to generation of incompletely degraded, C-terminally truncated α-synuclein species (Liu et al., 2005). Furthermore, it has been described that in LB diseases a modified form of α-synuclein of 22-24 kDa is the substrate of predominantly mono- or di-unbiquitination (Tofaris et al., 2003). Thus, ubiquitin-dependent degradation is probably not involved in the physiological degradation of α-synuclein but rather represents a disease specific pathway activated as a last attempt to unfold and/or degrade misfolded proteins either through the 26S proteasome via poly-ubiquitination, or the lysosome by mono-ubiquitination.

This notwithstandings, it has been showed that the direct expression of the chaperone Hsp70 prevents dopaminergic neuronal loss associated with α-synuclein toxicity in Drosophila (Auluck et al., 2002) like the overexpression of the co-chaperone carboxyl-terminus of Hsp70-interacting protein (CHIP) decreases the levels and the formations of intracellular α-synuclein inclusions via the proteasome and lysosome systems (Shin et al., 2005).

Interaction with lipid membranes could also play a role in the conversion of wild type α-synuclein to a pathogenic protein, as detergent stable oligomers of α-synuclein have been found in the brains of patients with PD and recombinant α-synuclein forms multimers "in vitro" upon exposure to vesicles polyunsaturated fatty acids (PUFA) acyl groups (Perrin et al., 2001). Moreover, exposure of mesencephalic neurons to PUFA increases α-synuclein oligomerisation "in vivo" (Sharon et al., 2003). These oligomers precede the formation of insoluble fibrillar aggregates and can bind and permeabilize membrane bilayers through electrostatic and hydrophobic interactions (Volles et al., 2001;Zhu et al., 2003). Conversely, more recent studies have shown that association of α-synuclein with biological membranes can also protect the protein from oxidation and nitrosylation, decreasing the formation of aggregates (Trostchansky et al., 2006) .

Finally, it has been found that overexpression of wild type and mutant α-synuclein in cells isolated from transgenic mice disrupted the vesicular pH and increased cytosolic catechol species, which in turn could trigger oxidative damage (Mosharov et al., 2006). Dopamine, on the other hand, has been found to stabilize oligomeric intermediates (Conway et al., 2001;Mazzulli et al., 2006) which can further disrupt the integrity of synaptic vesicles, thus initiating a vicious circle that eventually leads to aggregation and cell death. Dopamine overload can exacerbate the formation of insoluble α-synuclein-positive inclusions and cell death induced by nutrient starvation (Bellucci et al., 2008). Overexpression of wild type, A53T and A30P α-synuclein in human dopaminergic neurons led to 2-2.5-fold increase in apoptosis (Xu et al., 2002;Zhou et al., 2002). Thus, from these findings, it seems that dysregulation of dopamine homeostasis may underlie the vulnerability of dopaminergic neurons in PD. However, the possibility that post-translational modifications during disease process may at least partly be a secondary phenomena resulting from aggregation of α-synuclein cannot be excluded at present.

4. The α-synuclein synaptic proteome

Several lines of evidence indicate that α-synuclein is critically involved in the regulation of synaptic functions (Fortin et al., 2010;Bellani et al., 2010;Sousa et al., 2009;Tofaris and Spillantini, 2007). In particular, it has been shown that α-synuclein is loosely associated with the distal pool of synaptic vesicles (Kahle et al., 2000;Lee et al., 2008;Zhang et al., 2008) and with the lipid rafts of the plasma membrane (Fortin et al., 2004), thus indicating that the protein is able to associate with membranes, as confirmed by other studies (Chandra et al., 2003;Davidson et al., 1998;Eliezer et al., 2001;Jo et al., 2000). Nonetheless, it seems that the distribution of α-synuclein at synapses is very dynamic and dependent upon neuronal stimulation, with rapid exchanges taking place among neighbouring synapses (Fortin et al., 2005). The critical importance of α-synuclein in the modulation of synaptic functions is confirmed by numerous studies shading light upon the α-synuclein synaptic proteome. Numerous observations indicate that α-synuclein is crucially involved in the regulation of synaptic functions as it interacts with- and modulates key synaptic components including lipidic and protein molecules.

Yet, in 2003 Sharon and colleagues (2003) elegantly showed that α-synuclein accumulation can influence cellular and brain phospholipids levels, including certain PUFA, thus affecting membrane fluidity and synaptic membrane trafficking. Later on, Jo and coauthors (2004) found that wild type α-synuclein does not penetrate to the fatty acyl chains and in isolated synaptosomes, while the A53T mutated form of the protein binds to synaptosomal membranes, increases lipid headgroup packing, induces subtle changes in the lipid interfacial space and decreases the fluidity of the fatty acyl chains. However, a recent investigation concerning the lipidomic profiling of different mouse strains showed age and gender related differences that were poorly associated with α-synuclein genotype thus weakening the idea that α-synuclein-synaptic membrane interactions may underlie the onset of PD-related alterations (Rappley et al., 2009). However, these observations may be justified by the fact that α-synuclein is engaged in a foudamentally different mode of membrane interaction than the charge-dependent artificial membrane binding, and the mode of interaction is determined by the intrinsic properties of α-synuclein itself and by cytoplasmic context (Kim et al., 2006). Furthermore, it has been shown that nutrient starvation, a condition that mimics the impaired energy metabolism occurring in the aging brain (Bowling and Beal, 1995) induces α-synuclein pathological changes, that may lately affect the correct trafficking of synaptic proteins such as the DAT (Bellucci et al., 2008). Thus, we can't exclude that this effect can be related an α-synuclein accumulation-mediated change in synaptic membrane fluidity and composition.

This notwithstandings, the modulation of synaptic activity by α-synuclein is not solely mediated by the fact that the protein regulates some of the lipidic components of synaptic membrane. Hence, α-synuclein has been found to interact with numerous synaptic proteins, and it seems that this critical interaction may affect their specific localization and function. Indeed, α-synuclein binds to the actin cytoskeleton (Sousa et al., 2009) and modulates its dynamics, thus participating in the tuning of vesicle release process (Bellani et al., 2010). In 2007, Woods et al. described several new protein partners of α-synuclein by phage display and NMR spectroscopy, and among them a key protein implicated in the regulation synaptic vesicle release was identified: synapsin 1a. As a further indication of the occurrence of α-synuclein-synapsin 1 interaction, it has been shown that these two proteins are co-trasportated from the cell body to the axon by the slow component-b (Roy et al., 2007;Roy et al., 2008). These observations were lately confirmed by other findings indicating that α-synuclein transgenic overexpression results in a significant reduction of synapsin 1, thus impairing vesicle reclustering after exocytosis (Nemani et al., 2010). The authors elegantly discuss that since 1) synapsin 1 and 2 knock out mice show a reduction of the total number of synaptic vesicles, distinct from the primary defect in recycling pool size observed with α-synuclein overexpression, and 2) the overexpression of α-synuclein causes a more severe defect in recycling pool than the complete loss of synapsins and what's more, the transgenic mice only show a partial loss of synapsins, the effect of α-synuclein is unlikely to reflect the sole loss of synapsin. Rather, the inhibitory effect exerted by α-synuclein, may be related also to the modulation of other proteins, such as complexins, proteins involved in a step at or close to fusion with the plasma membrane (Sudhof and Rothman 2009), which have also been found to be reduced by α-synuclein overexpression. However, complexins levels are moderately changed in α- and β-synuclein knockout mice (Chandra et al., 2004), implying that α-synuclein is not strikingly involved in their physiological regulation at synaptic sytes. Thus, besides synapsin 1, the expression and subcellular localization of other proteins seem to be affected by α-synuclein accumulation. Remarkably, it has been shown that α-synuclein is able to restore N-ethylmaleimide sensitive fusion attachment protein receptor (SNARE) proteins (SNAREs) assembly induced by the cysteine-string protein-α (CSP-α) knockout by acting through a downstream mechanism that requires phospholipids binding, thus protecting nerve terminals against CSP-α deletion-induced injury (Chandra et al., 2005). The modulation of SNARE complex formation by α-synuclein likely occur through a direct interaction with synaptobrevin-2, which involves the C-terminal portion of α-synuclein as recently postulated by Burrè et al. (2010). Therefore, C-terminally truncated α-synuclein is likely unable to interact with synaptobrevin-2, and to regulate SNARE complex assembly. Furthermore, α-synuclein can indirectly affect SNAREs activation by sequestering arachidonic acid (Darios et al., 2010). Another study showed that transgenic overexpression of α-synuclein resulted in the selective reduction of synaptobrevin-2 and synapsin 1 as well as of other synaptic proteins playing a role in exocytosis and endocytosis such as piccolo or endocytosis-regulating proteins such as amphiphysin (Scott et al., 2010).

Synphilin, an adaptor molecule which anchors α-synuclein to intracellular proteins involved in vesicle transport and cytoskeletal functions (Lee et al., 2004), is another protein member of the synaptic proteome (Engelender et al., 1999;Neystat et al., 2002;Alvarez-Castelao and Castano, 2010). In particular, it has been shown that synphilin-1 binds to α-synuclein thus promoting the formation of cytosolic inclusions (Engelender et al., 1999). This effect may be due to the fact that the interaction of the central region of synphilin-1 with the N-terminal region of α-synuclein prevents α-synuclein degradation by the proteasome (Alvarez-Castelao and Castano, 2010).

More recently, a broad proteomic analysis investigated the serine 129 and serine 125 phosphorylation-dependent α-synuclein interactions (McFarland et al., 2008). In this paper, authors singled out several other synaptic protein partners such as synaptophysin, SNAP-25-interacting protein, vesicle-associated membrane protein-associated protein (VAPA) A and B and syntaxin-binding protein 1.

Finally, it has been shown that α-synuclein interacts with and modulate the membrane trafficking of several neuron-specific transporters implicated in neurotransmitter re-uptake from synaptic clefts, among them the DAT (Sidhu et al., 2004;Lee et al., 2001a;Bellucci et al., 2008) as well as the noradrenalin transporter (NET) (Wersinger et al., 2006a) and serotonine transporter (SERT) (Wersinger et al., 2006b). Remarkably, besides dopaminergic neurons of the substantia nigra, the noradrenergic locus ceruleus (oral parts) and motor vagal nucleus as well as serotonergic neurons of the Raphe nuclei are among the most vulnerable neurons in the PD brain (Jellinger, 1991), thus, a loss of DAT, NET or SERT synaptic membrane content, may critically be involved in the onset of PD.

5. Alpha-synuclein-related synaptic pathology at the synapse: Biochemical characteristics and functional consequences

Since many recent reports have highlighted that α-synuclein plays a crucial role in the regulation of synaptic functions by modulating lipid synaptic membrane composition and fluidity as well as the trafficking and function of several key synaptic proteins, it has been hypothesized that α-synuclein loss of function at the synapse may be one of the pathophysiological mechanisms of PD. Thus, many post-mortem studies on the brain of PD patients as well as investigations on "in vitro" and "in vivo" models of PD showing α-synuclein accumulation have been focused on the evaluation of the biochemical and functional consequences of α-synuclein accumulation at synaptic sites.

Numerous findings indicate that transgenic overexpression of wild type, A53T, A30P and truncated α-synuclein results in the degeneration of TH-positive terminals with a reduction of striatal dopamine levels (Rockenstein et al., 2002;Fernagut et al., 2007;Ono et al., 2009;Gao et al., 2008;Gomez-Isla et al., 2003;Nieto et al., 2006;Chen et al., 2006). Interestingly, a couple of these reports described specific alterations of crucial synaptic proteins for dopaminergic neuronal functions such as the DAT (Chen et al., 2006;Magen and Chesselet, 2010). However, results of these studies had different conclusions, with the first one showing a reduction of DAT levels in the striatum and nucleus accumbens while the second one demonstrating an increase in DAT density. More recently, it was shown that DAT co-immunoprecipitates with both full length and C-terminally truncated α-synuclein in dopaminergic differentiated SH-SY5Y cells and its membrane levels are decreased in parallel with an increase of α-synuclein levels and aggregation (Bellucci et al., 2008). In this same research report, authors described that the DAT is retained into α-synuclein-immunopositive inclusions following α-synuclein aggregation. In addition, the DAT is specifically redistributed in striatal synapses in the brain of a human (1-120) C-terminally-truncated transgenic mouse model of PD (Garcia-Reitbock et al., 2010), thus suggesting that alterations in its subcellular distribution, mediated by the pathological aggregation of α-synuclein within striatal dopaminergic synapses, may underlie the beginning of the nigro-striatal dopaminergic loss of function. Hence, a decrease of DAT membrane content due to the fact that the protein is retained into α-synuclein intracellular inclusions, may be one of the first central pathologic events leading to dopaminergic neuron loss of function and degeneration. Most importantly, a reduction of the membrane content of the DAT may underlie the onset of PD-related motor symptoms. The critical relevance of α-synuclein in modulating DAT levels is also confirmed by recent findings describing that DAT expression is specifically decreased in fetal embryonic nigral grafts showing LB-like pathology, while TH and VMAT2 expression are unaffected (Kordower et al., 2008a). Thus, it emerges that the DAT is one of the protein member of the α-synuclein-related synaptic proteome which could be pivotally involved in the onset of PD-related synaptic dysfunctions.

However, alterations in other neurotransmitter systems relevant for PD, such as reductions in striatal serotonin (5-HT) or cortical noradrenalin (NE) levels, as well as increased cortical 5-HT and NE levels have also been detected in several α-synuclein transgenic mouse models (Magen and Chesselet, 2010). This is a crucial point, as cell loss in PD occurs not only in basal ganglia circuits. Indeed, changes in both 5-HT and NE levels are thought to underlie the manifestation of early symptoms of PD (Simola et al., 2010;Barone, 2010). Furthermore, α-synuclein knock out has been demonstrated to impair mobilization of glutamate from the reserve pool, thus confirming that the protein may play a role in the regulation of synaptic exocytotic mechanisms (Gureviciene et al., 2007). However, transgenic overexpression of either wild type or A30P mutated α-synuclein does not perturbe the functions of endogenous mouse α-synuclein in glutamate mobilization (Gureviciene et al., 2007), thus indicating that the effect of α-synuclein-mediated synaptic control is specific for each neurotransmitter pathway, and that monoaminergic neurons are significantly more sensitive to its pathological changes and accumulation. This notwithstandings, it emerges that α-synuclein is critically involved in the induction of synaptic dysfunctions not necessarily implicating a direct correlation with the dopaminergic system, because it could affect the basal molecular machinery involved in synaptic release. Remarkably, Garcia-Reitböck and colleagues (2010) have shown that overexpression of C-terminally truncated (1-120) human α-synuclein (hsyn120) impaired synaptic vesicle release "in vitro". In parallel, they found that transgenic overexpression of hsyn120 resulted in the redistribution of SNARE proteins at striatal dopaminergic terminals and coincided with a reduction of dopamine release (Garcia-Reitböck et al., 2010) further supporting that α-synuclein can regulate SNARE complex assembly. SNAREs are pivotally involved in synaptic vesicles release. In particular, vesicular (synaptobrevin-2 and synaptotagmin) SNAREs (V-SNAREs) and target membrane-localized (SNAP-25 and syntaxin-1) SNAREs (T-SNAREs) zipper up into an α-helical bundle that pulls the two membranes tightly together to exert the force required for fusion, thus leading to neurotransmitter release (Sudhof and Rothman, 2009). Authors found a co-localization between truncated α-synuclein-immunopositive aggregates and SNARE proteins and they showed that both the target-membrane localized SNAREs SNAP-25 and syntaxin-1 were accumulated in the striatum of PD patients, thus indicating that the observations in the SYN120 transgenic mice are of significance for human disease. In line with these findings, Burrè and coauthors (2010) found that triple-knockout mice lacking synucleins develop age dependent neurological impairments, exhibit decreased SNARE-complex assembly, and die prematurely, suggesting that synucleins may function to sustain normal SNARE-complex assembly in presynaptic terminals during aging. However, these results are in conflict with other findings by Darios and colleagues (2010) which showed an inhibitory action of α-synuclein on SNAREs which is mediated by its sequestration of arachidonic acid. Indeed, arachidonic acid–stimulated glutamate release from isolated synaptosomes is enhanced in α-synuclein C57BL/6S null mice. Thus, these latter two findings display controversial conclusions, although it is clear that, since hsyn120 overexpression results in a redistribution of SNAREs, the formation of these species of the protein may contribute to the induction of synaptic hypofunctions in α-synuclein-related diseases.

5.1 Putative pharmacological interventions for α-synuclein-related synaptic dysfunctions

It has to be taken into account that the identification of a disease modifying therapy to slow, delay or stop the progression of pathology is one of the unmet needs in the management of PD. Multiple candidate targets and neuroprotective drugs have been proposed in recent years as disease-modifying agents by the analysis of their potential functions in experimental models of PD (Olanow and Kieburtz, 2010). Among these agents, molecules acting at synaptic sites have been investigated. In recent years, much research has been dedicated to dopaminergic agonists that have been hypothesized to possess disease-modifying actions. In particular, several studies in experimental models of PD have shown that, beside their dopamine-like effect on striatal neurons, they may display neuroprotective actions on dopaminergic neurons (Sethy et al., 1997;Le and Jankovic, 2001;Schapira, 2002), and they are also able to block α-synuclein aggregation "in vitro" (Ono et al., 2007;Bellucci et al., 2008). In particular, we recently showed that dopamine D2/D3 receptor agonists can reduce the formation of α-synuclein+DAT-immunopositive inclusions in experimental models of PD (Bellucci et al., 2008) an effect which may be due to the fact that D2 receptors are able to stimulate DAT membrane translocation (Bolan et al., 2007). Thus, it emerges that the critical interaction of α-synuclein with synaptic proteins in dopaminergic terminals may underlie the specificity of α-synuclein toxicity in PD. On this line, in the above cited research report we found that cocaine is also able to prevent the formation of α-synuclein+DAT-immunopositive inclusions likely acting through three possible mechanisms: 1) the block of dopamine uptake and the consequent formation of dopamine-toxic metabolites that can exacerbate α-synuclein aggregation, 2) the increase of extracellular dopamine that may result in an higher stimulation of D2/D3 receptors or 3) the direct stimulation of the membrane translocation of DAT and α-synuclein. Indeed, increased DAT and α-synuclein membrane translocation occur in the striatum of cocaine abusers, thus indicating that DAT blockers can modulate the trafficking of both proteins and confirming that α-synuclein plays a key role in the control of dopamine synaptic tone (Qin et al., 2005). Interestingly, DAT inhibitors have been shown to be able to alleviate specific parkinsonian motor deficits in 1-

methyl-4-phenyl-1,2,3,6-tetrahydropyridine-treated monkeys (Madras et al., 2006). Thus, drugs acting on protein members of the α-synuclein synaptic proteome may be effective for PD. However, the risk for abuse liability strongly unwarrant the establishment of clinical trials with DAT inhibitors. Furthermore, positive trial results with dopaminergic agonists using surrogate neuroimaging biomarkers as primary endpoints could not determinate with certainty if reduced rate of decline of the biomarker was due to a drug-mediated protective effect on dopamine neurons or pharmacologic effects on the biomarker that had nothing to do with their integrity (Rascol and Montastruc, 2000). In addition, a recent clinical report, has shown that dopamine agonist treatment of PD carries a substantial risk of pathological behaviors (Hassan et al., 2011;Ceravolo et al., 2009). These evidences are complicated by the fact that these drugs are usually associated with a wide panel of unwanted side effects such as cardiovascular and gastrointestinal troubles, fibrosis and sudden sleep attacks (Simola et al., 2010).

Among the PD-related therapeutic agents monoamine oxidases-B (MAO-B) inhibitors are widely used to attenuate dopamine catabolism and increase dopaminergic tone (Magyar et al., 2004;Simola et al., 2010). Selegiline is the most used MAO-B inhibitor since it can ameliorate motor impairments in early and moderate PD although its efficacy is weaker than L-DOPA (Caslake et al., 2009;Simola et al., 2010) and it has been recently shown to prevent α-synuclein aggregation (Ono et al., 2007;Braga et al., 2011), thus opening the way to the possibility that this agent may effectively display disease modifying properties by slowing α-synuclein-aggregation and the related synaptic pathology.

Entacapone and tolcapone, two Catechol-O-Methyl Transferase (COMT) inhibitors that also counteract dopamine metabolism, have shown to be effective as L-DOPA adjuvant for the control of motor symptoms and of the wearing off on fluctuations phases of PD. Remarkably, both these drugs are able to block fibril formation of α-synuclein (Di Giovanni et al., 2010) and therefore could display some beneficial effects by slowing α-synuclein-related pathology. However, a strong limitation for the employment of these drugs derives from the fact that they display a wide panel of untoward effects such as vomiting, nausea and hypotension, or in the sole case of tolcapone, hepatotoxicity (Simola et al., 2010).

Finally, in line with previously cited evidences indicating that cholesterol metabolites can accelerate α-synuclein fibril formation, cholesterol lowering agents have been shown to reduce α-synuclein accumulation and the associated neuronal pathology "in vitro" and "in vivo" (Koob et al., 2010). Thus it is likely that these compounds may be able to exert their effects by lowering the α-synuclein-related pathology at the synapse, but further investigation is needed in order to clarify these aspects.

Nonetheless, these considerations leave us with the simple conclusion that none of the compounds which has been shown to be effective in reducing PD symptoms could slow or delay disease progression. In particular, alternative therapeutic strategies aimed at counteracting the α-synuclein-related derangement of dopaminergic synapses may represent a powerful tool to slow or delay PD progression and correct the related simptomathology.

Finally, numerous agents have been shown to counteract α-synuclein aggregation, ranging from antioxidants, sex hormones or receptor agonists such as nicortine. Thus, it can be hypothesized that these compounds may affect the related synaptic pathology in PD. However, at present, none of these molecules has been demonstrated to be effective in modifying or slowing disease progression.

5.2 Gene-based strategies to block or delay synaptic dysfunctions in PD

Since dopaminergic neuronal dysfunctions are central to the pathogenesis of PD, it has been recently hypothesized that a restoration of the correct function of dopamine neurons may be achieved by the employment of gene based strategies. In particular, a multicistronic lentiviral vector encoding three crucial genes involved in dopamine synthesis: TH, aromatic L-amino acid decarboxylase and guanosine 5'-triphosphate cyclohydrolase has been produced and tested in experimental models of PD, including MPTP-treated primates. Results of these studies indicate that this gene-based dopamine replacement may be able to correct motor deficits. However, the models used to test these compounds do not exactly reproduce all the features of PD. Indeed, toxin-based models don't show α-synuclein inclusions, or at least significant pathological modifications of α-synuclein has been reported only by one group in MPTP-treated squirrel monkeys (McCormack et al 2008). This is not surprising, as mitochondrial dysfunctions have been linked to the induction of α-synuclein aggregation, but these features doesn't necessarily resemble the disease. Indeed, dopaminergic degeneration in toxin-based models is achieved through methods that rapidly and drastically lead to neuronal death and thus they don't reproduce the exact pathological series of event that leads to this phenomenon in PD patients. Therefore, whether PD onset and progression are dependent on the pathological accumulation of α-synuclein at striatal terminals, the gene-based dopamine replacement approach may reproduce the effect of L-DOPA therapy without affectively modifying the pathophysiological aspects of the disease. Indeed, in light of the relevant role played by α-synuclein in the control of synaptic activity, a putative disease modifying intervention for PD should block α-synuclein-related synaptic dysfunctions. Indeed, its pathological accumulation impairs synaptic release through multiple mechanisms (Figure 2), thus implying that even in the presence of dopamine, the synaptic terminals containing α-synuclein aggregates still don't act.

A concept that is reinforced by the fact that α-synuclein can be transmitted from cell to cell, thus implying that correction of dopamine deficiency may be uneffective also because of the spreading of α-synuclein through adjacent synapses. Thus, again, targeting the α-synuclein-related synaptic proteome may represent a powerful tool to block or delay disease progression. As previously described, α-synuclein is able to interact with key synaptic proteins, such as DAT and synapsin 1. The synapsins are a family of neuron-associated proteins involved in the regulation of synaptic vesicle release (Cesca et al., 2010;Kile et al., 2010). Synapsin 3 is likely the only isoform which is present in striatal dopaminergic terminals. Indeed, synapsin 1 and 2 have been found to miscolocalize with VMAT2 in the neostriatum of mice (Bogen et al., 2006) although the mRNA for either forms is present in the striatum (Kile et al., 2010). Remarkably, synapsin 3 is a negative regulator of striatal dopamine release (Kile et al., 2010). Although studies reporting a possible involvement of synapsin 3 in the pathogenesis of α-synuclein-related disease are lacking, previous studies (Galvin et al., 1999) have shown that synapsin 1 appears to accumulate in α-synuclein-immunopositive lesions in axon terminals of the hippocampus of PD patients. Furthermore, synapsin 1 and α-synuclein share numerous functional and biochemical similarities. Indeed, besides being both part of the DAT (Maiya et al., 2007) and synaptic proteome (Burre and Volknandt, 2007), they are co-transported from the cell body to the axon by the slow component b as multiprotein complexes without being affected by actin depletion (Roy et al., 2007;Roy et al., 2008) and they can bind to synaptic vesicles and interact with presynaptic membranes and actin cytoskeleton, modulating the dynamics of the actin-based network during the exo-endocytotic cycle (Cesca et al., 2010;Tofaris and Spillantini, 2007).

Noteworthy, despite their different localization in subregions of the adult brain (Pieribone et al., 2002;Cesca et al., 2010) synapsin 1 and 3 share a strong structural homology in their functional domains (Hosaka and Sudhof, 1998), suggesting that they may likely interact with similar proteins and cytoskeletal components, although they differentially regulate neurotransmitter release (Kile et al., 2010;Feng et al., 2002;Cesca et al., 2010).

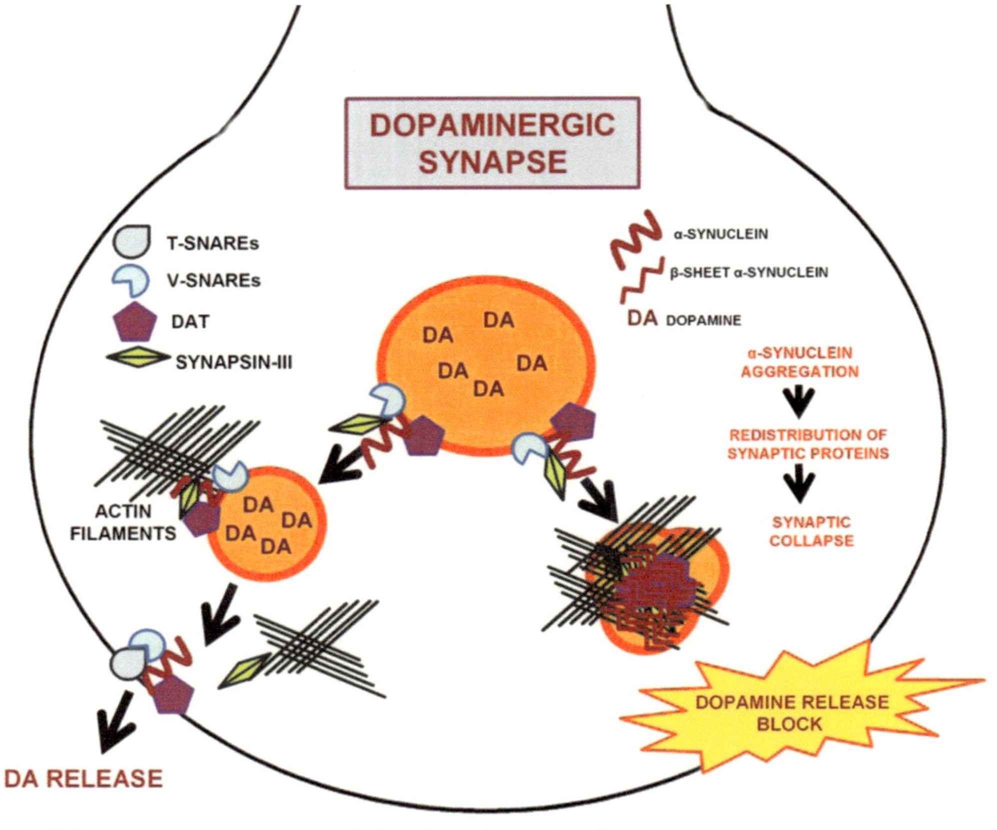

Fig. 2. Schematic representation of the physiological and pathological localization of α-synuclein within dopaminergic synapses. Alpha-synuclein aggregation may compromise dopaminergic synaptic release by altering the subcellular localization of key proteins involved in this process.

Thus, it is likely that α-synuclein can also interact with- and modulate synapsin 3. As a support to this notion, previous reports have shown that synapsin 1 levels in the striatum of PD patients are comparable to those of control subjects (Girault et al., 1989), thus suggesting that synapsin 1 is not specifically implicated in the pathophysiology of nigrostriatal dopamine deficiency in PD. Thus, α-synuclein and synapsin 3 likely share common regulatory roles in nigrostriatal dopaminergic synapses suggesting that α-synuclein accumulation may critically affect the function of synapsin 3 by altering its levels and distribution. In particular, an increase and redistribution of α-synuclein and synapsin 3 complexes in striatal dopaminergic synapses could be associated to deregulation or loss of dopamine release as both proteins are negative regulators of this event. Furthermore,

synapsin 3 increase and redistribution may mechanistically induce the misregulation of other α-synuclein/synapsin 3 protein partners such as DAT and synaptobrevin-2 as suggested by recent findings.
Therefore, in the scenario of the dopaminergic synapse, deregualtion of synapsin 3 by the pathological aggregation of α-synuclein may be a key event compromising synaptic functions as well as the correct tethering and fusion of synaptic vesicles.
Another way to improve dopaminergic neuronal functions in relation to α-synuclein toxicity at the synapse could be the gene-based delivery of the DAT. Nonetheless, it should be taken into account that, since the DAT can precipitate with α-synuclein within intracellular inclusions, delivery of this protein may also foster the pathological aggregation of α-synuclein, an event which may be controlled by the administration of dopaminergic agonists which are known to prevent the formation of DAT/α-synuclein-immunopositive inclusions.

6. Conclusions

A large body of evidence strikingly indicate that α-synuclein pathology at the synapse may be crucially involved in PD pathophysiology. Indeed, α-synuclein accumulation, pathological modifications and aggregation are able to significantly impair synaptic functions in experimental models of PD. In particular, it appears that α-synuclein aggregation at dopaminergic synaptic sites may damage neuronal functions by affecting the correct subcellular distribution of several molecular members of its lipidome and proteome, thus leading to synaptic vesicle stall and to the consequent block of synaptic release. This event may underlie the onset of a perilous axonal degeneration which may retrogradely compromise neuronal resilience, thus leading to dopaminergic cell dysfunctions and death. This view opens the way to the discovery and characterization of novel possible targets to develop drug- and gene-based therapeutical strategies to cure the disease, possibly by modifying and/or slowing disease progression. This is a crucial point, as current therapeutical approaches for PD are aimed at ameliorating disease simptomathology, but none of the present known agent is able to block the progression of the disease. Targeting the α-synuclein-related synaptic proteome by drug-based or gene-based therapeutical interventions may thus represent a new frontier to develop disease modifying strategies for PD and other α-synucleinopathies.

7. Acknowledgements

We are grateful to Dr. Laura Navarria and Michela Zaltieri for technical assistance and insightful discussion.

8. References

Abeliovich A, Schmitz Y, Farinas I, Choi-Lundberg D, Ho WH, Castillo PE, Shinsky N, Verdugo JM, Armanini M, Ryan A, Hynes M, Phillips H, Sulzer D, Rosenthal A (2000) Mice lacking alpha-synuclein display functional deficits in the nigrostriatal dopamine system. Neuron 25:239-252.

Albani D, Peverelli E, Rametta R, Batelli S, Veschini L, Negro A, Forloni G (2004) Protective effect of TAT-delivered alpha-synuclein: relevance of the C-terminal domain and involvement of HSP70. FASEB J 18:1713-1715.

Alvarez-Castelao B, Castano JG (2010) Synphilin-1 inhibits alpha-synuclein degradation by the proteasome. Cell Mol Life Sci. 68:2643-2654.

Alves da Costa C, Ancolio K, Checler F (2000) Wild-type but not Parkinson's disease-related ala-53 --> Thr mutant alpha -synuclein protects neuronal cells from apoptotic stimuli. J Biol Chem 275:24065-24069.

Antony T, Hoyer W, Cherny D, Heim G, Jovin TM, Subramaniam V (2003) Cellular polyamines promote the aggregation of alpha-synuclein. J Biol Chem 278:3235-3240.

Auluck PK, Chan HY, Trojanowski JQ, Lee VM, Bonini NM (2002) Chaperone suppression of alpha-synuclein toxicity in a Drosophila model for Parkinson's disease. Science 295:865-868.

Azzouz M, Martin-Rendon E, Barber RD, Mitrophanous KA, Carter EE, Rohll JB, Kingsman SM, Kingsman AJ, Mazarakis ND (2002) Multicistronic lentiviral vector-mediated striatal gene transfer of aromatic L-amino acid decarboxylase, tyrosine hydroxylase, and GTP cyclohydrolase I induces sustained transgene expression, dopamine production, and functional improvement in a rat model of Parkinson's disease. J Neurosci 22:10302-10312.

Baba M, Nakajo S, Tu PH, Tomita T, Nakaya K, Lee VM, Trojanowski JQ, Iwatsubo T (1998) Aggregation of alpha-synuclein in Lewy bodies of sporadic Parkinson's disease and dementia with Lewy bodies. Am J Pathol 152:879-884.

Barone P (2010) Neurotransmission in Parkinson's disease: beyond dopamine. Eur J Neurol 17:364-376.

Batelli S, Albani D, Rametta R, Polito L, Prato F, Pesaresi M, Negro A, Forloni G (2008) DJ-1 modulates alpha-synuclein aggregation state in a cellular model of oxidative stress: relevance for Parkinson's disease and involvement of HSP70. PLoS One 3:e1884.

Bayer TA, Jakala P, Hartmann T, Egensperger R, Buslei R, Falkai P, Beyreuther K (1999) Neural expression profile of alpha-synuclein in developing human cortex. Neuroreport 10:2799-2803.

Beach TG, Adler CH, Lue L, Sue LI, Bachalakuri J, Henry-Watson J, Sasse J, Boyer S, Shirohi S, Brooks R, Eschbacher J, White CL, III, Akiyama H, Caviness J, Shill HA, Connor DJ, Sabbagh MN, Walker DG (2009a) Unified staging system for Lewy body disorders: correlation with nigrostriatal degeneration, cognitive impairment and motor dysfunction. Acta Neuropathol 117:613-634.

Beach TG, White CL, III, Hladik CL, Sabbagh MN, Connor DJ, Shill HA, Sue LI, Sasse J, Bachalakuri J, Henry-Watson J, Akiyama H, Adler CH (2009b) Olfactory bulb alpha-synucleinopathy has high specificity and sensitivity for Lewy body disorders. Acta Neuropathol 117:169-174.

Belin AC, Westerlund M (2008) Parkinson's disease: a genetic perspective. FEBS J 275:1377-1383.

Bellani S, Sousa VL, Ronzitti G, Valtorta F, Meldolesi J, Chieregatti E (2010) The regulation of synaptic function by alpha-synuclein. Commun Integr Biol 3:106-109.

Bellucci A, Collo G, Sarnico I, Battistin L, Missale C, Spano P (2008) Alpha-synuclein aggregation and cell death triggered by energy deprivation and dopamine overload are counteracted by D2/D3 receptor activation. J Neurochem 106:560-577.

Bellucci A, Navarria L, Zaltieri M, Falarti E, Bodei S, Sigala S, Battistin L, Spillantini M, Missale C, Spano P (2011) Induction of the unfolded protein response by alpha-synuclein in experimental models of Parkinson's disease. J Neurochem 116:588-605.

Bence NF, Sampat RM, Kopito RR (2001) Impairment of the ubiquitin-proteasome system by protein aggregation. Science 292:1552-1555.

Bergeron C, Petrunka C, Weyer L, Pollanen MS (1996) Altered neurofilament expression does not contribute to Lewy body formation. Am J Pathol 148:267-272.

Bjorklund A, Bjorklund T, Kirik D (2009) Gene therapy for dopamine replacement in Parkinson's disease. Sci Transl Med 1:2ps2.

Bjorklund T, Kirik D (2009) Scientific rationale for the development of gene therapy strategies for Parkinson's disease. Biochim Biophys Acta 1792:703-713.

Bogen IL, Boulland JL, Mariussen E, Wright MS, Fonnum F, Kao HT, Walaas SI (2006) Absence of synapsin I and II is accompanied by decreases in vesicular transport of specific neurotransmitters. J Neurochem 96:1458-1466.

Bolan EA, Kivell B, Jaligam V, Oz M, Jayanthi LD, Han Y, Sen N, Urizar E, Gomes I, Devi LA, Ramamoorthy S, Javitch JA, Zapata A, Shippenberg TS (2007) D2 receptors regulate dopamine transporter function via an extracellular signal-regulated kinases 1 and 2-dependent and phosphoinositide 3 kinase-independent mechanism. Mol Pharmacol 71:1222-1232.

Bonini NM, Giasson BI (2005) Snaring the function of alpha-synuclein. Cell 123:359-361.

Bowling AC, Beal MF (1995) Bioenergetic and oxidative stress in neurodegenerative diseases. Life Sci 56:1151-1171.

Braak H, Del TK, Rub U, de Vos RA, Jansen Steur EN, Braak E (2003) Staging of brain pathology related to sporadic Parkinson's disease. Neurobiol Aging 24:197-211.

Braga CA, Follmer C, Palhano FL, Khattar E, Freitas MS, Romao L, Di GS, Lashuel HA, Silva JL, Foguel D (2011) The anti-Parkinsonian drug selegiline delays the nucleation phase of alpha-synuclein aggregation leading to the formation of nontoxic species. J Mol Biol 405:254-273.

Burre J, Sharma M, Tsetsenis T, Buchman V, Etherton MR, Sudhof TC (2010) Alpha-synuclein promotes SNARE-complex assembly in vivo and in vitro. Science 329:1663-1667.

Burre J, Volknandt W (2007) The synaptic vesicle proteome. J Neurochem 101:1448-1462.

Campbell BC, McLean CA, Culvenor JG, Gai WP, Blumbergs PC, Jakala P, Beyreuther K, Masters CL, Li QX (2001) The solubility of alpha-synuclein in multiple system atrophy differs from that of dementia with Lewy bodies and Parkinson's disease. J Neurochem 76:87-96.

Caslake R, Macleod A, Ives N, Stowe R, Counsell C (2009) Monoamine oxidase B inhibitors versus other dopaminergic agents in early Parkinson's disease. Cochrane Database Syst RevCD006661.

Ceravolo R, Frosini D, Rossi C, Bonuccelli U (2009) Impulse control disorders in Parkinson's disease: definition, epidemiology, risk factors, neurobiology and management. Parkinsonism Relat Disord 15 Suppl 4:S111-S115.

Cesca F, Baldelli P, Valtorta F, Benfenati F (2010) The synapsins: key actors of synapse function and plasticity. Prog Neurobiol 91:313-348.
Chandra S, Chen X, Rizo J, Jahn R, Sudhof TC (2003) A broken alpha -helix in folded alpha -Synuclein. J Biol Chem 278:15313-15318.
Chandra S, Fornai F, Kwon HB, Yazdani U, Atasoy D, Liu X, Hammer RE, Battaglia G, German DC, Castillo PE, Sudhof TC (2004) Double-knockout mice for alpha- and beta-synucleins: effect on synaptic functions. Proc Natl Acad Sci U S A 101:14966-14971.
Chandra S, Gallardo G, Fernandez-Chacon R, Schluter OM, Sudhof TC (2005) Alpha-synuclein cooperates with CSPalpha in preventing neurodegeneration. Cell 123:383-396.
Chen L, Thiruchelvam MJ, Madura K, Richfield EK (2006) Proteasome dysfunction in aged human alpha-synuclein transgenic mice. Neurobiol Dis 23:120-126.
Choi W, Zibaee S, Jakes R, Serpell LC, Davletov B, Crowther RA, Goedert M (2004) Mutation E46K increases phospholipid binding and assembly into filaments of human alpha-synuclein. FEBS Lett 576:363-368.
Clayton DF, George JM (1998) The synucleins: a family of proteins involved in synaptic function, plasticity, neurodegeneration and disease. Trends Neurosci 21:249-254.
Conway KA, Harper JD, Lansbury PT (1998) Accelerated in vitro fibril formation by a mutant alpha-synuclein linked to early-onset Parkinson disease. Nat Med 4:1318-1320.
Conway KA, Lee SJ, Rochet JC, Ding TT, Harper JD, Williamson RE, Lansbury PT, Jr. (2000) Accelerated oligomerization by Parkinson's disease linked alpha-synuclein mutants. Ann N Y Acad Sci 920:42-45.
Conway KA, Rochet JC, Bieganski RM, Lansbury PT, Jr. (2001) Kinetic stabilization of the alpha-synuclein protofibril by a dopamine-alpha-synuclein adduct. Science 294:1346-1349.
Cookson MR (2005) The biochemistry of Parkinson's disease. Annu Rev Biochem 74:29-52.
Cookson MR, van der BM (2008) Cell systems and the toxic mechanism(s) of alpha-synuclein. Exp Neurol 209:5-11.
Crowther RA, Jakes R, Spillantini MG, Goedert M (1998) Synthetic filaments assembled from C-terminally truncated alpha-synuclein. FEBS Lett 436:309-312.
Darios F, Ruiperez V, Lopez I, Villanueva J, Gutierrez LM, Davletov B (2010) Alpha-synuclein sequesters arachidonic acid to modulate SNARE-mediated exocytosis. EMBO Rep 11:528-533.
Davidson WS, Jonas A, Clayton DF, George JM (1998) Stabilization of alpha-synuclein secondary structure upon binding to synthetic membranes. J Biol Chem 273:9443-9449.
Desplats P, Lee HJ, Bae EJ, Patrick C, Rockenstein E, Crews L, Spencer B, Masliah E, Lee SJ (2009) Inclusion formation and neuronal cell death through neuron-to-neuron transmission of alpha-synuclein. Proc Natl Acad Sci U S A 106:13010-13015.
Dufty BM, Warner LR, Hou ST, Jiang SX, Gomez-Isla T, Leenhouts KM, Oxford JT, Feany MB, Masliah E, Rohn TT (2007) Calpain-cleavage of alpha-synuclein: connecting proteolytic processing to disease-linked aggregation. Am J Pathol 170:1725-1738.
Elbaz A, Moisan F (2008) Update in the epidemiology of Parkinson's disease. Curr Opin Neurol 21:454-460.

Eliezer D, Kutluay E, Bussell R, Jr., Browne G (2001) Conformational properties of alpha-synuclein in its free and lipid-associated states. J Mol Biol 307:1061-1073.

Engelender S, Kaminsky Z, Guo X, Sharp AH, Amaravi RK, Kleiderlein JJ, Margolis RL, Troncoso JC, Lanahan AA, Worley PF, Dawson VL, Dawson TM, Ross CA (1999) Synphilin-1 associates with alpha-synuclein and promotes the formation of cytosolic inclusions. Nat Genet 22:110-114.

Feany MB, Bender WW (2000) A Drosophila model of Parkinson's disease. Nature 404:394-398.

Feng J, Chi P, Blanpied TA, Xu Y, Magarinos AM, Ferreira A, Takahashi RH, Kao HT, McEwen BS, Ryan TA, Augustine GJ, Greengard P (2002) Regulation of neurotransmitter release by synapsin III. J Neurosci 22:4372-4380.

Fernagut PO, Hutson CB, Fleming SM, Tetreaut NA, Salcedo J, Masliah E, Chesselet MF (2007) Behavioral and histopathological consequences of paraquat intoxication in mice: effects of alpha-synuclein over-expression. Synapse 61:991-1001.

Fernandez CO, Hoyer W, Zweckstetter M, Jares-Erijman EA, Subramaniam V, Griesinger C, Jovin TM (2004) NMR of alpha-synuclein-polyamine complexes elucidates the mechanism and kinetics of induced aggregation. EMBO J 23:2039-2046.

Forno LS (1996) Neuropathology of Parkinson's disease. J Neuropathol Exp Neurol 55:259-272.

Fortin DL, Nemani VM, Nakamura K, Edwards RH (2010) The behavior of alpha-synuclein in neurons. Mov Disord 25 Suppl 1:S21-S26.

Fortin DL, Nemani VM, Voglmaier SM, Anthony MD, Ryan TA, Edwards RH (2005) Neural activity controls the synaptic accumulation of alpha-synuclein. J Neurosci 25:10913-10921.

Fortin DL, Troyer MD, Nakamura K, Kubo S, Anthony MD, Edwards RH (2004) Lipid rafts mediate the synaptic localization of alpha-synuclein. J Neurosci 24:6715-6723.

Fujiwara H, Hasegawa M, Dohmae N, Kawashima A, Masliah E, Goldberg MS, Shen J, Takio K, Iwatsubo T (2002) alpha-Synuclein is phosphorylated in synucleinopathy lesions. Nat Cell Biol 4:160-164.

Gai WP, Yuan HX, Li XQ, Power JT, Blumbergs PC, Jensen PH (2000) In situ and in vitro study of colocalization and segregation of alpha-synuclein, ubiquitin, and lipids in Lewy bodies. Exp Neurol 166:324-333.

Galvin JE, Lee VM, Trojanowski JQ (2001) Synucleinopathies: clinical and pathological implications. Arch Neurol 58:186-190.

Galvin JE, Uryu K, Lee VM, Trojanowski JQ (1999) Axon pathology in Parkinson's disease and Lewy body dementia hippocampus contains alpha-, beta-, and gamma-synuclein. Proc Natl Acad Sci U S A 96:13450-13455.

Gao HM, Kotzbauer PT, Uryu K, Leight S, Trojanowski JQ, Lee VM (2008) Neuroinflammation and oxidation/nitration of alpha-synuclein linked to dopaminergic neurodegeneration. J Neurosci 28:7687-7698.

Garcia-Reitbock P, Anichtchik O, Bellucci A, Iovino M, Ballini C, Fineberg E, Ghetti B, Della CL, Spano P, Tofaris GK, Goedert M, Spillantini MG (2010) SNARE protein redistribution and synaptic failure in a transgenic mouse model of Parkinson's disease. Brain 133:2032-2044.

George JM, Jin H, Woods WS, Clayton DF (1995) Characterization of a novel protein regulated during the critical period for song learning in the zebra finch. Neuron 15:361-372.

Giasson BI, Duda JE, Murray IV, Chen Q, Souza JM, Hurtig HI, Ischiropoulos H, Trojanowski JQ, Lee VM (2000) Oxidative damage linked to neurodegeneration by selective alpha-synuclein nitration in synucleinopathy lesions. Science 290:985-989.

Giasson BI, Duda JE, Quinn SM, Zhang B, Trojanowski JQ, Lee VM (2002) Neuronal alpha-synucleinopathy with severe movement disorder in mice expressing A53T human alpha-synuclein. Neuron 34:521-533.

Girault JA, Raisman-Vozari R, Agid Y, Greengard P (1989) Striatal phosphoproteins in Parkinson disease and progressive supranuclear palsy. Proc Natl Acad Sci U S A 86:2493-2497.

Goedert M (1999) Filamentous nerve cell inclusions in neurodegenerative diseases: tauopathies and alpha-synucleinopathies. Philos Trans R Soc Lond B Biol Sci 354:1101-1118.

Goers J, Uversky VN, Fink AL (2003) Polycation-induced oligomerization and accelerated fibrillation of human alpha-synuclein in vitro. Protein Sci 12:702-707.

Gomez-Isla T, Irizarry MC, Mariash A, Cheung B, Soto O, Schrump S, Sondel J, Kotilinek L, Day J, Schwarzschild MA, Cha JH, Newell K, Miller DW, Ueda K, Young AB, Hyman BT, Ashe KH (2003) Motor dysfunction and gliosis with preserved dopaminergic markers in human alpha-synuclein A30P transgenic mice. Neurobiol Aging 24:245-258.

Greenbaum EA, Graves CL, Mishizen-Eberz AJ, Lupoli MA, Lynch DR, Englander SW, Axelsen PH, Giasson BI (2005) The E46K mutation in alpha-synuclein increases amyloid fibril formation. J Biol Chem 280:7800-7807.

Gureviciene I, Gurevicius K, Tanila H (2007) Role of alpha-synuclein in synaptic glutamate release. Neurobiol Dis 28:83-89.

Halliday GM, McCann H (2010) The progression of pathology in Parkinson's disease. Ann N Y Acad Sci 1184:188-195.

Han H, Weinreb PH, Lansbury PT, Jr. (1995) The core Alzheimer's peptide NAC forms amyloid fibrils which seed and are seeded by beta-amyloid: is NAC a common trigger or target in neurodegenerative disease? Chem Biol 2:163-169.

Hashimoto M, Hsu LJ, Rockenstein E, Takenouchi T, Mallory M, Masliah E (2002) alpha-Synuclein protects against oxidative stress via inactivation of the c-Jun N-terminal kinase stress-signaling pathway in neuronal cells. J Biol Chem 277:11465-11472.

Hashimoto M, Hsu LJ, Xia Y, Takeda A, Sisk A, Sundsmo M, Masliah E (1999) Oxidative stress induces amyloid-like aggregate formation of NACP/alpha-synuclein in vitro. Neuroreport 10:717-721.

Hassan A, Bower JH, Kumar N, Matsumoto JY, Fealey RD, Josephs KA, Ahlskog JE (2011) Dopamine agonist-triggered pathological behaviors: Surveillance in the PD clinic reveals high frequencies. Parkinsonism Relat Disord 17:260-264.

Hill WD (1996) Altered neurofilament expression does not contribute to Lewy body formation. Am J Pathol 149:728-729.

Hodara R, Norris EH, Giasson BI, Mishizen-Eberz AJ, Lynch DR, Lee VM, Ischiropoulos H (2004) Functional consequences of alpha-synuclein tyrosine nitration: diminished binding to lipid vesicles and increased fibril formation. J Biol Chem 279:47746-47753.

Hosaka M, Sudhof TC (1998) Synapsins I and II are ATP-binding proteins with differential Ca2+ regulation. J Biol Chem 273:1425-1429.

Iwai A, Masliah E, Yoshimoto M, Ge N, Flanagan L, de Silva HA, Kittel A, Saitoh T (1995) The precursor protein of non-A beta component of Alzheimer's disease amyloid is a presynaptic protein of the central nervous system. Neuron 14:467-475.

Jakes R, Spillantini MG, Goedert M (1994) Identification of two distinct synucleins from human brain. FEBS Lett 345:27-32.

Jarraya B, Boulet S, Ralph GS, Jan C, Bonvento G, Azzouz M, Miskin JE, Shin M, Delzescaux T, Drouot X, Herard AS, Day DM, Brouillet E, Kingsman SM, Hantraye P, Mitrophanous KA, Mazarakis ND, Palfi S (2009) Dopamine gene therapy for Parkinson's disease in a nonhuman primate without associated dyskinesia. Sci Transl Med 1:2ra4.

Javoy-Agid F, Hirsch EC, Dumas S, Duyckaerts C, Mallet J, Agid Y (1990) Decreased tyrosine hydroxylase messenger RNA in the surviving dopamine neurons of the substantia nigra in Parkinson's disease: an in situ hybridization study. Neuroscience 38:245-253.

Jellinger KA (1991) Pathology of Parkinson's disease. Changes other than the nigrostriatal pathway. Mol Chem Neuropathol 14:153-197.

Jellinger KA (2009) A critical evaluation of current staging of alpha-synuclein pathology in Lewy body disorders. Biochim Biophys Acta 1792:730-740.

Jenco JM, Rawlingson A, Daniels B, Morris AJ (1998) Regulation of phospholipase D2: selective inhibition of mammalian phospholipase D isoenzymes by alpha- and beta-synucleins. Biochemistry 37:4901-4909.

Jo E, Darabie AA, Han K, Tandon A, Fraser PE, McLaurin J (2004) alpha-Synuclein-synaptosomal membrane interactions: implications for fibrillogenesis. Eur J Biochem 271:3180-3189.

Jo E, McLaurin J, Yip CM, St George-Hyslop P, Fraser PE (2000) alpha-Synuclein membrane interactions and lipid specificity. J Biol Chem 275:34328-34334.

Kahle PJ, Neumann M, Ozmen L, Muller V, Jacobsen H, Schindzielorz A, Okochi M, Leimer U, van Der PH, Probst A, Kremmer E, Kretzschmar HA, Haass C (2000) Subcellular localization of wild-type and Parkinson's disease-associated mutant alpha - synuclein in human and transgenic mouse brain. J Neurosci 20:6365-6373.

Kaplitt MG (2010) Parkinson disease: Another player in gene therapy for Parkinson disease. Nat Rev Neurol 6:7-8.

Kile BM, Guillot TS, Venton BJ, Wetsel WC, Augustine GJ, Wightman RM (2010) Synapsins differentially control dopamine and serotonin release. J Neurosci 30:9762-9770.

Kim YS, Laurine E, Woods W, Lee SJ (2006) A novel mechanism of interaction between alpha-synuclein and biological membranes. J Mol Biol 360:386-397.

Kirik D, Rosenblad C, Burger C, Lundberg C, Johansen TE, Muzyczka N, Mandel RJ, Bjorklund A (2002) Parkinson-like neurodegeneration induced by targeted overexpression of alpha-synuclein in the nigrostriatal system. J Neurosci 22:2780-2791.

Klein RL, King MA, Hamby ME, Meyer EM (2002) Dopaminergic cell loss induced by human A30P alpha-synuclein gene transfer to the rat substantia nigra. Hum Gene Ther 13:605-612.

Koob AO, Ubhi K, Paulsson JF, Kelly J, Rockenstein E, Mante M, Adame A, Masliah E (2010) Lovastatin ameliorates alpha-synuclein accumulation and oxidation in transgenic mouse models of alpha-synucleinopathies. Exp Neurol 221:267-274.

Kordower JH, Chu Y, Hauser RA, Freeman TB, Olanow CW (2008a) Lewy body-like pathology in long-term embryonic nigral transplants in Parkinson's disease. Nat Med 14:504-506.

Kordower JH, Chu Y, Hauser RA, Olanow CW, Freeman TB (2008b) Transplanted dopaminergic neurons develop PD pathologic changes: a second case report. Mov Disord 23:2303-2306.

Kramer ML, Behrens C, Schulz-Schaeffer WJ (2008) Selective detection, quantification, and subcellular location of alpha-synuclein aggregates with a protein aggregate filtration assay. Biotechniques 44:403-411.

Le WD, Jankovic J (2001) Are dopamine receptor agonists neuroprotective in Parkinson's disease? Drugs Aging 18:389-396.

Lee FJ, Liu F, Pristupa ZB, Niznik HB (2001a) Direct binding and functional coupling of alpha-synuclein to the dopamine transporters accelerate dopamine-induced apoptosis. FASEB J 15:916-926.

Lee G, Tanaka M, Park K, Lee SS, Kim YM, Junn E, Lee SH, Mouradian MM (2004) Casein kinase II-mediated phosphorylation regulates alpha-synuclein/synphilin-1 interaction and inclusion body formation. J Biol Chem 279:6834-6839.

Lee HJ, Lee SJ (2002) Characterization of cytoplasmic alpha-synuclein aggregates. Fibril formation is tightly linked to the inclusion-forming process in cells. J Biol Chem 277:48976-48983.

Lee M, Hyun D, Halliwell B, Jenner P (2001b) Effect of the overexpression of wild-type or mutant alpha-synuclein on cell susceptibility to insult. J Neurochem 76:998-1009.

Lee MK, Stirling W, Xu Y, Xu X, Qui D, Mandir AS, Dawson TM, Copeland NG, Jenkins NA, Price DL (2002) Human alpha-synuclein-harboring familial Parkinson's disease-linked Ala-53 --> Thr mutation causes neurodegenerative disease with alpha-synuclein aggregation in transgenic mice. Proc Natl Acad Sci U S A 99:8968-8973.

Lee SJ, Jeon H, Kandror KV (2008) Alpha-synuclein is localized in a subpopulation of rat brain synaptic vesicles. Acta Neurobiol Exp (Wars) 68:509-515.

Lee VM, Trojanowski JQ (2006) Mechanisms of Parkinson's disease linked to pathological alpha-synuclein: new targets for drug discovery. Neuron 52:33-38.

Li JY, Englund E, Holton JL, Soulet D, Hagell P, Lees AJ, Lashley T, Quinn NP, Rehncrona S, Bjorklund A, Widner H, Revesz T, Lindvall O, Brundin P (2008) Lewy bodies in grafted neurons in subjects with Parkinson's disease suggest host-to-graft disease propagation. Nat Med 14:501-503.

Lindersson E, Beedholm R, Hojrup P, Moos T, Gai W, Hendil KB, Jensen PH (2004) Proteasomal inhibition by alpha-synuclein filaments and oligomers. J Biol Chem 279:12924-12934.

Liu CW, Giasson BI, Lewis KA, Lee VM, Demartino GN, Thomas PJ (2005) A precipitating role for truncated alpha-synuclein and the proteasome in alpha-synuclein aggregation: implications for pathogenesis of Parkinson disease. J Biol Chem 280:22670-22678.

Lo BC, Ridet JL, Schneider BL, Deglon N, Aebischer P (2002) alpha -Synucleinopathy and selective dopaminergic neuron loss in a rat lentiviral-based model of Parkinson's disease. Proc Natl Acad Sci U S A 99:10813-10818.

Madras BK, Fahey MA, Goulet M, Lin Z, Bendor J, Goodrich C, Meltzer PC, Elmaleh DR, Livni E, Bonab AA, Fischman AJ (2006) Dopamine transporter (DAT) inhibitors alleviate specific parkinsonian deficits in monkeys: association with DAT occupancy in vivo. J Pharmacol Exp Ther 319:570-585.

Magen I, Chesselet MF (2010) Genetic mouse models of Parkinson's disease The state of the art. Prog Brain Res 184:53-87.

Magyar K, Palfi M, Tabi T, Kalasz H, Szende B, Szoko E (2004) Pharmacological aspects of (-)-deprenyl. Curr Med Chem 11:2017-2031.

Maiya R, Ponomarev I, Linse KD, Harris RA, Mayfield RD (2007) Defining the dopamine transporter proteome by convergent biochemical and in silico analyses. Genes Brain Behav 6:97-106.

Mak SK, McCormack AL, Langston JW, Kordower JH, Di Monte DA (2009) Decreased alpha-synuclein expression in the aging mouse substantia nigra. Exp Neurol 220:359-365.

Maroteaux L, Campanelli JT, Scheller RH (1988) Synuclein: a neuron-specific protein localized to the nucleus and presynaptic nerve terminal. J Neurosci 8:2804-2815.

Mazzulli JR, Mishizen AJ, Giasson BI, Lynch DR, Thomas SA, Nakashima A, Nagatsu T, Ota A, Ischiropoulos H (2006) Cytosolic catechols inhibit alpha-synuclein aggregation and facilitate the formation of intracellular soluble oligomeric intermediates. J Neurosci 26:10068-10078.

McCormack AL, Mak SK, Shenasa M, Langston WJ, Forno LS, DiMonte DA (2008) Pathological modifications of α-synuclein in 1-Methyl-4-Phenyl-1,2,3,6-Tetrahydropyridine (MPTP)-Treated Squirrel Monkeys. J. Neuropathol. Exp. Neurol. 67(8): 793-802.

McFarland MA, Ellis CE, Markey SP, Nussbaum RL (2008) Proteomics analysis identifies phosphorylation-dependent alpha-synuclein protein interactions. Mol Cell Proteomics 7:2123-2137.

McKeith IG (2006) Consensus guidelines for the clinical and pathologic diagnosis of dementia with Lewy bodies (DLB): report of the Consortium on DLB International Workshop. J Alzheimers Dis 9:417-423.

McKeith IG, et al. (2005) Diagnosis and management of dementia with Lewy bodies: third report of the DLB Consortium. Neurology 65:1863-1872.

McKeith IG, et al. (1996) Consensus guidelines for the clinical and pathologic diagnosis of dementia with Lewy bodies (DLB): report of the consortium on DLB international workshop. Neurology 47:1113-1124.

Michell AW, Tofaris GK, Gossage H, Tyers P, Spillantini MG, Barker RA (2007) The effect of truncated human alpha-synuclein (1-120) on dopaminergic cells in a transgenic mouse model of Parkinson's disease. Cell Transplant 16:461-474.

Mishizen-Eberz AJ, Norris EH, Giasson BI, Hodara R, Ischiropoulos H, Lee VM, Trojanowski JQ, Lynch DR (2005) Cleavage of alpha-synuclein by calpain: potential role in degradation of fibrillized and nitrated species of alpha-synuclein. Biochemistry 44:7818-7829.

Mosharov EV, Staal RG, Bove J, Prou D, Hananiya A, Markov D, Poulsen N, Larsen KE, Moore CM, Troyer MD, Edwards RH, Przedborski S, Sulzer D (2006) Alpha-synuclein overexpression increases cytosolic catecholamine concentration. J Neurosci 26:9304-9311.

Murphy DD, Rueter SM, Trojanowski JQ, Lee VM (2000) Synucleins are developmentally expressed, and alpha-synuclein regulates the size of the presynaptic vesicular pool in primary hippocampal neurons. J Neurosci 20:3214-3220.

Murray IV, Giasson BI, Quinn SM, Koppaka V, Axelsen PH, Ischiropoulos H, Trojanowski JQ, Lee VM (2003) Role of alpha-synuclein carboxy-terminus on fibril formation in vitro. Biochemistry 42:8530-8540.

Nakajo S, Tsukada K, Omata K, Nakamura Y, Nakaya K (1993) A new brain-specific 14-kDa protein is a phosphoprotein. Its complete amino acid sequence and evidence for phosphorylation. Eur J Biochem 217:1057-1063.

Negro A, Brunati AM, Donella-Deana A, Massimino ML, Pinna LA (2002) Multiple phosphorylation of alpha-synuclein by protein tyrosine kinase Syk prevents eosin-induced aggregation. FASEB J 16:210-212.

Nemani VM, Lu W, Berge V, Nakamura K, Onoa B, Lee MK, Chaudhry FA, Nicoll RA, Edwards RH (2010) Increased expression of alpha-synuclein reduces neurotransmitter release by inhibiting synaptic vesicle reclustering after endocytosis. Neuron 65:66-79.

Neumann M, Kahle PJ, Giasson BI, Ozmen L, Borroni E, Spooren W, Muller V, Odoy S, Fujiwara H, Hasegawa M, Iwatsubo T, Trojanowski JQ, Kretzschmar HA, Haass C (2002) Misfolded proteinase K-resistant hyperphosphorylated alpha-synuclein in aged transgenic mice with locomotor deterioration and in human alpha-synucleinopathies. J Clin Invest 110:1429-1439.

Neystat M, Rzhetskaya M, Kholodilov N, Burke RE (2002) Analysis of synphilin-1 and synuclein interactions by yeast two-hybrid beta-galactosidase liquid assay. Neurosci Lett 325:119-123.

Nieto M, Gil-Bea FJ, Dalfo E, Cuadrado M, Cabodevilla F, Sanchez B, Catena S, Sesma T, Ribe E, Ferrer I, Ramirez MJ, Gomez-Isla T (2006) Increased sensitivity to MPTP in human alpha-synuclein A30P transgenic mice. Neurobiol Aging 27:848-856.

Norris EH, Giasson BI, Hodara R, Xu S, Trojanowski JQ, Ischiropoulos H, Lee VM (2005) Reversible inhibition of alpha-synuclein fibrillization by dopaminochrome-mediated conformational alterations. J Biol Chem 280:21212-21219.

Okochi M, Walter J, Koyama A, Nakajo S, Baba M, Iwatsubo T, Meijer L, Kahle PJ, Haass C (2000) Constitutive phosphorylation of the Parkinson's disease associated alpha-synuclein. J Biol Chem 275:390-397.

Olanow CW, Kieburtz K (2010) Defining disease-modifying therapies for PD--a road map for moving forward. Mov Disord 25:1774-1779.

Ono K, Hirohata M, Yamada M (2007) Anti-fibrillogenic and fibril-destabilizing activities of anti-Parkinsonian agents for alpha-synuclein fibrils in vitro. J Neurosci Res 85:1547-1557.

Ono K, Ikemoto M, Kawarabayashi T, Ikeda M, Nishinakagawa T, Hosokawa M, Shoji M, Takahashi M, Nakashima M (2009) A chemical chaperone, sodium 4-phenylbutyric acid, attenuates the pathogenic potency in human alpha-synuclein A30P + A53T transgenic mice. Parkinsonism Relat Disord 15:649-654.

Ostrerova N, Petrucelli L, Farrer M, Mehta N, Choi P, Hardy J, Wolozin B (1999) alpha-Synuclein shares physical and functional homology with 14-3-3 proteins. J Neurosci 19:5782-5791.

Oueslati A, Fournier M, Lashuel HA (2010) Role of post-translational modifications in modulating the structure, function and toxicity of alpha-synuclein: implications for Parkinson's disease pathogenesis and therapies. Prog Brain Res 183:115-145.

Patt S, Gertz HJ, Gerhard L, Cervos-Navarro J (1991) Pathological changes in dendrites of substantia nigra neurons in Parkinson's disease: a Golgi study. Histol Histopathol 6:373-380.

Perrin RJ, Woods WS, Clayton DF, George JM (2001) Exposure to long chain polyunsaturated fatty acids triggers rapid multimerization of synucleins. J Biol Chem 276:41958-41962.

Piccini P, Brooks DJ, Bjorklund A, Gunn RN, Grasby PM, Rimoldi O, Brundin P, Hagell P, Rehncrona S, Widner H, Lindvall O (1999) Dopamine release from nigral transplants visualized in vivo in a Parkinson's patient. Nat Neurosci 2:1137-1140.

Pieribone VA, Porton B, Rendon B, Feng J, Greengard P, Kao HT (2002) Expression of synapsin III in nerve terminals and neurogenic regions of the adult brain. J Comp Neurol 454:105-114.

Polymeropoulos MH, Lavedan C, Leroy E, Ide SE, Dehejia A, Dutra A, Pike B, Root H, Rubenstein J, Boyer R, Stenroos ES, Chandrasekharappa S, Athanassiadou A, Papapetropoulos T, Johnson WG, Lazzarini AM, Duvoisin RC, Di IG, Golbe LI, Nussbaum RL (1997) Mutation in the alpha-synuclein gene identified in families with Parkinson's disease. Science 276:2045-2047.

Pronin AN, Morris AJ, Surguchov A, Benovic JL (2000) Synucleins are a novel class of substrates for G protein-coupled receptor kinases. J Biol Chem 275:26515-26522.

Qin Y, Ouyang Q, Pablo J, Mash DC (2005) Cocaine abuse elevates alpha-synuclein and dopamine transporter levels in the human striatum. Neuroreport 16:1489-1493.

Rappley I, Myers DS, Milne SB, Ivanova PT, Lavoie MJ, Brown HA, Selkoe DJ (2009) Lipidomic profiling in mouse brain reveals differences between ages and genders, with smaller changes associated with alpha-synuclein genotype. J Neurochem 111:15-25.

Rascol O, Montastruc JL (2000) [Role of dopaminergic agonists]. Rev Neurol (Paris) 156 Suppl 2 Pt 2:98-104.

Rockenstein E, Mallory M, Hashimoto M, Song D, Shults CW, Lang I, Masliah E (2002) Differential neuropathological alterations in transgenic mice expressing alpha-synuclein from the platelet-derived growth factor and Thy-1 promoters. J Neurosci Res 68:568-578.

Roy S, Winton MJ, Black MM, Trojanowski JQ, Lee VM (2007) Rapid and intermittent cotransport of slow component-b proteins. J Neurosci 27:3131-3138.

Roy S, Winton MJ, Black MM, Trojanowski JQ, Lee VM (2008) Cytoskeletal requirements in axonal transport of slow component-b. J Neurosci 28:5248-5256.

Schapira AH (2002) Dopamine agonists and neuroprotection in Parkinson's disease. Eur J Neurol 9 Suppl 3:7-14.

Schneider BL, Seehus CR, Capowski EE, Aebischer P, Zhang SC, Svendsen CN (2007) Overexpression of alpha-synuclein in human neural progenitors leads to specific changes in fate and differentiation. Hum Mol Genet 16:651-666.

Schulz-Schaeffer WJ (2010) The synaptic pathology of alpha-synuclein aggregation in dementia with Lewy bodies, Parkinson's disease and Parkinson's disease dementia. Acta Neuropathol 120:131-143.

Scott DA, Tabarean I, Tang Y, Cartier A, Masliah E, Roy S (2010) A pathologic cascade leading to synaptic dysfunction in alpha-synuclein-induced neurodegeneration. J Neurosci 30:8083-8095.

Serpell LC, Berriman J, Jakes R, Goedert M, Crowther RA (2000) Fiber diffraction of synthetic alpha-synuclein filaments shows amyloid-like cross-beta conformation. Proc Natl Acad Sci U S A 97:4897-4902.

Sethy VH, Wu H, Oostveen JA, Hall ED (1997) Neuroprotective effects of the dopamine agonists pramipexole and bromocriptine in 3-acetylpyridine-treated rats. Brain Res 754:181-186.

Sharon R, Bar-Joseph I, Frosch MP, Walsh DM, Hamilton JA, Selkoe DJ (2003) The formation of highly soluble oligomers of alpha-synuclein is regulated by fatty acids and enhanced in Parkinson's disease. Neuron 37:583-595.

Shin Y, Klucken J, Patterson C, Hyman BT, McLean PJ (2005) The co-chaperone carboxyl terminus of Hsp70-interacting protein (CHIP) mediates alpha-synuclein degradation decisions between proteasomal and lysosomal pathways. J Biol Chem 280:23727-23734.

Sidhu A, Wersinger C, Vernier P (2004) alpha-Synuclein regulation of the dopaminergic transporter: a possible role in the pathogenesis of Parkinson's disease. FEBS Lett 565:1-5.

Simola N, Pinna A, Fenu S (2010) Pharmacological therapy of Parkinson's disease: current options and new avenues. Recent Pat CNS Drug Discov 5:221-238.

Sousa VL, Bellani S, Giannandrea M, Yousuf M, Valtorta F, Meldolesi J, Chieregatti E (2009) {alpha}-synuclein and its A30P mutant affect actin cytoskeletal structure and dynamics. Mol Biol Cell 20:3725-3739.

Spillantini MG, Crowther RA, Jakes R, Hasegawa M, Goedert M (1998) alpha-Synuclein in filamentous inclusions of Lewy bodies from Parkinson's disease and dementia with lewy bodies. Proc Natl Acad Sci U S A 95:6469-6473.

Spillantini MG, Goedert M (2000) The alpha-synucleinopathies: Parkinson's disease, dementia with Lewy bodies, and multiple system atrophy. Ann N Y Acad Sci 920:16-27.

Spillantini MG, Schmidt ML, Lee VM, Trojanowski JQ, Jakes R, Goedert M (1997) Alpha-synuclein in Lewy bodies. Nature 388:839-840.

Sudhof TC, Rothman JE (2009) Membrane fusion: grappling with SNARE and SM proteins. Science 323:474-477.

Tofaris GK, Garcia RP, Humby T, Lambourne SL, O'Connell M, Ghetti B, Gossage H, Emson PC, Wilkinson LS, Goedert M, Spillantini MG (2006) Pathological changes in dopaminergic nerve cells of the substantia nigra and olfactory bulb in mice transgenic for truncated human alpha-synuclein(1-120): implications for Lewy body disorders. J Neurosci 26:3942-3950.

Tofaris GK, Razzaq A, Ghetti B, Lilley KS, Spillantini MG (2003) Ubiquitination of alpha-synuclein in Lewy bodies is a pathological event not associated with impairment of proteasome function. J Biol Chem 278:44405-44411.

Tofaris GK, Spillantini MG (2005) Alpha-synuclein dysfunction in Lewy body diseases. Mov Disord 20 Suppl 12:S37-S44.

Tofaris GK, Spillantini MG (2007) Physiological and pathological properties of alpha-synuclein. Cell Mol Life Sci 64:2194-2201.

Tompkins MM, Hill WD (1997) Contribution of somal Lewy bodies to neuronal death. Brain Res 775:24-29.

Tritschler HJ, Packer L, Medori R (1994) Oxidative stress and mitochondrial dysfunction in neurodegeneration. Biochem Mol Biol Int 34:169-181.

Trojanowski JQ, Lee VM (2003) Parkinson's disease and related alpha-synucleinopathies are brain amyloidoses. Ann N Y Acad Sci 991:107-110.

Trostchansky A, Lind S, Hodara R, Oe T, Blair IA, Ischiropoulos H, Rubbo H, Souza JM (2006) Interaction with phospholipids modulates alpha-synuclein nitration and lipid-protein adduct formation. Biochem J 393:343-349.

Ueda K, Fukushima H, Masliah E, Xia Y, Iwai A, Yoshimoto M, Otero DA, Kondo J, Ihara Y, Saitoh T (1993) Molecular cloning of cDNA encoding an unrecognized component of amyloid in Alzheimer disease. Proc Natl Acad Sci U S A 90:11282-11286.

Uversky VN (2007) Neuropathology, biochemistry, and biophysics of alpha-synuclein aggregation. J Neurochem 103:17-37.

Venkatraman P, Wetzel R, Tanaka M, Nukina N, Goldberg AL (2004) Eukaryotic proteasomes cannot digest polyglutamine sequences and release them during degradation of polyglutamine-containing proteins. Mol Cell 14:95-104.

Volles MJ, Lee SJ, Rochet JC, Shtilerman MD, Ding TT, Kessler JC, Lansbury PT, Jr. (2001) Vesicle permeabilization by protofibrillar alpha-synuclein: implications for the pathogenesis and treatment of Parkinson's disease. Biochemistry 40:7812-7819.

Wakabayashi K, Tanji K, Mori F, Takahashi H (2007) The Lewy body in Parkinson's disease: molecules implicated in the formation and degradation of alpha-synuclein aggregates. Neuropathology 27:494-506.

Weinreb PH, Zhen W, Poon AW, Conway KA, Lansbury PT, Jr. (1996) NACP, a protein implicated in Alzheimer's disease and learning, is natively unfolded. Biochemistry 35:13709-13715.

Wersinger C, Banta M, Sidhu A (2004) Comparative analyses of alpha-synuclein expression levels in rat brain tissues and transfected cells. Neurosci Lett 358:95-98.

Wersinger C, Jeannotte A, Sidhu A (2006a) Attenuation of the norepinephrine transporter activity and trafficking via interactions with alpha-synuclein. Eur J Neurosci 24:3141-3152.

Wersinger C, Rusnak M, Sidhu A (2006b) Modulation of the trafficking of the human serotonin transporter by human alpha-synuclein. Eur J Neurosci 24:55-64.

Wislet-Gendebien S, D'Souza C, Kawarai T, St George-Hyslop P, Westaway D, Fraser P, Tandon A (2006) Cytosolic proteins regulate alpha-synuclein dissociation from presynaptic membranes. J Biol Chem 281:32148-32155.

Wislet-Gendebien S, Visanji NP, Whitehead SN, Marsilio D, Hou W, Figeys D, Fraser PE, Bennett SA, Tandon A (2008) Differential regulation of wild-type and mutant alpha-synuclein binding to synaptic membranes by cytosolic factors. BMC Neurosci 9:92.

Woods WS, Boettcher JM, Zhou DH, Kloepper KD, Hartman KL, Ladror DT, Qi Z, Rienstra CM, George JM (2007) Conformation-specific binding of alpha-synuclein to novel protein partners detected by phage display and NMR spectroscopy. J Biol Chem 282:34555-34567.

Xie W, Li X, Li C, Zhu W, Jankovic J, Le W (2010) Proteasome inhibition modeling nigral neuron degeneration in Parkinson's disease. J Neurochem 115:188-199.

Xiong N, Huang J, Zhang Z, Zhang Z, Xiong J, Liu X, Jia M, Wang F, Chen C, Cao X, Liang Z, Sun S, Lin Z, Wang T (2009) Stereotaxical infusion of rotenone: a reliable rodent model for Parkinson's disease. PLoS One 4:e7878.

Xu J, Kao SY, Lee FJ, Song W, Jin LW, Yankner BA (2002) Dopamine-dependent neurotoxicity of alpha-synuclein: a mechanism for selective neurodegeneration in Parkinson disease. Nat Med 8:600-606.

Zhang L, Zhang C, Zhu Y, Cai Q, Chan P, Ueda K, Yu S, Yang H (2008) Semi-quantitative analysis of alpha-synuclein in subcellular pools of rat brain neurons: an immunogold electron microscopic study using a C-terminal specific monoclonal antibody. Brain Res 1244:40-52.

Zhou W, Schaack J, Zawada WM, Freed CR (2002) Overexpression of human alpha-synuclein causes dopamine neuron death in primary human mesencephalic culture. Brain Res 926:42-50.

Zhu M, Li J, Fink AL (2003) The association of alpha-synuclein with membranes affects bilayer structure, stability, and fibril formation. J Biol Chem 278:40186-40197.

8

Effects of Alpha-Synuclein on Cellular Homeostasis

Kostas Vekrellis, Georgia Minakaki and Evangelia Emmanouilidou
Department of Neurosciences, Biomedical Research Foundation of the Academy of Athens
Greece

1. Introduction

1.1 α-synuclein: A "leading act" in the synapse

α-Synuclein is a relatively abundant 140-residue neuronal protein physiologically found in presynaptic neuronal terminals (Abeliovich et al., 2000; Spillantini, Crowther, Jakes, Hasegawa, & Goedert, 1998; Wacker, Zareie, Fong, Sarikaya, & Muchowski, 2004). α-synuclein belongs to a highly conserved family of proteins which includes β- and γ-synucleins. It is an intrinsically unfolded, or natively unfolded, protein, meaning that in its purified form at neutral pH it lacks an ordered secondary or tertiary structure (Trojanowski & Lee, 1998). Three missense point mutations (A53T, A30P and E46K) have been identified in families with autosomal dominant Parkinson's disease (PD) (Figure 1) (Chartier-Harlin et al., 2004; Kruger et al., 1998; Polymeropoulos et al., 1997). In addition, duplications and triplications in the gene encoding for α-synuclein have been shown to cause rare familial forms of PD, suggesting that the levels of the protein are critical in the pathogenesis of the disease (Singleton et al., 2003; Zarranz et al., 2004). Over-expression of mutant α-synuclein in transgenic mice under various promoters presents only certain aspects of PD and some have been shown to lead to neurodegeneration (reviewed in Sulzer, 2010). Knockout mice for α-synuclein do not exhibit severe neuropathological alterations but, at least in the nigrostriatal dopaminergic system, they show an enhancement of response to paired electrical stimuli, suggesting that α-synuclein, normally, negatively controls neurotransmitter release.

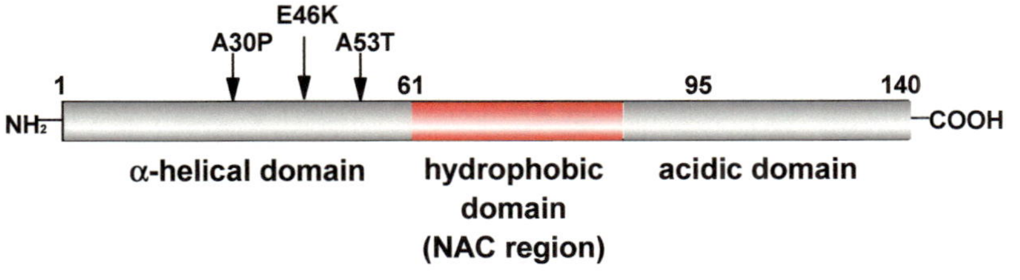

Fig. 1. Schematic representation of α-synuclein showing the basic regions of the protein and the point mutations that have been linked with familial PD.

With respect to neurotransmission, it has been recently reported that excessive α-synuclein induces a series of pathologic changes, including deficits in neurotransmitter release. In a recent study, Nemani et al. (2010) showed that following only modest increases in α-synuclein, an inhibition of neurotransmitter release was observed in glutamatergic hippocampal pyramidal neurons and mesencephalic dopaminergic neurons (Nemani et al., 2010). This inhibition appeared to be a consequence of the failure to get recycling vesicles clustered near synaptic release sites. In a different study, Scott et al. (2010) demonstrated that α-synuclein can reduce the levels of several critical presynaptic proteins involved in exocytosis and endocytosis (Scott et al., 2010). The group further observed significant reductions in miniEPSC frequency, diminished presynaptic exocytosis and altered vesicle size by EM in α-synuclein-overexpressing neurons.

A role of α-synuclein in the integrity of the SNARE complex was also reported by Darios et al., (2010) who showed that α-synuclein sequesters arachidonic acid and thereby blocks the activation of SNARE protein interactions (Darios et al., 2010). Precisely how increased α-synuclein expression impairs clustering of vesicles near the synapse remains to be elucidated. However, α-synuclein has been found to rescue the disassembly of the SNARE complex and the degeneration of neuritic terminals associated with lack of the presynaptic protein Cystein String Protein-α (CSP- α), by facilitating the assembly of SNARE complexes that mediate vesicle fusion at presynaptic terminals. By directly examining SNARE assembly, Burré et al (2010) showed that this facilitating process depends on synaptic activity and propose that the association of α-synuclein with VAMP may ultimately mediate the process (Burré et al., 2010). Furthermore, the same group generated α-, β-, and γ-synuclein triple knockout mice, which as they aged, made SNARE complexes less, displayed a significant age-dependent decrease in synaptobrevin-2 and perished prematurely. The role of synucleins was fully dispensable in young animals but became essential in aged ones, which suggests that α-synuclein maintains normal synaptic function during aging. Moreover, the authors found that restoring expression of α-synuclein in cultured neurons from the triple knockout mice helped re-establish SNARE complexes, and did so in a dose-dependent way.

Further arguing for a physiological role of synucleins in synaptic transmission, synuclein null mice lacking α-, β-, and γ-synucleins generated by Greten–Harison et al. (2010), exhibited prominent age-dependent changes in synaptic protein composition and axonal structure that led to severe neuronal dysfunction in the central nervous system and neuronal death (Greten-Harrison et al., 2010). Importantly, in the hippocampus, young synuclein null mice exhibited increased basic transmission which could be rescued with both mouse and human α-synuclein transgenes, confirming that synucleins affect basal neurotransmission. In agreement with a role for α-synuclein in synaptic function, Keri et al. (2010) reported impaired learning in people who have two copies of the α-synuclein gene but lack PD-like symptoms (Keri, Moustafa, Myers, Benedek, & Gluck, 2010). Compared to age-matched volunteers whose α-synuclein was normal, the group reported that the gene duplication carriers showed defects in learning. α-Synuclein also binds and inactivates phospholipase D2, and could thus influence synaptic membrane biogenesis through phosphatidic acid metabolism.

Overall, distinct α-synuclein concentration thresholds seem to be permissive for synapse function, raising the question of whether early signs of neurodegenerative pathology reflect a disturbance in synaptic density homeostasis. Targeting synaptic membrane proteins that tend to interact with α-synuclein and affect membrane trafficking under physiological conditions, could present a pool of potential molecular therapeutic targets.

1.2 α-Synuclein toxic species: The search goes on

The feature of α-synuclein that has attracted the most attention is its distinctive propensity to aggregate *in vitro*, through a sequence of conversion from a natively unfolded monomeric form to a fibrillar form; a phenomenon associated with a conformational change from random coil to β-pleeted sheet. Aggregated insoluble α-synuclein is the major constituent of cytoplasmic inclusions termed Lewy bodies and Lewy neurites, which are the pathological hallmarks of inherited and sporadic PD (Spillantini et al., 1998). The presence of Lewy Bodies in the substantia nigra is diagnostic for PD, but α-synuclein pathology is also encountered in other brain regions and may account for the wide range of non-motor symptoms observed (Bate, Gentleman, & Williams, 2010).

Although the exact aberrant function of α-synuclein that links it to neurodegeneration is not known, the weight of the evidence suggests that the process of its conversion to toxic oligomers is involved, hence has been the subject of extensive research. Similar to amyloid beta (Aβ), attention has recently shifted from the insoluble amyloid fibrils to the soluble oligomeric intermediates, or protofibrils, in the α-synuclein aggregation process. There is evidence that the soluble oligomeric protofibrils, and not the mature fibrils, are the toxic species. Although the question is still open (Waxman & Giasson, 2009), data obtained in three established model systems for PD, such as primary neurons, C. elegans, and Drosophila, show a strong correlation between α-synuclein oligomers, neuronal toxicity, and behavioral defects (Karpinar et al., 2009), further sustaining a pathogenic role for α-synuclein oligomers in PD. The A30P and A53T mutations of α-synuclein associated with familial forms of PD both promote protofibril formation relative to wild type α-synuclein (J. Li, Uversky, & Fink, 2001; Rochet, Conway, & Lansbury, 2000). The A30P mutation was also shown to delay the formation of amyloid fibrils relative to the wild type protein, suggesting that α-synuclein protofibrils rather than fibrils may be the pathogenic species (Conway et al., 2000). In addition, the presence of soluble protofibrilar species, when compared to frank fibrillar inclusions or monomers, correlates better temporally with death in cellular and *in vivo* models (Danzer et al., 2007; Emmanouilidou, Stefanis, & Vekrellis, 2010; Kayed et al., 2003).

Several α-synuclein post-translational modifications lead to the formation of stable oligomers. These include nitration, oxidation, phosphorylation, and interaction with iron. Oxidative modification of α-synuclein via dopamine adducts may facilitate aggregation (Conway, Rochet, Bieganski, & Lansbury, 2001). Dopamine and its metabolites modulate differently the stability of soluble oligomers and mature fibrils and act as inhibitors of the conversion of protofibrils to fibrils, thus favouring protofibril accumulation (Follmer et al., 2007; Sultzer, Gray, Gunay, Wheatley, & Mahler, 2001). In a recent report Tsika et al. (2010) showed that, despite similarities in basic biochemical properties, α-synuclein oligomeric intermediates obtained from different neural regions demonstrated unexpected divergence in promoting α-synuclein amyloid fibril formation and toxicity (Tsika et al., 2010). This is in agreement with the fact that despite the ubiquitous expression of α-synuclein throughout the CNS, Lewy bodies are found in certain susceptible neuronal subtypes of specific brain nuclei (Braak, Rub, & Del Tredici, 2003).

A possible mechanism by which oligomers could be toxic is through the disruption and permeabilization of cellular membranes (Lashuel et al., 2002; Volles et al., 2001). Oligomeric α-synuclein has been shown to permeabilize negatively charged synthetic phospholipid vesicles (Volles et al., 2001; Zhu, Li, & Fink, 2003). Soluble oligomers are considered to be cytotoxic and to disrupt cellular membranes, by forming pore-like complexes in the bilayer in a manner similar to bacterial pore forming toxins (Lashuel & Hirling, 2006). The pore formation, inducing disruption of cellular ion homeostasis, may be responsible for the neurotoxic effect (Volles et al., 2001). So far, it has been demonstrated that α-synuclein regulates calcium entry pathways and, consequently, that abnormal α-synuclein levels may promote neuronal damage through disregulation of calcium homeostasis. However, to date, there has been very limited evidence that supports the pore formation by cell-produced α-synuclein oligomers.

Studies aiming to identify the potential toxic species are also based primarily on experiments in which oligomerization of the protein is forced *in vitro* (Danzer et al., 2007; Goldberg & Lansbury, 2000). Recently, a study by the Masliah group in UCSD (2011) using a rat lentiviral system showed that only those mutations of α-synuclein that could cause the formation of soluble oligomers could also confer toxicity to dopaminergic neurons by disturbing the plasma membrane (Winner et al., 2011). Other proposed mechanisms through which these oligomers can confer cell death include alterations in the lysosomal-dependent autophagy pathway (Xilouri, Vogiatzi, Vekrellis, & Stefanis, 2008) and mitochondrial dysfunction (Martin et al., 2006). Evidence on a role of phosphorylation in the oligomerization and neurotoxicity of α-synuclein has also been provided (Cavallarin, Vicario, & Negro 2010). It has been shown that α-synuclein is heavily phosphorylated in Lewy bodies found in patients with synucleinopathies but studies have disagreed about whether this phosphorylation promotes or prevents neurotoxicity (Azeredo da Silveira et al., 2009) because α-synuclein carries a number of potential phosphorylation sites. Phosphorylation of α-synuclein at Ser129 strongly modulates interactions between α-synuclein and synphilin-1 and the formation of inclusions. Soluble α-synuclein oligomeric species are increased by phosphorylation at Ser129 (Chen et al., 2009). Recently, Paleologou et al., (2010) demonstrated that phosphorylation of α-synuclein at Ser87 is elevated in brain extracts from cases of dementia with Lewy bodies (DLB), multiple system atrophy, and from several mouse models of synucleinopathy where most of the modified protein was associated with membranes (Paleologou et al., 2010). The authors also showed that modifications at Ser87 affect both α-synuclein's pathological aggregation and its normal interaction with cell membranes.

Finally, oligomeric α-synuclein can induce microglia activation (Zhang et al., 2005) and cause subsequent neuro-inflammation which aggravates DA neuronal loss (Koprich, Reske-Nielsen, Mithal, & Isacson, 2008).

2. Effects of intracellular α-synuclein on cellular homeostasis

Physiologic function of the cell requires proper and continuous functioning of cellular surveillance mechanisms that identify and clear unwanted adducts in the cell interior. Intracellular buildup of aberrant components disturbs cellular homeostasis ultimately leading to cell death. Chaperones and proteolytic systems are responsible for cellular quality control, and defects in both systems have been involved in PD pathogenesis. Molecular chaperones is a highly conserved class of proteins that are responsible for the proper folding of macromolecules and the refolding of proteins that have become misfolded as a result of cellular stress (Muchowski & Wacker, 2005). As mentioned above, PD is characterized by the accumulation of misfolded α-synuclein in intraneuronal inclusions called Lewy bodies, and several studies have suggested that failure of chaperone-mediated protection may enhance α-synuclein aggregation and neurotoxicity (Ali, Kitay, & Zhai; Muchowski & Wacker, 2005). Changes in the two major intracellular proteolytic systems, the ubiquitin-proteasome system (UPS) and the lysosome-autophagy system, are widely considered to contribute to the accumulation of aggregated α-synuclein species that in turn affect vital cellular pathways and lead to cell death. Dysfunctions in macroautophagy and chaperone-mediated autophagy, the two main lysosomal degradation systems, have been linked with intracellular α-synuclein accumulation in several studies using both cellular and animal models (Cuervo, Wong, & Martinez-Vicente, 2010; Xilouri & Stefanis, 2011). In this manuscript, we will preferentially focus on the impact of α-synuclein burden on the UPS as a potential pathway to neurodegeneration.

2.1 The proteasome: Structure, regulation and proteolytic function

The ubiquitin-proteasome system (UPS) is a major system for intracellular protein degradation, a complex and tightly regulated process (Goldberg et al., 2003). Protein degradation through the UPS pathway consists of two discrete and successive steps. The first step is ubiquitylation, a process through which the small protein ubiquitin is covalently attached to surface-exposed lysine residues of the target protein to be degradated (Glickman & Ciechanover, 2002). Ubiquitin is a highly evolutionarily conserved 76-residue polypeptide that is abundantly found in the cell cytoplasm. Ubiquitylation is accomblished via a three-step cascade mechanism where each step is catalyzed by ubiquitin-activating (E1), ubiquitin-conjugating (E2) and ubiquitin-ligase (E3) enzymes. Once the initial ubiquitin is conjugated, polyubiquitylation of the substrate occurs through the sequential transfer of ubiquitin molecules, thus forming an ubiquitin chain. The minimum signal for UPS-mediated proteolytic degradation is a chain of four ubiquitin moieties (Gallastegui & Groll; Glickman & Ciechanover, 2002; Layfield et al., 2001). In the second step of the degradation process, this poly-ubiquitin chain is recognized by the proteolytic core engine of the UPS, the 26S proteasome complex, which in turn degrades the substrate protein into defined oligopeptides with release of free and reusable ubiquitin. The removal of the ubiquitin tag is mediated by ubiquitin recycling enzymes (Ardley & Robinson, 2005; Glickman & Ciechanover, 2002).

The 26S proteasome is a 2-2.5 MDa proteolytic enzyme that is highly conserved among eukaryotes (Besche, Haas, Gygi, & Goldberg, 2009). It comprises two multimeric protein complexes, the 20S core particle, where actual proteolysis occurs, and two 19S regulatory particles, that regulate the function of the 20S (Benaroudj, Zwickl, Seemuller, Baumeister, & Goldberg, 2003; Crews, 2003; Goldberg et al., 2003). Each one of the two regulatory units attach to the outer surface of the core particle. The 20S core complex is a ~700 kDa barrel-shaped structure made up of four stacked hetero-heptameric rings: two identical outer rings consisting of α-type subunits and two identical inner rings consisting of β-type subunits. Each of the β-rings possesses three different catalytic activities for cleavage after specific amino acids. The 19S regulatory particle, also known as the PA700 particle, caps one or both ends of the 20S cylinder and is itself composed of two subcomplexes, the lid and the base, that have distinct regulatory functions. The base complex is thought to mediate the ATP-dependent unfolding of protein substrates and their translocation to the 20S chamber through a narrow gated pore channel. This gate is formed by the interlacing N-termini of the α subunits thereby preventing nonspecific degradation of cellular proteins. The lid complex

is responsible for the initial recognition, binding and de-ubiquitination of the ubiquitin-tagged polypeptides (Benaroudj et al., 2003; Besche et al., 2009; Glickman & Ciechanover, 2002).
Perhaps the most intriguing question is how the proteasome achieves its high specificity and selectivity. Collective data suggest that two distinct groups of proteins, the E3 ligases and the proteasome ancillary proteins, determine the proteasome specificity through control of the substrate recognition process (Glickman & Ciechanover, 2002). As already mentioned, E3s catalyze substrate recognition prior to their ubiquitination. Such recognition can be accomplished by direct binding of substrates to the appropriate E3 enzyme via their NH_2-terminal residue (the N-end rule pathway). However, in most cases indirect pathways facilitate protein recognition. Alternative modes of recognition include post-translational modifications or allosteric activation of the E3 enzyme, phosphorylation of the substrate and/or E3s, or changes in the conformation state of the substrate protein. Ancillary proteins, such as chaperone proteins or transcription factors, also facilitate substrate recognition through a variety of mechanisms (Glickman & Ciechanover, 2002).
Proteasome regulation is tightly controlled by the 19S complex. The base subcomplex of the 19S particle consists of six different ATPase subunits (Rpts1-6) that promote gate opening upon ATP binding (Demartino & Gillette, 2007). This process also requires binding of the C-terminal tails of Rpt1, Rpt3 and Rpt5 to the 20S through a specific conserved sequence motif (HbYX motif). Interestingly, binding of the C-terminus of Rpt2 acts as a potent repressor of substrate accessibility into the 20S particle. The ATPases Rpt4 and Rpt6 are not involved in gate opening; rather they are thought to regulate the ordered assembly of the 19S complex via binding of their C-terminus tail with external chaperone proteins. Finally, the UPS system can also be regulated at the level of proteasomal activity either by enhancing the catalytic activities or by altering the specificity of the cleavage sites (Gallastegui & Groll, 2010). Alternatively, regulator non-ATPase complexes, such as the PA28 activator, can interact with the one end of the 20S enhancing the overall proteolytic activity of the proteasome, possibly by removing the occlusion at the chamber pore. Since these activators do not bind to polyubiquitin chains, their assembly into the 19S/20S complex results in ubiquitin-independent proteolysis (Demartino & Gillette, 2007).

2.2 The impact of protein aggregation on the UPS

Neurodegenerative diseases like Parkinson's disease, Alzheimer's disease, Huntington's disease and others share a common neuropathological characteristic which is the aggregation of abnormal proteins that fold improperly and impair neuronal function. Accumulation of aberrant proteins could be achieved by several mechanisms including mutations, overproduction or impairment of their clearance. Clearly, such accumulations are indicative of a malfunction of the process of protein turnover since they are not found in healthy individuals. Proteolysis is an important cellular process which involves the tightly regulated removal of unwanted proteins. The ubiquitin-proteasome system (UPS) eliminates mutated or abnormally folded proteins by degradation to prevent their accumulation in the cell and the subsequent formation of inclusion bodies. Most likely, dysfunction of the UPS contributes to the neuropathogenesis of various types of conformational diseases such as the ones mentioned above. It is plausible that failure of protein degradation from the UPS can lead to imbalance in protein homeostasis that could in turn promote the toxic accumulation of proteins which is detrimental for neuronal viability (Sherman & Goldberg, 2001). It is interesting that in postmortem studies proteasomal activity was significantly reduced in the brain of PD patients (McNaught, Perl, Brownell, & Olanow, 2004).

A rather important question still under investigation is why protein quality control mechanisms, such as the UPS, fail to keep cells free from misfolded proteins. Recent evidence clearly suggests that there is a reciprocal relationship between protein aggregation and the UPS, meaning that one can influence the other. The selective accumulation of oligomeric-prone proteins could be explained by the inability of the UPS to cope with these proteins once their levels have been increased as a consequence of cellular stress. In an elegant study, Bence, et al. reported that protein aggregation directly impaired the function of the UPS (Bence, Sampat, & Kopito, 2001). They demonstrated that expression of two aggregation-prone proteins, the DF508 mutant of cystic fibrosis conductance regulator (CFTR) and an N-terminal fragment of Huntingtin with an expanded polyglutamine repeat (Q103), in Human Embruonic Kidney (HEK) cells was associated with accumulation of the artificial fluorescent proteasome substrate GFPu. Moreover, the authors reported that fluorescence was proportional to the inclusion size, indicating that larger inclusions were associated with more intense proteasome dysfunction. Transient expression of two unrelated aggregation-prone proteins, a huntingtin fragment containing a pathogenic polyglutamine repeat and a folding mutant of cystic fibrosis transmembrane conductance regulator, caused nearly complete inhibition of the UPS.

Because of the central role of ubiquitin-dependent proteolysis in regulating fundamental cellular events such as cell division and apoptosis, these data suggest a potential mechanism linking protein aggregation to cellular disregulation and cell death. The exact species of the aggregate-prone proteins responsible for the dysfunction of the proteasome are unknown. For example, we have not found evidence for accumulation of total α-synuclein after proteasomal inhibition following either pharmacologic treatment or overexpression of the protein, in the cellular systems that we have used (Emmanouilidou, Stefanis et al., 2010; Rideout, Larsen, Sulzer, & Stefanis, 2001; Rideout & Stefanis, 2002). However, α-synuclein does seem to be turned over by the proteasome in other experimental settings (Tofaris, Razzaq, Ghetti, Lilley, & Spillantini, 2003; Webb, Ravikumar, Atkins, Skepper, & Rubinsztein, 2003). Similarly, studies suggest that expanded polyglutamine regions are by themselves intrinsically resistant to degradation by purified proteasomes (Venkatraman, Wetzel, Tanaka, Nukina, & Goldberg, 2004), although not all studies agree to that (Michalik & Van Broeckhoven, 2004).

Although these results suggest that inclusions are the primary deleterious species causing proteasomal dysfunction, it is also possible that other species of the aggregation process, rather than the inclusions themselves, are responsible for inhibition especially if proteasome inhibition itself accelerates inclusion formation. In this respect, *in vitro* studies show that α-synuclein, especially the oligomeric-aggregated conformation, can directly inhibit proteasomal function (Lindersson et al., 2004). These data suggest that the inhibition of proteasomal function observed in the cellular systems with mutant α-synuclein overexpression, are likely due to soluble oligomeric forms of the protein. Clearly, well-formed inclusions are unlikely to interact with the proteasome as substrates. They may, however, sequester chaperones and proteasomes that are recruited during the increased effort of the cell to degrade the misfolded proteins. This may eventually lead to the depletion of the proteasome and of other UPS components from their usual site of action and subsequent UPS dysfunction. Consistent with this idea, Jana NR., et al. 2001 showed that expression of N-terminal Huntingtin with expanded polyglutamine repeats in cells and in transgenic animals led to the incorporation of the 20S proteasome in inclusions (Jana, Zemskov, Wang, & Nukina, 2001). Although the UPS appears as a very attractive option for therapeutic intervention in neurodegenerative diseases, the confirmation of the identity of the toxic proteins species involved remain unresolved. Importantly, as yet there are no strong *in vivo* data linking proteasome inhibition to cellular toxicity.

2.3 α-synuclein impairs UPS function

Several lines of evidence suggest that dysfunction of protein degradation through the UPS may be involved in PD-related neurodegeneration (Lang-Rollin, Rideout, & Stefanis, 2003). *In vivo,* data from studies using the *gad* mouse model directly support this statement. The *gad* mouse lacks expression of murine UCH-L1, a deubiquitinating E3 ligase that is highly abundant in neuronal cells. UCH-L1 has been found in Lewy inclusions which characterize the PD pathology (Lowe, McDermott, Landon, Mayer, & Wilkinson, 1990). These mice display neuronal degeneration with progressive accumulation of ubiquitin-positive inclusions into sensory and motor neurons (Saigoh et al., 1999). The two components of the UPS, UCH-L1 and parkin, are genetically implicated with familial PD (Kitada et al., 1998). Additionally, α-synuclein and DJ-1, two key proteins in PD pathogenesis, have been shown to be degraded by the UPS (Ardley & Robinson, 2005; Miller & Wilson, 2003; Snyder et al., 2003).

A great number of studies propose a link between α-synuclein and the UPS system, although it remains controversial whether the proteasome is responsible for the degradation of this protein (Bennett et al., 1999; Rideout et al., 2001). *In vitro* work has demonstrated that the expression of mutant or wild type α-synuclein is sufficient to cause proteasomal inhibition in neuronal cell culture systems (Petrucelli et al., 2002; Smith et al., 2005; Snyder et al., 2003; Stefanis, Larsen, Rideout, Sulzer, & Greene, 2001; Tanaka et al., 2001). In accordance with these data, α-synuclein can directly bind to Rpt5 *in vitro,* a subunit of the 19S regulatory particle (Ghee, Melki, Michot, & Mallet, 2005). In most of the cases, aggregated or oligomeric α-synuclein had a stronger effect on proteasome function compared with the monomeric form of the protein (Lindersson et al., 2004; Snyder et al., 2003). However, Martin-Clemente *et al.* failed to show UPS inhibition in PC12 cells overexpressing mutant α-synuclein or in α-synuclein transgenic mice (Martin-Clemente et al., 2004).

Given the complexity of the mechanism through which α-synuclein affects proteasome function, we have addressed, in a cellular context, the identity of α-synuclein species that are implicated in UPS dysfunction (Emmanouilidou, Stefanis et al., 2010). We have shown that stable overexpression of wild type or A53T mutant α-synuclein in PC12 cells significantly reduces all proteasome activities (chymotrypsin-like, trypsin-like and caspase-like activities). In this study, the assessment of proteasome activity was performed in functional 26S proteasomes isolated by size exclusion chromatography (SEC) from cell extracts rather than analysing crude cell lysates. This method provides increased accuracy in the measurement of enzymatic activity since it precludes any interference from other common proteinases present in the cell lysate (Rodgers & Dean, 2003). The observed proteasome inhibition was not due to decreased levels of proteasome subunits or abnormal assembly of the complex. Separation of cytosolic proteins by SEC showed that a small amount of α-synuclein (corresponding only to 0.5% of the total α-synuclein contained in the lysate) co-eluted in the 26S proteasome-containing fractions. Ultrafiltration experiments verified the presence of α-synuclein in these high MW fractions. This co-elution was shown to be specific for α-synuclein and not an artifact of mere protein overexpression or the result of producing high levels of an aggregation-prone protein in the cell model used (Emmanouilidou, Stefanis et al., 2010).

Non-denaturing gel electrophoresis revealed that the α-synuclein co-eluting with the 26S proteasome was oligomeric in nature, migrating between 150 and 450 kDa (Emmanouilidou, Stefanis et al., 2010). Importantly, these species were detected in the cortex homogenates of homozygous transgenic mice which express the human A53T α-synuclein under the control of the prion promoter (Giasson et al., 2002). Further proving the oligomeric state of these specific species, treatment of the cell lysates with Congo Red (CR), a compound known to disrupt preformed oligomeric/aggregated forms of various proteins (Carter & Chou, 1998), significantly reduced α-synuclein burden in the 26S proteasome fractions. In doing so, CR treatment restored the proteasome activity without interfering with the assembly of the 26S complex. In another approach, treatment with the heat shock protein inducer, geldanamycin, resulted in the reduction of α-synuclein species from the proteasome fractions. Again, removal of the proteasome-associated oligomeric α-synuclein led to restoration of proteasome activity (Emmanouilidou, Stefanis et al., 2010). Application of selective proteasomal and lysosomal inhibitors further demonstrated that these specific α-synuclein oligomers are indeed degraded by the proteasome but not the lysosome. Overall, these data indicated that specific oligomeric α-synuclein species of intermediate size are targeted to, and impair the 26S proteasome possibly through a functional interaction.

What this interaction involves is still unclear (Figure 2). One possibility could be the direct binding of α-synuclein oligomers to the active sites of the 20S β-subunits. However, this mechanism would require translocation of the oligomers into the catalytic cylinder through a narrow open-gated channel (Pickart & Cohen, 2004). Alternatively, α-synuclein oligomers may interfere with processes controlled by the 19S complex. Our data (Emmanouilidou, Stefanis et al., 2010) show that proteasome assembly is not affected by the presence of such species. 19S inhibition may involve a physical interaction between α-synuclein and a 19S subunit (Ghee et al., 2005). It is possible that α-synuclein oligomers are targeted to the 26S proteasome by means of their aberrant conformation. In line with this notion, α-synuclein present in the proteasome-enriched fractions lacks ubiquitylation, the targeting signal for degradation via the UPS system (Emmanouilidou, Stefanis et al.). As reported previously, misfolded polypeptides are recognized by the 26S proteasome by the help of certain molecular chaperones (Benaroudj et al., 2003; Glickman & Ciechanover, 2002). In this context, the bulky α-synuclein oligomers may prevent 19S-mediated protein unfolding and translocation due to steric hindrance preventing further interactions of other substrates with the proteasome. Such an idea has also been suggested in the case of oligomeric PrP (Kristiansen et al., 2007). Recently, Machiya Y et al. (2010) showed that Ser-129-phosphorylated α-synuclein is targeted to the proteasome pathway in an ubiquitin-independent manner, in addition to undergoing dephosphorylation (Machiya et al., 2010). Thus, the proteasome pathway may also have a role in the biogenesis of Ser-129-phosphorylated α-synuclein-rich LBs.

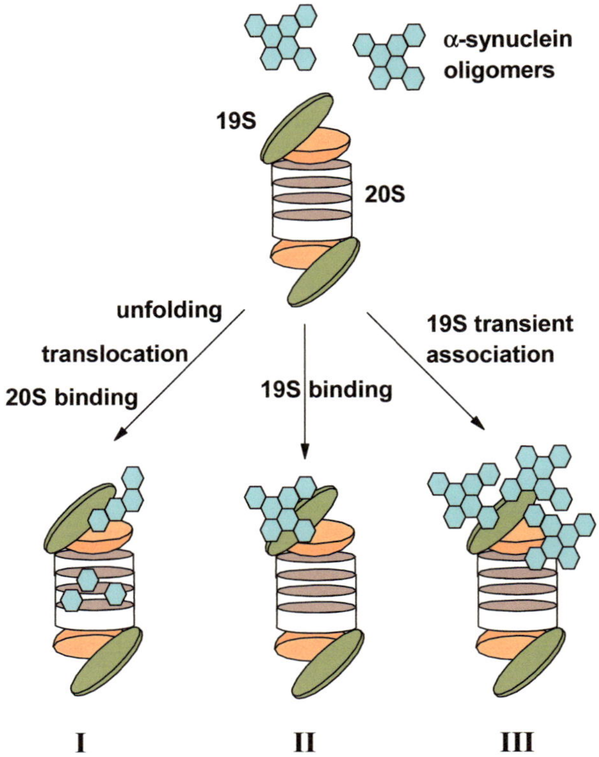

Fig. 2. Schematic illustration of the possible interaction between α-synuclein and the 26S proteasome. α-synuclein can gain access into the interior of the 20S champer and bind to one or more of the catalytic β-subunits. Such changes would interfere with the active site(s) thus decreasing the overall proteolytic activity of the proteasome (I). Alternatively, oligomeric α-synuclein can directly bind to a subunit of the 19S complex thereby inhibiting substrate recognition or gate opening (II). Finally, α-synuclein oligomers can transiently interact with the 19S particle and its function possibly by preventing 19S subunits from obtaining the appropriate conformation. This "clogging" of the 19S cap would result in the cytoplasmic accumulation of other proteins due to their deficient degradation (III).

3. Effects of extracellular α-synuclein on cellular homeostasis

3.1 α-synuclein is detected in biological fluids

Since α-synuclein lacks a signal peptide targeting the protein for ER-mediated exocytosis, it was considered to be primarily localized in the cytoplasm where it would exert its pathogenic effects. However, a number of studies suggest that α-synuclein can be secreted in the medium of cultured cells and is detectable in human biological fluids such as CSF and plasma of PD patients and controls. The first studies to demonstrate detection of α-synuclein in the CSF and plasma utilized biochemical techniques such as immunoprecipitation and western blotting in a small number of human samples (Borghi et al., 2000; El-Agnaf et al., 2003). However, these initial studies failed to show a significant difference in the levels of α-synuclein between PD and healthy subjects.

In an attempt to assess the applicability of α-synuclein concentration in biological fluids as a biomarker for PD, α-synuclein was measured by specific ELISAs that provide higher sensitivity and accuracy. Some of these studies (Mollenhauer et al., 2008; Tokuda et al., 2006), but not all (Ohrfelt et al., 2009), reported significant differences in the levels of α-synuclein in PD and control samples. Since there is substantial evidence indicating that α-synuclein aggregation is central in PD pathogenesis, some other studies focus on the quantification of α-synuclein oligomers in CSF (Tokuda et al., 2010) or plasma (El-Agnaf et al., 2006) using oligomer-specific ELISAs. Overall, there is great variability in the amount of α-synuclein quantified in either blood plasma or CSF. Two basic reasons could account for this discrepancy. First, the ELISA system employed for the measurement of α-synuclein varies between groups in terms of both the antibodies and the detection method used. This results in differences in the specificity and the sensitivity of the measurement. Second, each group does not follow similar protocols for sample collection and processing. Protein integrity and erythrocyte contamination are important parameters related to sample acquisition and processing and should be carefully monitored to assure valid assessment of α-synuclein in biological fluids. While future work is required to establish a correlation between disease and α-synuclein levels in biological fluids, α-synuclein remains an appealing protein to be used as a diagnostic marker for PD.

3.2 Mechanism of α-synuclein release

Numerous studies employing a variety of cell systems reveal a dynamic network of molecular communication between cells, involving secretion. Deciphering the components of this network as well as their biological significance represents a major challenge in the field of neurodegeneration in particular.

In this respect, α-synuclein has been shown to be released from neuronal cells in culture independently of the expression method used; stable overexpression (El-Agnaf et al., 2003), inducible overexpression (Emmanouilidou, Melachroinou et al., 2010), transient transfection (Sung et al., 2005) or viral-mediated expression (H. J. Lee, Patel, & Lee, 2005). The presence of α-synuclein in the conditioned media (CM) of the α-synuclein-expressing cells reflects physiologic secretion of the protein and not an artifact of membrane leakage, since other abundant cytoplasmic proteins are not detected in the CM. The secretion of α-synuclein has been reported to be insensitive to brefeldin A (H. J. Lee et al., 2005), suggesting that it is secreted via an ER/Golgi-independent pathway. In accordance with a vesicular mechanism of secretion, a portion of intracellular α-synuclein has been found in the lumen of vesicles from rat brain homogenates, rat embryonic cortical neurons and human neuroblastoma cells (H. J. Lee et al., 2005). Electron microscopy and density gradient ultracentrifugation suggested that the vesicles containing α-synuclein have morphologies and sedimentation properties similar to the dense core vesicles (H. J. Lee et al., 2005), but their exact identities remain unknown.

In a recent study, treatment of MES cells in culture with aggregated recombinant α-synuclein results in the internalization of the protein which is subsequently released in the extracellular space by rab11a/HSP90-mediated exocytosis (Liu et al., 2009). The mechanism of exocytosis was found to be temperature-sensitive and time-dependent. Part of this internalized protein is also degraded through the lysosomal-endosomal pathway (Liu et al., 2009). Indeed, we recently demonstrated that a non-classical secretory pathway is involved in the physiological and constitutive release of α-synuclein in the extracellular space

(Emmanouilidou, Melachroinou et al., 2010). In this study, α-synuclein was exported in a calcium-dependent manner in association with externalized membrane vesicles that involved in the endocytic pathway (Figure 3).

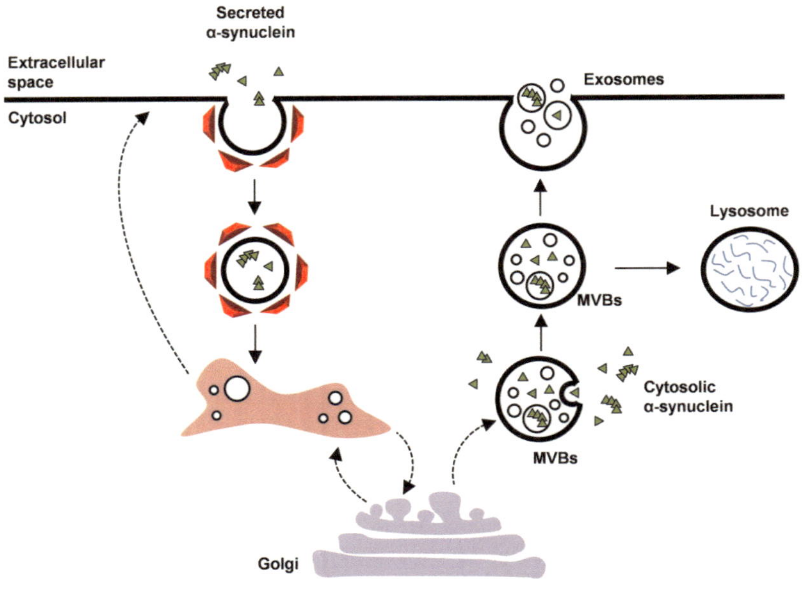

Fig. 3. α-Synuclein transportation through the endocytic pathway. Along with membrane proteins, secreted α-synuclein can enter the cell via endocytosis of clathrin-coated vesicles which fuse with early endosomes. In early endosomes, protein material is either recycled back to the plasma membrane or sorted to MVBs. Cytoplasmic α-synuclein can also enter MVBs at this point via inward budding of the limiting membrane of these vesicles. For protein degradation, MVBs fuse with lysosomes. Alternatively, MVBs can fuse with the plasma membrane releasing their content in the extracellular space as exosomes.

In the first step of the endocytic pathway (Figure 3) internalized proteins via clathrin-coated vesicles are delivered to early endosomes. Proteins are then either recycled back to the plasma membrane or accumulate in multivesicular endosomes, commonly called multivesicular bodies (MVBs). Proteins destined for degradation are sorted into small (40-100 nm in diameter) intraluminal vesicles (ILVs) that are generated by inward budding from the limiting membrane of MVBs (Fevrier & Raposo, 2004; Keller, Sanderson, Stoeck, & Altevogt, 2006). Degradation of the vesicle-associated proteins and lipids is achieved upon fusion of the MVBs with lysosomes. This process allows the cell to remove certain transmembrane proteins and excessive membranes. Alternatively, MVBs can fuse with the plasma membrane releasing ILVs in the extracellular environment as exosomes (Fevrier & Raposo, 2004; Keller et al., 2006).

Exosomal protein content includes cytosolic proteins, heat shock proteins, tetraspanins and transmembrane proteins; proteins originating from mitochondria, ER or nucleus are excluded (Thery, Zitvogel, & Amigorena, 2002). Exosomes share common characteristics, most important of which is that they are delimited in a cholesterol-rich lipid bi-layer containing cytosolic compounds. Most secreted exosomes contain lipid rafts, a characteristic which signifies selectivity of protein sequestration (Vella, Sharples, Nisbet, Cappai, & Hill, 2008). Interestingly, this bi-layer also carries transmembrane cell adhesion molecules such as integrins, which enable the dynamic communication of the cytoskeleton with the extracellular matrix (ECM) and neighboring cells. The origin of exosomes led to the suggestion that this mechanism was an alternative to autophagic degradation, another means of "discarding" unwanted cytosolic material. Recently, it was found that under certain conditions, exosomes can be biologically active entities, important for intercellular communication (Valadi et al., 2007) and key players in significant biological processes. They are secreted by most cells that have been examined so far including primary neurons (Lachenal et al., 2010). Furthermore, exosomal release by neurons was shown to be dependent on synaptic activity. It is suggested that exosomes could be a mechanism of releasing proteins in the extracellular space in order to be proteolytically processed. Alternatively, exosomes can mediate cell-to-cell communication since they can attach and fuse with membranes of neighbouring target cells transferring exosomal molecules from one cell to another (Thery et al., 2002; Vella et al., 2008). The exosomal pathway thus seems to represent a well-designed mechanism for local and systemic inter-neuronal transfer of information (Smalheiser, 2007).

Several groups have reported that exosomes contain pathological proteins. Biochemical studies from L. Rajendran et al. in 2006 reported that Aβ peptides were indeed found on vesicles positive for specific markers of exosomal identity (Rajendran et al., 2006). This suggested that toxic species of processed Amyloid beta Precursor Protein (APP) are also excreted via exosomes. Most importantly, neuritic plaques are co-localized with exosomal markers, indicating that exosomes are able to act at a distance from their source of generation like amyloidogenic fragments of the APP (Rajendran et al., 2006). Similarly, Fevrier and Raposo demonstrated association of prion protein with exosomes (Fevrier & Raposo, 2004). In this sense, exosomes are the central component of a theory that is starting to gain scientific traction over the past few years. The "Trojan horse" hypothesis is an appealing hypothesis according to which, toxic protein contents of a cell are packed into exosomes, shipped extracellularly and are subsequently received by neighboring cells in the context of cell-to-cell communication (Ghidoni, Benussi, & Binetti, 2008). Upon membrane fusion, exosomal cargo is released and causes spread of disease. Up-regulation of exosome secretion is correlated with conditions that promote protein misfolding and impair proteolysis (Alvarez-Erviti et al.; Eldh et al.; Jang et al.), hence, increase cytosolic cargo of a particular protein. In our study, α-synuclein was shown to be associated with both the exosomal membrane and lumen. Importantly, not only monomeric α-synuclein but also oligomeric forms of the protein were found in our exosomal preparations (Emmanouilidou, Melachroinou et al., 2010), further suggesting that exosomes can indeed carry "potentially toxic" cargo. The finding that α-synuclein can be partly externalized via the exosomal pathway provides a common mechanism for the delivery of a potentially cytotoxic protein in the extracellular space (Figure 3).

Undoubtedly, deciphering networks of intercellular communication is a fascinating field of research. Understanding the physiological mechanisms of exchanging information between cells will allow the identification of new, effective therapeutic targets for late-onset neurodegenerative diseases, including Parkinson's disease. The dynamic nature of neuron-to-neuron interactions leads us to the thought that more enlightening answers are to come from the field of synaptic plasticity and function. So far, data interpretation in most studies focuses on cell-autonomous effects and networks. Perhaps, data interpretation should be realized under the scope of a three-dimensional neuronal interface in order to uncover the moving forces underlying cell content alterations and communication at a systemic level. The exact role and contribution of exosomes in this dynamic interplay remains to be elucidated.

3.3 Pathologic neuronal interplay mediated by α-synuclein?

Recent studies by Desplats et al. demonstrated that neurons overexpressing α-synuclein can transmit the protein to neural precursor cells in tissue culture and in transgenic animals (Desplats et al., 2009). Interestingly, the precursors were shown to readily uptake and propagate α-synuclein oligomers leading to cellular dysfunction as well as to inflammatory responses. Therapeutic strategies directed at reducing the formation and propagation of α-synuclein oligomers might be critical in developing new treatments for PD and DLB. Among them, considerable effort has been devoted in the last few years to promoting the clearance. This can be achieved by increasing lysosomal activity (autophagy) or degradation with immunotherapy or by pharmacologically blocking α-synuclein aggregation with small organic molecules.

Host-to-graft propagation of α-synuclein pathology has recently been demonstrated with the discovery that fetal dopaminergic neurons (derived from multiple, genetically unrelated donors) that had been implanted into PD patients 11–14 years earlier developed Lewy body pathology immunopositive for α-synuclein and thioflavin-S (Kordower, Chu, Hauser, Freeman, & Olanow, 2008; J. Y. Li et al., 2008). It is possible that these inclusions were formed as a result of the "disease environment" of the PD brain. One plausible explanation is that oligomeric α-synuclein was transmitted from the already affected host neurons to healthy implanted fetal neurons, and induced endogenous α-synuclein to misfold. Such an infective process mechanism is supported by the Desplats et al., data and could be an explanation of the step-wise progression of the disease pathology and the involvement of specific neural pathways as suggested by the Braak staging of PD progression (Braak, Del Tredici et al., 2003). Importantly, Patric Brundin and his group recently demonstrated that this process may be indeed involved in the spread of aggregated synuclein in a manner similar to that suggested for prion diseases (J. Y. Li et al., 2008). The group showed *in vivo* and *in vitro* that α-synuclein not only can transfer from one cell to another, but also that the transferred protein can seed aggregation of α-synuclein in recipient cells. Alternatively, the source of "seeding" might be microparticles, like exosomes containing α-synuclein, which following uptake by healthy "acceptors" accelerate aggregation of endogenous α-synuclein.

Collectively, recent data provide good evidence to speculate that α-synuclein exhibits prion-like behaviour. For example, oligomers from both misfolded prion and α-synuclein can "instruct" the misfolding of the normal proteins (Ferreon, Gambin, Lemke, & Deniz, 2009). Therefore it is possible, that α-synuclein is a prion itself that in a misfolded oligomeric conformation can be transmitted to neighbouring healthy neurons, thus extending the disease process. However, the cause of such an infectious spread has to be more multifactorial. The parkinsonian milieu that causes α-synuclein accumulation and extension of pathology is not yet known and could be the result, of a combination of factors. For example, aging, oxidative stress, and inflammation, may contribute to altered metabolism of α-synuclein, resulting in the pathogenesis of sporadic PD. Furthermore, continuous accumulation of misfolded proteins ,which is a common pathological phenomenon in various neurodegenerative disorders, compromises the ability of the cell's proteolytic systems. Impairement of lysosomal and proteasomal protein degradation increases the burden of uncleared, unwanted proteins thus promoting their further accumulation and the development of a self-propagating cycle that eventually leads to cell death. Lysosomal function has been reported to decrease in PD patients (Alvarez-Erviti et al.; Chu, Dodiya, Aebischer, Olanow, & Kordower, 2009) and α-synuclein has been shown to be degraded by the lysosome specific mechanism of chaperone mediated autophagy (Cuervo, Stefanis, Fredenburg, Lansbury, & Sulzer, 2004; Xilouri et al., 2008).

Interestingly, Alvarez-Erviti et al. (2010), recently demonstrated that lysosomal inhibition in cells dramatically increased the intracellular and secreted pools of α-synuclein (Alvarez-Erviti et al.). The group further demonstrated a neuron-to-neuron exchange of cytosolic content via exosomes. It could be that under conditions which promote the intracellular accumulation of misfolded proteins, such as lysosomal and proteasomal dysfunction, the homeostatic mechanisms favor the secretion of aggregated forms of α-synuclein. Although the evidence for extracellular α-synuclein internalization in Emmanouilidou (2010) and Alvarez-Erviti (2010) studies are slightly debatable, there are strong indications at both that exosomes are an important mediator of intercellular communication. Exosome exchange between neurons might also represent a way for propagating pathological alterations throughout the brain during neurodegenerative diseases (Aguzzi & Rajendran, 2009; Smalheiser, 2007).

A demonstration that exosomes allow exchange of proteinaceaous or genetic material within the nervous system would provide an an explanation of how pathologies like Alzheimer's Creuzfeld Jacob or Parkinson's diseases, which begin in discrete regions spread overtime to connected regions of the central nervous system. This idea proposes that drugs directed toward reducing the formation and/or facilitating the clearance of misfolded α-synuclein, in order to arrest or reverse the self-propagation process, might represent novel therapeutic interventions for the treatment of PD. In addition, understanding how the neuropathology spreads throughout the nervous system in Parkinson's disease, will open up avenues for new treatments.

3.4 Effects of extracellular α-synuclein on cellular homeostasis

There are several studies addressing the role of extracellular α-synuclein especially in the context of PD pathology. The first indications that high levels of extracellular α-synuclein can impact cell viability came from studies using the recombinant protein. Exogenous addition of recombinant α-synuclein to the cultured medium of neuronal cells significantly decreased the viability of the recipient cells. Cell death was linearly correlated with the concentration of exogenous α-synuclein and was amplified when the applied protein also contained soluble oligomers (Albani et al., 2004; Du et al., 2003; Sung et al., 2001; Zhang et al., 2005). Application of recombinant monomeric or aggregated α-synuclein also revealed that this protein can be readily be uptaken by neuronal cells or even neural stem cells in culture (Ahn, Kim, Kang, Ryu, & Kim, 2006; Desplats et al., 2009; H. J. Lee et al., 2008; Luk et al., 2009; Sung et al., 2001). It has been suggested that the mechanism for α-synuclein internalization involves receptor-mediated endocytosis of the protein (Desplats et al., 2009; H. J. Lee et al., 2008; Sung et al., 2001). It has been proposed that this mechanism specifically mediates the uptake of oligomeric and fibrillar α-synuclein whereas monomeric α-synuclein enters cells via simple diffusion across the plasma membrane. Following internalization, extracellular α-synuclein was shown to move through the endosomal compartment and finally, to be degraded by lysosomes (H. J. Lee et al., 2008). However, these results were obtained by using very high concentrations of recombinant α-synuclein and cationic liposomes to assist the uptake.

Importantly, recent data using cell-secreted α-synuclein have verified its impact on neuronal survival. Application of conditioned medium containing cell-secreted α-synuclein to neuronal cells induced cell death to the recipient cells (Emmanouilidou, Melachroinou et al., 2010). This toxic effect was concentration-dependent and was conferred synergistically by both oligomeric and monomeric α-synuclein species present in the conditioned medium. In this study, however, there was evidence of very low, if any, α-synuclein uptake by neuronal cells (Emmanouilidou, Melachroinou et al., 2010). Similarly, apoptotic death of neurons, both *in vitro* and *in vivo*, was observed upon their exposure to cell-derived extracellular α-synuclein (Desplats et al., 2009). Secreted α-synuclein, that was readily endocytosed by neurons, was transmitted from one cell to another thereby supporting the idea of a mechanism of pathological propagation in PD (Desplats et al., 2009). Cell-to-cell transfer of α-synuclein was also demonstrated using co-culture systems (Hansen et al., 2010). In fact, this transfer did not require cell contact and was independent of the aggregation state of the protein. Fluorescently-labeled recombinant α-synuclein was uptaken by neuronal cells *in vitro* and *in vivo* via an endocytic mechanism. Altogether, these data demonstrated that endocytosed extracellular α-synuclein can be internalized by recipient cells, interact with the pool of intracellular α-synuclein and seed aggregation (Hansen et al., 2010).

An alternative mechanism of neurodegeneration induced by extracellular α-synuclein may involve the initiation of neuroinflammatory responses. Microglia are resident immune cells that are sensitive to even minor disturbances in the homeostasis of the central nervous system (Soulet & Rivest, 2008). Activation of microglia results in a change in cell morphology (from a ramified to amoeboid shape) accompanied by alterations in surface receptor expression, production of reactive oxygen species (ROS) and release of chemokines and cytokines (Kim & Joh, 2006; Soulet & Rivest, 2008). There is increasing evidence suggesting that extracellularly added recombinant α-synuclein can trigger microglia activation which induces the production of various cytokines, such as IL1β and IL6, and inflammation-related enzymes (Su et al., 2008; Zhang et al., 2005). In fact, microglia activation has been shown to be one of the mechanisms by which α-synuclein induces dopaminergic neurodegeneration, rather than being an epiphenomenon following cell death (Zhang et al., 2007). Further dissection of the pathway of microglia activation, suggested that α-synuclein potentially binds to Mac-1 receptors which subsequently activate PHOX, a ROS-generating enzyme, to produce $O_2^{\bullet}$ ultimately leading to neurotoxicity. Importantly, microglia activation did not require internalization/phagocytosis of α-synuclein by microglial cells (Zhang et al., 2007).To this end, microglial prostaglandin E_2 receptor subtype 2 (EP2) plays a critical role in α-synuclein-induced neurotoxicity partly by decreasing PHOX activation (Jin et al., 2007). Cell-produced α-synuclein also resulted in the activation of primary microglia, leading to the induction of inflammatory signaling pathways (E. J. Lee et al., 2010). It was suggested that α-synuclein-induced microglia activation involves the secretion of MMPs which in turn activate PAR-1 receptor (E. J. Lee et al.). Alternatively, recent data indicate that cell-released α-synuclein can also be internalized by astrocytes thereby producing inflammatory responses both *in vitro* and *in vivo* (E. J. Lee et al., 2010).

4. Conclusion

α-Synuclein is genetically linked to PD. Maintenance of intracellular steady-state concentration of α-synuclein is considered to be a key challenge for neuronal homeostasis and total levels of the protein have been directly linked with PD pathogenesis. Importantly, Genome-Wide association Studies (GWAS) have provided a strong genetic link between α-synuclein and sporadic PD, and clearly point to α-synuclein as being one of the very few genetic loci consistently associated with disease progression. The physiological and aberrant functions of α-synuclein are still under investigation. However, cytoplasmic soluble oligomers/protofibrils of the protein appear to be one of the primary "suspects" in the pathogenesis of PD. Therefore, prevention of α-synuclein aggregation and intervention in the mechanisms of abnormal protein turnover appears to be a highly promising therapeutic target for the treatment of PD as well as other synucleinopathies.

From a therapeutic standpoint, it follows that enhancement of α-synuclein clearance via proteasomal or lysosomal degradation may represent a valid therapeutic intervention for PD. New evidence, suggests that α-synuclein is also physiologically secreted, and as such, it can exert as yet unknown paracrine effects in the brain. Still, the presence and exact levels of α-synuclein in the interstitial fluid in the brain remain to be clarified. Recent clinical observations have suggested that secreted α-synuclein may aggravate PD pathology via a mechanism that underlies cell-to-cell propagation of the protein. It is possible that a dynamic equilibrium between intracellular and extracellular α-synuclein exists, ensuring normal function of neuronal cells. In this respect, dysfunctions in the mechanism(s) regulating extracellular α-synuclein levels, such as mechanisms of secretion or extracellular clearance, may affect neuronal survival. Increases in extracellular α-synuclein may trigger the formation of toxic oligomers in neighbouring neurons and in the extracellular space, and result in inflammatory glia activation, utterly leading to a vicious cycle of neurodegeneration. Along these lines, compounds which block other signalling pathways - switched on as a consequence of microglial activation which may ultimately lead to neuronal death- might also represent new targets for therapeutic intervention. Under this scope, manipulation of regulatory mechanisms that alleviate the extracellular α-synuclein "burden" represents a potential target for the development of novel treatment strategies for PD. It is obvious that α-synuclein can affect neuronal cell homeostasis in numerous ways and at multiple levels. The intrinsic complexity of the neuronal interface may suggest that its actions be considered within the context of non cell-autonomous models and thus be interpreted by taking into account that the nature of communication between brain cells is indeed very dynamic.

5. Acknowledgments

KV and EE acknowledge support from the MJF Foundation and the EU 7th Framework Program MEFOPA.

6. References

Abeliovich, A., Schmitz, Y., Farinas, I., Choi-Lundberg, D., Ho, W. H., Castillo, P. E., et al. (2000). Mice lacking alpha-synuclein display functional deficits in the nigrostriatal dopamine system. *Neuron, 25*(1), 239-252.

Aguzzi, A., & Rajendran, L. (2009). The transcellular spread of cytosolic amyloids, prions, and prionoids. *Neuron, 64*(6), 783-790.

Ahn, M., Kim, S., Kang, M., Ryu, Y., & Kim, T. D. (2006). Chaperone-like activities of alpha-synuclein: alpha-synuclein assists enzyme activities of esterases. *Biochem Biophys Res Commun, 346*(4), 1142-1149.

Albani, D., Peverelli, E., Rametta, R., Batelli, S., Veschini, L., Negro, A., et al. (2004). Protective effect of TAT-delivered alpha-synuclein: relevance of the C-terminal domain and involvement of HSP70. *FASEB J, 18*(14), 1713-1715.

Ali, Y. O., Kitay, B. M., & Zhai, R. G. Dealing with misfolded proteins: examining the neuroprotective role of molecular chaperones in neurodegeneration. *Molecules, 15*(10), 6859-6887.

Alvarez-Erviti, L., Seow, Y., Schapira, A. H., Gardiner, C., Sargent, I. L., Wood, M. J., et al. Lysosomal dysfunction increases exosome-mediated alpha-synuclein release and transmission. *Neurobiol Dis.*

Ardley, H. C., & Robinson, P. A. (2005). E3 ubiquitin ligases. *Essays Biochem, 41*, 15-30.

Azeredo da Silveira, S., Schneider, B. L., Cifuentes-Diaz, C., Sage, D., Abbas-Terki, T., Iwatsubo, T., et al. (2009). Phosphorylation does not prompt, nor prevent, the formation of alpha-synuclein toxic species in a rat model of Parkinson's disease. *Hum Mol Genet, 18*(5), 872-887.

Bate, C., Gentleman, S., & Williams, A. alpha-synuclein induced synapse damage is enhanced by amyloid-beta1-42. *Mol Neurodegener, 5*, 55.

Benaroudj, N., Zwickl, P., Seemuller, E., Baumeister, W., & Goldberg, A. L. (2003). ATP hydrolysis by the proteasome regulatory complex PAN serves multiple functions in protein degradation. *Mol Cell, 11*(1), 69-78.

Bence, N. F., Sampat, R. M., & Kopito, R. R. (2001). Impairment of the ubiquitin-proteasome system by protein aggregation. *Science, 292*(5521), 1552-1555.

Bennett, M. C., Bishop, J. F., Leng, Y., Chock, P. B., Chase, T. N., & Mouradian, M. M. (1999). Degradation of alpha-synuclein by proteasome. *J Biol Chem, 274*(48), 33855-33858.

Besche, H. C., Haas, W., Gygi, S. P., & Goldberg, A. L. (2009). Isolation of mammalian 26S proteasomes and p97/VCP complexes using the ubiquitin-like domain from HHR23B reveals novel proteasome-associated proteins. *Biochemistry, 48*(11), 2538-2549.

Borghi, R., Marchese, R., Negro, A., Marinelli, L., Forloni, G., Zaccheo, D., et al. (2000). Full length alpha-synuclein is present in cerebrospinal fluid from Parkinson's disease and normal subjects. *Neurosci Lett, 287*(1), 65-67.

Braak, H., Del Tredici, K., Rub, U., de Vos, R. A., Jansen Steur, E. N., & Braak, E. (2003). Staging of brain pathology related to sporadic Parkinson's disease. *Neurobiol Aging, 24*(2), 197-211.

Braak, H., Rub, U., & Del Tredici, K. (2003). Involvement of precerebellar nuclei in multiple system atrophy. *Neuropathol Appl Neurobiol, 29*(1), 60-76.

Burre, J., Sharma, M., Tsetsenis, T., Buchman, V., Etherton, M. R., & Sudhof, T. C. Alpha-synuclein promotes SNARE-complex assembly in vivo and in vitro. *Science, 329*(5999), 1663-1667.

Carter, D. B., & Chou, K. C. (1998). A model for structure-dependent binding of Congo red to Alzheimer beta-amyloid fibrils. *Neurobiol Aging, 19*(1), 37-40.

Cavallarin, N., Vicario, M., & Negro, A. The role of phosphorylation in synucleinopathies: focus on Parkinson's disease. *CNS Neurol Disord Drug Targets, 9*(4), 471-481.

Chartier-Harlin, M. C., Kachergus, J., Roumier, C., Mouroux, V., Douay, X., Lincoln, S., et al. (2004). Alpha-synuclein locus duplication as a cause of familial Parkinson's disease. *Lancet, 364*(9440), 1167-1169.

Chen, L., Periquet, M., Wang, X., Negro, A., McLean, P. J., Hyman, B. T., et al. (2009). Tyrosine and serine phosphorylation of alpha-synuclein have opposing effects on neurotoxicity and soluble oligomer formation. *J Clin Invest, 119*(11), 3257-3265.

Chu, Y., Dodiya, H., Aebischer, P., Olanow, C. W., & Kordower, J. H. (2009). Alterations in lysosomal and proteasomal markers in Parkinson's disease: relationship to alpha-synuclein inclusions. *Neurobiol Dis, 35*(3), 385-398.

Conway, K. A., Lee, S. J., Rochet, J. C., Ding, T. T., Williamson, R. E., & Lansbury, P. T., Jr. (2000). Acceleration of oligomerization, not fibrillization, is a shared property of both alpha-synuclein mutations linked to early-onset Parkinson's disease: implications for pathogenesis and therapy. *Proc Natl Acad Sci U S A, 97*(2), 571-576.

Conway, K. A., Rochet, J. C., Bieganski, R. M., & Lansbury, P. T., Jr. (2001). Kinetic stabilization of the alpha-synuclein protofibril by a dopamine-alpha-synuclein adduct. *Science, 294*(5545), 1346-1349.

Crews, C. M. (2003). Feeding the machine: mechanisms of proteasome-catalyzed degradation of ubiquitinated proteins. *Curr Opin Chem Biol, 7*(5), 534-539.

Cuervo, A. M., Stefanis, L., Fredenburg, R., Lansbury, P. T., & Sulzer, D. (2004). Impaired degradation of mutant alpha-synuclein by chaperone-mediated autophagy. *Science, 305*(5688), 1292-1295.

Cuervo, A. M., Wong, E. S., & Martinez-Vicente, M. Protein degradation, aggregation, and misfolding. *Mov Disord, 25 Suppl 1*, S49-54.

Danzer, K. M., Haasen, D., Karow, A. R., Moussaud, S., Habeck, M., Giese, A., et al. (2007). Different species of alpha-synuclein oligomers induce calcium influx and seeding. *J Neurosci, 27*(34), 9220-9232.

Darios, F., Ruiperez, V., Lopez, I., Villanueva, J., Gutierrez, L. M., & Davletov, B. Alpha-synuclein sequesters arachidonic acid to modulate SNARE-mediated exocytosis. *EMBO Rep, 11*(7), 528-533.

Demartino, G. N., & Gillette, T. G. (2007). Proteasomes: machines for all reasons. *Cell, 129*(4), 659-662.

Desplats, P., Lee, H. J., Bae, E. J., Patrick, C., Rockenstein, E., Crews, L., et al. (2009). Inclusion formation and neuronal cell death through neuron-to-neuron transmission of alpha-synuclein. *Proc Natl Acad Sci U S A, 106*(31), 13010-13015.

Du, H. N., Tang, L., Luo, X. Y., Li, H. T., Hu, J., Zhou, J. W., et al. (2003). A peptide motif consisting of glycine, alanine, and valine is required for the fibrillization and cytotoxicity of human alpha-synuclein. *Biochemistry, 42*(29), 8870-8878.

El-Agnaf, O. M., Salem, S. A., Paleologou, K. E., Cooper, L. J., Fullwood, N. J., Gibson, M. J., et al. (2003). Alpha-synuclein implicated in Parkinson's disease is present in extracellular biological fluids, including human plasma. *FASEB J, 17*(13), 1945-1947.

El-Agnaf, O. M., Salem, S. A., Paleologou, K. E., Curran, M. D., Gibson, M. J., Court, J. A., et al. (2006). Detection of oligomeric forms of alpha-synuclein protein in human plasma as a potential biomarker for Parkinson's disease. *FASEB J, 20*(3), 419-425.

Eldh, M., Ekstrom, K., Valadi, H., Sjostrand, M., Olsson, B., Jernas, M., et al. Exosomes communicate protective messages during oxidative stress; possible role of exosomal shuttle RNA. *PLoS One, 5*(12), e15353.

Emmanouilidou, E., Melachroinou, K., Roumeliotis, T., Garbis, S. D., Ntzouni, M., Margaritis, L. H., et al. Cell-produced alpha-synuclein is secreted in a calcium-dependent manner by exosomes and impacts neuronal survival. *J Neurosci, 30*(20), 6838-6851.

Emmanouilidou, E., Stefanis, L., & Vekrellis, K. Cell-produced alpha-synuclein oligomers are targeted to, and impair, the 26S proteasome. *Neurobiol Aging, 31*(6), 953-968.

Ferreon, A. C., Gambin, Y., Lemke, E. A., & Deniz, A. A. (2009). Interplay of alpha-synuclein binding and conformational switching probed by single-molecule fluorescence. *Proc Natl Acad Sci U S A, 106*(14), 5645-5650.

Fevrier, B., & Raposo, G. (2004). Exosomes: endosomal-derived vesicles shipping extracellular messages. *Curr Opin Cell Biol, 16*(4), 415-421.

Follmer, C., Romao, L., Einsiedler, C. M., Porto, T. C., Lara, F. A., Moncores, M., et al. (2007). Dopamine affects the stability, hydration, and packing of protofibrils and fibrils of the wild type and variants of alpha-synuclein. *Biochemistry, 46*(2), 472-482.

Gallastegui, N., & Groll, M. The 26S proteasome: assembly and function of a destructive machine. *Trends Biochem Sci, 35*(11), 634-642.

Ghee, M., Melki, R., Michot, N., & Mallet, J. (2005). PA700, the regulatory complex of the 26S proteasome, interferes with alpha-synuclein assembly. *FEBS J, 272*(16), 4023-4033.

Ghidoni, R., Benussi, L., & Binetti, G. (2008). Exosomes: the Trojan horses of neurodegeneration. *Med Hypotheses, 70*(6), 1226-1227.

Giasson, B. I., Duda, J. E., Quinn, S. M., Zhang, B., Trojanowski, J. Q., & Lee, V. M. (2002). Neuronal alpha-synucleinopathy with severe movement disorder in mice expressing A53T human alpha-synuclein. *Neuron, 34*(4), 521-533.

Glickman, M. H., & Ciechanover, A. (2002). The ubiquitin-proteasome proteolytic pathway: destruction for the sake of construction. *Physiol Rev, 82*(2), 373-428.

Goldberg, M. S., Fleming, S. M., Palacino, J. J., Cepeda, C., Lam, H. A., Bhatnagar, A., et al. (2003). Parkin-deficient mice exhibit nigrostriatal deficits but not loss of dopaminergic neurons. *J Biol Chem, 278*(44), 43628-43635.

Goldberg, M. S., & Lansbury, P. T., Jr. (2000). Is there a cause-and-effect relationship between alpha-synuclein fibrillization and Parkinson's disease? *Nat Cell Biol, 2*(7), E115-119.

Greten-Harrison, B., Polydoro, M., Morimoto-Tomita, M., Diao, L., Williams, A. M., Nie, E. H., et al. alphabetagamma-Synuclein triple knockout mice reveal age-dependent neuronal dysfunction. *Proc Natl Acad Sci U S A, 107*(45), 19573-19578.

Hansen, C., Angot, E., Bergstrom, A. L., Steiner, J. A., Pieri, L., Paul, G., et al. alpha-Synuclein propagates from mouse brain to grafted dopaminergic neurons and seeds aggregation in cultured human cells. *J Clin Invest, 121*(2), 715-725.

Jana, N. R., Zemskov, E. A., Wang, G., & Nukina, N. (2001). Altered proteasomal function due to the expression of polyglutamine-expanded truncated N-terminal huntingtin induces apoptosis by caspase activation through mitochondrial cytochrome c release. *Hum Mol Genet, 10*(10), 1049-1059.

Jang, A., Lee, H. J., Suk, J. E., Jung, J. W., Kim, K. P., & Lee, S. J. Non-classical exocytosis of alpha-synuclein is sensitive to folding states and promoted under stress conditions. *J Neurochem, 113*(5), 1263-1274.

Jin, J., Shie, F. S., Liu, J., Wang, Y., Davis, J., Schantz, A. M., et al. (2007). Prostaglandin E2 receptor subtype 2 (EP2) regulates microglial activation and associated neurotoxicity induced by aggregated alpha-synuclein. *J Neuroinflammation, 4*, 2.

Karpinar, D. P., Balija, M. B., Kugler, S., Opazo, F., Rezaei-Ghaleh, N., Wender, N., et al. (2009). Pre-fibrillar alpha-synuclein variants with impaired beta-structure increase neurotoxicity in Parkinson's disease models. *EMBO J, 28*(20), 3256-3268.

Kayed, R., Head, E., Thompson, J. L., McIntire, T. M., Milton, S. C., Cotman, C. W., et al. (2003). Common structure of soluble amyloid oligomers implies common mechanism of pathogenesis. *Science, 300*(5618), 486-489.

Keller, S., Sanderson, M. P., Stoeck, A., & Altevogt, P. (2006). Exosomes: from biogenesis and secretion to biological function. *Immunol Lett, 107*(2), 102-108.

Keri, S., Moustafa, A. A., Myers, C. E., Benedek, G., & Gluck, M. A. {alpha}-Synuclein gene duplication impairs reward learning. *Proc Natl Acad Sci U S A, 107*(36), 15992-15994.

Kim, Y. S., & Joh, T. H. (2006). Microglia, major player in the brain inflammation: their roles in the pathogenesis of Parkinson's disease. *Exp Mol Med, 38*(4), 333-347.

Kitada, T., Asakawa, S., Hattori, N., Matsumine, H., Yamamura, Y., Minoshima, S., et al. (1998). Mutations in the parkin gene cause autosomal recessive juvenile parkinsonism. *Nature, 392*(6676), 605-608.

Koprich, J. B., Reske-Nielsen, C., Mithal, P., & Isacson, O. (2008). Neuroinflammation mediated by IL-1beta increases susceptibility of dopamine neurons to degeneration in an animal model of Parkinson's disease. *J Neuroinflammation, 5*, 8.

Kordower, J. H., Chu, Y., Hauser, R. A., Freeman, T. B., & Olanow, C. W. (2008). Lewy body-like pathology in long-term embryonic nigral transplants in Parkinson's disease. *Nat Med, 14*(5), 504-506.

Kristiansen, M., Deriziotis, P., Dimcheff, D. E., Jackson, G. S., Ovaa, H., Naumann, H., et al. (2007). Disease-associated prion protein oligomers inhibit the 26S proteasome. *Mol Cell, 26*(2), 175-188.

Kruger, R., Kuhn, W., Muller, T., Woitalla, D., Graeber, M., Kosel, S., et al. (1998). Ala30Pro mutation in the gene encoding alpha-synuclein in Parkinson's disease. *Nat Genet, 18*(2), 106-108.

Lachenal, G., Pernet-Gallay, K., Chivet, M., Hemming, F. J., Belly, A., Bodon, G., et al. Release of exosomes from differentiated neurons and its regulation by synaptic glutamatergic activity. *Mol Cell Neurosci, 46*(2), 409-418.

Lang-Rollin, I., Rideout, H., & Stefanis, L. (2003). Ubiquitinated inclusions and neuronal cell death. *Histol Histopathol, 18*(2), 509-517.

Lashuel, H. A., & Hirling, H. (2006). Rescuing defective vesicular trafficking protects against alpha-synuclein toxicity in cellular and animal models of Parkinson's disease. *ACS Chem Biol, 1*(7), 420-424.

Lashuel, H. A., Petre, B. M., Wall, J., Simon, M., Nowak, R. J., Walz, T., et al. (2002). Alpha-synuclein, especially the Parkinson's disease-associated mutants, forms pore-like annular and tubular protofibrils. *J Mol Biol, 322*(5), 1089-1102.

Layfield, R., Tooth, D., Landon, M., Dawson, S., Mayer, J., & Alban, A. (2001). Purification of poly-ubiquitinated proteins by S5a-affinity chromatography. *Proteomics, 1*(6), 773-777.

Lee, E. J., Woo, M. S., Moon, P. G., Baek, M. C., Choi, I. Y., Kim, W. K., et al. Alpha-synuclein activates microglia by inducing the expressions of matrix metalloproteinases and the subsequent activation of protease-activated receptor-1. *J Immunol, 185*(1), 615-623.

Lee, H. J., Patel, S., & Lee, S. J. (2005). Intravesicular localization and exocytosis of alpha-synuclein and its aggregates. *J Neurosci, 25*(25), 6016-6024.

Lee, H. J., Suk, J. E., Bae, E. J., Lee, J. H., Paik, S. R., & Lee, S. J. (2008). Assembly-dependent endocytosis and clearance of extracellular alpha-synuclein. *Int J Biochem Cell Biol, 40*(9), 1835-1849.

Li, J., Uversky, V. N., & Fink, A. L. (2001). Effect of familial Parkinson's disease point mutations A30P and A53T on the structural properties, aggregation, and fibrillation of human alpha-synuclein. *Biochemistry, 40*(38), 11604-11613.

Li, J. Y., Englund, E., Holton, J. L., Soulet, D., Hagell, P., Lees, A. J., et al. (2008). Lewy bodies in grafted neurons in subjects with Parkinson's disease suggest host-to-graft disease propagation. *Nat Med, 14*(5), 501-503.

Lindersson, E., Beedholm, R., Hojrup, P., Moos, T., Gai, W., Hendil, K. B., et al. (2004). Proteasomal inhibition by alpha-synuclein filaments and oligomers. *J Biol Chem, 279*(13), 12924-12934.

Liu, G., Zhang, C., Yin, J., Li, X., Cheng, F., Li, Y., et al. (2009). alpha-Synuclein is differentially expressed in mitochondria from different rat brain regions and dose-dependently down-regulates complex I activity. *Neurosci Lett, 454*(3), 187-192.

Lowe, J., McDermott, H., Landon, M., Mayer, R. J., & Wilkinson, K. D. (1990). Ubiquitin carboxyl-terminal hydrolase (PGP 9.5) is selectively present in ubiquitinated inclusion bodies characteristic of human neurodegenerative diseases. *J Pathol, 161*(2), 153-160.

Luk, K. C., Song, C., O'Brien, P., Stieber, A., Branch, J. R., Brunden, K. R., et al. (2009). Exogenous alpha-synuclein fibrils seed the formation of Lewy body-like intracellular inclusions in cultured cells. *Proc Natl Acad Sci U S A, 106*(47), 20051-20056.

Machiya, Y., Hara, S., Arawaka, S., Fukushima, S., Sato, H., Sakamoto, M., et al. Phosphorylated alpha-synuclein at Ser-129 is targeted to the proteasome pathway in a ubiquitin-independent manner. *J Biol Chem, 285*(52), 40732-40744.

Martin-Clemente, B., Alvarez-Castelao, B., Mayo, I., Sierra, A. B., Diaz, V., Milan, M., et al. (2004). alpha-Synuclein expression levels do not significantly affect proteasome function and expression in mice and stably transfected PC12 cell lines. *J Biol Chem, 279*(51), 52984-52990.

Martin, L. J., Pan, Y., Price, A. C., Sterling, W., Copeland, N. G., Jenkins, N. A., et al. (2006). Parkinson's disease alpha-synuclein transgenic mice develop neuronal mitochondrial degeneration and cell death. *J Neurosci, 26*(1), 41-50.

McNaught, K. S., Perl, D. P., Brownell, A. L., & Olanow, C. W. (2004). Systemic exposure to proteasome inhibitors causes a progressive model of Parkinson's disease. *Ann Neurol, 56*(1), 149-162.

Michalik, A., & Van Broeckhoven, C. (2004). Proteasome degrades soluble expanded polyglutamine completely and efficiently. *Neurobiol Dis, 16*(1), 202-211.

Miller, R. J., & Wilson, S. M. (2003). Neurological disease: UPS stops delivering! *Trends Pharmacol Sci, 24*(1), 18-23.

Mollenhauer, B., Cullen, V., Kahn, I., Krastins, B., Outeiro, T. F., Pepivani, I., et al. (2008). Direct quantification of CSF alpha-synuclein by ELISA and first cross-sectional study in patients with neurodegeneration. *Exp Neurol, 213*(2), 315-325.

Muchowski, P. J., & Wacker, J. L. (2005). Modulation of neurodegeneration by molecular chaperones. *Nat Rev Neurosci, 6*(1), 11-22.

Nemani, V. M., Lu, W., Berge, V., Nakamura, K., Onoa, B., Lee, M. K., et al. Increased expression of alpha-synuclein reduces neurotransmitter release by inhibiting synaptic vesicle reclustering after endocytosis. *Neuron, 65*(1), 66-79.

Ohrfelt, A., Grognet, P., Andreasen, N., Wallin, A., Vanmechelen, E., Blennow, K., et al. (2009). Cerebrospinal fluid alpha-synuclein in neurodegenerative disorders-a marker of synapse loss? *Neurosci Lett, 450*(3), 332-335.

Paleologou, K. E., Oueslati, A., Shakked, G., Rospigliosi, C. C., Kim, H. Y., Lamberto, G. R., et al. Phosphorylation at S87 is enhanced in synucleinopathies, inhibits alpha-synuclein oligomerization, and influences synuclein-membrane interactions. *J Neurosci, 30*(9), 3184-3198.

Petrucelli, L., O'Farrell, C., Lockhart, P. J., Baptista, M., Kehoe, K., Vink, L., et al. (2002). Parkin protects against the toxicity associated with mutant alpha-synuclein: proteasome dysfunction selectively affects catecholaminergic neurons. *Neuron, 36*(6), 1007-1019.

Pickart, C. M., & Cohen, R. E. (2004). Proteasomes and their kin: proteases in the machine age. *Nat Rev Mol Cell Biol, 5*(3), 177-187.

Polymeropoulos, M. H., Lavedan, C., Leroy, E., Ide, S. E., Dehejia, A., Dutra, A., et al. (1997). Mutation in the alpha-synuclein gene identified in families with Parkinson's disease. *Science, 276*(5321), 2045-2047.

Rajendran, L., Honsho, M., Zahn, T. R., Keller, P., Geiger, K. D., Verkade, P., et al. (2006). Alzheimer's disease beta-amyloid peptides are released in association with exosomes. *Proc Natl Acad Sci U S A, 103*(30), 11172-11177.

Rideout, H. J., Larsen, K. E., Sulzer, D., & Stefanis, L. (2001). Proteasomal inhibition leads to formation of ubiquitin/alpha-synuclein-immunoreactive inclusions in PC12 cells. *J Neurochem, 78*(4), 899-908.

Rideout, H. J., & Stefanis, L. (2002). Proteasomal inhibition-induced inclusion formation and death in cortical neurons require transcription and ubiquitination. *Mol Cell Neurosci, 21*(2), 223-238.

Rochet, J. C., Conway, K. A., & Lansbury, P. T., Jr. (2000). Inhibition of fibrillization and accumulation of prefibrillar oligomers in mixtures of human and mouse alpha-synuclein. *Biochemistry, 39*(35), 10619-10626.

Rodgers, K. J., & Dean, R. T. (2003). Assessment of proteasome activity in cell lysates and tissue homogenates using peptide substrates. *Int J Biochem Cell Biol, 35*(5), 716-727.

Saigoh, K., Wang, Y. L., Suh, J. G., Yamanishi, T., Sakai, Y., Kiyosawa, H., et al. (1999). Intragenic deletion in the gene encoding ubiquitin carboxy-terminal hydrolase in gad mice. *Nat Genet, 23*(1), 47-51.

Scott, D. A., Tabarean, I., Tang, Y., Cartier, A., Masliah, E., & Roy, S. A pathologic cascade leading to synaptic dysfunction in alpha-synuclein-induced neurodegeneration. *J Neurosci, 30*(24), 8083-8095.

Sherman, M. Y., & Goldberg, A. L. (2001). Cellular defenses against unfolded proteins: a cell biologist thinks about neurodegenerative diseases. *Neuron, 29*(1), 15-32.

Singleton, A. B., Farrer, M., Johnson, J., Singleton, A., Hague, S., Kachergus, J., et al. (2003). alpha-Synuclein locus triplication causes Parkinson's disease. *Science, 302*(5646), 841.

Smalheiser, N. R. (2007). Exosomal transfer of proteins and RNAs at synapses in the nervous system. *Biol Direct, 2*, 35.

Smith, W. W., Jiang, H., Pei, Z., Tanaka, Y., Morita, H., Sawa, A., et al. (2005). Endoplasmic reticulum stress and mitochondrial cell death pathways mediate A53T mutant alpha-synuclein-induced toxicity. *Hum Mol Genet, 14*(24), 3801-3811.

Snyder, H., Mensah, K., Theisler, C., Lee, J., Matouschek, A., & Wolozin, B. (2003). Aggregated and monomeric alpha-synuclein bind to the S6' proteasomal protein and inhibit proteasomal function. *J Biol Chem, 278*(14), 11753-11759.

Soulet, D., & Rivest, S. (2008). Microglia. *Curr Biol, 18*(12), R506-508.

Spillantini, M. G., Crowther, R. A., Jakes, R., Hasegawa, M., & Goedert, M. (1998). alpha-Synuclein in filamentous inclusions of Lewy bodies from Parkinson's disease and dementia with lewy bodies. *Proc Natl Acad Sci U S A, 95*(11), 6469-6473.

Stefanis, L., Larsen, K. E., Rideout, H. J., Sulzer, D., & Greene, L. A. (2001). Expression of A53T mutant but not wild-type alpha-synuclein in PC12 cells induces alterations of the ubiquitin-dependent degradation system, loss of dopamine release, and autophagic cell death. *J Neurosci, 21*(24), 9549-9560.

Su, X., Maguire-Zeiss, K. A., Giuliano, R., Prifti, L., Venkatesh, K., & Federoff, H. J. (2008). Synuclein activates microglia in a model of Parkinson's disease. *Neurobiol Aging, 29*(11), 1690-1701.

Sultzer, D. L., Gray, K. F., Gunay, I., Wheatley, M. V., & Mahler, M. E. (2001). Does behavioral improvement with haloperidol or trazodone treatment depend on psychosis or mood symptoms in patients with dementia? *J Am Geriatr Soc, 49*(10), 1294-1300.

Sulzer, D. Clues to how alpha-synuclein damages neurons in Parkinson's disease. *Mov Disord, 25 Suppl 1*, S27-31.

Sung, J. Y., Kim, J., Paik, S. R., Park, J. H., Ahn, Y. S., & Chung, K. C. (2001). Induction of neuronal cell death by Rab5A-dependent endocytosis of alpha-synuclein. *J Biol Chem, 276*(29), 27441-27448.

Sung, J. Y., Park, S. M., Lee, C. H., Um, J. W., Lee, H. J., Kim, J., et al. (2005). Proteolytic cleavage of extracellular secreted {alpha}-synuclein via matrix metalloproteinases. *J Biol Chem, 280*(26), 25216-25224.

Tanaka, Y., Engelender, S., Igarashi, S., Rao, R. K., Wanner, T., Tanzi, R. E., et al. (2001). Inducible expression of mutant alpha-synuclein decreases proteasome activity and increases sensitivity to mitochondria-dependent apoptosis. *Hum Mol Genet, 10*(9), 919-926.

Thery, C., Zitvogel, L., & Amigorena, S. (2002). Exosomes: composition, biogenesis and function. *Nat Rev Immunol, 2*(8), 569-579.

Tofaris, G. K., Razzaq, A., Ghetti, B., Lilley, K. S., & Spillantini, M. G. (2003). Ubiquitination of alpha-synuclein in Lewy bodies is a pathological event not associated with impairment of proteasome function. *J Biol Chem, 278*(45), 44405-44411.

Tokuda, T., Qureshi, M. M., Ardah, M. T., Varghese, S., Shehab, S. A., Kasai, T., et al. Detection of elevated levels of alpha-synuclein oligomers in CSF from patients with Parkinson disease. *Neurology, 75*(20), 1766-1772.

Tokuda, T., Salem, S. A., Allsop, D., Mizuno, T., Nakagawa, M., Qureshi, M. M., et al. (2006). Decreased alpha-synuclein in cerebrospinal fluid of aged individuals and subjects with Parkinson's disease. *Biochem Biophys Res Commun, 349*(1), 162-166.

Trojanowski, J. Q., & Lee, V. M. (1998). Aggregation of neurofilament and alpha-synuclein proteins in Lewy bodies: implications for the pathogenesis of Parkinson disease and Lewy body dementia. *Arch Neurol, 55*(2), 151-152.

Tsika, E., Moysidou, M., Guo, J., Cushman, M., Gannon, P., Sandaltzopoulos, R., et al. Distinct region-specific alpha-synuclein oligomers in A53T transgenic mice: implications for neurodegeneration. *J Neurosci, 30*(9), 3409-3418.

Valadi, H., Ekstrom, K., Bossios, A., Sjostrand, M., Lee, J. J., & Lotvall, J. O. (2007). Exosome-mediated transfer of mRNAs and microRNAs is a novel mechanism of genetic exchange between cells. *Nat Cell Biol, 9*(6), 654-659.

Vella, L. J., Sharples, R. A., Nisbet, R. M., Cappai, R., & Hill, A. F. (2008). The role of exosomes in the processing of proteins associated with neurodegenerative diseases. *Eur Biophys J, 37*(3), 323-332.

Venkatraman, P., Wetzel, R., Tanaka, M., Nukina, N., & Goldberg, A. L. (2004). Eukaryotic proteasomes cannot digest polyglutamine sequences and release them during degradation of polyglutamine-containing proteins. *Mol Cell, 14*(1), 95-104.

Volles, M. J., Lee, S. J., Rochet, J. C., Shtilerman, M. D., Ding, T. T., Kessler, J. C., et al. (2001). Vesicle permeabilization by protofibrillar alpha-synuclein: implications for the pathogenesis and treatment of Parkinson's disease. *Biochemistry, 40*(26), 7812-7819.

Wacker, J. L., Zareie, M. H., Fong, H., Sarikaya, M., & Muchowski, P. J. (2004). Hsp70 and Hsp40 attenuate formation of spherical and annular polyglutamine oligomers by partitioning monomer. *Nat Struct Mol Biol, 11*(12), 1215-1222.

Waxman, E. A., & Giasson, B. I. (2009). Molecular mechanisms of alpha-synuclein neurodegeneration. *Biochim Biophys Acta, 1792*(7), 616-624.

Webb, J. L., Ravikumar, B., Atkins, J., Skepper, J. N., & Rubinsztein, D. C. (2003). Alpha-Synuclein is degraded by both autophagy and the proteasome. *J Biol Chem, 278*(27), 25009-25013.

Winner, B., Jappelli, R., Maji, S. K., Desplats, P. A., Boyer, L., Aigner, S., et al. In vivo demonstration that {alpha}-synuclein oligomers are toxic. *Proc Natl Acad Sci U S A, 108*(10), 4194-4199.

Xilouri, M., & Stefanis, L. Autophagic pathways in Parkinson disease and related disorders. *Expert Rev Mol Med, 13*, e8.

Xilouri, M., Vogiatzi, T., Vekrellis, K., & Stefanis, L. (2008). alpha-synuclein degradation by autophagic pathways: a potential key to Parkinson's disease pathogenesis. *Autophagy, 4*(7), 917-919.

Zarranz, J. J., Alegre, J., Gomez-Esteban, J. C., Lezcano, E., Ros, R., Ampuero, I., et al. (2004). The new mutation, E46K, of alpha-synuclein causes Parkinson and Lewy body dementia. *Ann Neurol, 55*(2), 164-173.

Zhang, W., Dallas, S., Zhang, D., Guo, J. P., Pang, H., Wilson, B., et al. (2007). Microglial PHOX and Mac-1 are essential to the enhanced dopaminergic neurodegeneration elicited by A30P and A53T mutant alpha-synuclein. *Glia, 55*(11), 1178-1188.

Zhang, W., Wang, T., Pei, Z., Miller, D. S., Wu, X., Block, M. L., et al. (2005). Aggregated alpha-synuclein activates microglia: a process leading to disease progression in Parkinson's disease. *FASEB J, 19*(6), 533-542.

Zhu, M., Li, J., & Fink, A. L. (2003). The association of alpha-synuclein with membranes affects bilayer structure, stability, and fibril formation. *J Biol Chem, 278*(41), 40186-40197.

9

Actions of GDNF on Midbrain Dopaminergic Neurons: The Signaling Pathway

Dianshuai Gao, Yi Liu, Shen Sun, Li Li and Ye Xiong
Xuzhou Medical College
China

1. Introduction

Parkinson's disease (PD) is a degenerative disease of the central nervous system (CNS) predominantly occurring in older adults, and is particularly common after the age of 60. The primary pathologic characteristics of PD are neuronal degeneration and cell death of dopaminergic (DA-ergic) neurons, leading to a decrease in the dopamine (DA) level in the striatum. Originally extracted and purified in 1993, glial cell line-derived neurotrophic factor (GDNF) is a novel neurotrophic factor which exerts neurotrophic effects upon DA-ergic neurons in the midbrain, sympathetic neurons in the superior cervical ganglion and motor neurons in the spinal cord. Specially, GDNF protects midbrain DA-ergic neurons, and promotes their differentiation and survival (Lin *et al.*, 1993). These studies provide impetus to delve more deeply into the underlying mechanisms of GDNF, and suggest potential future applications of GDNF. The present review focuses on the correlates of neurotrophic factors and PD treatments, and the mechanisms of action of GDNF.

2. Parkinson's disease and neurotrophic factors

2.1 Parkinson's disease

Parkinson's disease (PD) is also known as paralysis agitans. As a degenerative disease of the central nervous system (CNS), PD is characterized by static tremors, bradykinesia, myotonia and unstable posture. It is a disease normally occurring in older adults, especially after the age of 60. Thus far, the etiology and mechanisms underlying this disease have not been fully elucidated (Daly *et al.*, 1999), though most scholars support the dopamine hypothesis and the oxidative stress hypothesis of PD. According to the dopamine hypothesis, dopamine synthesis decreases following the pathologic degeneration of DA-ergic neurons in the substantia nigra pars compacta (SNpc), leading to a decrease in inhibition of acetylcholine in the corpus striatum and a relative increasing excitability of acetylcholine. The disequilibrium between dopamine and acetylcholine results in the hyper-functioning of the extrapyramidal system, thus leading to paralysis agitans. The oxidative stress hypothesis explains the causes of degeneration of DA-ergic neurons in the SNpc. In PD, hydrogen peroxide (H_2O_2) and superoxide anions, produced during the process of oxidative metabolism under oxidative stress, are catalyzed by Fe^{2+} in the SNpc, and then formed into hydroxy radicals with more significant noxious properties. Meanwhile, the activity of complex I of the mitochondrial respiratory chain in DA-ergic neurons decreases, causing antioxidants (esp. glutathione) to disappear. At this point, the free radicals can no longer be removed. Thus, by oxidizing the lipoids of neurilemma, destroying the functions of the membranes and directly demolishing DNA in DA-ergic neurons, the free radicals cause the degeneration and death of the neurons.

2.2 Neurotrophic factors

Neurotrophic factors (NTFs), discovered at the end of the 20th century, are dissoluble polypeptides derived from tissues (e.g. muscles) which are innervated by nerves, or from astrocytes. They can promote and maintain the growth, survival and differentiation of specific neurons, as well as influence synaptic plasticity. More than twenty NTFs are known to exist, including brain-derived neurotrophic factor (BDNF), nerve growth factor (NGF) and glial cell line-derived neurotrophic factor (GDNF). Sharing as much as 50 - 60% homology in amino acid sequence, NTFs are quite congenerous. In general, the NTFs enter the nerve terminal through receptor-mediated endocytosis, then transport to the cell soma by retrograde axoplasmic transport. There, they promote the synthesis of numerous proteins supporting the growth, development and functional integrity of neurons. Recently, some NTFs were found to be produced by neurons and transported to nerve endings by anterograde axoplasmic transport, where they play a role in supporting the integrity of shape and function in postsynaptic neurons.

Neurotrophic factors, especially GDNF, exert protective effects on DA-ergic neurons, correlating with the etiology of PD. Some studies have demonstrated that the amount of NTFs is decreased in PD patients, compared with control. It is highly likely that this decrease could lead to the degeneration and death of DA-ergic neurons and induce the clinical symptoms of PD. In addition, some scholars propose that the apoptosis of numerous neurons during the process of development may be related to a decrease in NTFs. Studies based on animal models have demonstrated that the application of NTFs-medium can increase the survival rate of fetal DA-ergic neurons and reduce apoptosis *in vitro* (Siegel & Chauhan, 2000). Currently, no evidence exists addressing whether defects of NTFs or decreased expression of receptors for NTFs occur during the pathogenic progress of PD.

3. The structure, expression and basic physiological properties of GDNF

3.1 The structure of GDNF

The GDNF family ligands (GFLs) belong to the transforming growth factor-β (TGF-β) super-family, and include four neurotrophic factors: glial cell line-derived neurotrophic factor (GDNF), neurturin (NRTN), artemin (ARTN) and persephin (PSPN). These factors possess structures similar to other factors in the TGF-β super-family, and function as homodimers (Ibáñez, 1998). GFLs transduce signals through a receptor system, which is a protein complex consisting of RET tyrosine protein kinase and the GFRα family of proteins, playing an important role in the biological processes of cell survival, differentiation and migration.

The GFLs are secretory proteins, derived from the precursor preproGFL. ProGFLs can be activated by proteolytic cleavage. The diffusion and local concentration of proGFLs are influenced by the combination of GFLs and the lateral chain of heparan sulfate in the extracellular matrix (Hamilton *et al.*, 1998). Despite the fact that the binding sites for the GFLs have been extensively studied, the gene regulation, mechanisms of secretion and the precursors leading to the activation of GFLs have not been fully elucidated (Golden *et al.*,

1999). Similarly, the protease responsible for the breakdown and activation of the GFL precursor has yet to be revealed. Recent evidence has uncovered the biological activities for the precursor of secretory neurotrophic factors (Lee *et al.*, 2001). The secreted NGF and BDNF are sheared outside the cell by serine protein kinases and selective matrix metalloproteinases. ProNGF has a high affinity for p75NTR, a receptor responsible for the apoptosis of neurons in culture media, and maintains mild activation of the pathway, accompanied by differentiation and survival of cells mediated by TrkA. Whether the proteolytic cleavage mediates the biological activities of the GFLs, and whether the functional GFLs are different from other ligands, are major areas of interest to current scholars.

Of the 4 members of the GFLs, GDNF and NRTN were the first to be extracted. Subsequently, ARTN and PSPN were identified through basic data analysis and the use of homogeneous clones (Baloh *et al.*, 2000). The GDNF gene for both humans and mice has been cloned and expressed in prokaryotic and eukaryotic vectors. The human GDNF gene is located on chromosome 5p13. 1-13. 3, and is composed of two exons and one intron. In humans and mice, two types of GDNF mRNA with different lengths exist: a large fragment of 633bp and small fragment of 555bp, encoding for polypeptides of GDNF precursors with 211 amino acids and 185 amino acids, respectively. After the removal of 26 amino acids in the N terminal, the large fragment becomes smaller and the two fragments (large and small) are eventually transformed into polypeptides consisting of 134 amino acids (Trupp *et al.*, 1995). The mature protein of GDNF consists of 7 cysteine residues, and as such, 3 intrachain disulfide bonds are formed between the sites of amino acids 41 and 102, 68 and 131 and 72 and 133. The cysteine residues in the side chain of amino acid 101 form interchain disulfide bonds, thus forming the structure of the homodimer of GDNF (Haniu *et al.*, 1996). The structural features are quite similar to that of the TGF-β family members. Two glycosylation sites lie in the polypeptide chain, which has a molecular weight of 20 kD. The molecular weight of the natural GDNF dimer, which contains a heparan biding site, is 40 - 45 kD. X-ray methods have demonstrated that the structure of rat GDNF contains two finger-like structures lying in the rostral and caudal parts. Additionally, the amino acids in the middle form a helical structure; two monomers are connected by a pair of disulfide bonds, and the four finger-like structures form a plane (Eigenbrot *et al.*, 1997) (Figure 1). GDNF has conservation in evolution, as evidenced by the significant similarities between humans and mice in amino acid sequences in the mature proteins of GDNF (as high as 93%). Human GDNF, produced by genetic engineering, exerts activities on murine DA-ergic neurons. These lines of evidence indicate that GDNF has cross-species activity.

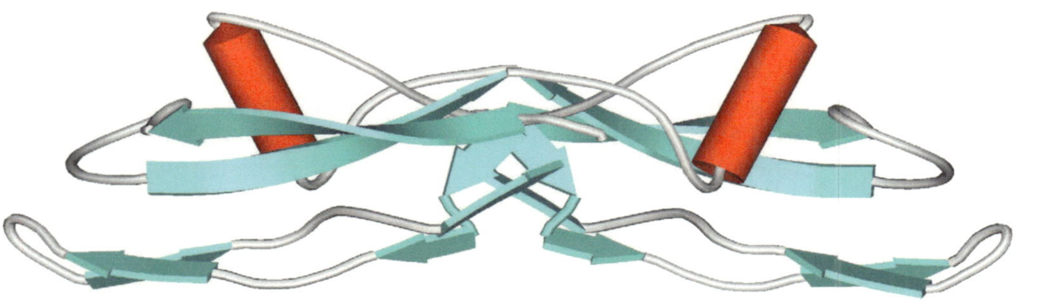

Fig. 1. The molecular structure for the crystal monomer of GDNF.

The monomer structure of GDNF includes a central α-spiral and β-fold (A and B). The amino acids of A include two reverse and parallel β-folds. The C-terminal of B contains four β-folds. The dimer, with a reverse and parallel structure, presents a symmetrical receptor binding site. A and B are crucial binding sites for GFRα1.

3.2 GDNF distribution and expression

In mammalian brains, GDNF is mainly expressed in the target cells of DA-ergic neurons in the midbrain substantia nigra, such as granular cells in the corpora striatum, nucleus accumbens, thalamic nuclei, tuber olfactorium, hippocampus, cerebellum, callosal gyrus and olfactory bulb, where it acts as the original neurotrophic factor (Sonntag *et al.*, 2005). In the kidneys and gastrointestinal tract, GDNF is expressed in media cells and smooth muscle cells, respectively. Additionally, GDNF induces the differentiation of neural crest cells and Wolffian ducts in intestinal neurons and renal ducts, respectively (Bohn *et al.*, 2000). The peripheral expression of GDNF can also been seen in tissues innervated by sensory neurons (trigeminal ganglion, nodosal ganglion and dorsal root ganglion) and autonomic neurons. The distribution of GDNF in the human brain, which is identical to that in the rat brain, includes high expression in the caudate nucleus (innervated by the substantia nigra), low expression in the dorsal caudate putamen and no expression in the substantia nigra (Schaar *et al.*, 1994). GDNF has also been reported to be expressed in the hippocampus, cortex and spinal cord (Springer *et al.*, 1994). In general, the GDNF expression in peripheral organs is higher than that of neuronal tissues.

3.3 The functions of GDNF

In the CNS, GFLs maintain the survival and activity of DA-ergic neurons in the midbrain and motor neurons of the cornu anterius medullae spinalis. In addition, GDNF, NRTN and ARTN maintain the differentiation and survival of some peripheral neurons, such as sympathetic neurons, parasympathetic neurons, sensory neurons and neurons in the intestinal wall. Outside of the nervous system, GDNF plays vital roles in the processes of kidney development and spermatic production, along with many other processes in the body (Airaksinen & Saarma, 2002; Manié *et al.*, 2001; Airaksinen *et al.*, 1999).
In the midbrain of adult animals, GDNF promotes the survival of DA-ergic neurons (Springer *et al.*, 1994). Some scholars have proposed that GDNF plays an essential role in supporting the survival and maintenance of mature DA-ergic neurons (Pascual *et al.*, 2008). Microinjection of 6-OHDA into the corpora striatum leads to the degeneration of DA-ergic neurons in the substantia nigra. This degeneration can be attenuated by pretreatment with GDNF in the substantia nigra, thus abrogating the injury induced by 6-OHDA and hindering the death of DA-ergic neurons. Other evidence has confirmed that GDNF promotes the regeneration of DA-ergic neurons after brain injury (Beck *et al.*, 1995; Tomac *et al.*, 1995; Hou *et al.*, 1996), which correlates with the fact that GDNF promotes the differentiation of DA-ergic neurons after brain injury. For example, GDNF promotes increase of the cell body, prolongation of axons and an increase in dopamine synthesis. Additionally, studies have demonstrated that GDNF can selectively protect DA-ergic neurons against the neurotoxic effects exerted by methylamphetamine (Cass, 1996). Thus far, GDNF, as a potential therapeutic agent for PD, has been studied extensively (Azzouz *et al.*, 2004; Eslamboli *et al.*, 2005). Further research has demonstrated that GDNF can modulate neuronal excitability and transmitter release (Wang *et al.*, 2003; Kobori *et al.*, 2004). For

example, *in vitro*, GDNF can rapidly activate the MAPK signaling pathway after acting on midbrain DA-ergic neurons, and increase neuronal excitability (Yang *et al.*, 2001). In addition, the GDNF signaling system can mediate the migration and chemotaxis of neurons (Tang *et al.*, 1998). Some researchers have also demonstrated that GDNF can potentiate analgesia in neuropathic pain (Sakai *et al.*, 2008). Further, GDNF plays critical roles in the neuronal development of sympathetic and motor neurons, and synapse formation in the hippocampus (Moore *et al.*, 1996; Ledda *et al.*, 2007).

4. The signal pathway for GDNF activation

4.1 GDNF receptors and structures

4.1.1 GFRα

The biological actions exerted by GDNF on cells must be mediated via trans-membrane signal transmission, i.e. membrane receptors, as GDNF is a secreted protein (Josso & di Clemente, 1997). The receptor system for GFLs is divided into two parts. One part, a binding receptor, anchors to the cell surface via GPI and binds to GDNF directly. The identified GFLs include GFRα1, GFRα2, GFRα3 and GFRα4, each with its own binding receptor. For example, GDNF binds to GFRα1, NRTN binds to GFRα2, ARTN binds to GFRα3 and PSPN binds to GFRα4. The other part of the GFLs receptor system consists of the trans-membrane signal transduction receptor, RET, as well as a tyrosine kinase receptor. In the process of signal transduction, the members of the GDNF family share the same RET, but a distinct GFRα (Airaksinen *et al.*, 1999). The homology between GFRα1 and GFRα2 is as high as 48%, and both are expressed in the neurons and tissues of the superior cervical ganglion and dorsal root ganglion (Baloh *et al.*, 1997). The expression of GFRα3 is strictly limited, and is not seen in the CNS (Widenfalk *et al.*, 1998). In contrast, GFRα1 and GFRα2 are widely expressed in the CNS and peripheral organs (Nomoto *et al.* 1998). The expression of GFRα4 has only been observed in avian cells (Saarma & Sariola, 1999). In addition, GFRα contains three corresponding cysteine-rich domains, with different lengths for three structural domains. The second domain binds to GFL, while the functions of the first and third domains are not clear. The first domain is not involved in the binding of RET and GFRα1, and is not expressed in GFRα4.

4.1.2 RET

RET is a trans-membrane tyrosine kinase receptor encoded by the oncogene *Ret*. *Ret* was first discovered in mice NIH/3T3 cells. Identical to other tyrosine kinase receptors, the RET protein is composed of an extracellular ligand-binding domain, a trans-membrane domain and an intracellular functional tyrosine kinase domain. The RET protein contains 21 exons and many spliceosomes, with four cadherin-like domains and a cysteine-rich domain.

RET can be expressed as many sub-types based on the selective splicing of the primary *Ret* transcript (Tahira *et al.*, 1990; Lorenzo *et al.*, 1995). Two subtypes, RET9 and RET51, have been further studied, and the functional difference between the two is ascribed mainly to structural differences in the tails. The C-terminal end of RET9 contains nine amino acids, and the entire protein consists of 1072 amino acids. RET51 is longer than RET9, with a total of 1114 amino acids, including 51 amino acids in the tail. Both RET9 and RET51 have Tyr1062 in their C-terminal. Tyr1062 is phosphorylated during RET activation and anchoring of the receptor protein. Some researchers have demonstrated the regulation of lateral sequences in the C-terminal of Tyr 1062, which leads to different activities of the two subtypes (Wong *et al.*, 2005). Moreover, RET51 contains two tyrosine residues, Tyr 1090 and Tyr1096, which interact with SHC and GRB2, respectively (Lorenzo *et al.*, 1997; Alberti *et al.*, 1998; Borrello *et al.*, 2002).

RET, a common signal transduction receptor for GFLs, mediates many signal pathways for GDNF and induces apoptosis (Bordeaux *et al.*, 2000), and also inhibits tumor growth (Cañibano *et al.*, 2007) when GDNF is absent. The mutation of *Ret* may lead to diseases with functional depletion. Activating mutations correlate with thyroid cancer and type-II familial polyendocrine adenomatosis. A deactivating mutation of *Ret* is the cause of Hirchsprung disease. In adult animals, the depletion of RET leads to the depletion of DA-ergic cells in the nigrostriatal system. This indicates that RET is a key factor in maintaining the nigrostriatal system. The degradation of RET occurs through Cb-1 ubiquitin ligase mediated receptor recruitment and ubiquitination in the proteasome pathway.

4.1.3 NCAM

In the CNS, the regions of expression of GFRα1 and RET are not identical, e.g. GFRα1, but not RET, is expressed in the cortex and hippocampus (Trupp *et al.*, 1997; Glazner *et al.*, 1998; Golden *et al.*, 1998; Burazin & Gundlach, 1999; Golden *et al.*, 1999). The absence of RET expression in these regions indicates the existence of RET-independent GDNF signal pathways. In 2003, Paratcha *et al.* demonstrated that GDNF has the ability to transmit signals through directly binding to NCAM (Paratcha *et al.*, 2003). NCAM belongs to the cell adhesion molecule super family, and is encoded by a singular gene consisting of 26 exons (Lin *et al.*, 1993). The selective splicing of the gene can produce almost 120 NCAM subtypes, three of which are named NCAM-120, NCAM-140 and NCAM-180. These three subtypes possess an identical extracellular N-terminus, which contains five immunoglobulin-like domains and two domains located on the cell surface that are homologous with type-III fibronectin. Both NCAM-140 and NCAM-180 are trans-membrane proteins possessing the same trans-membrane domains but different intracellular domains. NCAM-120 has no trans-membrane or intracellular domains, and anchors to the extracellular surface via GPI. NCAM-180 and NCAM-120 are expressed predominantly in fetal neurons and neuroglia, respectively, while NCAM-140 is expressed in both (Noble *et al.*, 1985). Further research has demonstrated that the NCAM-140 subtype mediates the biological activities of GDNF. NCAM is not only involved in the adherence of cells, but also induces the intracellular signal transduction, and thus promotes axon growth and neuronal survival (Ditlevsen *et al.*, 2008) and inhibits the proliferation of astrocytes (Krushel *et al.*, 1998). The action of GDNF on DA-ergic neurons in the midbrain can be attenuated by blocking the function of NACM using anti-NACM antibodies, indicating that GDNF is activated via an NACM-transmitted signaling pathway, even in brain regions that express RET (Chao *et al.*, 2003).

4.1.4 Integrins and N-cadherin

Integrins are a family of cell surface receptors of cell adhesion molecules (CAMs). As a transmembrane glycoprotein, integrin is distributed on many types of cells, and can interact with extracellular ligands, the intracellular cystoskeleton and signal molecules to integrate the intra-with the extracellular environmental signals. Integrin is a heterodimer composed of an α and a β subunit, coupled by non-covalent bonds. Studies have indicated that integrin assembles some protein complexes via its β subunit, which is responsible for the specificity of those proteins and the subsequent signals. FAK, a non-receptor tyrosine kinase, plays an important role in this process. First, FAK binds to corresponding proteins in the C terminus and phosphorylates itself. The phosphorylated tyrosine then binds to an SH2 domain in Src. Next, many amino acids sites in FAK are phosphorylated by Src which initiates a series of signals. The extracellular segment of the α subunit can bind to other proteins on the membrane, which would, in turn, bind to other SHCs. The phosphorylated tyrosines in SHC then bring the Grb2-SOS complex to the cell membrane and activate Ras. Integrins can bind to many extracellular matrix proteins, including laminin and fibronectin, which play vital roles in cell movement, adherence, synaptogenesis, proliferation, apoptosis, neural development and the inflammatory response (Chao *et al.*, 2003; Anton *et al.*, 1999). Some studies have indicated that GDNF is effective at increasing the expression of integrin αV, and the trans-membrane signal may include integrin β1. Hence, integrin αV and integrin β1 are thought to be candidate receptors for GDNF (Cao *et al.*, 2008).

N-cadherin, a member of the cadherin (cell adhesion molecule) super-family, is widely distributed in the CNS, and has a molecular weight of 130 kD. Cadherin super-family molecules are cell surface glucoproteins whose main functions include the regulation of calcium-mediated cell adhesion, cell polarity and morphogenesis, and involvement in the mechanisms underlying intercellular recognition and signal transduction. The recognition of N-cadherin is derived from its actions on cellular differentiation and growth in the CNS. N-cadherin is a canonical trans-membrane protein, with five extracellular segments (cadherin domains) composed of 110 amino acid residues. Research has demonstrated that the entire extracellular segment of N-cadherin is very similar to that of RET (Anders *et al.*, 2001) (Figure 2). The extracellular segments of N-cadherin can interact with catenin and other proteins, so as to regulate intracellular adhesion and recombination, and promote the survival and migration of cells.

Accumulating evidence has demonstrated that both fibroblast growth factor (FGF) and epidermal growth factor (EGF) can exert their actions by binding to N-cadherin via their receptors. Recently, our studies (using plasmid construction and cell transfection) have demonstrated that inhibition of the biological functions of N-cadherin may influence the protective effects exerted by GDNF upon DA-ergic neurons. At the same time, we discovered that GDNF can bind to N-cadherin or RET directly (data not shown). Further studies should be undertaken to determine whether GDNF activation of downstream signal pathways is dependent on the interaction of its receptor and N-cadherin (a process that is identical to FGF and EGF).

The distance from the neuronal adherent proteins' domain to the cell membrane is similar to that of RET. The encoding of the RET residues is consistent with the naïve RET molecule. The black solid line indicates the inserted sequence for the RET extracellular segment. The black solid circle indicates coherent calcium binding sites. CD = binding site for cadherin, TK = tyrosine kinase, Cys = cysteine-rich domain, Cyt = cytoplasmic domain (adapted from Anders *et al.*,,2001)

4.1.5 Heparan sulfate glycosaminoglycans

Aside from RET and GFRα1, heparan sulfate proteoglycans, including syndecan and glypican, are essential in mediating the signal pathway of GDNF (Barnett *et al.*, 2002). Bespalov *et al.* demonstrated that syndecan, exerts its function via binding to heparan sulfate with high affinity (Bespalov *et al.*, 2011).

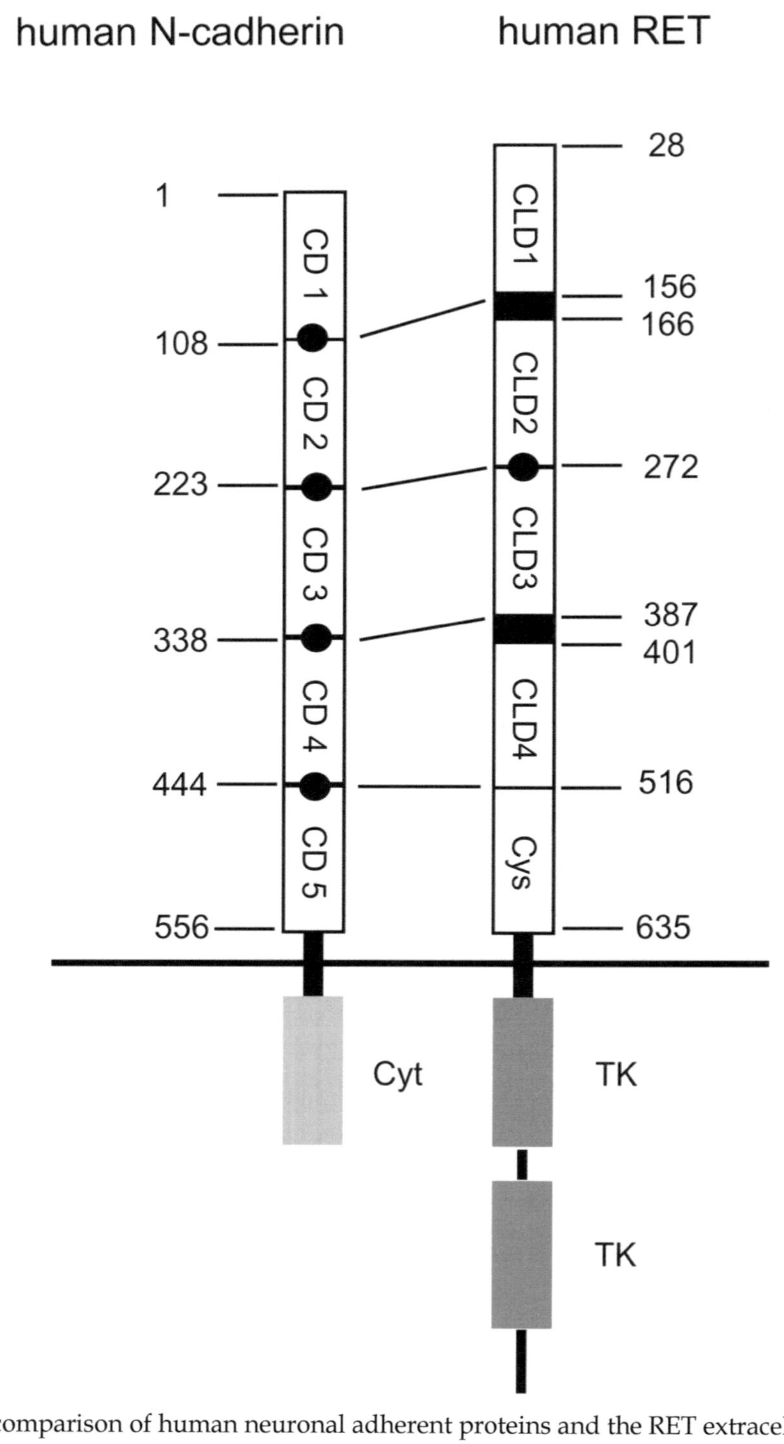

Fig. 2. The comparison of human neuronal adherent proteins and the RET extracellular segment.

GDNF mediates axonal growth and promotes neuronal migration via binding to syndecan 3. Of course, syndecan 3 may mediate the GFL signaling pathway, or may submit GFLs to the RET receptor pathway. With regard to other receptors, activation of the MET tyrosine kinase receptor by heparan sulfate proteoglycans is essential for the NCAM mediated GDNF pathway (Sariola & Saarma, 2003). The effects of heparan sulfate proteoglycans on the integrin αV/β1 and N-cadherin mediated GDNF signal pathway is under investigation.

The paucity of heparan sulfate proteoglycans may inhibit GDNF-dependent RET phosphorylation, GDNF mediated axon growth and differentiation of endothelial cells (Barnett *et al.*, 2002). Substantial evidence in mice indicates that a lack of syndecan or GDNF may lead to a decrease in GABA-releasing neurons, which implies that the two molecules are involved in cortex development.

4.1.6 Heat shock protein 27

Heat shock protein 27 (HSP27) is a protein with high conservation that is selectively synthesized after being stimulated. It resides ubiquitously in the cell membrane, cytoplasm and nucleus of all prokaryotes and eukaryotes. HSP27 is involved in maintaining microfilaments, signal transduction of cytokines, maintaining the integrity of the cell membrane under stimuli and protection of cells against some stress injuries (Nakamoto & Vígh L, 2007). In 2009, Hong Z *et al.* discovered that 92 proteins were altered under the action of GDNF; among the altered proteins, the phosphorylation of HSP27 significantly increased, accompanied by nuclear translocation. The GDNF induced axonal growth of PC 12 cells is significantly inhibited by interference of HSP27 mRNA, which implies that many proteins are involved in GDNF-mediated neuronal differentiation of DA-ergic neurons. HSP27 is a novel signaling molecule involved in GDNF-mediated axon growth of DA-ergic neurons (Hong *et al.*, 2009).

4.2 RET-dependent signaling pathway

GFRα1 and RET are expressed in the DA-ergic neurons of the substantia nigra and ventral tegmental area, as well as in the α-motor neurons of the ventral spine and motor nuclei in the brain stem, such as the hypoglossal nucleus, facial nucleus, nuclei of the trigeminal nerve and the nucleus nervi abducentis (Glazner *et al.*, 1998). RET is mainly located in non-lipid regions where GDNF action is absent (Paratcha *et al.*, 2001).

GDNF activates RET via two pathways, in cis and in trans. When expressed in the same cell, the combination of GFRα1-RET is mediated by a cis signaling system (Yu *et al.*, 1998; Paratcha *et al.*, 2001), delineated as: (1) activation of the cis system, (2) GDNF binds to GPI-anchored GFRα1 on the membrane, (3) c-RET is recruited and activated, which is independent of tyrosine kinase activity. On the other hand, when GFRα1 is dissoluble, its binding to GFRα1-RET via a trans signaling system is delineated as: (1) GDNF and dissoluble GFRα1 (sGFRα1) are released from consecutive cells, (2) activation of extracellular c-RET, (3) the activated receptors couple and phosphorylate SHC, (4) c-RET is recruited to the membrane via activation of its tyrosine kinase and phosphorylation of Tyr-1062. Compared with the cis system, the recruitment of RET to the membrane mediated by dissoluble GFRα1 is delayed and persistent, and is dependent on the activation of domains of the RET self-kinase (Yu *et al.*, 1998; Paratcha *et al.*, 2001).

RET is recruited to the membrane and binds to GDNF-GFRα1 via the two pathways mentioned above. After recruitment to the membrane, a dimer is formed, which is followed by self-phosphorylation of RET intracellular segments (rendered as tyrosine kinase activity), recruitment of downstream signal molecules and activation of several intracellular signal pathways via a series of enzymatic reactions (Airaksinen *et al.*, 1999). In this way, cell survival, differentiation, proliferation, migration and chemotaxis are regulated. The binding site of SHC receptor proteins, tyrosine 1062, plays vital roles in the activated intracellular signal cascade reactions. After binding to the intracellular tyrosine of RET, SHC forms a complex with the GAB1/2 receptor protein and GRB2/SOS, and induces activation of the PI3K/Akt and RAS/ERK signaling pathways, respectively. After combination of tyrosine 1096 and GRB2, GAB1/2 binds to the p85 subunit of PI3K, causing the activation of PI3K (Airaksinen & Saarma, 2002). GDNF induces the formation of neuronal lamellar parapodia, which is related to the formation of the neural axis (Van Weering & Bos, 1997) and DA-ergic differentiation *in vitro* (Pong *et al.*, 1998). Jun N-terminal Kinase (JNK) is activated by Rhc/Ras-related small molecules (Chiariello *et al.*, 1998), such as GTPase and CDC42. As key regulatory factors for survival of neurotrophin-dependent neurons, JNK and PI3K/Akt may be involved in the trophic action of GDNF (Kaplan & Miller, 1997). Tyrosine 981 binds to Src, and activated p60Src is a key factor for GFL-induced signal cascade reactions. The GDNF signaling pathway regulates axonal epitaxy, distribution of ureters and neural survival (Airaksinen & Saarma, 2002). After binding to tyrosine 1015, PLC is activated and hydrolyzes the second messenger produced by IP_3, which increases intracellular calcium and activates multi-signal transmissions such as gene expression. The Ras-MAPK and PI3K/Akt signal pathways are involved in DA-ergic neurons, and GDNF activates cAMP/PKA/CREB in brain neurons in the fetus. The activation of Src kinase and PLC is involved in sensory neurons (Sariola & Saarma, 2003) (Figure 3). RET possesses other tyrosine residues, including Tyr687, Tyr826 and Tyr 1029, which correlate with GFL binding. The mechanisms involved in signal transmission, however, are still unclear.

RET, but not GFR, is expressed in the cerebellum, olfactory tubercles and nuclei in the hypothalamus. This could be explained by the hypothesis that the actions of GFR are independent on RET, and GFR is only active in trans-formation (Saarma & Sariola, 1999).

The extracellular domain of RET contains four cadherin-like structures and a cysteine-rich region. Phosphorylated Y1062 is the binding site for several proteins, which subsequently activates the RAS/ERK, JNK and PI3K/Akt signal pathways via binding to SHC, FRS2, IRS1/2, Dok1-5 and Enigma. Phosphorylated Y905, Y981, Y1015 and 1096 bind to GRB7/10, Src, PLCγ and GRB2, respectively, and mediate a series of signal pathways. (Adapted from Wells & Santoro, 2009).

4.3 RET-independent signaling pathway

In spite of the vital roles played by RET-mediated signaling pathways, the GFRα1-RET signal system is not an essential pathway for neuronal development (demonstrated in knockout mice). Recently, a series of studies has demonstrated that GDNF may exert its biological actions via RET-independent signaling pathways.

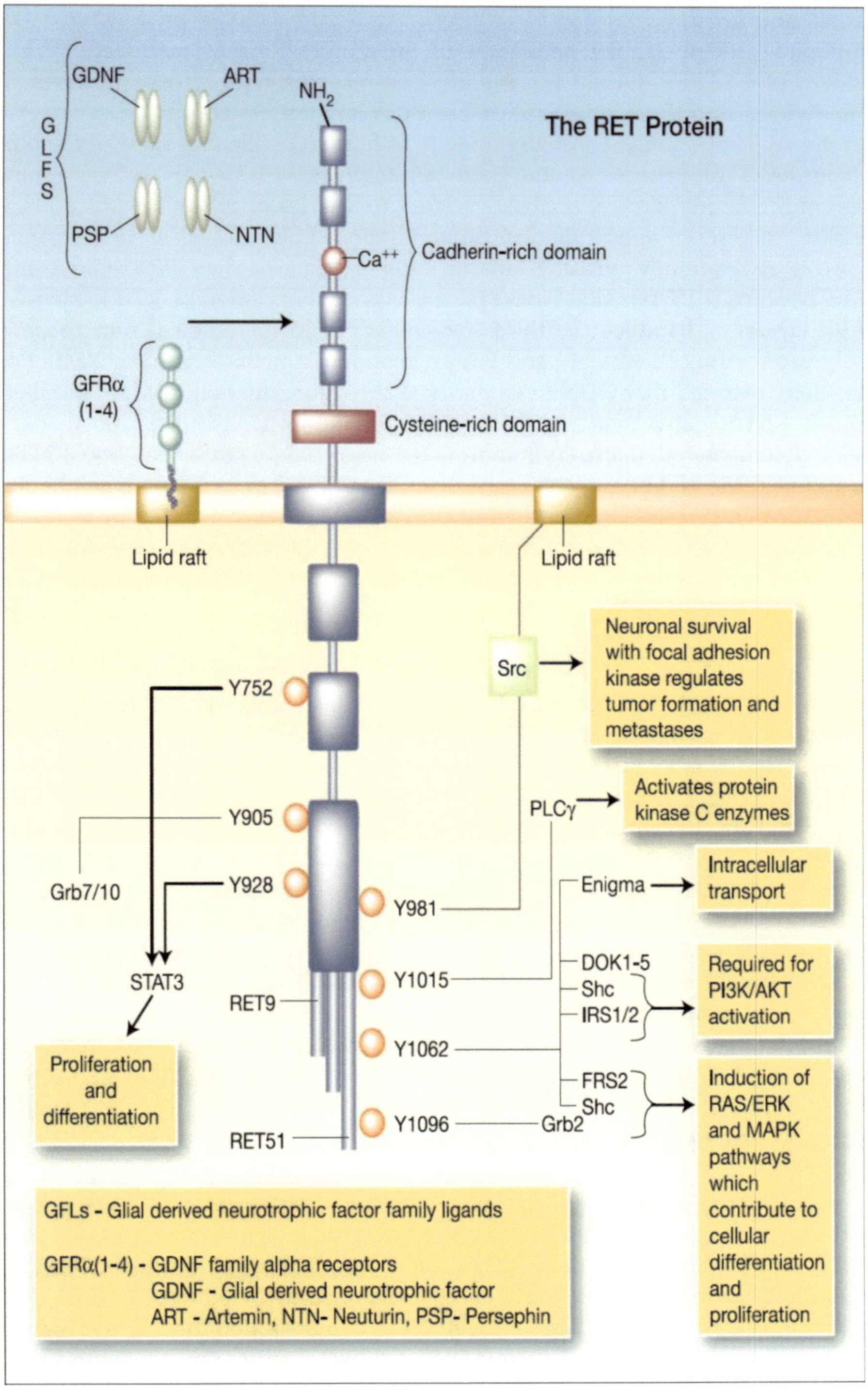

Fig. 3. The structure of RET and its signal pathway mediation.

4.3.1 GDNF and Src

As mentioned previously, the activation of Src family kinases mediated by GDNF is independent of RET. Src family kinases are non-receptor type tyrosine kinases. The Src family is divided into three sub-families: the SrcA sub-family, consisting of Src, Yes, Fyn, and Fgr; the SrcB sub-family, consisting mainly of Lck, Hck, Blk, and Lyn; and another sub-family composed of Frk. SrcA and SrcB sub-families are specific to vertebrates. The activation of Src family kinases is closely related to a series of biological functions, such as cell division, migration, apoptosis and differentiation. Poteryaev *et al.* demonstrated that GDNF activates Src-family tyrosine kinases, after binding to the GFRα1-GPI complex, in mice DRG neurons (RET tyrosine kinase paucity); phosphorylation of MAPK kinase, PLC2γ and CREB ensue, and induce the third messenger IP_3 to increase calcium concentration, eventually promoting cell survival and Fos expression (Paratcha & Ibáñez, 2002). Popsueva *et al.* also demonstrated that GDNF can promote the differentiation of MDCK cells (GFRα1 positive and RET negative) via activation of the Src family kinases (Popsueva *et al.*, 2003). Trupp also demonstrated, using an immortalized neuronal precursor cell line, RN33B (high expression of GFRα1 and no expression of RET), that GDNF does not activate the Ras/ERK signaling pathway, in these cells; instead GDNF induces the activation of Src family kinases, rapid phosphorylation of CREB and up-regulation of c-fos mRNA (Trupp *et al.*, 1999). This study provides additional evidence supporting the notion that the functions of GDNF are independent of RET.

4.3.2 GDNF and MET

The differential expression models for GFR and RET indicate that: (1) GFR functions via signal transduction pathways that do not involve RET, and (2) other GDNF ligands (binding to GFR) are involved. MET is a hepatocyte growth factor receptor (HGFR) that is normally expressed in epithelium-derived cells. The expression of hepatocyte growth factor is limited in desmohemoblast-derived cells. The primary precursor proteins of MET are cleaved to produce α and β subunits. The mature receptor is formed via a disulfide bond, and plays preliminary roles in embryonic development and wound healing. After stimulating hepatocyte growth factor, MET induces several biological reactions. In many RET-absent but GFRα1-rich cells, GDNF induces the phosphorylation of MET, and then activates the Src family kinases. This provides impetus for research on a RET-independent GDNF signaling system. The RET-independent activation of Src and MET, induced by GDNF, may be regulated by heparan sulfate and NCAM. However, *in vivo* immunoprecipitation studies have demonstrated that MET does not bind to GDNF, implying an uncertain role for GDNF-induced MET activation.

4.3.3 GDNF and NCAM

The GFRα receptor is expressed more widely than RET in many regions of the nervous system, especially the procerebrum, cortex and internal ear (Trupp *et al.*, 1997; Kokaia *et al.*, 1999), indicating that the signal transduction in neurons and glials, and GLF-protein binding may not always be dependent on RET. Other studies demonstrated that GFRα1, but not RET, is expressed in the RN33B cell line, and the signal pathway induced by GDNF overlaps with that induced by NCAM. In 2003, Paratcha *et al.* demonstrated that NCAM may mediate actions via RET-independent trans-membrane signaling. Further studies demonstrated that NCAM is involved in the promotion effects, engendered by GDNF, affecting the survival of DA-ergic neurons (Paratcha *et al.*, 2003). When GFRα is absent, the binding between GFLs and NCAM is low. In contrast, GDNF binds to NCAM140 closely when GFRα1 binds to NCAM; this leads to the phosphorylation of Fyn, a molecule conjugated to the intracellular segments of NCAM, followed by phosphorylation of FAK, and eventually activation of the MAPK signal pathway via normal signal transduction. Interestingly, the combination of GFRα1 and NCAM may downregulate NCAM-mediated cellular adherence when GDNF is absent (Cao *et al.*, 2008). This regulation is indicative of the independent roles played by GFRα1-NCAM and the GDNF-GFRα1-NCAM signaling pathway. In the RET-independent model, GDNF stimulates the migration of neurilemma cells and the growth of synapses. This finding indicates that the GFRα protein, GFLs, or their combination with NCAM, activates distinct pathways to regulate differential signal pathways.

4.3.4 GDNF and integrins

GDNF is a crucial neurotrophic factor for DA-ergic neurons. Transmembrane signal transduction is mediated by a special receptor system, which includes GFRα, RET, and NCAM140. Thus far, we have identified that another transmembrane cell adhesion molecule, integrin (a heterodimer consisting of α and β subunits), can regulate the signal transduction of GDNF. Some studies have demonstrated that chronic injection of GDNF into the substantia nigra increases the expression of integrin αV and NCAM (Chao *et al.*, 2003). This implies that GDNF exerts special effects on the increase of integrin αV expression, and that integrin αV may be a selective receptor for functional GDNF.

Under the influence of GDNF, the combination of phosphorylated SHC and intracellular integrin β1 increases. Data from co-immunoprecipitation demonstrate that integrin β1 and GFRα1 form a complex. Additionally, phosphorylation of SHC in the cytoplasmic domain of integrin β1 was shown to increase after stimulation with GDNF. Other data from molecular models demonstrated the presence of four hydrogen bonds between integrin β1 and GFRα1. These data indicate that integrin β1 may be involved in the transmembrane signaling of GDNF, and that integrin β1 may even be a selective signal receptor for GDNF (Cao *et al.*, 2008).

4.3.5 GDNF and N-cadherin

N-cadherin is a transmembrane adhesion protein, whose cytoplasmic region can interact with various intracellular proteins (Drees *et al.*, 2005; Reynolds, 2007). When its extracellular domain binds a ligand, the intracellular domain of N-cadherin can activate the PI3K/Akt and Ras/Raf/MAPK signaling pathways (Hulit *et al.*, 2007). It is well-known that the structural and functional characteristics of N-cadherin are somewhat similar to that of NCAM and integrin β1, and that it mediates not only adherence, but also signal transduction. In addition, the binding site for the extracellular domains of RET and the GDNF/GFRα1 complex, is a cadherin-like domain. Our previous studies have demonstrated that N-cadherin can also bind to GDNF, and the phosphorylation of the N-cadherin intracellular domain (Tyr860) is mediated by GDNF. Further studies, using gene silencing and immunoblotting, have demonstrated that GDNF activates the intracellular PI3K/Akt signaling pathway via N-cadherin, thus protecting DA-ergic neurons. Results from studies, using flow cytometry and Hoechst 33258 staining, indicate that GDNF interferes with the expression of N-cadherin, and that the apoptosis of injured DA-ergic neurons increases. Additional results from immunoblotting indicate, under the same conditions, that phosphorylated Akt, but not total Akt, decreases in the cytoplasm. Results from immunohistochemistry indicate a decrease in total N-cadherin, phosphorylated N-cadherin (Tyr860) and phosphorylated Akt, however, total Akt does not change. Finally, through immunoblotting it was discovered that the levels of phosphorylated N-cadherin (Tyr860) and phosphorylated Akt are dose-dependent on GDNF, and that the peak levels of both occur at 50 ng/ml (*in vitro*) and 13 ng/μl (*in vivo*) of GDNF. The levels of phosphorylated N-cadherin (Tyr860) and phosphorylated Akt are also time-dependent, and the peak levels of both occur at 15 min (*in vitro*) and 30 min (*in vivo*) after GDNF actions. Statistical analyses show that the two phosphorylations are positively related. Thus, it may be concluded that GDNF activates the PI3K/Akt pathway via N-cadherin to protect DA-ergic neurons.

5. Effects of membrane lipid rafts on GDNF actions

Tiny regions in cell membrane exist that differ in composition from other parts of the membrane. In these regions, the extracellular lipids contain rich sphingolipids and cholesterol molecules, which gather and form a mobile platform of fluid double-lipids, i.e. lipid raft. The main components of lipid rafts include GPI-coupled proteins (extramembrane), trans-membrane tyrosine kinases (intermembrane) and two Src family tyrosine kinases (intramembrane) (Simons & Ikonen, 1997). The lipid raft is an essential structure in the membrane for signal transduction, and plays a vital role in cell adherence, axon guidance and synaptic transmission (Paratcha & Ibáñez, 2002).

Substantial studies have focused on GDNF and its receptors, but the studies on the function of lipid rafts and the relationship between GDNF and its receptors are few and far between. To determine whether receptor-mediated GDNF is dependent on the functional lipid rafts, we investigated four transmembrane proteins in the lipid rafts (RET, NCAM140, integrin β1 and N-cadherin) and their involvement in mediating GDNF signal pathways. To this end, the binding of these proteins and GDNF was analyzed, using co-immunoprecipitation, based on the integrity of the membrane lipid rafts. The results demonstrated that all proteins bound to GDNF when the lipid raft was complete, and only RET and N-cadherin bound to GDNF when the lipid raft was not complete. In addition, extraction tests for the membrane lipid rafts have demonstrated that RET and NCAM, but not N-cadherin and integrin β1, may be shifted to the lipid rafts by GDNF. This series of tests indicates the importance of lipid rafts in mediating the interaction of GDNF with its receptors (Figure 4).

RET can mediate the protective actions exerted by GDNF upon DA-ergic neurons (Trupp *et al.*, 1996; Durbec *et al.*, 1996). After GDNF stimulation, RET induces multiple signals to mediate the signal pathways of GDNF via two models (intra-lipid raft and extra-lipid raft) (Tansey *et al.*, 2000). Membrane lipid rafts are the basis for the shift and functional activation of RET (Poteryaev *et al.*, 1999). Activated RET influences different downstream targets in lipid rafts. The RET activated extra-raft preferentially binds to SHC, and the RET activated intra-raft binds preferentially to FRS2, thus mediating a series of signal pathways. The membrane lipid rafts provide abundant micro-environments for the binding of RET and kinases/receptor proteins in the raft, and is involved in the GFL signaling pathway. For example, Src family kinases, as proteins in the raft, mediate a series of functions of GDNF signal transduction, after binding to activated RET. In the lipid rafts rich in GFRα1 and Src, GDNF activates Src via a GFRα1 mediated pathway (Tansey *et al.*, 2000). Furthermore, the location of RET on the lipid raft enhances its binding to Src, whose activation is essential for GDNF mediated promotion of survival (Encinas *et al.*, 2001). In a lipid raft, RET cannot be degraded by proteases, and this protective effect may be related to its downstream actions of regulating receptor functions (Pierchala *et al.*, 2006).

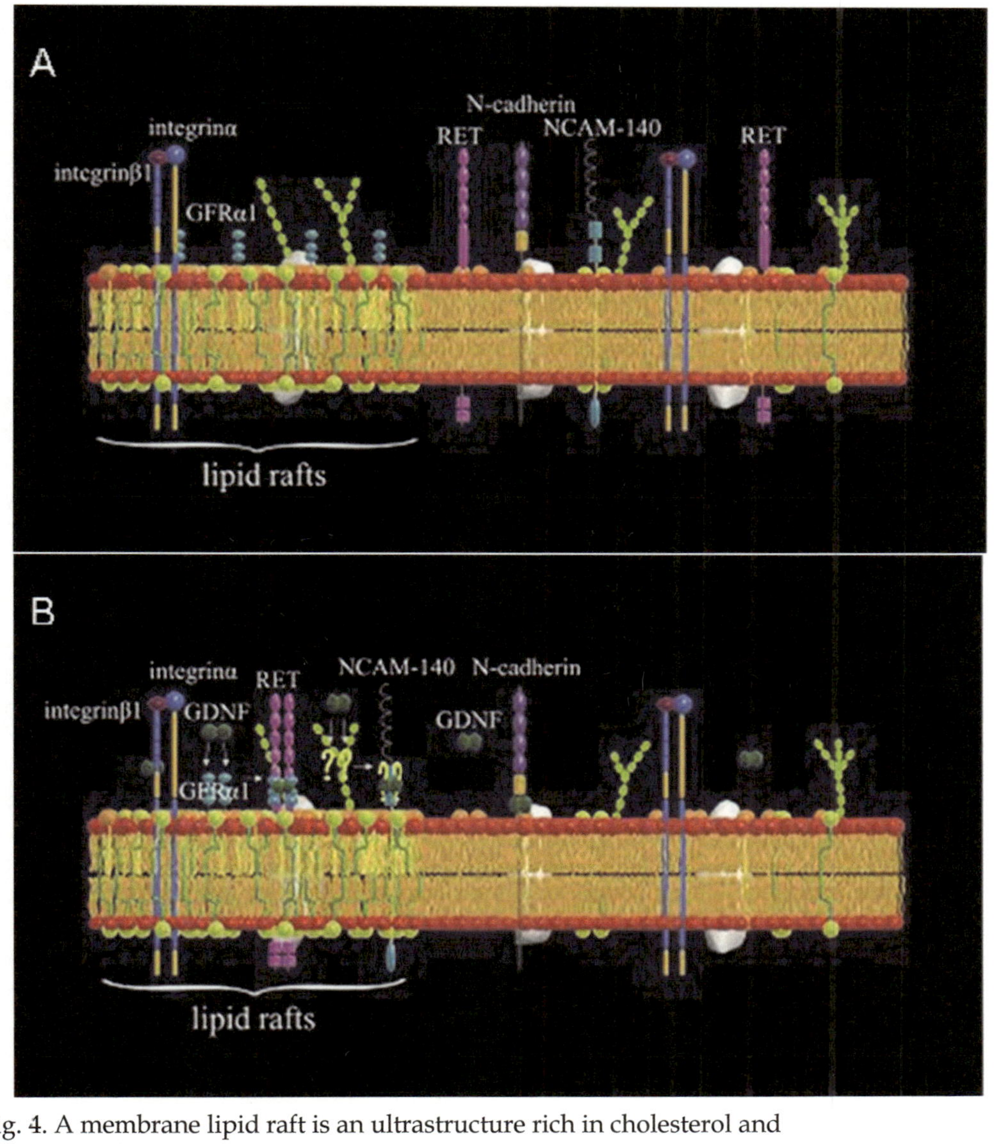

Fig. 4. A membrane lipid raft is an ultrastructure rich in cholesterol and phosphosphingolipids.

NCAM can function as a receptor of GDNF signal transduction (Sjöstrand *et al.*, 2007; Sjöstrand & Ibáñez, 2008). Under the influence of GDNF, NCAM140 binds to Fyn and is recruited to lipid rafts, followed by stimulation of the migration of Schwann cells and promotion of neuronal axonal growth (Paratcha *et al.*, 2003). In membrane lipid rafts, the binding of NCAM and Fyn leads to recruitment of FAK and the activation of the Ras-Raf-ERK1/2 pathway (Beggs *et al.*, 1997; Niethammer *et al.*, 2002).

Integrin β1 is a transmembrane cell adhesion molecule, which is expressed in DA-ergic neurons in the substantia nigra of adult mice (Cao *et al.*, 2008). Inhibitory antibodies can counteract the effects of GDNF on the promotion of survival and growth of DA-ergic

neurons (Chao *et al.*, 2003). Some reports have demonstrated that the membrane lipid rafts provide a perfect environment for the activation of integrins, mediated by growth factors, in the system of survival for oligodendrocytes. The shift of activated integrin to membrane lipid rafts is an important cue, which provides rationale for the actions of functional T cells and the basis for the study of integrin in other cells (Leitinger & Hogg, 2002).
N-cadherin, a calcium dependent cell adhesion molecule similar to NCAM140 and integrin β1, is a trans-membrane protein that mediates the axonal growth of astrocytes and Schwann cells. As mentioned above, the intracellular domain of N-cadherin is similar to the extra-domain of RET. Additionally, N-cadherin can activate the PI3K/Akt and Ras/Raf/MAPK signal pathways (*et al.*,) [(73)], which provides the rationale for further delving into GDNF and its function.
It is closely related to signal transduction in the membrane and provides a platform for anchoring proteins. A: GFRα1 and integrin β1 integrate into the membrane lipid raft of DA-ergic neurons, but RET, N-cadherin, and NCAM-140 are outside of the raft. B: A GDNF dimer combines with GFRα1 and forms a GDNF-GFRα1 complex, which binds to RET and gathers in the membrane lipid raft. The combination of the GDNF dimer and NCAM dimer requires another substance. N-cadherin and integrin do not gather in the membrane lipid raft, but N-cadherin can bind to GDNF outside of the raft.

6. GDNF treatment in Parkinson's disease

The degeneration of DA-ergic neurons in the substantia nigra of the midbrain is the main pathological characteristic of PD. Based on this characteristic, the most predominant therapeutic strategies are to administer DOPA agents to supply dopamine to the brain, or to employ dopamine agonists to activate the DA-receptor directly. However, the efficacies of these drugs tend to wane because the residual DA-ergic neurons decrease during the progression of PD. In 1993, GDNF, as a growth factor that promotes the survival and growth of DA-ergic neurons in the midbrain, was extracted and qualified (Lin *et al.*, 1993). Early studies demonstrated that GDNF elevates the affinity of neurons to DA, increases the uptake of DA and the expression of tyrosine hydroxylase and promotes the growth of neurapophysis in cultured midbrain DA-ergic neurons. In addition, GDNF was demonstrated to act as neurotrophic factor in spinal motor neurons (Henderson *et al.*, 1994) and noradrenergic neurons (Arenas *et al.*, 1995) in the CNS. Further, GDNF was found to maintain a low level in PD patients and in elder rodents (Yurek & Fletcher-Turner, 2000; Jenner and Olanow, 1998). Thus, this neurotrophic factor is viewed as a potential treatment for neurodegenerative disease.
In cultured embryonic DA-ergic neurons, the paucity of GDNF initiates a novel non-classical death pathway in which the mitochondria does not release cytochrome to the cytoplasm, Bax is not activated and over-expressed Bcl-xL does not inhibit death. However, death is inhibited by the caspase inhibitor BAF, and mutants of caspase-9, caspase-3 and caspase-7, indicating that caspases are essential for the process. Another study demonstrated that in the MLK-c-Jun pathway, caspase-2 and caspase-7 are essential for GDNF-paucity-induced death. In neuroblastoma cells, the GDNF response is similar.
Based on this principle, researchers have adopted different models to supply GDNF in PD animal models. The results demonstrated that GDNF inhibits the variation of Bcl-2 and Bax, up-regulates Bcl-XL, inhibits the combination of CYT-C and Apaf-1 as well as the activity of caspase-3 (Ghribi *et al.*, 2001) reverses the death of DA-ergic neurons induced by

neurotoxins and stimulates functional recovery. In the presence of Aβ peptide, GDNF can inhibit Aβ neurotoxin via blocking the activation of gad153, JNK and ERK induced by ER stress, and promote cell survival. In granular cells of the cerebellum, GDNF inhibits the activation of p38-MAPK via PI3K, and prevents the injury induced by TGF-β in the protoplasmic membrane (Subramaniam *et al.*, 2008).

The summary of research progress on different GDNF supplementation methods is as follows:

Direct injection of GDNF: Some studies have demonstrated that injection of GDNF into the substantia nigra only decreases the apoptosis of DA-ergic neurons, but injection into the striatum corpora repairs the neuronal process of TH-positive neurons and improves the PD symptoms (Bohn *et al.*, 2000). Injection of GDNF into the striatum corpora can decrease the death rate of DA-ergic neurons up to 60%, as well as increase the ispilateral TH-positive immunoreactivity and synaptic growth in the nigrostriatal system. Additionally, injection of GDNF into the striatum corpora can increase the amount, volume and synaptic length of DA-ergic neurons as well as the uptake of dopamine.

Injection of GDNF via virus vehicle: This method can transfer the neurotrophic factors into the CNS (Figure 5). In 1-methyl-4-phenyl-1,2,3,6-tetrahydropyridine (MPTP) animal models, a lentivirus encoding GDNF was injected into the caudate nucleus, putamen and substantia nigra; a lentivirus encoding for the β-galactosidase enzyme was injected in the control group. Three months later, the PD system scores in the test groups were improved compared to that of the control group (Kordower *et al.*, 2000). Bowenkamp *et al.* used 6-OHDA animal models and obtained similar results (Bowenkamp *et al.*, 1996). These findings indicate that GDNF plays a positive role in neuronal reconditioning and synaptic growth in the substantia nigra. However, over-expressed GDNF may also play a negative role in PD treatment. Eslamboli *et al.* reported that high levels of GDNF expression altered bilateral DA transport and synthesis, and produced toxic or adverse effects (Eslamboli *et al.*, 2003; Eslamboli *et al.*, 2005). Thus, low and sustained expression seems to be most prudent. In Huntington's disease, the repeated gene amplification of the huntingtin protein leads to neurological disorders, which can be attenuated by adenovirus-vehicle mediated GDNF expression.

Injection of GDNF via cell mediation: Researchers are searching for other efficacious ways to import GDNF. For example, the BHK-21 cell, transformed by genetic engineering, can persistently express GDNF in neural stem cells (Behrstock & Svendsen, 2004). Here, we introduce a method of delivering GDNF termed encapsulated cell delivery (ECD). This method requires a catheter-like device with a diameter of no more than 1 mm, which is used to inject agents into the striatum corpora. A mobile device, made up of a hollow fiber membrane (< 1.5 cm), is used to control the diffusion of nutrients and injected GDNF. Cell lines of high quality are selected via this fiber membrane. In the process, the membrane is a barrier preventing immunological rejection of allogenic cells.

GDNF permeable to the blood-brain barrier: Recently, a novel GDNF was developed. It is a fusion protein formed by the combination of GDNF and cell perforin mediated by the trans-activator of the HIV virus. Diez *et al.* demonstrated, in the mouse PD model (i.p. injection), that Tat-GDNF could cross the blood-brain barrier and enter into the nigrostriatal system (Dietz *et al.*, 2006). Unfortunately, Tat -GDNF could not protect injured DA-ergic neurons or improve PD symptoms in MPTP models.

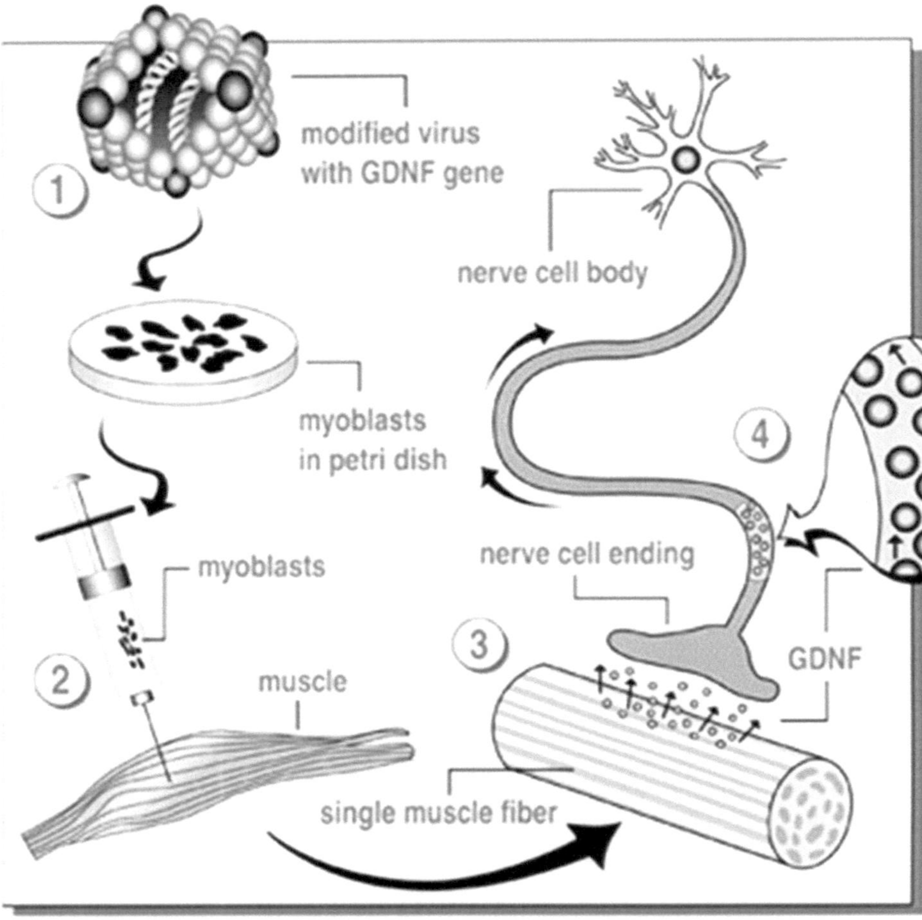

1. Immature myogenous cells are infected by improved GDNF-carrier genes.
2. The infected myogenous cells are injected into muscle in amyotrophic lateral sclerosis (ALS) mice
3. The infected cells mix with myogenous cells, and produce and secrete GDNF, which is absorbed by nerve fibers.
4. GDNF is transferred into the body of neurons and maintains the survival of the cells.

(Figure source: www.epfl.ch)

Fig. 5. Injection of GDNF into the CNS to transfer neurotrophic factors via virus-vehicle.

Results from animal models provide invaluable information for clinical research. In 2002, Steven Gill and colleagues injected GDNF directly into the brain of PD patients, which significantly attenuated the PD symptoms (Gill *et al.*, 2003). The purpose of this Phase I clinic trial was to evaluate the safety of GDNF injections. Previous data, based on animal models, showed that GDNF can prolong the survival time of DA-ergic neurons and enhance their functions. In this study, researchers pumped GDNF into the striatum corpora of five PD patients at dose of 40 mg/d, for 18 months. These researchers believed that the cells closest to tip of the catheter absorbed the GDNF first. After permeating the brain tissues, GDNF reached the DA-ergic cells. The results demonstrated that the symptoms were attenuated, the motor functions were elevated by 39%, the quality of life was improved and daily activities were increased by 61%; no adverse effects were reported up to one year later. Results from PET scans demonstrated that GDNF enhanced dopamine in brain. This therapy also attenuated L-dopa induced tremors. Unfortunately, in 2004, Amgen conducted a larger-scale trial, and GDNF did not exert effects as expected. Further, the company expressed concern over the safety of GDNF. After that, the direct application of GDNF was all but abandoned. However, exploration into mechanisms of action of GDNF is an alternative avenue that may aid in the development of new therapies for PD treatment.

7. Conclusion

After the identification of GDNF, three other family members (NTN, PSP and ART) were identified, and as further studies are undertaken, more family members may be uncovered. The receptors of these factors are composed of two parts: the GDNF family receptor and the transmembrane tyrosine kinase RET. The GPI-coupled GFR determines their specific signal transduction.

Initially, researchers assumed that only one signal pathway for GDNF existed: via GFRα1/2, anchored by receptor tyrosine kinase RET and glycosyl-phosphatidyl inositol. In 2003, *in vitro* studies demonstrated that the adhesion molecule NCAM was a receptor for GFLs that was independent of RET signaling. Recently, studies have indicated that integrin αV/β1 and N-cadherin may also be selective receptors for GDNF. As more evidence comes to light, it is evident that the signal pathway for GDNF protection of DA-ergic neurons is a complex one.

In DA-ergic neurons, GDNF activated Ras-MAPK and PI3K/Akt signaling pathways play vital roles in neuronal survival and axon growth. Present studies indicate that NCAM, a new GFI receptor, is also involved in the signaling pathways of GDNF-GFRα1-MET and NGF-TrkA-RET, which also makes the biological characteristics of GDNF complex.

Some progress has been made in therapeutic trials for neuronal degenerative diseases based on the neurotrophic actions of GDNF. Repeated, direct injection of GDNF is especially valuable for treating myeleterosis such as amyotrophic lateral sclerosis (ALS). Because of the features of the blood-brain barrier and brain tissues, direct injections of GDNF to treat PD and other neurodegenerative diseases have limited use. Thus, direct GDNF gene injection mediated by vehicle or transgenic cellular transplant is a promising alternative. Currently, the challenge lies in the development of a safe, novel vehicle for the delivery of genes that can be specially expressed in tissues, can induce gene expression and can replace the virus vehicle.

In the management of PD, the application of drugs with low molecular weights is another choice for recombining neurotrophic factors. Other GFLs may be of potential value for treatment. Present studies demonstrate that, in murine PD models, PSPN, which is transferred into brains via neuronal stem cells, exerts effects as well as GDNF, on the survival of DA-ergic neurons in the midbrain (Akerud *et al.*, 2002). As we know, the expression of GFRα4, which is the receptor of PSPN, is more limited than that of GFRα1, the receptor of GDNF. Thus, we can propose that, even if high concentrations of PSPN are used, the adverse effects may be fewer than using GDNF (Lindahl *et al.*, 2000). The next challenge is to identify novel drugs, with low molecular weights and natural neurotrophic properties, to influence intracellular signal transduction. These explorations should be based on the comprehensive recognition of GFLs and the 3D structure of its receptor, as well as molecules, cells and disease.

8. References

Airaksinen, MS. & Saarma, M. (2002). The GDNF family: signalling, biological functions and therapeutic value. Nat Rev Neurosci, Vol.3, No.5, pp.383-394, ISSN 1471-003X

Airaksinen, MS.; Titievsky, A. & Saarma, M. (1999). GDNF family neurotrophic factor signaling: four masters, one servant? Mol Cell Neurosci, Vol.13, No.5, pp.313-325, ISSN 1044-7431

Akerud, P.; Holm, PC.; Castelo-Branco, G.; Sousa, K.; Rodriguez, FJ. & Arenas, E. (2002). Persephin-overexpressing neural stem cells regulate the function of nigral dopaminergic neurons and prevent their degeneration in a model of Parkinson' s disease. Mol Cell Neurosci, Vol.21, No.2, pp.205-222, ISSN 1044-7431

Alberti, L.; Borrello, MG.; Ghizzoni, S.; Torriti, F.; Rizzetti, MG. & Pierotti, MA. (1998). Grb2 binding to the different isoforms of Ret tyrosine kinase. Oncogene, Vol.17, No.9, pp.1079-1087, ISSN 0950-9232

Anders, J.; Kjar, S. & Ibáñez, CF. (2001). Molecular modeling of the extracellular domain of the RET receptor tyrosine kinase reveals multiple cadherin-like domains and a calcium-binding site. J Biol Chem, Vol.276, No.38, pp.35808-35817, ISSN 0021-9258

Anton, ES.; Kreidberg, JA. & Rakic, P. (1999). Distinct functions of alpha3 and alpha(v) integrin receptors in neuronal migration and laminar organization of the cerebral cortex. Neuron, Vol.22, No.2, pp.277-289, ISSN 0896-6273

Arenas, E.; Trupp, M. & Akerud, P. (1995). GDNF prevents degeneration and promotes the phenotype of brain noradrenergic neurons in vivo. Neuron, Vol.15, No.6, pp.1465-1473, ISSN 0896-6273

Azzouz, M.; Ralph, S.; Wong, LF.; Day, D.; Askham, Z.; Barber, RD.; Mitrophanous, KA.; Kingsman, SM. & Mazarakis, ND. (2004). Neuroprotection in a rat Parkinson model by GDNF gene therapy using EIAV vector. Neuroreport, Vol.15, No.6, pp.985-990, ISSN 0959-4965

Baloh, RH.; Enomoto H.; Johnson, EM Jr. & Milbrandt, J. (2000). The GDNF family ligands and receptors-implications forneural development. Curr Opin Neurobiol, Vol.10, No.1, pp.103-110, ISSN 0959-4388

Baloh, RH.; Tansey, MG.; Golden, JP.; Creedon, DJ.; Heuckeroth, RO.; Keck, CL.; Zimonjic, DB.; Popescu, NC.; Johnson, EM Jr. & Milbrandt, J. (1997). TrnR2, a novel receptor that mediates neurturin and GDNF signaling through Ret. Neuron, Vol.18, No.5, pp.793-802, ISSN 0896-6273

Barnett, MW.; Fisher, CE.; Perona-Wright, G. & Davies, J. (2002). Signalling by glial cell line-derived neurotrophic factor (GDNF) requires heparan sulphate glycosaminoglycan. J Cell Sc, Vol.115, No.Pt23, pp.4495-4503, ISSN 0021-9533

Beck, KD.; Valverde, J.; Alexi, T.; Poulsen, K.; Moffat, B.; Vandlen, RA.; Rosenthal, A. & Hefti, F. (1995). Mesencephalic dopaminergic neurons protected by GDNF from axotomy-induced degeneration in the adult brain. Nature, Vol.373, No.6512, pp.339-341, ISSN 0028-0836

Beggs, HE.; Baragona, SC.; Hemperly, JJ. & Maness, PF. (1997). NCAM140 interacts with the focal adhesion kinase p125(fak) and the SRC-related tyrosine kinase p59(fyn). J Biol Chem, Vol.272, No.13, pp.8310-8319, ISSN 0021-9258

Behrstock, S. & Svendsen, CN. (2004). Combining growth factors, stem cells, and gene therapy for the aging brain. Ann N Y Acad Sci, Vol.1019, pp.5-14, ISSN 0077-8923

Bespalov, MM.; Sidorova, YA.; Tumova, S.; Ahonen-Bishopp, A.; Magalhães, AC.; Kulesskiy, E.; Paveliev, M.; Rivera, C.; Rauvala, H. & Saarma, M. (2011). Heparan sulfate proteoglycan syndecan-3 is a novel receptor for GDNF, neurturin, and artemin. J Cell Biol, Vol.192, No.1, pp.153-169, ISSN 0021-9525

Bohn, MC.; Kozlowski, DA. & Connor, B. (2000). G1ial cell line derived neurotrophic factors(GDNF) as a defensive molecule for neurodegenerative disease: a tribute to the studies of antonia vernadakis on neuronal-glial interactions. Int J Dev Neurosci, Vol.18, No.7, pp.679-684, ISSN 0736-5748

Bordeaux, MC.; Forcet, C.; Granger, L.; Corset, V.; Bidaud, C.; Billaud, M.; Bredesen, DE.; Edery, P. & Mehlen, P. (2000). The RET proto-oncogene induces apoptosis: a novel mechanism for Hirschsprung disease. EMBO J, Vol.19, No.15, pp.4056-4063, ISSN 0261-4189

Borrello, MG.; Mercalli, E.; Perego, C.; Degl'Innocenti, D.; Ghizzoni, S.; Arighi, E.; Eroini, B.; Rizzetti, MG. & Pierotti, MA. (2002). Differential interaction of Enigma protein with the two RET isoforms. Biochem Biophys Res Commun, Vol.296, No.3, pp.515-522, ISSN 0006-291X

Bowenkamp, KE.; David, D.; Lapchak, PL.; Henry, MA.; Granholm, AC.; Hoffer, BJ. & Mahalik, TJ. (1996). 6-hydroxydopamine induces the loss of the dopaminergic phenotype in substantia nigra neurons of the rat. A possible mechanism for restoration of the nigrostriatal circuit mediated by glial cell line-derived neurotrophic factor. Exp Brain Res, Vol.111, No.1, pp.1-7, ISSN 0014-4819

Burazin, TC. & Gundlach, AL. (1999). Localization of GDNF/neurturin receptor (c-ret, GFRalpha-1 and alpha-2) mRNAs in postnatal rat brain: differential regional and temporal expression in hippocampus, cortex and cerebellum. Brain Res Mol Brain Res, Vol.73, No.1-2, pp.151-171, ISSN 0169-328X

Cañibano, C.; Rodriguez, NL.; Saez, C.; Tovar, S.; Garcia-Lavandeira, M.; Borrello, MG.; Vidal, A.; Costantini, F.; Japon, M.; Dieguez, C. & Alvarez, CV. (2007). The dependence receptor Ret induces apoptosis in somatotrophs through a Pit-1/p53 pathway, preventing tumor growth. EMBO J, Vol.26, No.8, pp.2015-2028, ISSN 0261-4189

Cao, JP.; Yu, JK.; Li, C.; Sun, Y.; Yuan, HH.; Wang, HJ. & Gao, DS. (2008). Integrin $\beta 1$ is involved in the signaling of glial cell line-derived neurotrophic factor. J Comp Neurol, Vol.509, No.2, pp.203-210, ISSN 0021-9967

Cass, WA. (1996). GDNF selectively protects dopamine neurons over serotonin neurons against the neurotoxic effects of methamphetamine. J Neurosci, Vol.16, No.24, pp.8132-8139, ISSN 0270-6474

Chao, CC.; Ma, YL.; Chu, KY. & Lee, EH. (2003). Integrin αV and NCAM mediate the effects of GDNF on DA neuron survival, outgrowth, DA turnover and motor activity in rats. Neurobiol Aging, Vol.24, No.1, pp.105-111, ISSN 0197-4580

Chiariello, M.; Visconti R.; Carlomagno, F.; Melillo, RM.; Bucci, C.; de Franciscis, V.; Fox, GM.; Jing, S.; Coso, OA.; Gutkind, JS.; Fusco, A. & Santoro, M. (1998). Signalling of the Ret receptor tyrosine kinase through the c-jun NH2-terminal protein kinases

(JNKS): evidence for a divergence of the ERKs and JNKs pathways induced by Ret. Oncogene, Vol.16, No.19, pp.2435-2445, ISSN 0950-9232

Daly, TM.; Okuyama, T.; Vogler, C.; Haskins, ME.; Muzyczka, N. & Sands, MS. (1999). Neonatal intramuscular injection with recomb inant adeno-associated virus results in prolonged β-gluscuronidase expression in situ and correction of liver pathology inmucopolysac - charidosis type VII mice. Hum Gene Ther, Vol.10, No.1, pp.85-94, ISSN 1043-0342

Dietz, GP.; Valbuena, PC.; Dietz, B.; Meuer, K.; Müeller, P.; Weishaupt, JH. & Bähr, M. (2006). Application of a blood-brain-barrier-penetrating form of GDNF in a mouse model for Parkinson's disease. Brain Res, Vol.1082, No.1, pp.61-66, ISSN 0006-8993

Ditlevsen, DK.; Povlsen, GK.; Berezin, V. & Bock, E. (2008). NCAM-induced intracellular signaling revisited. J Neurosci Res, Vol.86, No.4, pp.727-743, ISSN 0270-6474

Drees, F.; Pokutta, S.; Yamada, S.; Nelson, WJ. & Weis, WI. (2005). Alpha-catenin is a molecular switch that binds E-cadherin - β-catenin and regulates actin-filament assembly. Cell, Vol.123, No.5, pp.903-915, ISSN 0092-8674

Durbec, P.; Marcos-Gutierrez, CV.; Kilkenny, C.; Grigoriou, M.; Wartiowaara, K.; Suvanto, P.; Smith, D.; Ponder, B.; Costantini, F.; Saarma, M. & Et, Al. (1996). GDNF signalling through the Ret receptor tyrosine kinase. Nature, Vol.381, No.6585, pp.789-793, ISSN 0028-0836

Eigenbrot, C. & Gerber, N. (1997). X-ray structure of glial cell line-derived neurotrophic factor at 1.9 A resolution and implications for receptor binding. Nat Struct Biol, Vol.4, No.6, pp.435-438, ISSN 1072-8368

Encinas, M.; Tansey, MG.; Tsui-Pierchala, BA.; Comella, JX.; Milbrandt, J. & Johnson, EM Jr. (2001). c-Src is required for glial cell line-derived neurotrophic factor (GDNF) family ligand-mediated neuronal survival via a phosphatidylinositol-3 kinase (PI-3K)-dependent pathway. J Neurosci, Vol.21, No.5, pp.1464-1472, ISSN 0270-6474

Eslamboli A.; Cummings RM.; Ridley RM.; Baker HF.; Muzyczka N.; Burger C.; Mandel RJ.; Kirik D. & Annett LE. (2003). Recombinant adeno-associated viral vector (rAAV) delivery of GDNF provides protection against 6-OHDA lesion in the common marmoset monkey (Callithrix jacchus). Exp Neuro, Vol.184, No.1, pp.536-548, ISSN 0014-4886

Eslamboli, A.; Georgievska, B.; Ridley, RM.; Baker, HF.; Muzyczka, N.; Burger, C.; Mandel ,RJ.; Annett, L. & Kirik, D. (2005). Continuous low-level glial cell line-derived neurotrophic factor delivery using recombinant adeno-associated viral vectors provides neuroprotection and induces behavioral recovery in a primate model of Parkinson's disease. J Neurosci, Vol.25, No.4, pp.769-777, ISSN 0270-6474

Ghribi, O.; Herman, MM.; Forbes, MS.; DeWitt, DA. & Savory, J. (2001). GDNF protects against aluminum-induced apoptosis in rabbits by upregulating Bcl-2 and Bcl-XL and inhibiting mitochondrial Bax translocation. Neurobiol Dis, Vol.8, No.5, pp.764-773, ISSN 0969-9961

Gill, SS.; Patel NK.; Hotton, GR.; O'Sullivan, K.; McCarter, R.; Bunnage, M.; Brooks, DJ.; Svendsen, CN. & Heywood, P. (2003). Direct brain infusion of glial cell line-derived neurotrophic factor in Parkinson disease. Nat Med, Vol.9, No.5, pp.589-595, ISSN 1078-8956

Glazner, GW.; Mu, X. & Springer, JE. (1998). Localization of glial cell line-derived neurotrophic factor receptor alpha and c-ret mRNA in rat central nervous system. J Comp Neurol, Vol.391, No.1, pp.42-49, ISSN 0021-9967

Golden, JP.; Baloh, RH.; Kotzbauer, PT.; Lampe, PA.; Osborne, PA.; Milbrandt, J. & Johnson, EM Jr. (1998). Expression of neurturin, GDNF, and their receptors in the adult mouse CNS. J Comp Neurol, Vol.398, No.1, pp.139-150, ISSN 0021-9967

Golden, JP.; DeMaro, JA.; Osborne, PA.; Milbrandt, J. & Johnson, EM, Jr. (1999). Expression of neurturin, GDNF, and GDNF family-receptor mRNA in the developing and mature mouse. Exp Neurol, Vol.158, No.2, pp.504-528, ISSN 0014-4886

Hamilton, JF.; Morrison, PF.; Chen, MY.; Harvey-White, J.; Pernaute, RS.; Phillips, H.; Oldfield, E. & Bankiewicz, KS. (2001). Heparin coinfusion during convectionenhanced delivery (CED) increases the distribution of the glial-derived neurotrophic factor (GDNF) ligand family in rat striatum and enhances the pharmacological activity of neurturin. Exp Neurol, Vol.168, No.1, pp.155-161, ISSN 0014-4886

Haniu, M.; Hui, J.; Young, Y.; Le, J.; Katta, V.; Lee, R.; Shimamoto, G. & Rohde, MF. (1996). Glial cell line-derived neurotrophic factor : selective reduction of the intermolecular disulfide linkage and characterizaion of its disulfide structure. Biochemistry, Vol.35, No.51, pp.16799-16805, ISSN 0006-2960

Henderson, CE.; Phillips, HS.; Pollock, RA.; Davies, AM.; Lemeulle, C.; Armanini, M.; Simmons, L.; Moffet, B.; Vandlen, RA.; Simmons, L. & Et, Al. (1994). GDNF: a potent survival factor for motoneurons present in peripheral nerve and muscle. Science, Vol.266, No.5187, pp.1062-1064, ISSN 0036-8075

Hong, Z.; Zhang, QY.; Liu, J.; Wang, ZQ.; Zhang, Y.; Xiao, Q.; Lu, J.; Zhou, HY. & Chen, SD. (2009). Phosphoproteome study reveals Hsp27 as a novel signaling molecule involved in GDNF-induced neurite outgrowth. J Proteome Res, Vol.8, No.6, pp.2768-2787, ISSN 1535-3893

Hou, JG.; Lin, LF. & Mytilineou, C. (1996). Glial cell line-derived neurotrophic factor exerts neurotrophic effects on dopaminergic neurons in vitro and promotes their survival and regrowth after damage by 1-methyl-4-phenylpyridinium. J Neurochem, Vol.66, No.1, pp.74-82, ISSN 0022-3042

Hulit, J.; Suyama K.; Chung, S.; Keren, R.; Agiostratidou, G.; Shan, W.; Dong, X.; Williams, TM.; Lisanti, MP.; Knudsen, K. & Hazan, RB. (2007). N-cadherin signaling potentiates mammary tumor metastasis via enhanced extracellular signal-regulated kinase activation. Cancer Res, Vol.67, No.7, pp.3106-3116, ISSN 0008-5472

Ibáñez, CF. (1998). Emerging themes in structural biology of neurotrophic factors. Trends Neurosci, Vol.21, No.10, pp.438-444, ISSN 0166-2236

Jenner, P. & Olanow, CW. (1998). Understanding cell death in Parkinson's disease. Ann Neuro, Vol.44, No.3 Suppl 1, pp.S72-S84, ISSN 0364-5134

Josso, N. & di Clemente, N. (1997). Serine/threonine kinase receptors and ligands. Curr Opin Genet Dev, Vol.7, No.3, pp.371-377, ISSN 0959-437X

Kaplan, DR. & Miller, FD. (1997). Signal transduction by the neurotrophin receptors. Curr Opin Cell Biol, Vol.9, No.2, pp.213-221, ISSN 0955-0674

Kobori, N.; Waymire, JC.; Haycock, JW.; Clifton, GL. & Dash, PK. (2004). Enhancement of tyrosine hydroxylase phosphorylation and activity by glial cell line-derived neurotrophic factor. J Biol Chem, Vol.279, No.3, pp.2182-2191, ISSN 0021-9258

Kokaia, Z.; Airaksinen, MS.; Nanobashvili, A.; Larsson, E.; Kujamäki, E.; Lindvall, O. & Saarma, M. (1999). GDNF family ligands and receptors are differentially regulated after brain insults in the rat. Eur J Neurosci, Vol.11, No.4, pp.1202-1216, ISSN 0953-816X

Kordower, JH.; Emborg, ME.; Bloch, J.; Ma, SY.; Chu, Y.; Leventhal, L.; McBride, J.; Chen, EY.; Palfi, S.; Roitberg, BZ.; Brown, WD.; Holden, JE.; Pyzalski, R.; Taylor, MD.; Carvey, P.; Ling, Z.; Trono, D.; Hantraye, P.; Déglon, N. & Aebischer, P. (2000). Neurodegeneration prevented by lentiviral vector delivery of GDNF in primate models of Parkinson's disease. Science, Vol.290, No.5492, pp.767-773, ISSN 0036-8075

Krushel, LA.; Tai, MH.; Cunningham, BA.; Edelman, GM. & Crossin, KL. (1998). Neural cell adhesion molecule (N-CAM) domains and intracellular signaling pathways involved in the inhibition of astrocyte proliferation. Proc Natl Acad Sci USA, Vol.95, No.5, pp.2592-2596, ISSN 0027-8424

Ledda, F.; Paratcha, G.; Sandoval-Guzmán, T. & Ibáñez, CF. (2007). GDNF and GFRalpha1 promote formation of neuronal synapses by ligand-induced cell adhesion. Nat Neurosci, Vol.10, No.3, pp.293-300, ISSN 1097-6256

Lee, R.; Kermani, P.; Teng, KK. & Hempstead, BL. (2001). Regulation of cell survival by secreted proneurotrophins. Science, Vol.294, No.5548, pp.1945-1948, ISSN 0036-8075

Leitinger, B. & Hogg, N. (2002). The involvement of lipid rafts in the regulation of integrin function. J Cell Sci, Vol.115, No.Pt 5, pp.963-972, ISSN 0021-9533

Lin, LF.; Doherty, DH.; Lile, JD.; Bektesh, S. & Collins, F. (1993). a glial cell line derived neurotrophic factor for midbrain dopaminergic neurons. Science, Vol.260, No.5111, pp.1130-1132, ISSN 0036-8075

Lindahl, M.; Timmusk, T.; Rossi, J.; Saarma, M. & Airaksinen, MS. (2000). Expression and alternative splicing of mouse GFRα4 suggest roles in endocrine cell development. Mol Cell Neurosci, Vol.15, No.6, pp.522-533, ISSN 1044-7431

Lorenzo, MJ.; Eng, C.; Mulligan, LM.; Stonehouse, TJ.; Healey, CS.; Ponder, BA. & Smith, DP. (1995). Multiple mRNA isoforms of the human RET proto-oncogene generated by alternate splicing. Oncogene, Vol.10, No.7, pp.1377-1383, ISSN 0950-9232

Lorenzo, MJ.; Gish, GD.; Houghton, C.; Stonehouse, TJ.; Pawson, T.; Ponder, BA. & Smith, DP. (1997). RET alternate splicing influences the interaction of activated RET with the SH2 and PTB domains of Shc, and the SH2 domain of Grb2. Oncogene, Vol.14, No.7, pp.763-771, ISSN 0950-9232

Manié, S.; Santoro, M.; Fusco, A. & Billaud, M. (2001). The RET receptor: function in development and dysfunction in congenital malformation. Trends Genet, Vol.17, No.10, pp.580-589, ISSN 0168-9525

Moore, MW.; Klein, RD.; Fariñas, I.; Sauer, H.; Armanini, M.; Phillips, H.; Reichardt, LF.; Ryan, AM.; Carver-Moore, K. & Rosenthal, A. (1996). Renal and neuronal abnormalities in mice lacking GDNF. Nature, Vol.382, No.6586, pp.76-79, ISSN 0028-0836

Nakamoto, H. & Vígh, L. (2007). The small heat shock proteins and their clients. Cell Mol Life Sci, Vol.64, No.3, pp.294-306, ISSN 1420-682X

Niethammer, P.; Delling, M.; Sytnyk, V.; Dityatev, A.; Fukami, K. & Schachner, M. (2002). Cosignaling of NCAM via lipid rafts and the FGF receptor is required for neuritogenesis. J Cell Biol, Vol.157, No.3, pp.521-532, ISSN 0021-9525

Noble, M.; Albrechtsen, M.; Møller, C.; Lyles, J.; Bock, E.; Goridis, C.; Watanabe, M. & Rutishauser, U. (1985). Glial cells express N-CAM/D2-CAM-like polypeptides in vitro. Nature, Vol.310, No.6030, pp.725-728, ISSN 0028-0836

Nomoto, S.; Ito, S.; Yang, LX. & Kiuchi, K. (1998). Molecular cloning and expression analysis of GFRα-3, a novel cDNA related to GDNFRα and NT NRα. Biochem Biophys Res Commu, Vol.244, No.3, pp.849-853, ISSN 0006-291X

Paratcha, G. & Ibáñez, CF. (2002). Lipid rafts and the control of neurotrophic factor signaling in the nervous system: variations on a theme. Curr Opin Neurobiol, Vol.12, No.5, pp.542-549, ISSN 0959-4388

Paratcha, G.; Ledda, F. & Ibáñez, CF. (2003). The neural cell adhesion molecule NCAM is an alternative signaling receptor for GDNF family ligands. Cell, Vol.113, No.7, pp.867-879, ISSN 0092-8674

Paratcha, G.; Ledda, F.; Baars, L.; Coulpier, M.; Besset, V.; Anders, J.; Scott, R. & Ibáñez, CF. (2001). Released GFRalpha1 potentiates downstream signaling, neuronal survival, and differentiation via a novel mechanism of recruitment of c-Ret to lipid rafts. Neuron, Vol.29, No.1, pp.171-184, ISSN 0896-6273

Pascual, A.; Hidalgo-Figueroa, M.; Piruat, JI.; Pintado, CO.; Gómez-Díaz, R. & López-Barneo, J. (2008). Absolute requirement of GDNF for adult catecholaminergic neuron survival. Nat Neurosci, Vol.11, No.7, pp.755-761, ISSN 1097-6256

Pierchala, BA.; Milbrandt, J. & Johnson, EM Jr. (2006). Glial cell line-derived neurotrophic factor-dependent recruitment of Ret into lipid rafts enhances signaling by partitioning Ret from proteasome-dependent degradation. J Neurosci, Vol.26, No.10, pp.2777-2787, ISSN 0270-6474

Pong, K.; Xu, RY.; Baron, WF.; Louis, JC. & Beck, KD. (1998). Inhibition of phosphatidylinositol 3-kinase activity blocks cellular differentiation mediated by glial cell line-derived neurotrophic factor in dopaminergic neurons. J Neurochem, Vol.71, No.5, pp.1912-1919, ISSN 0022-3042

Popsueva, A.; Poteryaev, D.; Arighi, E.; Meng, X.; Angers-Loustau, A.; Kaplan, D.; Saarma, M. & Sariola, H. (2003). GDNF promotes tubulogenesis of GFRα1-expressing MDCK cells by Src-mediated phosphorylation of Met receptor tyrosine kinase. J Cell Biol, Vol.161, No.1, pp.119-129, ISSN 0021-9525

Poteryaev, D.; Titievsky, A.; Sun, YF.; Thomas-Crusells, J.; Lindahl, M.; Billaud, M.; Arumäe, U. & Saarma, M. (1999). GDNF triggers a novel retindependent Src kinase family-coupled signaling via a GPI-linked GDNF receptor alpha1. FEBS Lett, Vol.463, No.1-2, pp.63-66, ISSN 0014-5793

Reynolds, AB. (2007). p120-catenin: Past and present. Biochim Biophys Acta, Vol.1773, No.1, pp.2-7, ISSN 0006-3002

Saarma, M. & Sariola, H. (1999). Other neurotrophic factors: glial cell line-derived neurotrophic factor (GDNF). Microsc Res Tech, Vol.45, No.4-5, pp.292-302, ISSN 1059-910X

Sakai, A.; Asada, M.; Seno, N. & Suzuki, H. (2008). Involvement of neural cell adhesion molecule signaling in glial cell line-derived neurotrophic factor-induced analgesia in a rat model of neuropathic pain. Pain, Vol.137, No.2, pp.378-388, ISSN 0304-3959

Sariola H. & Saarma M. (2003). Novel functions and signalling pathways for GDNF. J Cell Sci, Vol.116, No.Pt 19, pp.3855-3862, ISSN 0021-9533

Schaar, DG.; Sieber, BA.; Sherwood, AC.; Dean, D.; Mendoza, G.; Ramakrishnan, L.; Dreyfus, CF. & Black, IB. (1994). Multiple astrocyte transcripts encode nigral trophic factors in rat and human. Exp Neurol, Vol.130, No.2, pp.387-393, ISSN 0014-4886

Siegel, GJ. & Chauhan, NB. (2000). Neurotrophic factors in Alzheimer' s and Parkinson' s disease brain. Brain Res Rev, Vol.33, No.2-3, pp.199-227, ISSN 0165-0173

Simons, K. & Ikonen, E. (1997). Functional rafts in cell membranes. Nature, Vol.387, No.6633, pp.569-572, ISSN 0028-0836

Sjöstrand, D. & Ibáñez, CF. (2008). Insights into GFRalpha1 regulation of neural cell adhesion molecule (NCAM) function from structure-function analysis of the NCAM/GFRalpha1 receptor complex. J Biol Chem, Vol.283, No.20, pp.13792-13798, ISSN 0021-9258

Sjöstrand, D.; Carlsson, J.; Paratcha, G.; Persson, B. & Ibáñez, CF. (2007). Disruption of the GDNF binding site in NCAM dissociates ligand binding and homophilic cell adhesion. J Biol Chem, Vol.282, No.17, pp.12734-12740, ISSN 0021-9258

Sonntag, KC.; Simantov, R. & Isacson, O. (2005). Stem ceils may reshape the prospect of Parkinson' s disease therapy. Mol Brain Res, Vol.134, No.1, pp.34-51, ISSN 0169-328X

Springer, JE.; Mu, X.; Bergmann, LW. & Trojanowski, JQ. (1994). Expression of GDNF mRNA in rat and human nervous tissue. Exp Neurol, Vol.127, No.2, pp.167-170, ISSN 0014-4886

Subramaniam, S.; Strelau, J. & Unsicker, K. (2008). GDNF prevents TGF-β-induced damage of the plasma membrane in cerebellar granule neurons by suppressing activation of p38-MAPK via the phosphatidylinositol 3-kinase pathway. Cell Tissue Res, Vol.311, No.2, pp.373-383, ISSN 0302-766X

Tahira, T.; Ishizaka, Y.; Itoh, F.; Sugimura, T. & Nagao, M. (1990). Characterization of ret proto-oncogene mRNAs encoding two isoforms of the protein product in a human neuroblastoma cell line. Oncogene, Vol.5, No.1, pp.97-102, ISSN 0950-9232

Tang, MJ.; Worley, D.; Sanicola, M. & Dressler, GR. (1998). The RET-glial cell-derived neurotrophic factor (GDNF) pathway stimulates migration and chemoattraction of epithelial cells. J Cell Biol, Vol.142, No.5, pp.1337-1345, ISSN 0021-9525

Tansey, MG.; Baloh, RH.; Milbrandt, J. & Johnson, EM Jr. (2000). GFRalpha-mediated localization of RET to lipid rafts is required for effective downstream signaling, differentiation, and neuronal survival. Neuron, Vol.25, No.3, pp.611-623, ISSN 0896-6273

Tomac, A.; Lindqvist, E.; Lin, LF.; Ogren, SO.; Young, D.; Hoffer, BJ. & Olson, L. (1995). Protection and repair of the nigrostriatal dopaminergic system by GDNF in vivo. Nature, Vol.373, No.6512, pp.335-339, ISSN 0028-0836

Trupp, M.; Arenas, E.; Fainzilber, M.; Nilsson, AS.; Sieber, BA.; Grigoriou, M.; Kilkenny, C.; Salazar-Grueso, E.; Pachnis, V. & Arumäe, U. (1996). Functional receptor for GDNF encoded by the c-ret proto-oncogene. Nature, Vol.381, No.6585, pp.785-789, ISSN 0028-0836

Trupp, M.; Belluardo, N.; Funakoshi, H. & Ibáñez, CF. (1997). Complementary and overlapping expression of glial cell line-derived neurotrophic factor (GDNF), c-ret proto-oncogene, and GDNF receptor-alpha indicates multiple mechanisms of trophic actions in the adult rat CNS. J Neurosci, Vol.17, No.10, pp.3554-3567, ISSN 0270-6474

Trupp, M.; Rydén, M.; Jörnvall, H.; Funakoshi, H.; Timmusk, T.; Arenas, E. & Ibáñez, CF. (1995). Peripheral expression and biological activities of GDNF , a new neurotrophic factor for a vian and mammaliam peripheral neurons. J Cell Biol, Vol.130, No.1, pp.137-148, ISSN 0021-9525

Trupp, M.; Scott, R.; Whittemore, SR. & Ibáñez, CF. (1999). Ret-dependent and -independent mechanisms of glial cell line-derived neurotrophic factor signaling in neuronal cells. J Biol Chem, Vol.274, No.30, pp.20885-20894, ISSN 0021-9258

Van Weering, DH. & Bos, JL. (1997). Glial cell line-derived neurotrophic factor induces Ret-mediated lamellipodia formation. J Biol Chem, Vol.272, No.1, pp.249-254, ISSN 0021-9258

Wang, J.; Chen, G.; Lu, B. & Wu, CP. (2003). GDNF acutely potentiates Ca2+ channels and excitatory synaptic transmission in midbrain dopaminergic neurons. Neurosignals, Vol.12, No.2, pp.78-88, ISSN 1424-862X

Wells, SA Jr. & Santoro, M. (2009). Targeting the RET pathway in thyroid cancer. Clin Cancer Res, Vol.15, No.23, pp.7119-7123, ISSN 1078-0432

Widenfalk, J.; Tomac, A.; Lindqvist, E. & Olson, L. Hoffer, B. (1998). GFRalpha-3, a protein related to GFRalpha-1, is expressed in developing peripheral neurons and ensheathing cells. Eur J Neurosci, Vol.10, No.4, pp.1508-1517, ISSN 0953-816X

Wong, A.; Bogni, S.; Kotka, P.; de Graaff, E.; D'Agati, V.; Costantini, F. & Pachnis, V. (2005). Phosphotyrosine 1062 is critical for the in vivo activity of the Ret9 receptor tyrosine kinase isoform. Mol Cell Biol, Vol.25, No.21, pp.9661-9673, ISSN 0270-7306

Yang, F.; Feng, L.; Zheng, F.; Johnson SW.; Du, J.; Shen, L.; Wu, CP. & Lu, B. (2001). GDNF acutely modulates excitability and A-type K(+) channels in midbrain dopaminergic neurons. Nat Neurosci, Vol.4, No.11, pp.1071-1078, ISSN 1097-6256

Yu, T.; Scully, S.; Yu, Y.; Fox, GM.; Jing, S. & Zhou, R. (1998). Expression of GDNF family receptor components during development: implications in the mechanisms of interaction. J Neurosci, Vol.18, No.12, pp.4684-4696, ISSN 0270-6474

Yurek, DM. & Fletcher-Turner, A. (2000). Lesion-induced increase of BDNF is greater in the striatum of young versus old rat brain. Exp Neurol, Vol.161, No.1, pp.392-396, ISSN 0014-4886

10

The Hsp70 Chaperone System in Parkinson's Disease

Adahir Labrador-Garrido[1], Carlos W. Bertoncini[2] and Cintia Roodveldt[1]
[1]CABIMER-Andalusian Center for Molecular Biology & Regenerative Medicine CSIC-University of Seville-UPO-Junta de Andalucía, Seville,
[2]Laboratory of Molecular Biophysics, Institute for Research in Biomedicine (IRB), Barcelona,
Spain

1. Introduction

Several neurodegenerative diseases are associated with a build up of misfolded or abnormal proteins and the formation of distinct aggregates, resulting in a putative pathological protein load on the nervous system (Chiti & Dobson, 2006). This aberrant accumulation of amyloid or amyloid-like aggregates occurs in Parkinson's (PD), Alzheimer's (AD), and Huntington's (HD) diseases, amyotrophic lateral sclerosis, and frontotemporal dementia, among others. A broad array of cellular defence mechanisms operate to counteract this effect, including antioxidant proteins, the stress-inducible response and, in particular, molecular chaperones (Morimoto, 2008; Voisine et al., 2010). Molecular chaperones are responsible for maintaining normal protein homeostasis within the cell by assisting protein folding, inhibiting protein aggregation, and modulating protein degradation pathways (Hartl & Hayer-Hartl, 2009). Currently, there is substantial evidence supporting the involvement of these protein aggregational processes and a role of molecular chaperones, and especially of Hsp70, in PD pathogenesis (Bandopadhyay & de Belleroche, 2010; Broadley & Hartl, 2009; Witt, 2009). Firstly, extensive colocalization of Hsp70 with α-synuclein (αSyn), the major component of Lewy bodies (LBs) (Spillantini et al., 1998), within the intraneuronal inclusions in PD brains has been demonstrated (Auluck et al., 2002; McLean et al., 2002). Secondly, patients with PD show highly perturbed expression of different members of the Hsp70 family in the *substantia nigra pars compacta* (SN) of the brain, which is precisely the target of neurodegeneration (Grunblatt et al., 2001; Hauser et al., 2005). Finally, there is a considerable amount of data derived from studies performed *in vitro*, in cell culture and with animal models of PD (Arawaka et al., 2010; Witt, 2009), that support the protective effects of Hsp70 against αSyn aggregation and toxicity, considered to be central in the aetiology of the disease.

The discovery within the last few years of three different missense mutations (A30P, E46K and A53T) in the αSyn gene as causative of early onset PD unambiguously linked this protein to disease onset and progression (Kruger et al., 1998; Polymeropoulos et al., 1997; Zarranz et al., 2004). Additionally, a locus triplication causing an increased dosage of the wild-type (Wt) αSyn gene has been found to potentiate neurodegeneration (Singleton et al.,

2003). Finally, as mentioned above, αSyn is the major component of intracellular protein-rich aggregates found in the brain of post-mortem patients of PD, the LBs and Lewy neurites (LNs). The appealing hypothesis for LBs formation is that αSyn monomers combine to form oligomers (or protofibrils), which coalesce into fibrils and then co-aggregate with other proteins into (intracellular) inclusions (Conway et al., 1998; Wood et al., 1999). While the monomers and oligomers of αSyn are soluble, the fibrils and LBs are insoluble in the neuronal cytoplasm. Some controversy arises, however, from the roles of the various physical forms or species of αSyn in PD pathogenesis. LBs have been proposed to be both neurotoxic (El-Agnaf et al., 1998), and protective (Mouradian, 2002; Rochet et al., 2000). Other hypotheses state that the pre-fibrillar intermediates, composed of αSyn oligomers, are the main toxic species towards dopaminergic neurons (Conway et al., 2000; Volles & Lansbury, 2003). Lansbury and co-workers have shown that αSyn oligomers can form annular, elliptical, or circular amyloid pores in cell membranes (Lashuel et al., 2002a; Volles & Lansbury, 2003), and cell culture studies have demonstrated that αSyn oligomers reduce cell viability, disrupt lysosomes and induce Golgi fragmentation (Gosavi et al., 2002), as well as toxicity in animal models (Karpinar et al., 2009). In line with these findings, the more neurotoxic A30P and A53T mutants of αSyn share an increased tendency to form soluble oligomeric intermediates, whereas the E46K and A53T mutants fibrillate faster than the wild-type protein (Conway et al., 2000; Choi et al., 2004).

The heat-shock-protein 70 (Hsp70) family of chaperones (Mayer & Bukau, 2005; Young, 2010) is well conserved from bacteria to higher eukaryotes (where it is found within different organelles), having critical roles in a range of cellular processes such as promoting the folding of newly synthesized proteins and assisting the rescue of misfolded aggregated proteins. Hsp70 is highly relevant in the context of protein conformational diseases given that stress-induced cytosolic Hsp70 can prevent protein aggregation and enables the cell to avoid the accumulation of potentially toxic aggregates (Hartl, 1996).

The structures of several Hsp70 homologues are similar and consist of an actin-like ATPase domain (nucleotide-binding domain, NBD) and a and a C-terminal substrate-binding domain (SBD), which are connected by a short linker region (Mayer & Bukau, 2005). The substrate binding pocket recognizes and binds to unstructured or partially folded stretches within polypeptides (Bukau & Horwich, 1998), with the current view that Hsp70s could prevent misfolding by binding to certain patterns in the polypeptide chain of the substrate that are highly enriched in hydrophobic residues (Maeda et al., 2007; Rudiger et al., 1997). Even though most of our current understanding of the Hsp70 molecular mechanism has largely derived from studies performed with the bacterial orthologue (DnaK), the outlines of the mechanism appear conserved (Hartl & Hayer-Hartl, 2002; Young, 2010). The ATPase cycle of Hsp70 involves alternation between an ATP-bound state which has low affinity and fast exchange rates for peptide substrates ('open' state), and an ADP-bound state with high affinity and low exchange rates for substrates ('closed' state) (Mayer & Bukau, 2005). This alternation is achieved by a bidirectional structural communication between the NBD and the SBD domains, driven by a complex allosteric mechanism (Mayer & Bukau, 2005; Young, 2010).

The ATPase cycle is typically modulated by several co-chaperones, most notably the 'J-domain' protein Hsp40/DNAJB1 (or DnaJ, the bacterial orthologue), resulting in increase of the ATPase activity (Bukau & Horwich, 1998; Mayer & Bukau, 2005; Minami et al., 1996), and the BAG family of proteins which function as nucleotide-exchange factors (NEFs) and promote the ADP release from the the Hsp70 NBD (Takayama et al., 1999; Young, 2010). In addition to acting as enhancer of the basal ATPase rate of Hsp70, the Hsp40 family of co-chaperones has a key role in the canonical model of the Hsp70 machinery mechanism, given the ability of some of them to also recognize and bind to unfolded client proteins and 'deliver' them to Hsp70 (Kampinga & Craig, 2010). Other important co-chaperones are Hop, which binds to the C-termini of Hsp70 and Hsp90 and assists substrate transfer between the two chaperones (Scheufler et al., 2000), and Hip (ST13) which has been shown to specifically bind to and stabilize, the ADP-bound state of Hsp70 (Hohfeld et al., 1995; Prapapanich et al., 1996), and has been suggested to increase the half-life of Hsp70-substrate complexes (Hohfeld et al., 1995). Finally, CHIP (Ballinger et al., 1999) acts as an E3-ubiquitin ligase that ubiquitinates HSPA8/Hsc70/Hsp73 (i.e. the constitutive cytosolic Hsp70) substrates, promoting their degradation by the proteasome (Hohfeld et al., 2001).

2. Links between Hsp70 and the pathogenesis of PD

PD is currently thought to involve different pathogenic mechanisms that eventually lead to neurodegeneration, as discussed elsewhere in this book series.. There is substantial evidence supporting a prominent role in PD-related cell death of αSyn toxic oligomers. One hypothesis postulates that certain αSyn species can affect the homeostasis of cell membranes (Gupta et al., 2008; Lashuel et al., 2002b; Volles & Lansbury, 2002), and produce ER and oxidative stress, UPS and mitochondrial dysfunction (Gupta et al., 2008; Jellinger, 2010), as well as neuroinflammation (Jellinger, 2010; Roodveldt et al., 2008) processes, all of which have been linked, to a lower or larger extent, to the amyloid-like aggregation of αSyn. As will be described below, the Hsp70 system has been found to be a key player in counteracting most of these processes, not only by physically interacting with αSyn, but also by promoting aggregation clearance (Figure 1).

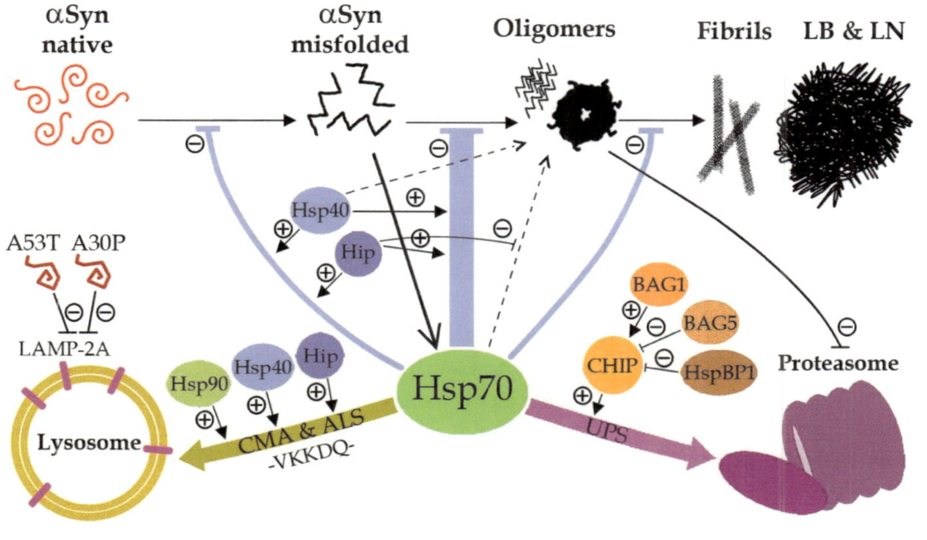

Fig. 1. Links between Hsp70 and the multiple αSyn-mediated processes in PD pathogenesis. CMA: chaperone-mediated autophagy; UPS: ubiquitin-proteasome system; LB: Lewy bodies; LN: Lewy neurites. Discontinuous lines depict the possible 'sequestration' of certain chaperones by αSyn aggregating species.

2.1 Hsp70 in modulation of αSyn aggregation and cytotoxicity

Heat-shock proteins (HSPs) prevent and reverse the misfolding and aggregation of proteins, and the Hsp70 family in particular is known to play important roles in protecting neurons from protein aggregation-derived stress (Lu et al., 2010). Therefore, it might not seem surprising that Hsp70 has been found to be linked to several neurodegenerative processes and 'conformational' disorders, including PD (Witt, 2009). Notably, Hsp70 has been shown to colocalize with aggregated αSyn within LBs in brains from PD patients (Auluck et al., 2002), strongly suggesting a role for this chaperone in managing αSyn aggregates in the context of PD (Figure 1). It is then that a substantial portion of the research in the field has focused on the effects of this major cytosolic chaperone on αSyn aggregation and cytotoxicity. Following the discovery that Hsp70 can abrogate the neurotoxicity of abnormal polyglutamine proteins (Warrick et al., 1999), it was shown that Hsp70 can also prevent dopaminergic neuronal loss associated with αSyn in a *Drosophila* PD model (Auluck et al., 2002). Numerous studies that followed have reported that over-expression of Hsp70 is able to reduce αSyn aggregation and/or toxicity in various cellular models (Danzer et al., 2011; Klucken et al., 2004b; McLean et al., 2004; Opazo et al., 2008; Outeiro et al., 2008; Zhou et al., 2004). In particular, McLean and co-workers (Outeiro et al., 2008) have found that Hsp70 rescues αSyn-linked toxicity by promoting the cellular clearance of αSyn oligomers, rather than monomers. Another study (Opazo et al., 2008) found that Hsp70 manages αSyn intracellular aggregation by increasing the clearing of aggregates primarily through the aggresome, and the subsequent removal of small aggregates and aggresomes from the cytosol. An interesting study by McLean and colleagues (Danzer et al., 2011) has recently shown that Hsp70 can also inhibit the formation of extracellular αSyn oligomers and rescue the cytotoxicity produced by such secreted oligomers, in a cellular model. Moreover, their data also indicates that Hsp70 is released to the extracellular medium together with secreted αSyn, adding to the accumulating evidence that Hsp70 can be released from cells by an active mechanism, with functionally relevant consequences.

Intriguingly, while it was found that over-expression of Hsp70 can prevent αSyn aggregation in a Wt αSyn transgenic mouse model (Klucken et al., 2004b), a recent work based on A53T-αSyn transgenic mice has failed to observe this effect (Shimshek et al., 2010), seeding some controversy. Could these findings reflect a difference in the nature of the aggregates generated by Wt and mutant αSyn, and therefore a differential ability of Hsp70 to cope with those aggregates? Even though there is compelling evidence demonstrating the important role of Hsp70 under physiological and pathological scenarios in modulating fibril formation based on *in vivo* and cellular models, the molecular mechanism underlying such anti-aggregation properties in the context of PD, is still not fully understood.

Unlike the many research works performed with PD cellular and animal models that have contributed to our understanding on Hsp70 function under physiological or pathological conditions, only a handful of studies have focused on the molecular mechanism and interactions that underlie the modulation of αSyn aggregation exerted by Hsp70. An in-cell fluorescence resonance energy transfer (FRET) study indicated that Hsp70 alters the conformation of αSyn, inducing it to adopt a more 'open' conformation, without affecting the αSyn-αSyn intermolecular interactions (Klucken et al., 2006). Similarly to what had been found *in vitro* for Hsp70 and the HD-related huntingtin protein (Muchowski et al., 2000; Wacker et al., 2004), several studies with αSyn have shown that Hsp70 is able to suppress αSyn fibril assembly. In this case, a variety of *in vitro* studies have shown that this efficient inhibition of amyloid assembly can occur in the absence of collaborating co-chaperones and in an ATP-independent manner (Ahmad, 2010; Dedmon et al., 2005; Huang et al., 2006; Luk et al., 2008; Roodveldt et al., 2009), while promoting formation of small oligomeric species of moderate toxicity (Roodveldt et al., 2009). However, our recent study demonstrates that, even though Hsp70 is indeed able to control αSyn fibrillation and its associated toxicity in an ATP-independent manner, it does so more efficiently in the presence of ATP (Roodveldt et al., 2009), consistent with the results obtained with a cellular model (Klucken et al., 2004a). Nevertheless, this ATP-dependent activity was found to require Hip co-chaperone activity, and not Hsp40 as observed in the case of mutant huntingtin protein (Lotz et al., 2010), suggesting that Hsp70 can function through different molecular mechanisms, depending on the nature of the aggregating client protein.

Interestingly, our study also showed that Hsp70 in the presence of ATP is prone to co-aggregate with aggregating αSyn, presumably caused by the formation of a highly insoluble (ADP)Hsp70/αSyn complex. Surprisingly, this co-aggregation can be prevented by the addition of the co-chaperone Hip (St13), which had been found to be under-expressed in serum of PD patients since the early stages of the disease (Scherzer et al., 2007). The relevance of Hip in assisting the suppression of αSyn aggregation in an Hsp70-dependent manner was further supported by a study we performed in a *C. elegans* model of PD (Roodveldt et al., 2009), in which knock-down of Hip produced a much stronger PD phenotype than knock-down of Hsp70, shown by higher levels of αSyn aggregation in the former condition. This finding indicates that Hip co-chaperone could be important not only in modulating the chaperone's molecular mechanism, but also in guarding the functionality and availability of Hsp70 under certain conditions.

One relevant question relates to the nature of the species along the aggregation pathway of αSyn that are specifically recognized and targeted by Hsp70. Initially, Hsp70 was reported to bind to αSyn filaments *in vitro* (Lindersson et al., 2004). However, it is currently understood that Hsp70 does not disaggregate or alter the structural properties of mature αSyn fibrils (Dedmon et al., 2005), but rather inhibits fibril formation via interactions with soluble pre-fibrillar forms of αSyn. A few studies performed with cell extracts (Zhou et al., 2004) and with live cells (Klucken et al., 2006), in addition to experiments with purified proteins (Dedmon et al., 2005; Huang et al., 2006; Roodveldt et al., 2009), demonstrate the existence of molecular interactions between Hsp70 and αSyn oligomeric species. Even though previous attempts to isolate such complexes by co-immunoprecipitation or pull-down experiments had failed (Luk et al., 2008), we have been able to probe the formation of a complex between Hsp70 and αSyn oligomeric species by FRET (Roodveldt et al., 2009), suggesting that these interactions are transient (Luk et al., 2008; Roodveldt et al., 2009), besides being highly dynamic (Luk et al., 2008; Roodveldt et al., 2009).

In addition, we have recently shown by FRET and nuclear magnetic resonance (NMR) analyses that, contrary to what was previously thought, Hsp70 can also interact with αSyn monomeric species (Roodveldt et al., 2009) with an affinity constant lying within the low micromolar range. Moreover, the fluorimetric study revealed the existence of diverse Hsp70/αSyn complexes that are formed depending on the nucleotide state of the chaperone, either nucleotide-free, or ATP- or ADP-bound, that are sampled along the ATPase cycle. Based on these structural studies, we have proposed that a particularly 'compact' Hsp70/αSyn complex in the ADP-state of Hsp70 that arises during the aggregation process of αSyn, leads to Hsp70 being entrapped or sequestered by the oligomers. However, we propose that this compact complex can be stabilized by the Hip co-chaperone and therefore the co-aggregation of the chaperone, and ultimately the formation of αSyn fibrils, can be prevented (Roodveldt et al., 2009). In other words, our findings indicated that a decreased expression of Hip could facilitate depletion of Hsp70 by amyloidogenic polypeptides, impairing chaperone proteostasis. Interestingly, another case of chaperone-inhibition/depletion by αSyn oligomers, but not by unstructured monomers, was recently reported for the Hsp70/Hsp40 system (Hinault et al., 2010). In this case, the authors found that the inhibition of the chaperone system was predominantly caused by the sequestration or incapacitation, by off-pathway αSyn oligomers, of the J-domain (Hsp40) co-chaperone (Hinault et al., 2010).

What is the region on the αSyn molecule thought to be recognized and bound by Hsp70? One study mapped this region as the broad segment between residues 21 and 110 (Luk et al., 2008). Based on a predictive algorithm for Hsp70-binding regions (Rudiger et al., 1997) and FRET analyses to probe Hsp70-αSyn interactions (Roodveldt et al., 2009), our results indicate that Hsp70 can bind to the N-terminus and the central NAC region of the protein. The first binding region is involved in functional lipid interactions, while the second one comprises the stretch of hydrophobic residues that readily forms fibrils *in vitro* and is generally assumed to be involved in initiating the fibrillation process (Giasson et al., 2001). In addition, our results suggest that Hsp70 also interacts with the negatively charged C-terminus of the αSyn molecule, especially in the nucleotide-free state. Taken together, the studies carried out thus far demonstrate that Hsp70 modulates αSyn aggregation by interacting with the protein at different stages of aggregation, by recognizing essentially two or three regions in the αSyn molecule, and forming different transient complexes with the substrate. The strong binding versatility displayed by Hsp70 with aggregating αSyn might be possible thanks to the large structural flexibility conferred by the lid subdomain within the SBD, that has been recently described by Mayer and colleagues (Schlecht et al., 2011).

2.2 Cooperation of Hsp70 with the ubiquitin-proteasome system (UPS)

2.2.1 Involvement of the ubiquitin-proteasome system in PD

The ubiquitin-proteasome system (UPS) is responsible for the degradation of vital regulatory proteins that control almost every cellular function (Hershko & Ciechanover, 1998). The UPS system is composed of three classes of ubiquitinating enzymes (E1, E2 and E3) that activate, transfer and attach the small protein ubiquitin to the Lys residues of proteins that are targeted for degradation. Conjugation of at least four ubiquitin moieties acts as the degradation signal in a process that is initiated by the recognition of the ubiquitin linkage by the proteasome, which first catalyzes the unfolding and then the proteolysis of the targeted protein (Hershko & Ciechanover, 1998).

Impairment in the UPS has been linked to many neurodegenerative disorders and indeed to contribute to disease progression in PD (Ciechanover & Brundin, 2003; Cook & Petrucelli, 2009; McNaught et al., 2001). The involvement of UPS in PD arouse major interest with the identification of mutations in the E3 ubiquitin ligase parkin protein as a cause of autosomal recessive PD (Kitada et al., 1998). Both the loss of E3 activity and the possibility of incomplete or aberrant ubiquitination are proposed as causes of parkin-related PD (Giasson & Lee, 2003). A second member of the UPS involved in PD is the ubiquitin carboxy-terminal hydrolase-L1 (UCH-L1), and mutations in the uchl-1 gene cause dysfunction of this enzyme and lead to accumulation of toxic products (Leroy et al., 1998).

Beyond the clear genetic association between the UPS and PD, several studies have demonstrated a reduced proteolytic activity in the SN of PD patients when compared with aged-matched controls (McNaught et al., 2003; McNaught & Jenner, 2001; McNaught & Olanow, 2006). In culture of rat primary neurons, treatment with proteasomal inhibitors has shown to lead to the formation of αSyn- and ubiquitin- positive proteinaceous inclusions, analogous to LBs found in PD patients (McNaught et al., 2002a; Rideout et al., 2005). Moreover, systemic administration of proteasomal inhibitors in rats produced a behavioural and pathological phenotype strongly reminiscent of PD (McNaught et al., 2004), although recently some controversy arose in this matter (Manning-Bog et al., 2006). Further support to the active role played by proteasomal impairment in PD progression originated from studies with pesticides, such as rotenone and paraquat (Cook & Petrucelli, 2009). Mice treated with such environmental toxins display a strong reduction in proteolytic activity that is dependent on the presence of αSyn (Fornai et al., 2005). All together, these data undoubtedly link αSyn aggregation with impairment of the UPS in PD progression.

In relation to protein misfolding and aggregation, it has been proposed that failure of the UPS to adequately remove misfolded or abnormal proteins may underlie demise of nigral cells in sporadic PD (McNaught et al., 2001). Furthermore, deficits in the 26/20S proteasome pathways are accompanied by protein accumulation and aggregation, which may also cause neurodegeneration (Chung et al., 2001), in line with recent findings that general intracellular aggregation of proteins into aggresomes can can inhibit the UPS (Bence et al., 2001). Moreover, chaperones of the heat-shock families, including HSP27, 40, 70, 60, 90, and 110, as well as components of the UPS, such as ubiquitin, UCH-L1 and parkin, are found in LBs extracted from PD patients *post mortem* (Shults, 2006). These combined pieces of evidence have attracted much attention lately as they imply that LBs could originate from ubiquitin-rich aggresomes that the proteasomal components may not be able to process (McNaught et al., 2002b). One plausible mechanism would involve αSyn adopting abnormal protein conformations and overwhelming the cellular protein degradation systems (Wong & Cuervo, 2010), whereas deficits in the UPS machinery would challenge the cell's ability to detect and degrade misfolded proteins that can result in the formation of toxic early aggregates (McNaught et al., 2002b). The common outcome of this failure at different levels is thus expected to be a cellular build-up of unwanted toxic species that should have been cleared in otherwise healthy conditions. Minimal defects in the crucial protein turnover machinery may suffice to cause a slow demise of dopaminergic neurons, which may explain the relentless, progressive nature of the disease (Vila & Przedborski, 2003).

Alpha-synuclein extracted from LBs in PD brains has been found to be mono- and di-ubiquitinated (Hasegawa et al., 2002), while soluble αSyn is mono-ubiquitinated by SIAH-1 and -2, but not by parkin (Liani et al., 2004; Rott et al., 2008). Instead, a modified, O-glycosylated, version of αSyn is a substrate for parkin-induced ubiquitination (Shimura et al., 2001), and it was shown that interaction of parkin with αSyn is mediated by synphilin-1 (Chung et al., 2001) as well as by the protein 14-3-3-η (Sato et al., 2006). Importantly, parkin has been shown to be able to rescue primary neurons from the toxic effects of αSyn (Petrucelli et al., 2002), suggesting that the two proteins share a common pathway that may determine the fate of dopaminergic neurons in PD. In addition, UCH-L1 may be involved in regulating the cytoplasmic abundance of αSyn, as it displays unexpected ubiquitin ligase activity that is also able to polyubiquitinate mono- and diubiquitinated αSyn (Liu et al., 2002). Since attachment of at least four ubiquitin molecules is known to be required for protein degradation via the UPS (Hershko & Ciechanover, 1998), it is likely that mono-, di-, and aberrant poly-ubiquitinated αSyn could have a pathogenic impact (Rott et al., 2008; Sun & Chen, 2004).

2.2.2 Role of the C-terminus Hsp70-interacting protein (CHIP) in PD

Hsp70 and Hsp90 family members as well as small HSPs all take part in the degradation of protein substrate and are able to cooperate with the UPS towards this goal (Patterson & Hohfeld, 2006). Notably, protein homeostasis thus appears to be tightly controlled by interplay between the protein folding and protein degradation systems. Hsp70 takes part in the degradation of immature and aberrant forms of certain proteins, particularly ER-bound membrane proteins (Taxis et al., 2003), but also some cytosolic and nuclear proteins (Bercovich et al., 1997). For example, Hsp70 assists in the folding of the aggregation prone cystic fibrosis transmembrane conductance regulator (CFTR); however, Hsp70 is also able to present CFTR to the UPS and thus to control precisely the abundance of this protein, which is known to accumulate in aggresome and to cause cystic fibrosis (Zhang et al., 2001). Indeed, Hsp70 is actively recruited to aggresome and it has been proposed that this chaperone can reduce aggresome formation by stimulating proteasomal degradation of misfolded proteins (Dul et al., 2001; Garcia-Mata et al., 1999). The proposed mechanism for chaperone-UPS cooperation is that both systems compete for the same misfolded and aggregation-prone substrate proteins, and that the efficiency of chaperones in maintaining these proteins in solution increments the probability of the UPS to degrade aberrant polypeptides. Conversely, failure of chaperones to keep misfolded proteins in a soluble state gives rise to aggregates that are not efficiently degraded by the UPS and, moreover, may inhibit UPS activity towards other protein targets, altering protein homeostasis (Figure 1).

Insights into the mechanism that enables the cooperation of protein chaperones with the UPS have been obtained from the identification and functional characterization of the C-terminal Hsp70 interacting protein (CHIP) co-chaperone (Ballinger et al., 1999; Hohfeld et al., 2001; McDonough & Patterson, 2003). CHIP contains three tetratricopeptide repeat (TPR) domains that recognize and bind to the EEVD motif in both Hsp70 and Hsp90 (Ballinger et al., 1999). CHIP-complexed Hsp70 displays reduced ATP hydrolysis *in vitro*, suggesting that the co-chaperone diminishes the on-rate of binding and release cycles in Hsp70 (Ballinger et al., 1999). In its C-terminus, CHIP possesses a ubiquitin ligase domain (U box) that is capable of targeting proteins to degradation, in a homologous manner to RING finger domains found in E3 ubiquitin ligase enzymes (Connell et al., 2001; Meacham et al., 2001).

CHIP has been shown to efficiently act as E3 ligase for several Hsp70 and Hsp90 substrates, such as the glucocorticoid receptor and Erb2 (Dickey et al., 2007; McDonough & Patterson, 2003; Murata et al., 2001). Proteins ubiquitinated by CHIP are efficiently targeted to the proteasome and subsequently degraded. Notably, the UbcH4/UbcH5 proteins are E2-conjugating enzymes (Demand et al., 2001) that are stress-activated, suggesting that upon stress CHIP furnishes the cell with chaperone-dependent ubiquitin ligases capable of ubiquitinating misfolded and aggregation-prone substrates.

The ubiquitinating activity of CHIP is regulated by two co-chaperones, BAG-1, which is an enhancer, and the Hsp70 binding protein 1 (HspBP1), which acts as a repressor. BAG-1 associates with the ATPase domain of Hsp70 and, in addition, possesses a ubiquitin-like domain that is efficiently recognized and bound by the proteasome (Luders et al., 2000). Thus, BAG-1 provides the proteasome with the capability to recruit Hsp70 and consequently degrade its cargo clients. A ternary complex involving BAG-1, Hsp70 and CHIP has been isolated, and BAG-1 is capable of stimulating CHIP mediated degradation of some proteins (Alberti et al., 2002). The co-chaperone HspBP1, in turn, competes with BAG-1 for binding to the ATPase domain of Hsp70 (Alberti et al., 2004). Notably, when in complex with HspBP1-bound Hsp70, CHIP shows a much reduced ubiquitin ligase activity and chaperone substrates are not longer ubiquitinated and targeted to the UPS (Alberti et al., 2004).

In the context of neurodegeneration, CHIP has been shown to intervene in the degradation of misfolded aggregation-prone proteins associated with AD, PD and HD, as well as with spinocerebellar ataxia and spinal bulbar muscle atrophy (Adachi et al., 2007; Al-Ramahi et al., 2006; Hatakeyama et al., 2004; Shin et al., 2005; Urushitani et al., 2004). Indeed, CHIP appears to play an active role in modulating αSyn aggregation and degradation (Kalia et al., 2011; Shin et al., 2005; Tetzlaff et al., 2008). It was shown that CHIP interacts with both soluble and aggregated αSyn, and its over-expression reduces αSyn abundance and aggregation (Shin et al., 2005). Interestingly, CHIP induces αSyn clearance via two alternative pathways, one involving Hsp70 and proteasomal degradation, and another Hsp70-independent route that targets αSyn to lysosomes (Shin et al., 2005). A fluorescence-complementation assay demonstrated that CHIP reduced significantly the abundance of αSyn toxic oligomers in cell culture, suggesting that this aberrant species is preferentially recognized by the co-chaperone (Tetzlaff et al., 2008). More recently, it was discovered that CHIP is an E3 ubiquitin ligase of αSyn since it efficiently conjugates ubiquitin moieties to this protein (Kalia et al., 2011). CHIP-catalyzed ubiquitinated forms of αSyn include mono- and poly-ubiquitinated species, and the activity of CHIP depends on the presence of Hsp70 and the co-chaperone BAG5. Contrary to the enhancer activity reported for BAG1, BAG5 reduces the ability of CHIP to ubiquitinate αSyn in and Hsp70-dependent manner (Kalia et al., 2011).

Additional pathogenic mechanisms in PD that involve the activity of CHIP relate to the ubiquitin ligase activity of parkin and the kinase activity of the leucine-rich repeat kinase-2 (LRRK2). It has been found that CHIP, Hsp70 and parkin form a ternary complex that promotes ubiquitination and degradation of the Pael receptor, a protein localized in the ER and whose accumulation has been linked to dopaminergic neuronal death (Imai et al., 2002), and CHIP has been proposed to enhance the activity of parkin, even in the absence of Hsp70 (Imai et al., 2002). Concerning LRRK2, CHIP regulates the ubiquitination, degradation, and toxicity mediated by pathogenic mutations of this kinase (Ko et al., 2009). Moreover, it has been shown that CHIP binds to LRRK2 via its TPR motifs and formation of this complex is protective in cell culture models, while in the presence of mutant LRKK2, knock-down of CHIP leads to cell death (Ko et al., 2009).

2.3 Hsp70 in chaperone-mediated autophagy (CMA)

Macroautophay and chaperone-mediated autophagy (CMA) are the two main lysosomal proteolytic systems in mammalian cells for the degradation of intracellular proteins (Xilouri & Stefanis, 2011). CMA is the process of degradation of intracellular components by lysosomes which selectively degrades cytotolic proteins containing a KFERQ-like motif (Koga & Cuervo, 2010). This process is known to involve binding of a complex of constitutive cytosolic Hsp70 (Hsc70) and co-chaperones (including Hsp40, Hip, Hsp90 and BAG1) to substrate proteins, and their subsequent targeting to lysosomes via the lysosomal surface receptor LAMP-2A (Xilouri & Stefanis, 2011). The substrate protein is subsequently degraded after unfolding and translocation into the lysosomal lumen, in a process involving lysosomal Hsc70 (Figure 1). It has been estimated that about 30% of cytosolic proteins could be subjected to degradation via CMA (Dice, 2007), and furthermore, this pathway may be a major route by which αSyn is degraded in neurons (Witt, 2009). Even though it is currently accepted that dysregulation of autophagy plays a role in neurodegeneration (Bandyopadhyay & Cuervo, 2007; Nixon, 2006; Rubinsztein, 2006; Xilouri & Stefanis, 2011), including the PD neurodegenerative process (Martinez-Vicente et al., 2008; Yang et al., 2009), the mechanism by which CMA modulates neuronal survival or death, is still unclear.

Given that pathologic accumulation of αSyn is a hallmark of PD, several recent studies have addressed the possible link between αSyn degradation, CMA dysfunction and the neurodegenerative process. Indeed, αSyn, which contains a pentapeptide sequence ($_{95}$VKKDQ$_{99}$) consistent with Hsc70 binding (Dice, 1990), has been shown to be degraded via CMA using isolated lysosomal preparations (Cuervo et al., 2004) and neuronal cells (Alvarez-Erviti et al., 2010; Martinez-Vicente et al.; Vogiatzi et al., 2008). On the contrary, the A30P and A53T αSyn variants were observed to bind strongly to LAMP-2A receptors but were not internalized, thus inhibiting the CMA degradation of other substrates (Cuervo et al., 2004). This CMA dysfunction was later shown to mediate αSyn toxicity in cellular models (Xilouri et al., 2009). Moreover, a recent study using both αSyn transgenic- and paraquat- PD mouse models (Mak et al., 2010), showed that αSyn can be degraded in the lysosome through CMA, *in vivo*. The study also revealed an up-regulation of LAMP-2A and lysosomal Hsc70 and an increase in Hsc70-αSyn interactions in brain lysosomes, relative to controls. On the other hand, a recent work work revealed a significant reduction of both LAMP-2A and Hsc70 levels in the SN and amygdala of PD brains, relative to age-matched Alzheimer's disease (AD) and healthy, brain controls (Alvarez-Erviti et al., 2010). Even though their results might initially appear contradictory, these findings support a key role for Hsc70 and the CMA system in maintaining intracellular general proteostasis, especially within the αSyn-overload scenario that is typically associated to PD and other α-synucleinopathies.

2.4 Emerging links between the Hsp70 system and neurodegeneration in PD

2.4.1 The CSPα-Hsc70-SGT complex and neurodegeneration in PD

Cysteine-string protein α (CSPα) is an abundant protein localized in synaptic vesicles that ameliorates neurodegeneration in cellular and animal models (Johnson et al., 2010). It contains a Dna-J domain and has been shown to interact with Hsc70 and to increase its ATPase activity (Braun et al., 1996). On the other hand, CSPα was shown to assemble into an enzymatically active ternary complex with Hsc70 and SGT (small glutamine-rich tetratricopeptide repeat domain protein) with a likely regulatory function in secretory vesicles (Tobaben et al., 2001). CSPα has also been reported to interact with other chaperones, including Hsp90 (Sakisaka et al., 2002), Hip, Hop (Rosales-Hernandez et al., 2009), and Hsp40 (Gibbs et al., 2009).

CSPα dysfunction has been implicated in various pathologies, including memory impairment, type-2 diabetes, cystic fibrosis, and HD (reviewed in (Johnson et al., 2010)). A few years ago, a link between CSPα and PD was also established (Chandra et al., 2005). The results of this study, performed using a transgenic mouse model, indicate that αSyn cooperates with CSPα in preventing neurodegeneration (Chandra et al., 2005). In a recent study (Sharma et al., 2011), the CSPα-Hsc70-SGT complex was found to bind to monomeric

SNAP-25, a pre-synaptic SNARE protein, and prevent its aggregation, thus promoting the formation of the SNARE complex involved in neuronal synapse. Interestingly, another recent study using a transgenic mouse model of αSyn aggregation with associated neurodegeneration, has shown that SNAP-25 is redistributed within synaptic terminals and the protein was found to colocalize with αSyn within intraneuronal aggregates (Garcia-Reitbock et al., 2010). These data raise the question whether aggregating αSyn might actually be sequestering CSPα involved in the CSPα-Hsc70-SGT complex, analogously to what was observed for aggregating huntingtin (Miller et al., 2003), and therefore enabling the aggregation of SNAP-25 in a PD scenario.

2.4.2 The unfolded protein response (UPR) in PD

The unfolded protein response (UPR) is a mechanism activated within the cell when the endoplasmic reticulum (ER) function is impaired and, as a result, unfolded proteins accumulate in the ER lumen (a process called 'ER stress'). The ER-resident Hsp70 family member GRP78 (HSPA5/BiP) recognizes and binds to such unfolded proteins, which causes the release of UPR-activating factors (Rutkowski & Kaufman, 2004). To restore ER function, the UPR reduces protein translation and enhances the folding and processing capacities within ER. However, if the stress overwhelms the cell restoring capacity, the UPR induces apoptosis (Paschen & Mengesdorf, 2005). A few years ago, a mutation in the parkin gene was found to be related to familiar PD due to the impairment of its ubiquitin ligase function which results in protein accumulation within the ER lumen and leads to ER stress and apoptosis (Imai et al., 2001). More recently, a strong correlation between UPR activation and PD pathogenesis in PD patients was established (Hoozemans et al., 2007), suggesting a functional connection between αSyn and ER stress. In addition, it was found that overexpression of (Wt) αSyn triggers UPR in yeast (Cooper et al., 2006). A recent study has shown that αSyn is also found aggregated and accumulated within the ER lumen and induces UPR by binding to GRP78/BiP in cells, which could lead to apoptosis (Bellucci et al., 2011). Clearly, supplementary investigations are needed to determine the exact role of the UPR in the pathophysiology of PD.

2.4.3 Mitochondrial dysfunction in PD

In both familial and sporadic forms of PD, several mitochondrial alterations and increase of oxidative species are well recorded (Jellinger, 2010). The important role of mitochondrial pathology in PD is reflected by the specific and selective loss of mitochondrial complex I activity in the SN of PD patients (Valente et al., 2004). Results from a study with neuronal cell cultures indicate that this impairment is dependent on αSyn mitochondrial import and accumulation (Devi et al., 2008). Interestingly, a recent proteomic study revealed that expression of mortalin (HSPA9/mtHSP70/GRP75), a mitochondrial stress protein and member of the Hsp70 chaperone family which binds to DJ-1 and αSyn (Jin et al., 2007), is significantly decreased in PD brains (De Mena et al., 2009; Jin et al., 2006) as well as in a cellular model of PD (Jin et al., 2006). Moreover, specific coding mutational variants of the mortalin gene have been recently discovered in a few PD patients (Burbulla et al., 2010; De Mena et al., 2009). Finally, differential levels of mitochondrial mortalin were measured in Wt and A53T cellular models of PD (Pennington et al., 2010), suggesting a possible involvement of αSyn aggregation in PD-related mitochondrial dysfunction (Xie et al., 2010).

3. The Hsp70 machinery members as biomarkers of PD

A biomarker is a naturally occurring molecule, gene, or characteristic by which a particular medical condition, disease, etc. can be identified. Despite the current relevance of identifying a biomarker for early diagnosis of PD and/or to follow up its progression, up to date there is no reliable biomarker available (Morgan et al., 2010; Nyhlen et al., 2010). Therefore, certain key proteins that are thought to be tightly linked to PD pathogenesis or progression, such as the members of the Hsp70 machinery discussed above, which could manifest changes in their expression levels in body fluids cells or alter their presence in body fluids in a PD scenario, could represent potential markers of disease development or predisposition.

Currently, it is well established the most promising biomarkers for PD in cerebrospinal fluidic (CSF) are αSyn, DJ-1, amyloid β, and the tau protein. These are the principal targets in the Parkinson's Progression Markers Initiative, a public-private, large-scale study project that aims to identify biological markers of disease progression (www.PPMI-info.org). DJ-1, which is the only chaperone to be included in this study, is a mitochondrial chaperone which has been one of the most studied proteins for its potential use as a PD biomarker. However, results published thus far from measurements of DJ-1 in CSF (Hong et al., 2010) and serum from PD patients (Hong et al., 2010; Shi et al., 2010; Waragai et al., 2007) are somewhat controversial or inconsistent, which could probably be explained by the high DJ-1 protein level present in blood cells (Shi et al., 2010).

Currently, it is well established that certain proteins, including members of the Hsp70 family such as Hsp701A and 1B, display perturbed expression levels in the SN of PD brains (Hauser et al., 2005); however, changes in tissue expression levels are in principle not useful for an application as biomarkers. Recently, a significant decrease in whole blood mRNA levels of St13/Hip co-chaperone was reported for early PD patients, but not for AD patients or healthy controls (Scherzer et al., 2007). However, a second group reported no significant differences in the expression pattern of ST13 in early-stage PD patients, as compared to controls (Shadrina et al., 2010). This discrepancy could be attributed, at least in part, to heterogeneity in the criteria of diagnosing and classifying the individuals into groups and to the difficulty in establishing the actual onset of the disease. Yet another study found differences in HSPA8 (Hsc70) and HIP2 expression levels between PD patients and controls (Grunblatt et al., 2010). Other members of the Hsp70 machinery are known to change their expression patterns in PD patients compared to healthy controls (Hauser et al., 2005). Unfortunately, these changes appear not specific or sufficient to differentiate between PD and other related neurodegenerative disorders (Hauser et al., 2005). This is probably due to the fact that the Hsp70 system plays a central role in maintaining cell proteostasis, which is perturbed in a variety of neurodegenerative diseases.

Considering that PD is a complex pathology that involves several systems such as the stress response, the UPS, the immune system, etc., a unique biomarker might not be enough as a tool for diagnosis or follow-up of disease progression. Instead, there is general consensus that the use of a set of distinct parameters, such as protein expression profiles, age, symptoms and others, would probably be the best approach (Fasano et al., 2008; Grunblatt et al., 2010; Scherzer et al., 2007).

4. The Hsp70 system as a therapeutic tool for PD

As described in this chapter, in the last few years it has become evident that HSPs play an important role in the initiation and progression of PD and other neurodegenerative diseases. This cumulative evidence has prompted the development of therapeutic tools based on the Hsp70 machinery. Different strategies have been tested to manipulate Hsp70 as a therapeutic approximation for PD and related neurodegenerative diseases (reviewed in Kalia 2010). Three general approaches have been explored, namely, to increase the intracellular activity of Hsp70, to overexpress Hsp70 and/or other co-chaperones, and to deliver chaperones or regulatory factors using cell-penetrating peptides (CPPs).

4.1 Increasing the intracellular activity of Hsp70

Theoretically, it should be feasible to control the activity of the cellular chaperone machinery by using different types of drugs. The mechanism of most of such chemical compounds is based on activating HSF-1, a key transcriptional regulator of the heat shock response (HSR) that activates the gene expression of inducible HSPs. One way of activating HSF-1 is by inhibiting Hsp90 activity; as a result, HSF-1 becomes active and increases the expression of inducible chaperones like HSPA1A/Hsp72 and others. Geldanamycin (GA) and its derivative 17-allylamino-17-demethoxygeldanamycin (17-AAG) are antibiotics with high affinity for the ATPase domain of Hsp90, which blocks its interaction with HSF-1 and subsequently allows its activation (Waza et al., 2006; Zou et al., 1998). GA prevents αSyn-induced dopaminergic cell loss in cell culture (McLean et al., 2004) and in animal models of PD (Auluck et al., 2005; Shen et al., 2005), while the less toxic 17-AAG has also proven to be neuroprotective in PD cellular models (Danzer et al., 2011; Riedel et al., 2010) and in two animal models of PD-related neurodegenerative diseases (Fujikake et al., 2008; Waza et al., 2005). Even though 17-AAG is currently under phase-II clinical trials as an anti-tumour drug (Pacey et al., 2010; Richardson et al., 2010; Solit et al., 2008), its use in patients with neurodegenerative diseases could be hampered by its toxicity and unavailability for oral administration (Pacey et al., 2010). Another family of inhibitors of Hsp90 activity, is SNX-2112 and its analogues, which are orally available and present improved blood brain barrier (BBB) permeability. In particular, SNX-0723 was shown to prevent αSyn oligomer formation and αSyn-induced toxicity in cell culture (Putcha et al., 2010), and preclinical studies for cancer therapy are proving their safety (Zhai et al., 2011), although similar studies in neurodegenerative animal models are still needed.

Other drugs are able to activate HSF-1 without inhibiting Hsp90 activity, which could represent a less toxic approximation for neurodegenerative pathologies. Arimoclomol, for example, has already been tested in phase I- and IIa-clinical trials for treating ALS, and shown to be safe and tolerable (Cudkowicz et al., 2008; Phukan, 2010). Another example is HSF-1A (Neef et al., 2010), shown to upregulate Hsp70 expression and to reduce poly-Q-citotoxicity in cell and fly models of poly-Q neurodegenerative disorders (Neef et al., 2010). Celastrol, yet a similar drug, and some structural relatives, appear as promising drugs due to their rapid kinetics and low EC_{50} (Westerheide et al., 2004), although further studies are needed.

Besides these approaches, HSF-1 co-inducers could represent more tolerable drugs for therapy. These are molecules that partially activate HSF-1, reducing its activation threshold and often working in conjunction with secondary stress signals to fully induce HSR. Non steroidal anti-inflammatory drugs (NSAIDs) are well known co-inducers of HSR. For example, Sodium salicylate and Indomethacin induce HSF-1 DNA binding and reduce the temperature required for triggering the HSR (Jurivich et al., 1995; Lee et al., 1995). The association of NSAIDs use with a lower risk of common neurodegenerative diseases such as AD and PD has been analysed in several studies (Etminan et al., 2008; Gagne & Power, 2010). According to one hypothesis, this negative correlation could be due to continuous up-regulation of HSR and consequently continued cytoprotection against neurodegenereration (Westerheide et al., 2004).

4.2 Overexpression of Hsp70 and/or related co-chaperones

In principle, it should be possible to design a gene therapy approach for the treatment of PD and other conformational neurodegenerative diseases based on HSPs, considering the substantial number of reports having characterized the molecular pathways by which Hsp70 acts in the context of disease. Intriguingly, even though overexpression of Hsp70 has been shown to be protective in animal models of PD (Dong et al., 2005; Jung et al., 2008), a recent study in mouse indicates otherwise (Shimshek et al.). Up to date, one phase-I study in PD patients using recombinant Adeno-Associated Virus (AAV) to deliver aromatic aminoacid decarboxylase enzyme into the putamen, supports the proof-of-principle for the use of gene therapy in PD (Christine et al., 2009). With this precedent, gene therapy could potentially be employed to overexpress other chaperones and co-chaperones that may improve Hsp70 function and its neuroprotective properties. Indeed, recombinant AAV has been already used to transduce Hsp104 (Vashist et al., 2010), a non-mammalian chaperone, in a rat model of PD and proven to be neuroprotective by disaggregating protein inclusions and synergizing with endogenous Hsp70 (Lo Bianco et al., 2008).

Given that co-chaperone BAG-5 is known as a negative regulator of Hsp70, downregulation of its expression has been tested in a mouse model of PD. In this study, direct expression in the SN by recombinant AAV delivery of BAG-5(DARA), a BAG-5 mutant which inhibits wild-type BAG-5 activity, resulted in increased dopaminergic neuron survival (Kalia et al., 2004). Another possible approach to increase Hsp70 function by using gene therapy techniques could be gene silencing by RNA interference to knockdown Hsp70 downregulators. Although these techniques have not been extensively tested for neurodegenerative therapy, they remain a potentially useful tool (Manfredsson et al., 2006).

4.3 Chaperones or regulatory factors delivery using CPPs

Cell penetrating peptides (CPPs) are the most recent approximation that shows promise towards increasing Hsp70 activity within cells. These are peptide motifs that allow cell transduction of macromolecules including functional full-length proteins. The basic domain of the trans-activator of transcription (TAT) from HIV-1 is the best known among CPPs and it has been shown that fusion with TAT allows proteins to penetrate cell membranes of several cell types and even to cross the BBB (Fawell et al., 1994; Schwarze et al., 1999). In the last few years, TAT-Hsp70 transduction has been reported to be neuroprotective against different kinds of stress in cell models (Lai et al., 2005; Nagel et al., 2008) as well as in a MPTP mouse model of PD (Nagel et al., 2008). In addition, transduction of TAT-Hsp40 has also been shown to be cytoprotective against oxidative stress in cells (Kim et al., 2008). Finally, transduction of HSF-1(+)-TAT, an HSF-1 mutant fused to TAT, capable of activating HSR by itself by itself, was demonstrated to induce to induce Hsp70 expression and to protect cells against heat stress *in vitro* (Hou & Zou, 2009). Although further investigation is needed, CPPs tagging could prove a powerful tool in therapy against neurodegenerative diseases by allowing the efficient transduction of cytoprotective proteins and factors.

5. Conclusions

There is strong experimental support to propose the Hsp70 chaperone system as a key player in pathogenesis and progression of PD. This central role seems to be especially linked to αSyn, although alternative connections between the Hsp70 machinery and different pathogenic mechanisms underlying PD might exist. Up to this point, there is substantial evidence supporting an active role of Hsp70 in well established PD-related processes. First, in the inhibition or modulation of αSyn aggregation pathway that results in the formation of LBs and the suppression of αSyn-mediated toxicity to cells that leads to neurodegeneration. Second, a prominent role in the control of the activity of the UPS machinery, the general protein degradation and disposal system in the cell. And third, a central role in CMA, which handles the lysosomal degradation of selected cytosolic proteins, including αSyn. In addition, emerging mechanisms for Hsp70 in relation to PD include its participation in the CSPα-Hsc70-SGT complex in the neuron, and the increasing attention paid to the UPR and mitochondrial dysfunction processes in PD, both of which rely on Hsp70.

The accumulated studies thus far suggest that Hsp70 chaperone is a highly versatile protein whose anti-aggregation activity seems to involve different interactions and the formation of transient and highly dynamic complexes with various αSyn species, presumably early oligomers and probably monomers, along the aggregation pathway. This activity can be certainly modulated by the presence of nucleotides and by certain co-chaperones, in particular, Hip. Clearly, further *in vitro* and in cell studies with Hsp70 and co-chaperones, to better understand the full molecular mechanism of mammalian Hsp70 in managing αSyn aggregation, are needed.

As a biomarker of PD, Hsp70 seems not to represent a good candidate itself, probably due to its central role in maintaining cellular proteostasis which is perturbed in several amyloidoses and related diseases. However, the Hsp70 co-chaperone Hip might represent a potentially useful biomarker for early diagnosis of PD, although more studies are needed in this direction. Given that PD is a complex disease, a 'complex biomarker' (i.e. composed of various markers) appears to be the only reliable option. Finally, the Hsp70 machinery can be indirectly enhanced by HSF-1 pharmacological activation, which represents one of the most promising therapeutic approaches for treating this complex and highly debilitating disease.

6. Acknowledgements

We acknowledge financial support provided by the Spanish Ministry of Health according to the 'Plan Nacional de I+D+I 2008-2011', Instituto Nacional Carlos III (ISCIII, project CP10/00527 to C.R.), and cofunding by FEDER funds., and the PAIDI Program from the Andalusian Government (CTS-677). A.L.G. holds a FPU Fellowship from the Spanish Ministry of Science (MICINN). C.W.B. acknowledges funding from the EU FP7 (MC-IEF 236721). The authors are grateful to Christopher M. Dobson (University of Cambridge, UK) and John Christodoulou (University College London, UK) for helpful and highly stimulating discussion of results.

7. References

Adachi, H., et al. (2007). CHIP overexpression reduces mutant androgen receptor protein and ameliorates phenotypes of the spinal and bulbar muscular atrophy transgenic mouse model. *J Neurosci*, 27, (19), pp. (5115-26).

Ahmad, A. (2010). DnaK/DnaJ/GrpE of Hsp70 system have differing effects on alpha-synuclein fibrillation involved in Parkinson's disease. *Int J Biol Macromol*, 46, (2), pp. (275-9).

Al-Ramahi, I., et al. (2006). CHIP protects from the neurotoxicity of expanded and wild-type ataxin-1 and promotes their ubiquitination and degradation. *J Biol Chem*, 281, (36), pp. (26714-24).

Alberti, S., et al. (2004). The cochaperone HspBP1 inhibits the CHIP ubiquitin ligase and stimulates the maturation of the cystic fibrosis transmembrane conductance regulator. *Mol Biol Cell*, 15, (9), pp. (4003-10).

Alberti, S., et al. (2002). Ubiquitylation of BAG-1 suggests a novel regulatory mechanism during the sorting of chaperone substrates to the proteasome. *J Biol Chem*, 277, (48), pp. (45920-7).

Alvarez-Erviti, L., et al. (2010). Chaperone-mediated autophagy markers in Parkinson disease brains. *Arch Neurol*, 67, (12), pp. (1464-72).

Arawaka, S., et al. (2010). Heat shock proteins as suppressors of accumulation of toxic prefibrillar intermediates and misfolded proteins in neurodegenerative diseases. *Curr Pharm Biotechnol*, 11, (2), pp. (158-66).

Auluck, P. K., et al. (2002). Chaperone suppression of alpha-synuclein toxicity in a Drosophila model for Parkinson's disease. *Science*, 295, (5556), pp. (865-8).

Auluck, P. K., et al. (2005). Mechanisms of Suppression of {alpha}-Synuclein Neurotoxicity by Geldanamycin in Drosophila. *J Biol Chem*, 280, (4), pp. (2873-8).

Ballinger, C. A., et al. (1999). Identification of CHIP, a novel tetratricopeptide repeat-containing protein that interacts with heat shock proteins and negatively regulates chaperone functions. *Mol Cell Biol*, 19, (6), pp. (4535-45).

Bandopadhyay, R.&J. de Belleroche (2010). Pathogenesis of Parkinson's disease: emerging role of molecular chaperones. *Trends Mol Med*, 16, (1), pp. (27-36).

Bandyopadhyay, U.&A. M. Cuervo (2007). Chaperone-mediated autophagy in aging and neurodegeneration: lessons from alpha-synuclein. *Exp Gerontol*, 42, (1-2), pp. (120-8).

Bellucci, A., et al. (2011). Induction of the unfolded protein response by alpha-synuclein in experimental models of Parkinson's disease. *J Neurochem*, 116, (4), pp. (588-605).

Bence, N. F., et al. (2001). Impairment of the ubiquitin-proteasome system by protein aggregation. *Science*, 292, (5521), pp. (1552-5).

Bercovich, B., et al. (1997). Ubiquitin-dependent degradation of certain protein substrates in vitro requires the molecular chaperone Hsc70. *J Biol Chem*, 272, (14), pp. (9002-10).

Braun, J. E., et al. (1996). The cysteine string secretory vesicle protein activates Hsc70 ATPase. *J Biol Chem*, 271, (42), pp. (25989-93).

Broadley, S. A.&F. U. Hartl (2009). The role of molecular chaperones in human misfolding diseases. *FEBS Lett*, 583, (16), pp. (2647-53).

Bukau, B.&A. L. Horwich (1998). The Hsp70 and Hsp60 chaperone machines. *Cell*, 92, (3), pp. (351-66).

Burbulla, L. F., et al. (2010). Dissecting the role of the mitochondrial chaperone mortalin in Parkinson's disease: functional impact of disease-related variants on mitochondrial homeostasis. *Hum Mol Genet*, 19, (22), pp. (4437-52).

Ciechanover, A.&P. Brundin (2003). The ubiquitin proteasome system in neurodegenerative diseases: sometimes the chicken, sometimes the egg. *Neuron*, 40, (2), pp. (427-46).

Connell, P., et al. (2001). The co-chaperone CHIP regulates protein triage decisions mediated by heat-shock proteins. *Nat Cell Biol*, 3, (1), pp. (93-6).

Conway, K. A., et al. (1998). Accelerated in vitro fibril formation by a mutant alpha-synuclein linked to early-onset Parkinson disease. *Nat Med*, 4, (11), pp. (1318-20).

Conway, K. A., et al. (2000). Acceleration of oligomerization, not fibrillization, is a shared property of both alpha-synuclein mutations linked to early-onset Parkinson's disease: implications for pathogenesis and therapy. *Proc Natl Acad Sci U S A*, 97, (2), pp. (571-6).

Cook, C.&L. Petrucelli (2009). A critical evaluation of the ubiquitin-proteasome system in Parkinson's disease. *Biochim Biophys Acta*, 1792, (7), pp. (664-75).

Cooper, A. A., et al. (2006). Alpha-synuclein blocks ER-Golgi traffic and Rab1 rescues neuron loss in Parkinson's models. *Science*, 313, (5785), pp. (324-8).

Cudkowicz, M. E., et al. (2008). Arimoclomol at dosages up to 300 mg/day is well tolerated and safe in amyotrophic lateral sclerosis. *Muscle Nerve*, 38, (1), pp. (837-44).

Cuervo, A. M., et al. (2004). Impaired degradation of mutant alpha-synuclein by chaperone-mediated autophagy. *Science*, 305, (5688), pp. (1292-5).

Chandra, S., et al. (2005). Alpha-synuclein cooperates with CSPalpha in preventing neurodegeneration. *Cell*, 123, (3), pp. (383-96).

Chiti, F.&C. M. Dobson (2006). Protein misfolding, functional amyloid, and human disease. *Annu Rev Biochem*, 75, pp. (333-66).

Choi, W., et al. (2004). Mutation E46K increases phospholipid binding and assembly into filaments of human alpha-synuclein. *FEBS Lett*, 576, (3), pp. (363-8).

Christine, C. W., et al. (2009). Safety and tolerability of putaminal AADC gene therapy for Parkinson disease. *Neurology*, 73, (20), pp. (1662-9).

Chung, K. K., et al. (2001). Parkin ubiquitinates the alpha-synuclein-interacting protein, synphilin-1: implications for Lewy-body formation in Parkinson disease. *Nat Med*, 7, (10), pp. (1144-50).

Danzer, K. M., et al. (2011). Heat-shock protein 70 modulates toxic extracellular alpha-synuclein oligomers and rescues trans-synaptic toxicity. *FASEB J*, 25, (1), pp. (326-36).

Danzer, K. M., et al. (2011). Heat-shock protein 70 modulates toxic extracellular alpha-synuclein oligomers and rescues trans-synaptic toxicity. *FASEB J*, 25, (1), pp. (326-36).

De Mena, L., et al. (2009). Mutational screening of the mortalin gene (HSPA9) in Parkinson's disease. *J Neural Transm*, 116, (10), pp. (1289-93).

Dedmon, M. M., et al. (2005). Heat shock protein 70 inhibits alpha-synuclein fibril formation via preferential binding to prefibrillar species. *J Biol Chem*, 280, (15), pp. (14733-40).

Demand, J., et al. (2001). Cooperation of a ubiquitin domain protein and an E3 ubiquitin ligase during chaperone/proteasome coupling. *Curr Biol*, 11, (20), pp. (1569-77).

Devi, L., et al. (2008). Mitochondrial import and accumulation of alpha-synuclein impair complex I in human dopaminergic neuronal cultures and Parkinson disease brain. *J Biol Chem*, 283, (14), pp. (9089-100).

Dice, J. F. (1990). Peptide sequences that target cytosolic proteins for lysosomal proteolysis. *Trends Biochem Sci*, 15, (8), pp. (305-9).

Dice, J. F. (2007). Chaperone-mediated autophagy. *Autophagy*, 3, (4), pp. (295-9).

Dickey, C. A., et al. (2007). Brain CHIP: removing the culprits in neurodegenerative disease. *Trends Mol Med*, 13, (1), pp. (32-8).

Dong, Z., et al. (2005). Hsp70 gene transfer by adeno-associated virus inhibits MPTP-induced nigrostriatal degeneration in the mouse model of Parkinson disease. *Mol Ther*, 11, (1), pp. (80-8).

Dul, J. L., et al. (2001). Hsp70 and antifibrillogenic peptides promote degradation and inhibit intracellular aggregation of amyloidogenic light chains. *J Cell Biol*, 152, (4), pp. (705-16).

El-Agnaf, O. M., et al. (1998). Aggregates from mutant and wild-type alpha-synuclein proteins and NAC peptide induce apoptotic cell death in human neuroblastoma cells by formation of beta-sheet and amyloid-like filaments. *FEBS Lett*, 440, (1-2), pp. (71-5).

Etminan, M., et al. (2008). Non-steroidal anti-inflammatory drug use and the risk of Parkinson disease: a retrospective cohort study. *J Clin Neurosci*, 15, (5), pp. (576-7).

Fasano, M., et al. (2008). Peripheral biomarkers of Parkinson's disease as early reporters of central neurodegeneration. *Biomark Med*, 2, (5), pp. (465-78).

Fawell, S., et al. (1994). Tat-mediated delivery of heterologous proteins into cells. *Proc Natl Acad Sci U S A*, 91, (2), pp. (664-8).

Fornai, F., et al. (2005). Parkinson-like syndrome induced by continuous MPTP infusion: convergent roles of the ubiquitin-proteasome system and alpha-synuclein. *Proc Natl Acad Sci U S A*, 102, (9), pp. (3413-8).

Fujikake, N., et al. (2008). Heat shock transcription factor 1-activating compounds suppress polyglutamine-induced neurodegeneration through induction of multiple molecular chaperones. *J Biol Chem*, 283, (38), pp. (26188-97).

Gagne, J. J.&M. C. Power (2010). Anti-inflammatory drugs and risk of Parkinson disease: a meta-analysis. *Neurology*, 74, (12), pp. (995-1002).

Garcia-Mata, R., et al. (1999). Characterization and dynamics of aggresome formation by a cytosolic GFP-chimera. *J Cell Biol*, 146, (6), pp. (1239-54).

Garcia-Reitbock, P., et al. (2010). SNARE protein redistribution and synaptic failure in a transgenic mouse model of Parkinson's disease. *Brain*, 133, (Pt 7), pp. (2032-44).

Giasson, B. I.&V. M. Lee (2003). Are ubiquitination pathways central to Parkinson's disease? *Cell*, 114, (1), pp. (1-8).

Giasson, B. I., et al. (2001). A hydrophobic stretch of 12 amino acid residues in the middle of alpha-synuclein is essential for filament assembly. *J Biol Chem*, 276, (4), pp. (2380-6).

Gibbs, S. J., et al. (2009). Hsp40 couples with the CSPalpha chaperone complex upon induction of the heat shock response. *PLoS One*, 4, (2), pp. (e4595).

Gosavi, N., et al. (2002). Golgi fragmentation occurs in the cells with prefibrillar alpha-synuclein aggregates and precedes the formation of fibrillar inclusion. *J Biol Chem*, 277, (50), pp. (48984-92).

Grunblatt, E., et al. (2001). Gene expression analysis in N-methyl-4-phenyl-1,2,3,6-tetrahydropyridine mice model of Parkinson's disease using cDNA microarray: effect of R-apomorphine. *J Neurochem*, 78, (1), pp. (1-12).

Grunblatt, E., et al. (2010). Pilot study: peripheral biomarkers for diagnosing sporadic Parkinson's disease. *J Neural Transm*, 117, (12), pp. (1387-93).

Gupta, A., et al. (2008). What causes cell death in Parkinson's disease? *Ann Neurol*, 64 Suppl 2, pp. (S3-15).

Hartl, F. U. (1996). Molecular chaperones in cellular protein folding. *Nature*, 381, (6583), pp. (571-9).

Hartl, F. U.&M. Hayer-Hartl (2002). Molecular chaperones in the cytosol: from nascent chain to folded protein. *Science*, 295, (5561), pp. (1852-8).

Hartl, F. U.&M. Hayer-Hartl (2009). Converging concepts of protein folding in vitro and in vivo. *Nat Struct Mol Biol*, 16, (6), pp. (574-81).

Hasegawa, M., et al. (2002). Phosphorylated alpha-synuclein is ubiquitinated in alpha-synucleinopathy lesions. *J Biol Chem*, 277, (50), pp. (49071-6).

Hatakeyama, S., et al. (2004). U-box protein carboxyl terminus of Hsc70-interacting protein (CHIP) mediates poly-ubiquitylation preferentially on four-repeat Tau and is involved in neurodegeneration of tauopathy. *J Neurochem*, 91, (2), pp. (299-307).

Hauser, M. A., et al. (2005). Expression profiling of substantia nigra in Parkinson disease, progressive supranuclear palsy, and frontotemporal dementia with parkinsonism. *Arch Neurol*, 62, (6), pp. (917-21).

Hershko, A.&A. Ciechanover (1998). The ubiquitin system. *Annu Rev Biochem*, 67, pp. (425-79).

Hinault, M. P., et al. (2010). Stable alpha-synuclein oligomers strongly inhibit chaperone activity of the Hsp70 system by weak interactions with J-domain co-chaperones. *J Biol Chem*, 285, (49), pp. (38173-82).

Hohfeld, J., et al. (2001). From the cradle to the grave: molecular chaperones that may choose between folding and degradation. *EMBO Rep*, 2, (10), pp. (885-90).

Hohfeld, J., et al. (1995). Hip, a novel cochaperone involved in the eukaryotic Hsc70/Hsp40 reaction cycle. *Cell*, 83, (4), pp. (589-98).

Hong, Z., et al. (2010). DJ-1 and alpha-synuclein in human cerebrospinal fluid as biomarkers of Parkinson's disease. *Brain*, 133, (Pt 3), pp. (713-26).

Hoozemans, J. J., et al. (2007). Activation of the unfolded protein response in Parkinson's disease. *Biochem Biophys Res Commun*, 354, (3), pp. (707-11).

Hou, Y.&J. Zou (2009). Delivery of HSF1(+) protein using HIV-1 TAT protein transduction domain. *Mol Biol Rep*, 36, (8), pp. (2271-7).

Huang, C., et al. (2006). Heat shock protein 70 inhibits alpha-synuclein fibril formation via interactions with diverse intermediates. *J Mol Biol*, 364, (3), pp. (323-36).

Imai, Y., et al. (2002). CHIP is associated with Parkin, a gene responsible for familial Parkinson's disease, and enhances its ubiquitin ligase activity. *Mol Cell*, 10, (1), pp. (55-67).

Imai, Y., et al. (2001). An unfolded putative transmembrane polypeptide, which can lead to endoplasmic reticulum stress, is a substrate of Parkin. *Cell*, 105, (7), pp. (891-902).

Jellinger, K. A. (2010). Basic mechanisms of neurodegeneration: a critical update. *J Cell Mol Med*, 14, (3), pp. (457-87).

Jin, J., et al. (2006). Proteomic identification of a stress protein, mortalin/mthsp70/GRP75: relevance to Parkinson disease. *Mol Cell Proteomics*, 5, (7), pp. (1193-204).

Jin, J., et al. (2007). Identification of novel proteins associated with both alpha-synuclein and DJ-1. *Mol Cell Proteomics*, 6, (5), pp. (845-59).

Johnson, J. N., et al. (2010). CSPalpha: the neuroprotective J protein. *Biochem Cell Biol*, 88, (2), pp. (157-65).

Jung, A. E., et al. (2008). HSP70 and constitutively active HSF1 mediate protection against CDCrel-1-mediated toxicity. *Mol Ther*, 16, (6), pp. (1048-55).

Jurivich, D. A., et al. (1995). Salicylate triggers heat shock factor differently than heat. *J Biol Chem*, 270, (41), pp. (24489-95).

Kalia, L. V., et al. (2011). Ubiquitinylation of alpha-Synuclein by Carboxyl Terminus Hsp70-Interacting Protein (CHIP) Is Regulated by Bcl-2-Associated Athanogene 5 (BAG5). *PLoS One*, 6, (2), pp. (e14695).

Kalia, S. K., et al. (2004). BAG5 inhibits parkin and enhances dopaminergic neuron degeneration. *Neuron*, 44, (6), pp. (931-45).

Kampinga, H. H. & E. A. Craig (2010). The HSP70 chaperone machinery: J proteins as drivers of functional specificity. *Nat Rev Mol Cell Biol*, 11, (8), pp. (579-92).

Karpinar, D. P., et al. (2009). Pre-fibrillar alpha-synuclein variants with impaired beta-structure increase neurotoxicity in Parkinson's disease models. *EMBO J*, 28, (20), pp. (3256-68).

Kim, S. A., et al. (2008). TAT-Hsp40 inhibits oxidative stress-mediated cytotoxicity via the inhibition of Hsp70 ubiquitination. *FEBS Lett*, 582, (5), pp. (734-40).

Kitada, T., et al. (1998). Mutations in the parkin gene cause autosomal recessive juvenile parkinsonism. *Nature*, 392, (6676), pp. (605-8).

Klucken, J., et al. (2006). Detection of novel intracellular alpha-synuclein oligomeric species by fluorescence lifetime imaging. *FASEB J*, 20, (12), pp. (2050-7).

Klucken, J., et al. (2004a). A single amino acid substitution differentiates Hsp70-dependent effects on alpha-synuclein degradation and toxicity. *Biochem Biophys Res Commun*, 325, (1), pp. (367-73).

Klucken, J., et al. (2004b). Hsp70 Reduces alpha-Synuclein Aggregation and Toxicity. *J Biol Chem*, 279, (24), pp. (25497-502).

Ko, H. S., et al. (2009). CHIP regulates leucine-rich repeat kinase-2 ubiquitination, degradation, and toxicity. *Proc Natl Acad Sci U S A*, 106, (8), pp. (2897-902).

Koga, H.&A. M. Cuervo (2010). Chaperone-mediated autophagy dysfunction in the pathogenesis of neurodegeneration. *Neurobiol Dis*, pp.

Kruger, R., et al. (1998). Ala30Pro mutation in the gene encoding alpha-synuclein in Parkinson's disease. *Nat Genet*, 18, (2), pp. (106-8).

Lai, Y., et al. (2005). Selectively increasing inducible heat shock protein 70 via TAT-protein transduction protects neurons from nitrosative stress and excitotoxicity. *J Neurochem*, 94, (2), pp. (360-6).

Lashuel, H. A., et al. (2002a). Neurodegenerative disease: amyloid pores from pathogenic mutations. *Nature*, 418, (6895), pp. (291).

Lashuel, H. A., et al. (2002b). Alpha-synuclein, especially the Parkinson's disease-associated mutants, forms pore-like annular and tubular protofibrils. *J Mol Biol*, 322, (5), pp. (1089-102).

Lee, B. S., et al. (1995). Pharmacological modulation of heat shock factor 1 by antiinflammatory drugs results in protection against stress-induced cellular damage. *Proc Natl Acad Sci U S A*, 92, (16), pp. (7207-11).

Leroy, E., et al. (1998). The ubiquitin pathway in Parkinson's disease. *Nature*, 395, (6701), pp. (451-2).

Liani, E., et al. (2004). Ubiquitylation of synphilin-1 and alpha-synuclein by SIAH and its presence in cellular inclusions and Lewy bodies imply a role in Parkinson's disease. *Proc Natl Acad Sci U S A*, 101, (15), pp. (5500-5).

Lindersson, E., et al. (2004). Proteasomal inhibition by alpha-synuclein filaments and oligomers. *J Biol Chem*, 279, (13), pp. (12924-34).

Liu, Y., et al. (2002). The UCH-L1 gene encodes two opposing enzymatic activities that affect alpha-synuclein degradation and Parkinson's disease susceptibility. *Cell*, 111, (2), pp. (209-18).

Lo Bianco, C., et al. (2008). Hsp104 antagonizes alpha-synuclein aggregation and reduces dopaminergic degeneration in a rat model of Parkinson disease. *J Clin Invest*, 118, (9), pp. (3087-97).

Lotz, G. P., et al. (2010). Hsp70 and Hsp40 functionally interact with soluble mutant huntingtin oligomers in a classic ATP-dependent reaction cycle. *J Biol Chem*, 285, (49), pp. (38183-93).

Lu, T. Z., et al. (2010). Multifaceted role of heat shock protein 70 in neurons. *Mol Neurobiol*, 42, (2), pp. (114-23).

Luders, J., et al. (2000). The ubiquitin-related BAG-1 provides a link between the molecular chaperones Hsc70/Hsp70 and the proteasome. *J Biol Chem*, 275, (7), pp. (4613-7).

Luk, K. C., et al. (2008). Interactions between Hsp70 and the hydrophobic core of alpha-synuclein inhibit fibril assembly. *Biochemistry*, 47, (47), pp. (12614-25).

Maeda, H., et al. (2007). Biological heterogeneity of the peptide-binding motif of the 70-kDa heat shock protein by surface plasmon resonance analysis. *J Biol Chem*, 282, (37), pp. (26956-62).

Mak, S. K., et al. (2010). Lysosomal degradation of alpha-synuclein in vivo. *J Biol Chem*, 285, (18), pp. (13621-9).

Manfredsson, F. P., et al. (2006). RNA knockdown as a potential therapeutic strategy in Parkinson's disease. *Gene Ther*, 13, (6), pp. (517-24).

Manning-Bog, A. B., et al. (2006). Lack of nigrostriatal pathology in a rat model of proteasome inhibition. *Ann Neurol*, 60, (2), pp. (256-60).

Martinez-Vicente, M., et al. (2008). Dopamine-modified alpha-synuclein blocks chaperone-mediated autophagy. *J Clin Invest*, 118, (2), pp. (777-88).

Martinez-Vicente, M., et al. Cargo recognition failure is responsible for inefficient autophagy in Huntington's disease. *Nat Neurosci*, 13, (5), pp. (567-76).

Mayer, M. P.&B. Bukau (2005). Hsp70 chaperones: cellular functions and molecular mechanism. *Cell Mol Life Sci*, 62, (6), pp. (670-84).

McDonough, H.&C. Patterson (2003). CHIP: a link between the chaperone and proteasome systems. *Cell Stress Chaperones*, 8, (4), pp. (303-8).

McLean, P. J., et al. (2002). TorsinA and heat shock proteins act as molecular chaperones: suppression of alpha-synuclein aggregation. *J Neurochem*, 83, (4), pp. (846-54).

McLean, P. J., et al. (2004). Geldanamycin induces Hsp70 and prevents alpha-synuclein aggregation and toxicity in vitro. *Biochem Biophys Res Commun*, 321, (3), pp. (665-9).

McNaught, K. S., et al. (2003). Altered proteasomal function in sporadic Parkinson's disease. *Exp Neurol*, 179, (1), pp. (38-46).

McNaught, K. S.&P. Jenner (2001). Proteasomal function is impaired in substantia nigra in Parkinson's disease. *Neurosci Lett*, 297, (3), pp. (191-4).

McNaught, K. S., et al. (2002a). Impairment of the ubiquitin-proteasome system causes dopaminergic cell death and inclusion body formation in ventral mesencephalic cultures. *J Neurochem*, 81, (2), pp. (301-6).

McNaught, K. S.&C. W. Olanow (2006). Proteasome inhibitor-induced model of Parkinson's disease. *Ann Neurol*, 60, (2), pp. (243-7).

McNaught, K. S., et al. (2001). Failure of the ubiquitin-proteasome system in Parkinson's disease. *Nat Rev Neurosci*, 2, (8), pp. (589-94).

McNaught, K. S., et al. (2004). Systemic exposure to proteasome inhibitors causes a progressive model of Parkinson's disease. *Ann Neurol*, 56, (1), pp. (149-62).

McNaught, K. S., et al. (2002b). Aggresome-related biogenesis of Lewy bodies. *Eur J Neurosci*, 16, (11), pp. (2136-48).

Meacham, G. C., et al. (2001). The Hsc70 co-chaperone CHIP targets immature CFTR for proteasomal degradation. *Nat Cell Biol*, 3, (1), pp. (100-5).

Miller, L. C., et al. (2003). Cysteine string protein (CSP) inhibition of N-type calcium channels is blocked by mutant huntingtin. *J Biol Chem*, 278, (52), pp. (53072-81).

Minami, Y., et al. (1996). Regulation of the heat-shock protein 70 reaction cycle by the mammalian DnaJ homolog, Hsp40. *J Biol Chem*, 271, (32), pp. (19617-24).

Morgan, J. C., et al. (2010). Biomarkers in Parkinson's disease. *Curr Neurol Neurosci Rep*, 10, (6), pp. (423-30).

Morimoto, R. I. (2008). Proteotoxic stress and inducible chaperone networks in neurodegenerative disease and aging. *Genes Dev*, 22, (11), pp. (1427-38).

Mouradian, M. M. (2002). Recent advances in the genetics and pathogenesis of Parkinson disease. *Neurology*, 58, (2), pp. (179-85).

Muchowski, P. J., et al. (2000). Hsp70 and hsp40 chaperones can inhibit self-assembly of polyglutamine proteins into amyloid-like fibrils. *Proc Natl Acad Sci U S A*, 97, (14), pp. (7841-6).

Murata, S., et al. (2001). CHIP is a chaperone-dependent E3 ligase that ubiquitylates unfolded protein. *EMBO Rep*, 2, (12), pp. (1133-8).

Nagel, F., et al. (2008). Tat-Hsp70 protects dopaminergic neurons in midbrain cultures and in the substantia nigra in models of Parkinson's disease. *J Neurochem*, 105, (3), pp. (853-64).

Neef, D. W., et al. (2010). Modulation of heat shock transcription factor 1 as a therapeutic target for small molecule intervention in neurodegenerative disease. *PLoS Biol*, 8, (1), pp. (e1000291).

Nixon, R. A. (2006). Autophagy in neurodegenerative disease: friend, foe or turncoat? *Trends Neurosci*, 29, (9), pp. (528-35).

Nyhlen, J., et al. (2010). Problems associated with fluid biomarkers for Parkinson's disease. *Biomark Med*, 4, (5), pp. (671-81).

Opazo, F., et al. (2008). Accumulation and clearance of alpha-synuclein aggregates demonstrated by time-lapse imaging. *J Neurochem*, 106, (2), pp. (529-40).

Outeiro, T. F., et al. (2008). Formation of toxic oligomeric alpha-synuclein species in living cells. *PLoS One*, 3, (4), pp. (e1867).

Pacey, S., et al. (2010). A Phase II trial of 17-allylamino, 17-demethoxygeldanamycin (17-AAG, tanespimycin) in patients with metastatic melanoma. *Invest New Drugs*, pp.

Paschen, W.&T. Mengesdorf (2005). Endoplasmic reticulum stress response and neurodegeneration. *Cell Calcium*, 38, (3-4), pp. (409-15).

Pennington, K., et al. (2010). Differential effects of wild-type and A53T mutant isoform of alpha-synuclein on the mitochondrial proteome of differentiated SH-SY5Y cells. *J Proteome Res*, 9, (5), pp. (2390-401).

Petrucelli, L., et al. (2002). Parkin protects against the toxicity associated with mutant alpha-synuclein: proteasome dysfunction selectively affects catecholaminergic neurons. *Neuron*, 36, (6), pp. (1007-19).

Phukan, J. (2010). Arimoclomol, a coinducer of heat shock proteins for the potential treatment of amyotrophic lateral sclerosis. *IDrugs*, 13, (7), pp. (482-96).

Polymeropoulos, M. H., et al. (1997). Mutation in the alpha-synuclein gene identified in families with Parkinson's disease. *Science*, 276, (5321), pp. (2045-7).

Prapapanich, V., et al. (1996). Molecular cloning of human p48, a transient component of progesterone receptor complexes and an Hsp70-binding protein. *Mol Endocrinol*, 10, (4), pp. (420-31).

Putcha, P., et al. (2010). Brain-permeable small-molecule inhibitors of Hsp90 prevent alpha-synuclein oligomer formation and rescue alpha-synuclein-induced toxicity. *J Pharmacol Exp Ther*, 332, (3), pp. (849-57).

Richardson, P. G., et al. (2010). Tanespimycin with bortezomib: activity in relapsed/refractory patients with multiple myeloma. *Br J Haematol*, 150, (4), pp. (428-37).

Rideout, H. J., et al. (2005). Dopaminergic neurons in rat ventral midbrain cultures undergo selective apoptosis and form inclusions, but do not up-regulate iHSP70, following proteasomal inhibition. *J Neurochem*, 93, (5), pp. (1304-13).

Riedel, M., et al. (2010). 17-AAG induces cytoplasmic alpha-synuclein aggregate clearance by induction of autophagy. *PLoS One*, 5, (1), pp. (e8753).

Rochet, J. C., et al. (2000). Inhibition of fibrillization and accumulation of prefibrillar oligomers in mixtures of human and mouse alpha-synuclein. *Biochemistry*, 39, (35), pp. (10619-26).

Roodveldt, C., et al. (2009). Chaperone proteostasis in Parkinson's disease: stabilization of the Hsp70/alpha-synuclein complex by Hip. *EMBO J*, 28, (23), pp. (3758-70).

Roodveldt, C., et al. (2008). Immunological features of alpha-synuclein in Parkinson's disease. *J Cell Mol Med*, 12, (5B), pp. (1820-9).

Rosales-Hernandez, A., et al. (2009). RDJ2 (DNAJA2) chaperones neural G protein signaling pathways. *Cell Stress Chaperones*, 14, (1), pp. (71-82).

Rott, R., et al. (2008). Monoubiquitylation of alpha-synuclein by seven in absentia homolog (SIAH) promotes its aggregation in dopaminergic cells. *J Biol Chem*, 283, (6), pp. (3316-28).

Rubinsztein, D. C. (2006). The roles of intracellular protein-degradation pathways in neurodegeneration. *Nature*, 443, (7113), pp. (780-6).

Rudiger, S., et al. (1997). Substrate specificity of the DnaK chaperone determined by screening cellulose-bound peptide libraries. *EMBO J*, 16, (7), pp. (1501-7).

Rutkowski, D. T.&R. J. Kaufman (2004). A trip to the ER: coping with stress. *Trends Cell Biol*, 14, (1), pp. (20-8).

Sakisaka, T., et al. (2002). Rab-alphaGDI activity is regulated by a Hsp90 chaperone complex. *EMBO J*, 21, (22), pp. (6125-35).

Sato, S., et al. (2006). 14-3-3eta is a novel regulator of parkin ubiquitin ligase. *EMBO J*, 25, (1), pp. (211-21).

Scherzer, C. R., et al. (2007). Molecular markers of early Parkinson's disease based on gene expression in blood. *Proc Natl Acad Sci U S A*, 104, (3), pp. (955-60).

Scheufler, C., et al. (2000). Structure of TPR domain-peptide complexes: critical elements in the assembly of the Hsp70-Hsp90 multichaperone machine. *Cell*, 101, (2), pp. (199-210).

Schlecht, R., et al. (2011). Mechanics of Hsp70 chaperones enables differential interaction with client proteins. *Nat Struct Mol Biol*, 18, (3), pp. (345-51).

Schwarze, S. R., et al. (1999). In vivo protein transduction: delivery of a biologically active protein into the mouse. *Science*, 285, (5433), pp. (1569-72).

Shadrina, M. I., et al. (2010). Expression analysis of suppression of tumorigenicity 13 gene in patients with Parkinson's disease. *Neurosci Lett*, 473, (3), pp. (257-9).

Sharma, M., et al. (2011). CSPalpha promotes SNARE-complex assembly by chaperoning SNAP-25 during synaptic activity. *Nat Cell Biol*, 13, (1), pp. (30-9).

Shen, H. Y., et al. (2005). Geldanamycin induces heat shock protein 70 and protects against MPTP-induced dopaminergic neurotoxicity in mice. *J Biol Chem*, 280, (48), pp. (39962-9).

Shi, M., et al. (2010). Significance and confounders of peripheral DJ-1 and alpha-synuclein in Parkinson's disease. *Neurosci Lett*, 480, (1), pp. (78-82).

Shimshek, D. R., et al. (2010). The HSP70 molecular chaperone is not beneficial in a mouse model of alpha-synucleinopathy. *PLoS One*, 5, (4), pp. (e10014).

Shimura, H., et al. (2001). Ubiquitination of a new form of alpha-synuclein by parkin from human brain: implications for Parkinson's disease. *Science*, 293, (5528), pp. (263-9).

Shin, Y., et al. (2005). The co-chaperone carboxyl terminus of Hsp70-interacting protein (CHIP) mediates alpha-synuclein degradation decisions between proteasomal and lysosomal pathways. *J Biol Chem*, 280, (25), pp. (23727-34).

Shults, C. W. (2006). Lewy bodies. *Proc Natl Acad Sci U S A*, 103, (6), pp. (1661-8).

Singleton, A. B., et al. (2003). alpha-Synuclein locus triplication causes Parkinson's disease. *Science*, 302, (5646), pp. (841).

Solit, D. B., et al. (2008). Phase II trial of 17-allylamino-17-demethoxygeldanamycin in patients with metastatic melanoma. *Clin Cancer Res*, 14, (24), pp. (8302-7).

Spillantini, M. G., et al. (1998). alpha-Synuclein in filamentous inclusions of Lewy bodies from Parkinson's disease and dementia with lewy bodies. *Proc Natl Acad Sci U S A*, 95, (11), pp. (6469-73).

Sun, L.&Z. J. Chen (2004). The novel functions of ubiquitination in signaling. *Curr Opin Cell Biol*, 16, (2), pp. (119-26).

Takayama, S., et al. (1999). An evolutionarily conserved family of Hsp70/Hsc70 molecular chaperone regulators. *J Biol Chem*, 274, (2), pp. (781-6).

Taxis, C., et al. (2003). Use of modular substrates demonstrates mechanistic diversity and reveals differences in chaperone requirement of ERAD. *J Biol Chem*, 278, (38), pp. (35903-13).

Tetzlaff, J. E., et al. (2008). CHIP targets toxic alpha-Synuclein oligomers for degradation. *J Biol Chem*, 283, (26), pp. (17962-8).

Tobaben, S., et al. (2001). A trimeric protein complex functions as a synaptic chaperone machine. *Neuron*, 31, (6), pp. (987-99).
Urushitani, M., et al. (2004). CHIP promotes proteasomal degradation of familial ALS-linked mutant SOD1 by ubiquitinating Hsp/Hsc70. *J Neurochem*, 90, (1), pp. (231-44).
Valente, E. M., et al. (2004). Hereditary early-onset Parkinson's disease caused by mutations in PINK1. *Science*, 304, (5674), pp. (1158-60).
Vashist, S., et al. (2010). Applying Hsp104 to protein-misfolding disorders. *Biochem Cell Biol*, 88, (1), pp. (1-13).
Vila, M.&S. Przedborski (2003). Targeting programmed cell death in neurodegenerative diseases. *Nat Rev Neurosci*, 4, (5), pp. (365-75).
Vogiatzi, T., et al. (2008). Wild type alpha-synuclein is degraded by chaperone-mediated autophagy and macroautophagy in neuronal cells. *J Biol Chem*, 283, (35), pp. (23542-56).
Voisine, C., et al. (2010). Chaperone networks: tipping the balance in protein folding diseases. *Neurobiol Dis*, 40, (1), pp. (12-20).
Volles, M. J.&P. T. Lansbury, Jr. (2002). Vesicle permeabilization by protofibrillar alpha-synuclein is sensitive to Parkinson's disease-linked mutations and occurs by a pore-like mechanism. *Biochemistry*, 41, (14), pp. (4595-602).
Volles, M. J.&P. T. Lansbury, Jr. (2003). Zeroing in on the pathogenic form of alpha-synuclein and its mechanism of neurotoxicity in Parkinson's disease. *Biochemistry*, 42, (26), pp. (7871-8).
Wacker, J. L., et al. (2004). Hsp70 and Hsp40 attenuate formation of spherical and annular polyglutamine oligomers by partitioning monomer. *Nat Struct Mol Biol*, 11, (12), pp. (1215-22).
Waragai, M., et al. (2007). Plasma levels of DJ-1 as a possible marker for progression of sporadic Parkinson's disease. *Neurosci Lett*, 425, (1), pp. (18-22).
Warrick, J. M., et al. (1999). Suppression of polyglutamine-mediated neurodegeneration in Drosophila by the molecular chaperone HSP70. *Nat Genet*, 23, (4), pp. (425-8).
Waza, M., et al. (2005). 17-AAG, an Hsp90 inhibitor, ameliorates polyglutamine-mediated motor neuron degeneration. *Nat Med*, 11, (10), pp. (1088-95).
Waza, M., et al. (2006). Modulation of Hsp90 function in neurodegenerative disorders: a molecular-targeted therapy against disease-causing protein. *J Mol Med*, 84, (8), pp. (635-46).
Westerheide, S. D., et al. (2004). Celastrols as inducers of the heat shock response and cytoprotection. *J Biol Chem*, 279, (53), pp. (56053-60).
Witt, S. N. (2009). Hsp70 molecular chaperones and Parkinson's disease. *Biopolymers*, 93, (3), pp. (218-28).
Wong, E.&A. M. Cuervo (2010). Autophagy gone awry in neurodegenerative diseases. *Nat Neurosci*, 13, (7), pp. (805-11).
Wood, S. J., et al. (1999). alpha-synuclein fibrillogenesis is nucleation-dependent. Implications for the pathogenesis of Parkinson's disease. *J Biol Chem*, 274, (28), pp. (19509-12).
Xie, W., et al. (2010). New insights into the role of mitochondrial dysfunction and protein aggregation in Parkinson's disease. *Biochim Biophys Acta*, 1802, (11), pp. (935-41).
Xilouri, M.&L. Stefanis (2011). Autophagic pathways in Parkinson disease and related disorders. *Expert Rev Mol Med*, 13, pp. (e8).

Xilouri, M., et al. (2009). Abberant alpha-synuclein confers toxicity to neurons in part through inhibition of chaperone-mediated autophagy. *PLoS One*, 4, (5), pp. (e5515).

Yang, Q., et al. (2009). Regulation of neuronal survival factor MEF2D by chaperone-mediated autophagy. *Science*, 323, (5910), pp. (124-7).

Young, J. C. (2010). Mechanisms of the Hsp70 chaperone system. *Biochem Cell Biol*, 88, (2), pp. (291-300).

Zarranz, J. J., et al. (2004). The new mutation, E46K, of alpha-synuclein causes Parkinson and Lewy body dementia. *Ann Neurol*, 55, (2), pp. (164-73).

Zhai, Q. Q., et al. (2011). Preclinical pharmacokinetic analysis of SNX-2112, a novel Hsp90 inhibitor, 3 in rats. *Biomed Pharmacother*, 65, (2), pp. (132-6).

Zhang, Y., et al. (2001). Hsp70 molecular chaperone facilitates endoplasmic reticulum-associated protein degradation of cystic fibrosis transmembrane conductance regulator in yeast. *Mol Biol Cell*, 12, (5), pp. (1303-14).

Zhou, Y., et al. (2004). Analysis of alpha-synuclein-associated proteins by quantitative proteomics. *J Biol Chem*, 279, (37), pp. (39155-64).

Zou, J., et al. (1998). Repression of heat shock transcription factor HSF1 activation by HSP90 (HSP90 complex) that forms a stress-sensitive complex with HSF1. *Cell*, 94, (4), pp. (471-80).

11

The Noradrenergic System is a Major Component in Parkinson's Disease

Patricia Szot[1], Allyn Franklin[1] and Murray A. Raskind[1,2]
[1]*Veterans Administration Northwest Network for Mental Illness Research, Education and Clinical Center and Puget Sound Health Care System, Seattle,*
[2]*Department of Psychiatry and Behavioral Science, University of Washington, Seattle*
USA

1. Introduction

1.1 Dopaminergic neuronal loss in Parkinson's disease

Parkinson's disease (PD) is a neurological disorder that affects approximately 2% of the elderly population, and as our population continues to age, the incidence will only increase (Singh et al., 2007). PD is commonly characterized by various motor deficits including tremor, rigidity and bradykinesia (Singh et al., 2007). The cause of these motor symptoms is the loss of dopaminergic neurons in the substantia nigra pars compacta (SN) and reduced dopamine (DA) levels in the striatum (Damier et al., 1999; Gibb, 1991; Gibb and Lee, 1991). However, the appearance of PD symptoms does not occur until 70-80% of the dopaminergic neurons are lost. In the progression of this disorder, the loss of dopaminergic neurons is not observed until Stage 3 (out of 6 Stages) of the disorder (Braak et al., 2003a, 2003b, 2006).

1.2 Noradrenergic neuronal loss in Parkinson's disease

Of course a great deal of research has focused on the dopaminergic system in PD because loss of neurons in the SN is responsible for PD symptoms; however, PD is represented by multiple systems failing. During the earlier stages of the disorder, non-motor preclinical symptoms are observed. These preclinical symptoms include hyposmia (Berendse et al., 2001, Ponsen et al., 2004), REM-sleep disorder (Boeve et al., 2003, Scheneck et al., 2003), depression (Leentjens et al., 2003; Mayeux et al., 1992; Slaughter et al., 2001) and autonomic dysfunction such as orthostatic hypotension (Mathias, 1998; Ziemssen & Reichmann, 2007). These preclinical symptoms are attributed to neuropathological changes in neurotransmitter systems other than the SN dopaminergic nervous system. One neurotransmitter system that may be responsible for these early non-motor symptoms is the noradrenergic nervous system (Goldstein et al., 2011; Itoi & Sugimoto, 2010; Lopez-Munoz & Alamo, 2009; Mathias, 1998; Osaka & Matsumura, 1994; Ziegler et al., 1977). The presence of these symptoms would indicate an alteration in the noradrenergic nervous system is occurring early in the progression of PD. Postmortem examination of PD tissue demonstrates a significant loss of noradrenergic neurons in the locus coeruleus (LC); this loss is equal to or greater than the neuronal loss observed in the SN (Bertrand et al., 1997; Cash et al., 1987; Chan-Palay & Asan, 1989; Hornykiewicz & Kish, 1987; Marien et al., 2004; McMillan et al., 2011; Patt & Gerhard,

1993; Zarow et al., 2003). The loss of LC noradrenergic neurons also precedes the loss of dopaminergic neurons in the progression of PD (Braak et al., 2003b, 2006), correlating to the time that preclinical noradrenergic non-motor symptoms appear.

2. Noradrenergic cell bodies

2.1 Anatomical

There are two major clusters of noradrenergic neurons in the central nervous system (CNS): the LC and the lateral tegmental neurons. In contrast to the significant loss of LC noradrenergic neurons in PD as indicated above, the lateral tegmental group does not appear to demonstrate much of a loss in PD (Saper et al., 1991). LC noradrenergic neurons send projections to forebrain regions via three different tracts: the central tegmental tract, the central gray dorsal longitudinal fasciculus tract, and the ventral tegmental-medial forebrain bundle. A fourth tract innervates the cerebellum, and a fifth tract innervates the spinal cord. The rostral portion of the LC innervates forebrain structures such as the hippocampus, whereas the caudal portion of the LC innervates hindbrain structures such as the cerebellum and spinal cord (Aston-Jones et al., 1995; Fallon & Loughlin, 1982; Loughin et al., 1982, 1986b). The degree of LC innervation to forebrain regions compared to the lateral tegmental neurons varies from region to region, but the hippocampus and cortex appear to receive sole innervation from the LC (Aston-Jones et al., 1995; Jones & Moore, 1977; Loughlin et al., 1986a, b; Mason & Fibiger, 1970; Moore & Bloom, 1979; Olsen & Fuxe, 1971; Ungerstedt, 1971; Waterhouse et al., 1983). Innervation from the LC to forebrain regions also appears to be ipsilateral for the majority of regions (Ader et al., 1980; Room et al., 1981). Since the LC contains more than half of all noradrenergic neurons in the CNS (Aston-Jones et al., 2000), a reduction in the number of these neurons could have major consequences on the activity of many forebrain regions.

2.2 Synthesis of norepinephrine

The major neurotransmitter localized to noradrenergic neurons is norepinephrine (NE). However, NE is not the only transmitter released from noradrenergic terminals. Noradrenergic neurons also co-localize and release several other neuropeptides such as galanin, enkepalin and neuropeptide Y. NE and DA share a common synthetic pathway. NE is synthesized by several enzymatic steps (Figure 1): tyrosine is converted to L-3, 4-dihydroxphenylalanine (L-DOPA) by tyrosine hydroxylase (TH); L-DOPA is converted to DA by aromatic amino acid decarboxylase (AADC), and then in noradrenergic neurons DA is converted to NE by dopamine β-hydroxylase (DBH). In adrenergic neurons, NE is then converted to epinephrine by phenylthanolamine-N-methyltransferase (PMNT). TH is considered the rate-limiting enzyme in the synthesis of NE and DA. However, there is evidence to indicate that DBH activity can affect NE levels in the CNS when DBH levels are altered genetically (Thomas et al., 1995, 1998; Bourdelat-Parks et al., 2005), with excessive stimulation of noradrenergic neurons (Scatton et al., 1984) or when DBH inhibitors such as disulfiram or nepicastat are administered (Goldstein, 1966; Musacchio et al., 1966; Bourdelat-Parks et al., 2005; Beliaev et al., 2006; Schroeder et al., 2010). DBH knockout mice lack the ability to convert DA to NE so the CNS levels of DA are elevated as compared to wild-type mice (Thomas et al., 1995, 1998). NE levels in the periphery and CNS can be restored in DBH knockout mice with the peripheral administration of L-3,4-dihydoxyphenylserine (DOPS). DOPS is converted to NE through AADC, in noradrenergic and non-noradrenergic neurons. TH knockout mice lack the ability to synthesize both DA and NE (Zhou & Palmiter, 1995).

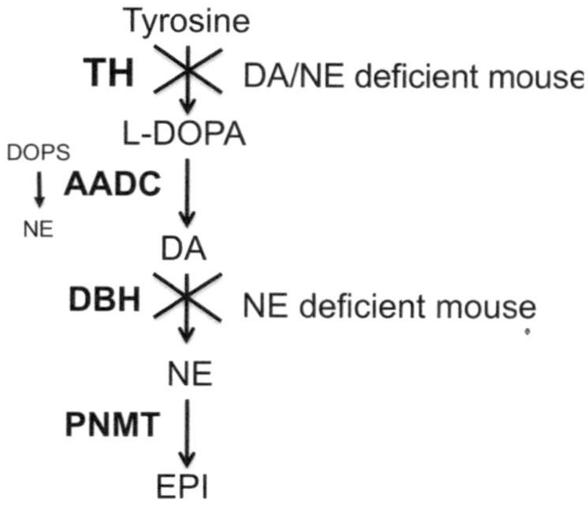

Fig. 1. Catecholamine biosynthesis and production of catecholamine knockout mice.

3. Consequence of LC neuronal loss in PD

3.1 Alterations in terminal noradrenergic markers

The loss of LC noradrenergic neurons in PD subjects should result in changes in NE levels at the various forebrain regions it innervates and the degree of loss should depend on the amount of LC innervation the region receives as compared to lateral tegmental groups. In PD subjects, there are reduced NE levels in the cortex, hypothalamus and cerebellum (Gasper et al., 1984, 1991; Kish et al., 1984; Shannak et al., 1994). TH- and DBH-immunoreactivity (IR) are also reduced in the cortex of PD subjects (Gasper et al., 1991). The reduction in neurotransmitter content and synthesizing enzymes in PD subjects can be attributed to the loss of noradrenergic innervation to these areas associated with the loss of LC noradrenergic neurons. The cortex, as indicated above, receives sole innervation from the LC, so changes in LC neuronal number would have a major impact in this region (Aston-Jones et al., 1995; Jones & Moore, 1977; Loughlin et al., 1986a, b; Mason & Fibiger, 1970; Moore & Bloom, 1979; Olsen & Fuxe, 1971; Ungerstedt, 1971; Waterhouse et al., 1983). Presently, the consequence of LC noradrenergic neuronal loss in PD on NE tissue content in the dopaminergic SN region is unknown.

3.2 Alterations in noradrenergic markers in LC

In contrast to terminal NE content in forebrain regions, NE levels in the LC of PD subjects does not appear to be different from controls (Cash et al., 1987). Examining different noradrenergic markers in the surviving LC neurons in PD subjects indicates the noradrenergic neurons are not compensating for the loss of surrounding neurons or terminal NE. The number of TH and DBH mRNA positively labeled neurons in the LC of PD subjects are significantly reduced as compared to age-matched control subjects (Szot, 2000, 2006; McMillan et al., 2011) and corresponds to the documented loss of noradrenergic neurons by other laboratories (Bertrand et al., 1997; Cash et al., 1987; Chan-Palay & Asan, 1989; Hornykiewicz & Kish, 1987; Marien et al., 2004; McMillan et al., 2011; Patt & Gerhard, 1993; Zarow et al., 2003). The degree of LC noradrenergic neuronal loss determined by TH and DBH mRNA expression in PD subjects is verified by counting the number of LC TH-IR positive labeled neurons (McMillan et al., 2011). TH mRNA expression/neuron of the surviving LC noradrenergic neurons in PD subjects did not differ from TH mRNA expression/neuron in age-matched control subjects, indicating a lack of compensation of the surviving LC neurons (McMillan et al., 2011). Another marker of noradrenergic neurons, NE transporter (NET), was measured in the LC of age-matched and PD subjects. NET's function is to remove released NE from the synapse. Therefore, NETs are localized only to noradrenergic cell bodies, dendrites (peri-LC dendritic zone), and axon terminals of noradrenergic neurons. NET binding over cell body region and peri-LC dendritic zone in PD subjects is significantly reduced compared to age-matched control subjects and the loss of NET binding over the cell body region corresponds to the number of LC noradrenergic neurons in the LC (McMillan et al., 2011). The loss of NET binding in the peri-LC dendritic zone in PD subjects indicates the surviving LC neurons are not compensating for neuronal loss by increasing dendritic innervation. The loss of dendritic innervation in PD subjects, as determined by NET binding, is supported by reduced dendritic TH-IR labeling in the LC region of PD subjects as compared to age-matched controls (McMillan et al., 2011). However, the surviving LC neurons in PD subjects do demonstrate compensation in the expression of DBH mRNA (McMillan et al., 2011). The increased DBH mRNA expression/neuron in the surviving LC neurons of PD subjects may not be a response to neuronal loss because DBH mRNA expression/neuron is not altered in another neurodegenerative disorder with a significant loss of LC noradrenergic neurons (see below). Therefore, the increase in DBH mRNA expression/neuron observed in the surviving LC neurons in PD subjects may be a response to some other factor particular to PD, although it is unclear what that factor might be. The consequence of increased DBH mRNA expression of surviving LC neurons on NE levels in PD subjects is also unclear. Studies measuring cerebral spinal fluid (CSF) NE levels in PD subjects are variable. CSF NE levels and metabolites vary from reduced to no difference in postmortem and alive PD subjects (withdrawn from L-DOPA treatment) as compared to control subjects (Chia et al., 1993, 1995; Mann et al., 1983; Scatton et al., 1986; Turkka et al., 1987). As indicated above, NE tissue content is reduced, but LC concentration is similar to control subjects. These data suggest that NE levels and function may be reduced in PD, similar to DA levels and function.

3.3 Effect of L-DOPA treatment on noradrenergic system

The "standard gold" treatment for PD is L-DOPA. Administration of L-DOPA alleviates the symptoms associated with the loss of dopaminergic neurons (Cotzias et al., 1969); however, L-DOPA does not necessarily alleviate the non-motor symptoms associated with the loss of noradrenergic neurons (Sethi, 2008). Chronic administration of L-DOPA to PD subjects significantly elevates CSF levels of L-DOPA, DA and the DA metabolite dihydroxyphenylacetic acid (DOPAC) from age-matched control subjects (Figure 2A, B and C). There is a positive correlation of CSF DA levels to CSF L-DOPA levels. CSF NE levels in PD subjects on chronic L- DOPA treatment are not statistically different from age-matched controls (Figure 2B), but the NE metabolite 3,4-dihydroxyphenylglycol (DHPG) is significantly elevated in PD patients on chronic L-DOPA (Figure 2C). It is unclear why NE levels do not correlate to CSF L-DOPA levels in PD subjects like DA. A possible reason for the discrepancy in NE and DA levels in PD subjects on chronic L-DOPA therapy may be because administered L-DOPA is decarboxylated to DA in striatal neurons (as compared to DA from SN terminals) and serotonergic neurons, not in the few remaining dopaminergic neurons (Huot & Parent, 2007; Yamada et al., 2007). Orthostatic hypotension, which is attributed to reduced CNS NE function, is relieved only with the administration of DOPS (Goldstein et al., 2011). DOPS is also used to normalize CNS levels of NE in the DBH knockout mouse that lacks the synthetic enzyme DBH that converts DA to NE (Figure 1) (Thomas et al., 1998). So these data would suggest that NE function in untreated PD and possibly treated subjects is reduced.

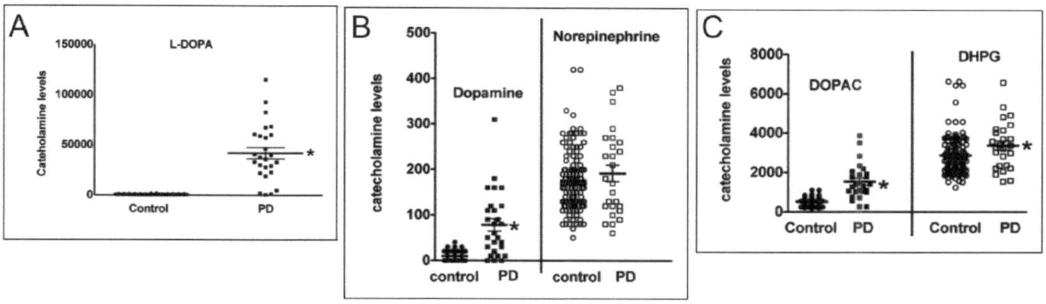

Fig. 2. CSF catecholamine levels in PD subjects on chronic L-DOPA treatment and age-matched control subjects. CSF spinal fluid was taken at the same time of day, approximately 4 hours after administration of L-DOPA. A) L-DOPA level, B) DA and NE levels and C) DOPAC and DHPG CSF levels in control and PD subjects on L-DOPA treatment. Catecholamine levels were extracted by alumina extraction and analyzed by high performance liquid chromatography (HPLC) as previously described (Szot et al., 2010). Each point represents a single individual catecholamine value for control and PD subjects, with average and standard error means (SEM) illustrated in bars for each catecholamine analyzed. * Indicates significant difference between control and PD subjects.

4. Comparison of the consequence of LC neuronal loss between PD and Alzheimer's disease (AD)

4.1 Alterations in terminal noradrenergic markers

Alzheimer's disease (AD), another neurodegenerative disorder, also exhibits significant LC noradrenergic neuronal loss (Bondareff et al., 1982; Chan-Palay & Asan, 1989; German et al., 1992; Mann et al., 1980; Marcyniuk et al., 1986; Szot et al., 2000, 2006; Tomlinson et al., 1981). However, unlike PD, in AD subjects the surviving LC noradrenergic neurons appear to be compensating for the loss. The content of NE in terminal regions of postmortem AD subjects is reduced, but the reduction does not correspond to the degree of neuronal loss (Adolfsson et al., 1979; Hoogendijk et al., 1999; Mann et al., 1981; Palmer et al., 1987; Reinikainen et al., 1988; Toghi et al., 1992; Tomlinson et al., 1981). Similar results were observed for IR of NE-synthesizing enzymes in the forebrain of postmortem AD subjects (Cross et al., 1981; Palmer et al., 1987; Perry et al., 1981; Russo-Neustadt et al., 1998). These data indicate that there is a reduction in NE function in forebrain regions of AD subjects, but it doesn't correlate to the degree of LC neuronal loss even in a region like the cortex which receives all of its innervation from the LC (Aston-Jones et al., 1995; Jones & Moore, 1977; Loughlin et al., 1986a, b; Mason & Fibiger, 1970; Moore & Bloom, 1979; Olsen & Fuxe, 1971; Ungerstedt, 1971; Waterhouse et al., 1983). These data suggest the surviving LC noradrenergic neurons in AD may be compensating for the lost neurons.

4.2 Alterations in noradrenergic markers in LC

To determine if the surviving LC noradrenergic neurons in AD subjects are demonstrating compensatory changes, several noradrenergic markers, similar to the markers used on the LC tissue of PD subjects, were assessed in the LC of subjects with AD. Work from my laboratory showed that the surviving noradrenergic neurons in the LC of AD and a related dementing disorder, dementia with Lewy body (DLB), showed compensatory changes. In subjects with dementia, the number of TH, DBH and NET mRNA positively labeled neurons in the LC are significantly reduced as compared to age-matched control subjects (Szot et al., 2000, 2006) and the degree of this LC neuronal loss corresponds to documented loss of noradrenergic neurons in AD by other laboratories (Bondareff et al., 1982; Chan-Palay & Asan, 1989; German et al., 1992; Mann et al., 1980; Marcyniuk et al., 1986; Tomlinson et al., 1981). The degree of LC noradrenergic neuronal loss determined by TH mRNA expression in AD subjects is verified by counting the number of TH-IR positive labeled neurons (McMillan et al., 2011).

	PD	AD
Neuronal Number	↓	↓
TH mRNA/neuron	—	↑
DBH mRNA/neuron	↑	—
NET cell body binding	↓	↓
NET peri-LC binding	↓	—
TH-IR surrounding LC	↓	—

Table 1. Changes in noradrenergic markers in the LC of PD subjects and subjects with dementia as compared to appropriate control groups.

However, in AD, the surviving LC noradrenergic neurons exhibit increased TH mRNA expression/neuron as compared to age-matched control subjects (Szot et al., 2000, 2006), suggesting compensation. NET binding over cell body region in the LC of AD subjects is significantly reduced as compared to age-matched control subjects, and the loss of NET binding over the cell body region corresponds to the number of LC noradrenergic neurons in the LC (Szot et al., 2006). However, NET binding sites over the peri-LC dendritic zone in AD subjects is not significantly different from age-matched control subjects, despite the reduction in LC noradrenergic neurons positively labeled for NET mRNA (Szot et al., 2000, 2006). The normal amount of NET binding in the peri-LC dendritic zone of AD subjects indicates dendritic sprouting of the surviving LC neurons. TH-IR labeling in dendritic region of AD supports the notion of enhanced dendritic innervation around LC noradrenergic neurons in AD subjects observed with NET binding (McMillan et al., 2011), again indicating compensation of the surviving LC neurons in AD. In addition to the sprouting in the LC, the surviving LC neurons in AD exhibit axonal sprouting into the hippocampus and prefrontal cortex (Szot et al., 2006, 2007). The difference in the response of the surviving LC noradrenergic neurons in PD and AD is observed even concerning DBH mRNA expression/neuron. In PD, DBH mRNA expression/neuron is elevated (as indicated above), but in subjects with dementia where TH mRNA expression/neuron is elevated, DBH mRNA expression/neuron is not different from controls (McMillan et al., 2011). This suggests that the loss of LC noradrenergic neurons does not necessarily result in increased DBH mRNA expression/neuron. Compensation of the LC noradrenergic nervous system in AD subjects is also observed in CSF NE levels, where CSF NE levels are similar to or elevated to age-matched control subjects (Elrod et al., 1997; Gottfries et al., 1983; Mann et al., 1981; Raskind et al., 1984; Toghi et al., 1992).

4.3 Summary

It appears then the response of surviving LC noradrenergic neurons in AD, in regards to the noradrenergic markers measured, is completely different from the response of surviving LC noradrenergic neurons in PD (Table 1). These noradrenergic markers in AD suggest that noradrenergic function in AD subjects may not be reduced and may even exceed function in normal subjects, while in PD subject's noradrenergic function is reduced. This hypothesis is supported clinically. Orthostatic hypotension, a common non-motor symptom observed in PD due to reduced noradrenergic function, is not observed in AD subjects despite a similar degree of LC noradrenergic neuronal loss. A progression of noradrenergic function can be drawn between these two neurodegenerative disorders; at one of the spectrum PD represents the loss of LC noradrenergic neurons with reduced noradrenergic function, while AD represents the other end of the spectrum with the loss of LC noradrenergic neurons but enhanced noradrenergic function.

5. LC innervation of dopaminergic regions

As indicated above, LC noradrenergic neurons are reduced early in the progression of PD (Braak et al., 2003b, 2006). However, for the noradrenergic system to be involved in the progression of PD, LC noradrenergic neurons need to innervate the regions involved in the symptoms of PD (i.e., striatum and SN). There is evidence to indicate that the LC noradrenergic nervous system can modulate dopaminergic activity at the level of the striatum and the SN as well as the ventral tegmental area (VTA) at the anatomical, electrophysiological, neurochemical, and behavioral levels.

5.1 LC innervation to striatum

LC noradrenergic neurons have direct projections to the striatum, though evidence indicates this innervation may be sparse (Aston-Jones et al., 1995; Jones & Moore, 1977; Jones & Yang, 1985; Mason & Fibiger, 1979; Swanson & Hartman, 1975). When measured, NE concentration in the striatum is low (especially compared to DA), while NET binding (a marker of noradrenergic terminals) is not detectable (Szot, Personal communication; Koob et al., 1975; Nomura et al., 1976). However, the striatum does contain a dense amount of beta-adrenergic receptors (β-AR) (Byland & Snyder, 1976; Dolphin et al., 1979; Rainbow et al., 1984; Strazielle et al., 1999), as well as alpha2-AR (α_2-AR) (Szot, Personal communication; Boyajian et al., 1987; Hudson et al., 1992; Nicholas et al., 1992; Scheinin et al., 1994; Strazielle et al., 1999; Zeng and Lynch, 1991) and alpha1-AR (α_1-AR) (Szot, Personal communication; Rommelfanger et al., 2009; Strazielle et al., 1999) binding sites. Direct application of NE or administration of AR agents can affect the activity of striatal neurons and release of DA in the striatum (Bevam et al., 1975; Fujimoto et al., 1981; Lategan et al., 1990).

5.2 LC innervation to midbrain dopaminergic neurons

The midbrain dopaminergic neurons in the SN and VTA also receive direct innervation from LC noradrenergic neurons (Fritschy & Grzanna, 1990; Jones & Moore, 1977; Jones & Yang, 1985; Phillipson, 1979; Simon et al., 1979; Swanson & Hartman, 1975). The SN and VTA regions have detectable levels of NET binding, also indicating direct noradrenergic innervation and some of the innervation is from the LC (Szot, Personal communications). The SN and VTA also have β-, α_1- and α_2-AR binding sites (Szot, Personal communication; Boyajian et al., 1987; Hudson et al., 1992; Lee et al., 1998; Rainbow et al., 1984; Rosin et al., 1996; Scheinin et al., 1994; Strazielle et al., 1999). The LC directly innervates and modifies the activity of midbrain dopaminergic neurons; the loss of LC noradrenergic neurons results in altered activity of dopaminergic neurons (Collingridge et al., 1979; Grenhoff et al., 1993, 1995; Grenhoff & Svensson, 1989, 1993; Guiard et al., 2008; Wang et al., 2010).

5.3 LC altered dopaminergic behavior

There have been several studies to indicate the ability of LC noradrenergic neurons to modulate dopamine-induced behavior, especially when LC noradrenergic neurons are reduced (Antelman & Caggiula, 1977; Archer & Fredriksson, 2006; Chopin et al., 1999; Grimbergen et al., 2009; Mavridis et al., 1991; Rommelfanger et al., 2007; Taylor et al., 2009; Villegier et al., 2003; Wang et al., 2010). In addition, reducing LC function alone by lesioning LC neurons can produce motor symptoms that are observed in PD (Grimbergen et al., 2009; Wang et al., 2010). In support of the LC lesion studies and the consequence of reduced NE content, DBH knockout mice, which do not synthesize NE, also exhibit PD motor symptoms with age (Rommelfanger et al., 2007). These data suggest the loss of LC noradrenergic function observed in PD may contribute to the motor symptoms of PD.

6. Neuroprotective effect of LC neurons on dopaminergic neurons

Since the noradrenergic nervous system experiences a loss of function before the dopaminergic system in PD (Braak et al., 2003b, 2006) and the noradrenergic nervous system innervates dopaminergic neurons in the SN and VTA (shown above); the noradrenergic nervous system could then affect the stability of dopaminergic neurons. There is data to support the hypothesis of a neuroprotective effect of the noradrenergic system upon dopaminergic neurons in animal models. To determine if the LC noradrenergic nervous system exerts a neuroprotective effect on dopaminergic neurons, a dopaminergic neurotoxin needs to be administered.

6.1 Animal models of PD

There are several different animal models of PD which have been described in detail elsewhere (Betarbet et al., 2002; Dauer & Przedborski, 2003; Jackson-Lewis & Przedborski, 2007; Luchtman et al., 2009) and are not the focus of this chapter. The classic PD symptoms induced by a variety of dopaminergic neurotoxins are reduced number of SN dopaminergic neurons and reduced amount of DA in the striatum. The most routinely used dopaminergic neurotoxins are 1-methyl-4-phenyl-1,2,3,6-tetrahydropyridine (MPTP) and 6-hydroxydopamine (6OHDA). The choice of neurotoxin depends on the species of animal to be studied. MPTP is typically the neurotoxin used to reduce the number of dopaminergic neurons in the SN (and to a lesser degree the VTA neurons) in mice and monkeys. MPTP is administered peripherally and depending on the dose and the number of times it is administered, a mild to severe degree of dopaminergic neuronal loss can be observed (Betarbet et al., 2002; Dauer & Przedborski, 2003; Jackson-Lewis & Przedborski, 2007; Luchtman et al., 2009). However, MPTP is not effective in rats (Jackson-Lewis & Przedborski, 2007). To reduce the number of SN dopaminergic neurons in rats, 6OHDA is administered directly into the medial forebrain bundle using stereotaxic surgery. The effect of 6OHDA in the SN is rapid and appears permanent (Walsh et al., 2011).

6.2 Enhanced LC function reduces dopaminergic neurotoxin-induced damage

6.2.1 Neuroprotective effect of enhanced noradrenergic function in tottering and NET transgenic mice

The tottering mouse has a mutation that results in hyperinnervation of noradrenergic terminals and increased concentration of NE throughout most regions of the forebrain. Administration of MPTP to these mutant mice has less of an effect on dopaminergic terminals in the striatum (i.e., loss of DA level) as compared to wild-type mice (Kilbourne et al., 1998). Another transgenic mouse that has enhanced noradrenergic function is the NET knockout mouse. NET knockout mice do not express the transporter protein for NE, which are localized specifically to noradrenergic neurons and responsible for removing NE from the synapse, resulting in enhanced NE in the synapse. Administration of MPTP to NET knockout mice, again, results in reduced damage to dopaminergic terminals in the striatum and DA levels in the striatum as compared to wild-type mice (Rommelfanger et al., 2004). These studies indicate that an enhanced noradrenergic system can protect dopaminergic neurons in the SN from damage.

6.2.2 Neuroprotective effect of AR agents

Another means of increasing noradrenergic function is to administer noradrenergic agonists. Administration of NET inhibitors to increase synaptic NE levels results in reduced dopaminergic damage on SN terminals in the striatum and DA levels, resembling the effect observed in the NET knockout mouse (Rommelfanger et al., 2004). Peripheral administration of α_2-AR agonists such as clonidine and detomidine also reduces MPTP-induced reduction in striatal DA levels, while administration of α_2-AR antagonists enhances MPTP-induced damage in mice (Fornai et al., 1995a). However, when 6OHDA is used as the dopaminergic neurotoxin in rats, the peripheral administration of α_2-AR antagonists reduces the loss of DA in the striatum (Srinivasan & Schmidt, 2004b, c), the opposite of what is observed in mice with MPTP. The ability of α_2-AR agents to either enhance or reduce damage on dopaminergic neurons could be attributed to the different species (rats versus mice) or the neurotoxin (MPTP versus 6OHDA) used. Another possible reason for the conflicting data of α_2-AR agents is the complexity of the α_2-AR. The α_2-AR receptor is composed of three different subtypes: α_{2A}-, α_{2B}-, and α_{2C}-AR. α_{2A}- and α_{2C}-ARs are localized on dendrites and terminals of noradrenergic neurons where they act as presynaptic autoreceptors to regulate the release of NE (L'Heureux et al., 1986; Van Gaalen et al., 1997; Kawahara et al., 1999), as well as postsynaptic receptors on dendrites and terminals of NE target cell that regulate the release of other neurotransmitters (heteroreceptors). α_{2A}-ARs are the most abundant α_2-AR subtype in the brain, comprising approximately 90% of all central α_2-ARs (Bucheler et al., 2002). The highest density of α_{2C}-AR is in the striatum, while α_{2B}-ARs have a very limited expression in the brain (Nicholas et al., 1993; Zeng & Lynch, 1991).

Clonidine and detomidine do not discriminate between the different subtypes, so it is unclear how these agonists affect noradrenergic function: reduced NE release and function by acting on presynaptic autoreceptors or enhancing NEs action at postsynaptic receptors. The same complexity exists for the effects of α_2-AR antagonists.

6.2.3 Summary

These studies indicate that increased noradrenergic function, either through genetic manipulation or pharmacologically, results in less damage to dopaminergic neurons by MPTP, indicating a neuroprotective effect of the noradrenergic nervous system on dopaminergic neurons. The major concern with these studies is that the enhanced noradrenergic function is not limited exclusively to the LC noradrenergic system. There is also the added complexity of the localization of the different noradrenergic receptors, pre- versus post-synaptically, and the differences in expression of AR between rats and mice (Szot, 2006) which may contribute to the conflicting results of α_2-AR agonists. Future studies could examine the ability of other AR agonists that act postsynaptically to modulate susceptibility of dopaminergic neurons to damage or determine if pharmacological agents produce a neuroprotective effect after direct administration into a specific brain region such as the striatum or SN.

6.3 Reduced LC function enhances susceptibility of dopaminergic neurons to damage

An easier approach in determining if the LC noradrenergic nervous system can affect the susceptibility of dopaminergic neurons to damage is to reduce the number of LC noradrenergic neurons and innervation to forebrain regions. This approach specifically targets the LC noradrenergic neurons, mimicking what is observed in PD. LC noradrenergic neuronal loss has been shown to occur with administration of 6OHDA directly into the LC and peripheral administration of N-(2-chloroethyl)-N-ethyl-2-bromobenzylamine (DSP4).

6.3.1 DSP4 enhances susceptibility of dopaminergic neurons to damage

DSP4 has been considered a LC selective noradrenergic neurotoxin since 1980s. The determination that DSP4 was a selective LC neurotoxin is based on documented changes in terminal noradrenergic fibers in regions innervated mainly by the LC. The appeal of DSP4 as a noradrenergic neurotoxin over other methods (like 6OHDA) is that DSP4 can produce this central affect by peripheral administration. DSP4 produces a rapid, though transient, reduction in terminal NE concentrations in the frontal cortex, hippocampus and cerebellum (Grzanna et al., 1989; Harro et al., 1999a, b; Hughes & Stanford, 1996, 1998; Jonsson et al., 1981; Kask et al., 1997; Ross, 1976; Szot et al., 2011; Theron et al., 1993; Wolfman et al., 1994). As indicated earlier, these regions receive sole innervation from the LC (Aston-Jones et al., 1995; Jones & Moore, 1977; Loughlin et al., 1986a, b; Mason & Fibiger, 1970; Moore & Bloom, 1979; Olsen & Fuxe, 1971; Ungerstedt, 1971; Waterhouse et al., 1983) so the original hypothesis was that DSP4 affected only LC neurons. NET binding sites are also reduced in specific forebrain regions, indicating a loss of innervation from the LC (Cheetham et al., 1996; Szot et al., 2010). The hypothesis that DSP4 was a neurotoxin was supported by TH-IR which demonstrated a gradual loss of LC noradrenergic neurons after by DSP4 administration (Grzanna et al., 1989). Since these initial descriptions of DSP4 as a noradrenergic neurotoxin, there have been other publications suggesting that DSP4 does not result in a loss of LC noradrenergic neurons (Booze et al., 1988; Lyon et al., 1983; Matsukawa et al., 2003; Robertson et al., 1993; Szot et al., 2010) and that DSP4 does not selectively affect LC noradrenergic terminals (Grzanna et al., 1989; Kask et al., 1997; Szot et al., 2010; Theron et al., 1993; Wolfman et al., 1994). Work in our laboratory indicated that DSP4 may affect noradrenergic terminals and specific ARs in many forebrain regions (not just regions innervated by the LC), but it does so without a loss of LC noradrenergic neurons (Szot et al., 2010). Despite the data that suggests DSP4 may not result in a loss of LC noradrenergic neurons, DSP4 does result in a temporary reduction in terminal NE levels in many forebrain regions.

Administration of DSP4 prior to methamphetamine, MPTP or 6OHDA into the medial forebrain bundle will increase the damage these dopaminergic neurotoxins exert on SN dopaminergic neurons and DA levels in the striatum (Fornai et al., 1995b, 1996, 1997; Marien et al., 1993; Srinivasan and Schmidt, 2003, 2004a). The enhanced susceptibility of dopaminergic neurons to damage from these dopaminergic neurotoxins is observed at a time when DSP4 results in a significant reduction in terminal NE levels. Administration of DSP4 after the dopaminergic neurotoxin does not enhance the susceptibility of dopaminergic neurons to damage (Fornai et al., 1997). These data indicate that a reduction in NE levels in forebrain regions will increase the susceptibility of dopaminergic neurons to damage. However, administration of MPTP to DBH knockout mice does not result in enhanced loss of SN neurons or DA levels in the striatum as compared to wild-type mice (Rommelfanger and Weinshenker, 2007). Administration of DSP4 prior to the administration of MPTP in the DBH knockout mouse does result in enhanced damage to dopaminergic neurons and terminals as compared to DBH knockout mice administered MPTP alone (Rommelfanger and Weinshenker, 2007).

6.3.2 6OHDA enhances susceptibility of dopaminergic neurons to damage

There are few studies examining the direct administration of the neurotoxin 6OHDA directly into those LC, though the few that do demonstrate a reduction in the number of LC noradrenergic neurons (Bing et al., 1991; Mavridis et al., 1991). Our laboratory has begun to examine the specificity of direct LC 6OHDA administration on LC neurons and lateral tegmental neurons as well as neurons in the SN and VTA. We have observed that direct administration of 6OHDA into the LC specifically reduces LC noradrenergic neurons, while there is no effect on SN or VTA dopaminergic neurons or on lateral tegmental neurons (data not shown).

There are two studies that have examined the ability of LC 6OHDA administration to increase MPTP-induced damage to dopaminergic neurons. Bing et al., (1994) examined the ability of LC 6OHDA to enhance MPTP-induced damage in the mouse, while Mavridis et al., (1991) examined LC 6OHDA in monkeys. Both of these studies demonstrated an enhanced susceptibility of dopaminergic neurons to damage following LC neuronal loss. Preliminary work in my laboratory has begun to examine the effects of 6OHDA administration into the LC of mice on the susceptibility of dopaminergic neurons to MPTP. We have examined the effect of MPTP (24 mg/kg, ip, twice, 2hrs apart) administered 3 days after bilateral administration of 6OHDA into the LC on LC, SN and VTA neurons. MPTP alone did not affect LC noradrenergic neurons, but MPTP alone significantly reduced DAergic neurons in the SN (28% reduced) with no effect on VTA neurons (7% reduced). However, the *combination* of 6OHDA + MPTP resulted in a further reduction in SN neurons (71% reduced) and a significant reduction in VTA neurons (54% reduced) (data not shown).

These data indicate that administration of the noradrenergic neurotoxin 6OHDA can increase the susceptibility of dopaminergic neurons to damage.

6.4 Summary
These data suggest that enhanced noradrenergic function can protect dopaminergic neurons from damage, while reducing noradrenergic function enhances the susceptibility of dopaminergic neurons to damage. The number of studies examining this important question are few, but the data indicates the LC noradrenergic nervous system can modulate the viability of dopaminergic neurons to damage. It is unknown why dopaminergic neurons in PD are reduced. The loss of dopaminergic neurons and the appearance of PD symptoms occur midway in the progression of the disorder, after the loss of LC noradrenergic neurons. Therefore, determining factors that can maintain the stability of dopaminergic neurons in the early stages of the disorder is imperative in preventing the loss of dopaminergic neurons and the onset of PD symptoms. Since LC neuronal loss occurs early in the progression of PD and is a prominent neuropathologic change in PD, an animal model examining the neuroprotective effect of the noradrenergic nervous system on dopaminergic neurons must exhibit reduced LC noradrenergic neuronal number, so DSP4 may not be the best animal model of LC neuronal loss. Future work will determine if there is a particular time following the loss of LC noradrenergic neurons that renders the dopaminergic neurons more susceptible to damage, or it may be that following administration of MPTP, animals with reduced LC function do not recover from the damage induced by MPTP.

7. Noradrenergic agents relieve L-DOPA-induced dyskinesia

7.1 Chronic L-DOPA therapy induces dyskinesia
In addition to the potential neuroprotective effect of the noradrenergic nervous system on dopaminergic neurons early in the progression of PD, the noradrenergic nervous system may also improve therapy of PD subjects. As indicated above, L-DOPA is the primary therapy in the treatment of PD motor symptoms. However, chronic treatment of L-DOPA in PD subjects results in permanent severe side effect, dyskinesia (abnormal involuntary movements). The incidence of dyskinesia in PD subjects increases with the length of time on L-DOPA therapy; 30% of patients experience dyskinesia after 4-6 years to 90% after 9 years (Rascol et al., 2000; Ahlskog & Muenter, 2001). The underlying mechanism behind L-DOPA-induced dyskinesia is thought to be extraphysiological DA release resulting in aberrant receptor signaling in the striatum; this enhanced dopaminergic signaling then dysregulates subsequent striatal output (Cenci, 2007, 2009; Winkler et al., 2002). Until a means of preventing the onset of PD occurs or a new treatment for PD that does not result in dyskinesia is found, adjunct pharmacological therapy with L-DOPA that prevents or reduces dyskinesia is the focus of future work in PD therapy.

7.2 AR antagonists reduce L-DOPA-induced dyskinesia
As indicated earlier, the different types of ARs (β-, α_1- and α_2-ARs) are localized to the striatum and AR agents can alter the activity of striatal neurons (see above). However, at the present time it is unclear if the loss of LC noradrenergic neurons early in the progression of PD contributes to the L-DOPA-induced overactivity of striatal neurons that ultimately results in dyskinesia (Marin et al., 2008) or how L-DOPA therapy affects noradrenergic

neurons (Figure 2). What is known is that α_2-AR agonists can facilitate movement by acting through the striatum (Hill and Brotchie, 1999). Therefore, α_2-AR antagonists have been studied as a potential adjunct therapy to reduce L-DOPA-induced dyskinesia. α_2-AR antagonists, yohimbine, idazoxan and fipamezole reduce L-DOPA dyskinesia in the MPTP and 6OHDA PD animal models and in Parkinsonian patients. These α_2-AR antagonists reduce L-DOPA-induced side effects without affecting the anti-parkinsonian effect of L-DOPA (Brotchie, 2005; Buck et al., 2010; Colosimo and Craus, 2003; Chopin et al., 1986; Gomez-Mancilla and Bedard, 1993; Grondin et al., 2000; Henry et al., 1999; Lundblad et al., 2002; Rascol et al., 2001; Savola et al., 2003). However, the anti-dyskinetic effect of α_2-AR antagonists may be limited to just L-DOPA; idazoxan did not reduce apomorphine-induced dyskinesia (Fox et al., 2001). The α_2-ARs are not the only receptor capable of modulating L-DOPA-induced dyskinesia. Because β-ARs are found in large concentrations in the striatum (see above), studies are now beginning to determine if β-AR antagonists, such as propranolol, can reduce L-DOPA-induced dyskinesia. These studies indicate that propranolol also reduces L-DOPA-induced dyskinesia (Goshima et al., 1991; Reisine et al., 1982; Carpentier et al., 1996; Dekundy et al., 2007). α_1-AR antagonist also reduces L-DOPA-induced dyskinesia; however, this receptor subtype has not been investigated to the same degree as α_2- and β-AR antagonists (Buck and Ferbeger, 2010).

8. Conclusion

The dopaminergic nervous system has been the major focus of research in PD for many years, and rightly so because it is the loss of dopaminergic neurons and function that is responsible for the appearance of the motor symptoms that define PD. However, the noradrenergic nervous system appears to play an important role in the progression of PD and in the therapy of PD. LC noradrenergic neurons are reduced early in the progression of PD, even before dopaminergic neurons. Animal models suggest that the loss of LC noradrenergic neurons will enhance the susceptibility of dopaminergic neurons to damage. Understanding the relationship of LC neuronal loss to enhanced dopaminergic susceptibility to damage introduces a time window in which pharmacological intervention could *prevent* the loss of dopaminergic neurons and the appearance of motor symptoms. But until this relationship is examined, the noradrenergic nervous system can be used to reduce Dyskinesia, the severe side effects of chronic L-DOPA therapy. These data indicate the importance of examining neurotransmitter systems other than DA and determining the role of transmitters, such as NE, in affecting PD.

9. Acknowledgement

This work was supported by the Department of Veterans Affairs Research and Development Services Northwest Network Mental Illness Research, Education and Clinical Center at the Seattle Puget Sound Health Care Center. The authors thank Dr. Charles Wilkinson and Carl Sikkema for CSF catecholamine analysis.

10. References

Ader, J.P., Room, P. & Postema, F. (1980). Bilaterally diverging axon collaterals and coutralateral projections from rat locus coeruleus neurons, demonstrated by fluorescent retrograde double labeling and norepinephrine metabolism. *J. Neural. Transm.* 49:207-218.

Adolfsson, R., Gottfries, C.G., Roos, B.E. & Winblad, B. (1979). Changes in the brain catecholamines in patients with dementia of Alzheimer's type. *Br. J. Psychiatry* 135: 216–223.

Ahlskog, J.E. & Muenter, M.D. (2001). Frequency of levodopa-related dyskinesias and motor fluctuations as estimated from the cumulative literature. *Mov. Disord.* 16:448-458.

Antelman, S.M. & Caggiula, A.R. (1977). Norepinephrine-dopamine interaction and behavior. *Science* 195:646-653.

Archer, T. & Fredriksson, A. (2006). Influence of noradrenaline denervation on MPTP-induced deficits in mice. *J. Neural. Trasm.* 113:1119-1129.

Aston-Jones, G., Rajkowski, J. & Kubiak, P. (2000). Locus coeruleus and regulation of behavioral flexibility and attention. *Prog. Brain Res.* 126:165-182.

Aston-Jones, G., Shipley, M. & Grzanna, R. (1995). The locus coeruleus, A5 and A7 noradrenergic cell groups, in: G. Paxinos (Ed.), *The Rat Nervous System*, Academic Press, Boca Raton, 1995, pp. 183-213.

Beliaev, A., Learmonth, D.A. & Soares-da-Silva, P. (2006). Synthesis and biological evaluation of novel, peripherally selective chromanyl imidazolethione-based inhibitors of dopamine β-hydroxylase. *J. Med. Chem.* 49: 1191–1197.

Berendse, H.W., Booij, J., Francot, C.M.J.E., Bergmans, P.L.M., Hijman, R., Stoof, J.C. & Wolters, E.C. (2001). Subclinical dopaminergic dysfunction in asymptomatic Parkinson's disease patients' relatives with a decreased sense of smell. *Ann. Neurol.* 50:34-41.

Bertrand, E., Lechowicz, W., Szpak, G.M. & Dynecki, J. (1997). Qualtitative and quantitative analysis of locus coeruleus neurons in Parkinson's disease. *Folia Neuropathol.* 35:80-86.

Betarbet, R., Sherer, T.B. & Greenamyre, J.T. (2002). Animal models of Parkinson's disease. *BioEssays* 24:308-318.

Bevan, P., Bradshaw, C.M. & Szabadi, E. (1975). Effects of desipramine on neuronal responses to dopamine, noradrenaline, 5-hydroxytryptamine and acetylcholine in the caudate nucleus of the rat. *Br. J. Pharmacol.* 54:285-293.

Bing, G., Zhang, Y., Watanabe, Y., McEwen, B.S. & Stone, E.A. (1994). Locus coeruleus lesions potentiate neurotoxic of MPTP in dopaminergic neurons of the substantia nigra. *Brain Res.* 668:261-265.

Boeve, B.F., Silber, M.H., Parisi, J.E., Dickson, D.W., Ferman, T.J., Benarroch, E.E., Schmeichel, A.M., Smith, G.E., Petersen, R.C., Ahlskog, J.E., Matsumoto, J.Y., Knopman, D.S., Schenck, C.H. & Mahowald, M.W. (2003). Synucleinopathy pathology and REM sleep behavior disorder plus dementia or parkinsonism. *Neurology* 61:40-45.

Bondareff, W., Mountjoy, C.Q. & Roth, M. (1982). Loss of neurons of origin of the adrenergic projection to cerebral cortex (nucleus locus ceruleus) in senile dementia. *Neurology* 32:164-168.

Booze, R.M., Hall, J.A., Cress, N.M., Miller, G.D. & Davis, J.N. (1988). DSP-4 treatment produces abnormal tyrosine hydroxylase immunoreactive fibers in rat hippocampus. *Exp. Neurol.* 101:75-86.

Bourdelat-Parks, B.N., Anderson, G.M., Donaldson, Z.R., Weiss, J.M., Bonsall, R.W., Emery, M.S., Liles, L.C. & Weinshenker, D. (2005). Effects of dopamine β-hydroxylase genotype and disulfiram inhibition on catecholamine homeostasis in mice. *Neuropharmacology* 183: 72–80.

Boyajian, C.L., Loughlin, S.E. & Leslie, F.M. (1987). Anatomical evidence for alpha-2 adrenoceptors heterogeneity: differential autoradiographic distributions of [^{3}H]rauwolscine and [^{3}H]idazoxan in rat brain. *J. Pharmacol. Expt. Therap.* 241:1079-1091.

Braak, H., Rub, U., Gai, W.P. & Tredici, K.D. (2003a). Idiopathic parkinson's disease: possible routes by which vulnerable neuronal types may be subject to neuroinvasion by an unknown pathogen. *J. Neural. Transm.* 110:517-536.

Braak, H., Rub, U. & Tredici, K.D. (2006). Cognitive decline correlates with neuropathological stage in Parkinson's disease. *J. Neurol. Sci.* 248:255-258.

Braak, H., Tredici, K.D., Rub, U., de Vos, R.A.I., Jansen Steur, E.N.H. & Braak, A. (2003b). Staging of brain pathology related to sporadic Parkinson's disease. *Neurobiol. Aging* 24:197-211.

Brotchie, J.M. (2005). Nondopaminergic mechanisms in levodopa-induced dyskinesia. *Mov. Disord.* 20:919-931.

Bucheler, M.M., Hadamek, K. & Hein, L. (2002). Two α_2-adrenergic receptor subtypes, α_{2A} and α_{2C}, inhibit transmitter release in the brain of gene-targeted mice. *Neuroscience* 109:819-826.

Buck, K., Voehringer, P. & Ferger, B. (2010) The α2 adrenoceptor antagonist idazoxan alleviates L-DOPA-induced dyskinesia by reduction of striatal dopamine levels: an in vivo microdialysis study in 6-hydroxydopamine-lesioned rats. *J. Neurochem.* 112:444-452.

Buck, K. & Ferger, B. (2010). The selective α1 adrenoceptor antagonist HEAT reduces LDOPA-induced dyskinesia in a rat model of Parkinson's disease. *Synapse* 64:117-126.

Bylund, D.B. & Snyder, S.H. (1976). Beta adrenergic receptor binding in membrane preparations from mammalian brain. *Mol. Pharmacol.* 12:568-580.

Carpentier, A.F., Bonnet ,A.M., Vidailhet, M. & Agid, Y. (1996). Improvement of levodopa induced dyskinesia by propranolol in Parkinson's disease. *Neurology,* 46:1548-1551.

Cash, R.,Dennis, T.,L'Heureux,R., Raisman, R., Javoy-Agid, F. & Scatton, B. (1987). Parkinson's disease and dementia: norepinephrine and dopamine in locus coeruleus. *Neurology* 37:42–46.

Cenci, M.A. (2007). Dopamine dysregulation of movement control in L-DOPA-induced dyskinesia. *Trends Neurosci.* 30:236-243.

Cenci, M.A., Ohlin, K.E. & Rylander, D. (2009). Plastic effects of L-DOPA treatment in the basal ganglia and their relevance to the development of dyskinesia. *Parkinsonism Rel. Beh.* 15S3:S59-S63.

Chan-Palay, V. & Asan, E. (1989). Alterations in catecholamine neurons of the locus coeruleus in senile dementia of the Alzheimer's type and in Parkinson's disease with and without dementia and depression. *J. Comp. Neurol.* 287:373-392.

Cheetham, S.C., Viggers, J.A., Butler, S.A., Prow, M.R. & Heal, D.J. (1996). [3H]Nisoxetine- a radioligand for noradrenaline reuptake sites: correlation with inhibition of [3H]noradrenaline uptake and effect of DSP-4 lesioning and antidepressant treatment. *Neuropharmacology* 35:63–70.

Chia, L.G., Cheng, L.J., Chuo, L.J., Cheng, F.C. & Cu, J.S. (1995). Studies of dementia, depression, electrophysiology and cerebrospinal fluid monoamine metabolites in patients with Parkinson's disease. *J. Neurol. Sci.* 133:73-78.

Chia, L.G., Cheng, F.C. & Kuo, J.S. (1993). Monoamines and their metabolites in plasma and lumbar cerebrospinal fluid of Chinese patients with Parkinson's disease. *J. Neurol. Sci.* 116:125-134.

Chopin, P., Colpaert ,F.C. & Marien, M. (1999). Effects of alpha-2-adrenoreceptor agonists and antagonists on circling behavior in rats with unilateral 6-hydroxydopamine lesions of the nigrostriatal pathway. *J. Pharmacol. Expt. Therap.* 288:798-804.

Chopin, P., Pellow, S. & File, S.E. (1986). The effects of yohimbine on exploratory and locomotor behavior are attributable to its effects at noradrenaline and not at benzodiazepine receptor. *Neuropharmacology* 25:53-57.

Collingridge, G.L., James, T.A. & MacLeod, N.K. (1979). Neurochemical and electrophysiological evidence for a projection from the locus coeruleus to the substantia nigra. *J. Physiol.* 290:44P.

Colosimo, C. & Craus, A. (2003). Noradrenergic drugs for levodopa-induced dyskinesia. *Clin. Neuropharmacol.* 26:299-305.

Cotzias, G.C., Papavasiliou, P.S. & Gellene, R. (1969). Modification of parkinsonism: Chronic treatment with L-DOPA. *N. Engl. J. Med.* 280:337-345.

Cross, A.J., Crow, T.J., Perry, E.K., Perry, R.H., Blessed, G. & Tomlinson, B.E. (1981). Reduced dopamine-beta-hydroxylase activity in Alzheimer's disease. *Br. J. Clin. Res. Ed.* 282, 93–94.

Damier, P., Hirsch, E.C., Agrid, Y. & Graybiel, A.M. (1999). The substantia nigra of the human brain. II. Patterns of loss of dopaminergic neurons in Parkinson's disease. *Brain* 122:1421-1236.

Dauer, W. & Przedborski, S. (2003). Parkinson's disease: Mechanisms and models. *Neuron* 39:889-909.

Dekundy, A., Lundblad, M., Danysz, W. & Cenci, M.A. (2007). Modulation of L-DOPA induced abnormal involuntary movements by clinically tested compounds: further validation of the rat dyskinesia model. *Behav. Brain Res.* 179:76-89.

Dolphin, A., Adrien, J., Hamon, M. & Bockaert, J. (1979). Identity of [3H]-dihydralprenolol binding sites and beta-adrenergic receptors coupled with adenylate cyclase in the central nervous system: pharmacological properties, distribution and adaptive responsiveness. *Mol. Pharmacol.* 15:1-15.

Elrod, R., Peskind, E.R., DiGiacomo, L., Brodkin, K.L., Veith, R.C. & Raskind, M.A. (1997). Effects of Alzheimer's disease severity on cerebrospinal fluid norepinephrine concentration. *Am. J. Psychiatry* 154:25-30.

Fallon, J.H. & Loughlin, S.E. (1982). Monoamine innervation of the forebrain: collateralization. *Brain Res. Bull.* 9:295-307.

Fornai, F., Alessandri, M.G., Fascetti, F., Vaglini, F. & Corsini, G.U. (1995a). Clonidine suppresses 1-methyl-4-phenyl-1,2,3,6-tetrahydropyridine-induced reductions of striatal dopamine and tyrosine hydroxylase activity in mice. *J. Neurochem.* 65:704-709.

Fornai, F., Alessandri, M.G., Torracca, M.T., Bassi, L. & Corsini, G.U. (1997). Effects of noradrenergic lesions on MPTP/MPP+ kinetics and MPTP-induced nigrostriatal dopamine depletions. *J. Pharmacol. Expt. Therap.* 283:100-107.

Fornai, F., Torracca, M.T., Bassi, L., D'Errigo, D.A., Scalori, V. & Corsini, G.U. (1996). Norepinephrine loss selectively enhances chronic nigrostriatal dopamine depletion in mice and rats. *Brain Res.* 735:349-353.

Fornai, F., Bassi, L., Torracca, M.T., Scalori, V. & Corsini, G.U. (1995b). Norepinephrine loss exacerbates methamphetamine-induced striatal dopamine depletion in mice. *Eur. J. Pharmacol.* 283:99-102.

Fox, S.H., Henry, B., Hill, M.P., Peggs, M.P., Crossman, A.R. & Brotchie, J.M. (2001). Neural mechanisms underlying peak-dose dyskinesia induced by L-DOPA and apomorphine are distinct: evidence from the effects of the alpha(2) adrenoceptor antagonist idazoxan. *Mov. Disord.* 16:642-650.

Fritschy, J.M. & Grzanna, R. (1990). Distribution of locus coeruleus axons within the rat brainstem demonstrated by Phaseolus vulgaris leucoagglutinin anterograde tracing in combination with dopamine-β-hydroxylase immunofluorescence. *J. Comp. Neurol.* 293:616-631.

Fujimoto, S., Sasa, M. & Takaori, S. (1981). Inhibition from locus coeruleus of caudate neurons activated by nigral stimulation. *Brain Res. Bull.* 6:267-274.

Gasper, P., Duyckaerts, C., Alvarez, C., Javoy-Agid, F. & Berger, B. (1991). Alterations of dopaminergic and noradrenergic innervation in motor cortex in Parkinson's disease. *Ann. Neurol.* 30:365-374.

Gasper, P. & Gray, F. (1984). Dementia in idiopathic Parkinson's disease. *Acta Neuropathol.* 64:43-52.

German, D.C., Manaye, K.F., White, C.L., Woodward, D.J., McIntire, D.D., Smith, W.K., Kalaria, R.N. & Mann, D.M. (1992). Disease-specific patterns of locus coeruleus cell. *Ann. Neurol.* 32: 667-676.

Gibb, W.R.G. (1991). Neuropathology of the substantia nigra. *Eur. Neurol.* 31(suppl):48-59.

Gibb, W.R.G. & Lees, A.J. (1991). Anatomy, pigmentation, ventral and dorsal subpopulations of the substantia nigra, and differential cell death in Parkinson's disease. *J. Neurol. Neurosurg. Psychiatry* 54:388-396.

Goldstein, M. (1966). Inhibition of norepinephrine biosynthesis at the dopamine-β-hydroxylation stage. *Pharmacol. Rev.* 18: 77–82.

Goldstein, D.S., Holmes, C., Sewell, L., Pechnik, S. & Kopin, I.J. (2011). Effects of carbidopa and entacapone on the metabolic fate of the norepinephrine prodrug L-DOPS. *J. Clin. Pharmacol.* 51:66-74.

Gomez-Mancilla, B. & Bedard, P.J. (1993). Effect of nondopaminergic drugs on L-DOPA-induced dyskinesias in MPTP-treated monkeys. *Clin. Neuropharmacol.* 16:418-427.

Goshima, Y., Misu, Y., Arai, N. & Misugi, K. (1991). Nanomolar L-dopa facilitates release of dopamine via presynaptic β-adrenoceptors: comparative studies on the actions in striatal slices from control and 1-methyl-4-phenyl-1,2,3,6-tetrahydropyridine (MPTP)-treated C57 black mice, an animal model for Parkinson's disease. *Jpn. J. Pharmacol.* 55:93-100.

Gottfries CG, Adolfsson R, Aquilonius SM, Carlsson A, Eckernas SA, Nordberg A, Oreland L, Svennerholm L, Wiberg A, Winblad B (1983) Biochemical changes in dementia disorders of Alzheimer's type (AD/SDAT). Neurobiol Aging 4:261-271.

Grenhoff, J., Nissel, M., Aston-Jones, G. & Svensson, T.H. (1993). Noradrenergic modulation of midbrain dopamine cell firing elicited by stimulation of the locus coeruleus in the rat. *J. Neural. Transm.* 93:11-25.

Grenhoff, J. & Svensson, T.H. (1989). Clonidine modulates dopamine cell firing in rat ventral tegmental area. *Eur. J. Pharmacol.* 165:11-18.

Grenhoff, J. & Svensson, T.H. (1993). Prazosin modulates the firing pattern of dopamine neurons in rat ventral tegmental area. *Eur. J. Pharmacol.* 233:79-8499)

Grenhoff, J., North, R.A. & Johnson, S.W. (1995). Alpha$_1$-adrenergic effects on dopamine neurons recorded intracellularly in the rat midbrain slice. *Eur. J. Neurosci.* 7:1707-1713.

Grimbergen, Y.A.M., Langston, J.W., Roos ,R.A.C. & Bloem, B. (2009). Postural instability in Parkinson's disease: the adrenergic hypothesis and the locus coeruleus. *Expert Rev. Neurotherap.* 9:279-290.

Grondin, R., Hadj Tahar, A., Doan, V.D., Ladure, P. & Bedard, P.J. (2000). Noradrenergic antagonism with idazoxan improves L-DOPA-induced dyskinesias in MPTP monkeys. *Naunyn Schmiedebergs Arch. Pharmacol.* 361:181-186.

Grzanna, R., Berger, U., Fritschy, J.-M. & Geffard, M. (1989). Acute action of DSP-4 on central norepinephrine axons: biochemical an immunohistochemical evidence for differential effects. *J. Histochem. Cytochem.* 37:1435–1442.

Guiard, B.P., Mansari, M.E., Merali, Z. & Blier, P. (2008). Functional interactions between dopamine, serotonin and norepinephrine neurons: an in-vivo electrophysiological study in rats with monoaminergic lesions. *Int. J. Neuropsychopharm.* 11:625-639.

Harro, J., Haidkind, R., Harro, M., Modiri, A.-R., Gillberg, P.-G., Pahkla, R., Matto, V. & Oreland, L. (1999a). Chronic mild unpredicatable stress after noradrenergic denervation: attenuation of behavioral and biochemical effects of DSP-4 treatment. *Eur. Neuropsychopharmacol.* 10:5–16.

Harro, J., Pahkla, R., Modiri, A.-R., Kask, A. & Oreland, L. (1999b). Dose dependent effects of noradrenergic denervation by DSP-4 treatment on forced swimming and β-adrenoceptor binding in the rat. *J. Neural. Transm.* 106:619–629.

Henry, B., Fox, S.H., Peggs, D., Crossman, A.R. & Brotchie, J.M. (1999). The alpha2-adrenergic receptor antagonist idazoxan reduces dyskinesia and enhances anti-parkinsonian actions of L-DOPA in the lesioned primate model of Parkinson's disease. *Mov. Disord.* 14:744-753.

Hill, M.P. & Brotchie, J.M. (1999). The adrenergic receptor agonist, clonidine, potentiates the anti-parkinsonian action of the selective kappa-opioid receptor agonist, enadoline, in the monoamine-depleted rat. *Br. J. Pharmacol.* 128:1577-1585.

Hoogendijk, W.J., Freenstra, M.G., Botterblom, M.H., Gilhuis, J., Sommer, I.E., Kamphorst, W., Eikelenboom, P. & Swaab, D.F. (1999). Increased activity of surviving locus coeruleus neurons in Alzheimer's disease. *Ann. Neurol.* 45, 82–91.

Hornykiewicz, O. & Kish, S.J. (1987). Biochemical pathophysiology of Parkinson's disease. *Adv. Neurol.* 45:19-34.

Hudson, A., Mallard, N., Tyacke, R. & Nutt, D. (1992). [3H]-RX821002: a highly selective ligand for the identification of alpha-2 adrenoceptors in the rat brain. *Mol. Neuropharmacol.* 1:219-229.

Hughes, Z.A. & Stanford, S.C. (1996). Increased noradrenaline efflux induced by local infusion of fluoxetine in the rat frontal cortex. *Eur. J. Pharmacol.* 317:83–90.

Hughes, Z.A. & Stanford, S.C. (1998). A partial noradrenergic lesion induced by DSP-4 increases extracellular noradrenaline concentration in rat frontal cortex: a microdialysis study in vivo. *Psychopharmacology* 136:299–303.

Huot, P. & Parent, A. (2007). Dopaminergic neurons intrinsic to the striatum. *J. Neurochem.* 101:1441-1447.

Itoi, K. & Sugimoto, N. (2010). The brainstem noradrenergic systems in stress, anxiety, and depression. *J. Neuroendocrinol.* 22:355-361.

Jackson-Lewis, V. & Przedborski, S. (2007). Protocol for the MPTP mouse model of Parkinson's disease. *Nature Protocols* 2:141-151.

Jones, B.E. & Moore, R.Y. (1977). Ascending projections of the locus coeruleus in the rat. II Autoradiographic study. *Brain Res.* 127:23-53.

Jones, B.E. & Yang, T.Z. (1985). The efferent projections from the reticular formation and the locus coeruleus studied by anterograde and retrograde axonal transport in the rat. *J. Comp. Neurol.* 242:56-92.

Jonsson, G., Hallman, H., Ponzio, F. & Ross, S. (1981). DSP4 (N-(2-chloroethyl)-N-ethyl-2-bromobenzylamine)—a useful denervation tool for central and peripheral noradrenaline neurons. *Eur. J. Pharmacol.* 72:173–188.

Kask, A., Harro, J., Tuomainen, P., Rago, L. & Mannisto, P.T. (1997). Overflow of noradrenaline and dopamine in frontal cortex after [N-(2-chloroethyl)- N-ethyl-2-bromobenzylamine] (DSP-4) treatment: in vivo microdialysis study in anaesthetized rats. *Naunyn Schmiedeberg Arch. Pharmacol.* 355:267–272.

Kawahara, Y., Kawahara, H. & Westernik, B.H.C. (1999). Tonic regulation of the activity of noradrenergic neurons in the locus coeruleus of the conscious rat studies by dual-probe microdialysis. *Brain Res.* 823:42-48.

Kilbourne, M.R., Sherman, P. & Abbott, L.C. (1998). Reduced MPTP neurotoxicity in striatum of the mutant mouse tottering. *Synapse* 30:205-210.

Kish, S.J., Shannak, K.S., Rajput, A.H., Gilbert, J.J. & Hornykiewicz, O. (1984). Cerebellar norepinephrine in patients with Parkinson's disease and control subjects. *Arch. Neurol.* 41:612-614.

Koob, G.F., Balcom, G.J. & Meyerhoff, J.L. (1975). Dopamine and norepinephrine levels in the nucleus accumbens, olfactory tubercle and corpus striatum following lesions in the ventral tegmental area. *Brain Res.* 94:45-55.

Lategan, A., Narien, M. & Colpaert, F. (1990). Effects of locus coeruleus lesions on the release of endogenous dopamine in the rat nucleus accumbens and caudate nucleus as determined by intracerebral microdialysis. *Brain Res.* 523:134-138.

Lee, A., Wissekerke, A.E., Rosin, D.L. & Lynch, K.R. (1998). Localization of α-2c-adrenergic receptor immunoreactivity in catecholaminergic neurons in the rat central nervous system. *Neuroscience* 84:1085-1096.

Leentjens, A.F., Van den Akker, M., Metsemakers, J.F.M., Lousberg R. & Verhey, F.R.J. (2003). Higher incidence of depression preceding the onset of Parkinson's disease: A register study. *Mov. Disord.* 18:414-418.

L'Heureux, R., Dennis, T., Curet, O. & Scatton, B. (1986). Measurement of endogenous noradrenaline release in the rat cerebral cortex in vivo by transcortical dialysis: effect of drugs affecting noradrenergic transmission. *J. Neurochem.* 46:1794-1801.

Lopez-Munoz, F. & Alamo, C. (2009). Monoaminergic neurotransmission: the history of the discovery of antidepressants from 1950s until today. *Curr. Pharm. Des.* 15:1563-1586.

Loughlin, S.E., Foote, S.L. & Bloom, F.E. (1986a). Efferent projections of nucleus locus coeruleus: topographic organization of cells of origin demonstrated by three-dimensional reconstruction. *Neuroscience* 18:291-306.

Loughlin, S.E., Foote, S.L. & Fallon, J.H. (1982). Locus coeruleus projections to cortex: topographic, morphology and collateralization. *Brain Res. Bull.* 9:287-294.

Loughlin, S.E., Foote, S.L. & Grzanna, R. (1986b). Efferent projections of nucleus locus coeruleus: morphologic sub-populations have different efferent's targets. *Neuroscience* 18:307-319.

Luchtman, D.W., Shao, D. & Song, C. (2009). Behavior, neurotransmitters and inflammation in three regimens of the MPTP mouse model of Parkinson's disease. *Physiol. Beh.* 98:130-138.

Lundblad, M., Andersson, M., Winkler, C., Kirk, D., Wierup, N. & Cenci, M.A. (2002). Pharmacological validation of behavioral measures of akinesia and dyskinesia in a rat model of Parkinson's disease. *Eur. J. Pharmacol.* 15:120-132.

Lyons, W.E., Fritschy, J.M. & Grzanna, R. (1989). The noradrenergic neurotoxin DSP-4 eliminates the coeruleospinal projection but spares projections of the A5 and A7 groups to the ventral horn of the rat spinal cord. *J. Neurosci.* 9:1481-1489.

Mann, D.M., Lincoln, J., Yates, .PO., Stamp, J.E. & Toper, S. (1980). Changes in the monoamine containing neurons of the human CNS in senile dementia. *Br. J. Psychiatry* 136:533-541.

Mann, J.J., Stanley, M., Kaplan, R.D., Sweeney, J. & Neophytides, A. (1983). Central catecholamine metabolism in vivo and the cognitive and motor deficits in Parkinson's disease. *J. Neurol. Neurosurg. Psychiatry* 46:905-910.

Mann, J.J., Stanley, M., Neophytides, A., de Leon, M.J., Ferris, S.H. & Gershon, S. (1981). Central amine metabolism in Alzheimer's disease: in vivo relationship to cognitive deficit. *Neurobiol. Aging* 2, 57–60.

Marcyniuk, B., Mann D.M. & Yates, P.O. (1986). Loss of nerve cells from locus coeruleus in Alzheimer's disease is topographically arranged. *Neurosci. Lett.* 64: 247-252.

Marien, M., Briley, M. & Colpaert, F. (1993). Noradrenaline depletion exacerbates MPTP-induced striatal dopamine loss in mice. *Eur. J. Pharmacol.* 236:487-489.

Marien, M.R., Colpaert, F.C. & Rosenquist, A.C. (2004). Noradrenergic mechanisms in neurodegenerative disease: a theory. Brain Res. Rev. 45:38-78.

Marin, C., Aguilar, E. & Bonastre, M. (2008). Effect of locus coeruleus denervation on levodopa-induced motor fluctuations in hemiparkinsonian rats. *J. Neural. Transm.* 115:1133-1139.

Mason, S.T. & Fibiger, H.C. (1979). Regional topography within noradrenergic locus coeruleus as revealed by retrograde transport of horseradish perixidase. *J. Comp. Neurol.* 187: 703-724.

Mathias, C.J. (1998). Cardiovascular autonomic function in parkinsonian patients. *Clin. Neurosci.* 5:153-166.

Matsukawa, M., Nakadate, K., Ishihara, I. & Okado, N. (2003). Synaptic loss following depletion of noradrenaline and/or serotonin in the rat visual cortex: a quantitative electron microscopic study. *Neuroscience* 122:627-635.

Mavridis, M., Colpaert, F.C. & Millan, M.J. (1991). Differential modulation of (+)-amphetamine-induced rotation in unilateral substanita nigra-lesioned rats by alpha 1 as compared to alpha 2 agonists and antagonists. *Brain Res.* 562: 216-224.

Mavridis, M., Degryse, A.D., Lategan, A., Marien, M. & Colpaert, F. (1991). Effects of locus coeruleus lesions on parkinsonian signs, striatal dopamine and substantia nigra cell loss after 1-methyl-4-phenyl-1,2,3,6-tetrahydropyridine in monkeys: a possible role for the locus coeruleus in the progression of Parkinson's disease. *Neuroscience* 41:507-523.

Mayeux, R., Denaro, J., Hemenegildo, N., Marder, K., Tang, M.X., Cote, L.J. & Stern, Y. (1992). A population-based investigation of Parkinson's disease with and without dementia. Relationship to age and gender. *Arch. Neurol.* 49:492-497.

McMillan, P.J., White, S.S., Franklin, A., Greenup, J.L., Leverenz, J.B., Raskind, M.A. & Szot, P. (2011). Differential response of the central noradrenergic nervous system to the loss of locus coeruleus neurons in Parkinson's disease and Alzheimer's disease. *Brain Res.* 1373:240-252.

Moore, R.Y. & Bloom, F.E. (1979). Central catecholamine neuron system: anatomy and physiology of the norepinephrine and epinephrine systems. *Ann. Rev. Neurosci.* 2:113-168.

Musacchio, J.M., Goldstein, M., Anagnoste, B., Poch, G. & Kopin, I.J. (1966). Inhibition of dopamine-β-hydroxylase by disufiram in vivo. *J. Pharmacol. Exp. Therap.* 152, 56–61.

Nicholas, A.P., Pieribone, V. & Hokfelt, T. (1993). Distribution of mRNA for alpha-2 adrenergic receptor subtypes in rat brain: an in situ hydridization study. *J. Comp. Neurol.* 328:575-594.

Nomura, Y., Naitoh, F. & Segawa, T. (1976). Regional changes in monoamine content and uptake of the rat brain during postnatal development. *Brain Res.* 101:305-315.

Osaka, T. & Matsumura, H. (1994). Noradrenergic inputs to sleep-related neurons in the preoptic area from the locus coeruleus and the ventrolateral medulla in the rat. *Neurosci. Res.* 19:39-50.

Palmer, A.M., Wilcock, G.K., Esiri, M.M., Francis, P.T. & Bowen, D.M. (1987). Monoaminergic innervation of the frontal and temporal lobes in Alzheimer's disease. *Brain Res.* 401, 231–238.

Patt, S. & Gerhard, L. (1993). A golgi study of human locus coeruleus in normal brains and in Parkinson's disease. *Neuropathol. Appl. Neurobiol.* 19: 519–523.

Perry, E.K., Blessed, G., Tomlinson, B.E., Perry, R.H., Crow, T.J., Cross, A.J., Dockray, G.J., Dimaline, R. & Arregui, A. (1981). Neurochemical activities in human temporal lobe related to aging and Alzheimer's-type changes. *Neurobiol. Aging* 2: 251–256.

Phillipson, O.T. (1979). Afferent projections to the ventral tegmental area of Tsai and interfascicular nucleus: a horseradish peroxidase study in the rat. *J. Comp. Neurol.* 187:117-144.

Ponsen, M.M., Stoffers, D., Booij, J., van Eck-Smit, B.L.F., Wolters, E.C. & Berendse, H.W. (2004). Idiopathic hyposmia as a preclinical sign of Parkinson's disease. *Ann. Neurol.* 56:173-181.

Rainbow, T.C., Parsons, B. & Wolfe, B.B. (1984). Quantitative autoradiography of β1- and β2-adrenergic receptors in rat brain. *Proc. Natl. Acad. Sci.* 81:1585-1589.

Rascol, O., Arnulf, I., Peyro-Saint Paul, H., Brefel-Courbon, C., Vidailhet, M., Thalamus, C., Bonnet, A.M., Descombes, S., Bejjani, B., Fabre, N., Montastruc, J.L. & Agid, Y. (2001). Idazoxan, an alpha-2 antagonist, and L-DOPA-induced dyskinesias in patients with Parkinson's disease. *Mov. Disord.* 16:708-713.

Rascol, O., Brooks, D.J., Korczyn, A.D., De Deyn, P.P., Clarke, C.E. & Lang, A.E. (2000). A five-year study of the incidence of dyskinesia in patients with early Parkinson's disease who were treated with ropinirole or levodopa. *N. Eng. J. Med.* 342:1484-1491.

Raskind, M.A., Peskind, E.R., Halter, J.B. & Jimerson, D.C. (1984). Norepinephrine and MHPG levels in CSF and plasma in Alzheimer's disease. *Arch. Gen. Psychiatry* 41:343-346.

Reinikainen, K.J., Paljarvi, L., Huuskonen, M., Soininen, H., Laakso, M. & Reikkinen, P. (1988). A post-mortem study of noradrenergic, serotonergic and GABAergic neurons in Alzheimer's disease. *J. Neurol. Sci.* 84, 101–116.

Reisine, T.D., Chesselet, M.F., Lubetzki, C., Chéramy, A. & Glowinsk, J. (1982). A role for striatal beta-adrenergic receptors in the regulation of dopamine release. *Brain Res.* 241:123-130.

Robertson, G.B., Fluharty, S.J., Zigmond, M.J., Sclabassi, R.J. & Berger, T.W. (1993). Recovery of hippocampal dentate gyrus granule cell responsiveness to entorhinal cortical input following norepinephrine depletion. *Brain Res.* 61:21-28.

Room, P., Postema, F., Korf, J. (1981). Divergent axon collaterals of rat locus coeruleus neurons: demonstration by a fluorescent double labeling technique. *Brain Res.* 221: 219-230.

Rommelfanger, K.S., Edwards, G.L., Freeman, K.G., Liles, L.C., Miller, G.W. & Weinshenker, D. (2007). Norepinpehrine loss produces more profound motor deficits than MPTP treatment in mice. *Proc. Natl. Acad. Sci.* 104:13804-13809.

Rommelfanger, K.S., Mitrano, D.A., Smith, Y. & Weinshenker, D. (2009). Light and electron microscopic localization of alpa-1 adrenergic receptor immunoreactivity in the rat striatum and ventral midbrain. *Neuroscience* 158:1530-1540.

Rommelfanger, K.S. & Weinshenker, D. (2007). Norepinephrine: the redheaded stepchild of Parkinson's disease. *Biochem. Pharmacol.* 74: 177-190.

Rommelfanger, K.S., Weinshenker, D. & Miller, G.W. (2004). Reduced MPTP toxicity in noradrenaline transporter knockout mice. *J. Neurochem.* 91:1116-1124.

Rosin, D.L., Talley, E.M., Lee, A., Stornetta, R.L., Gaylinn, B.D. & Guyenet, P.G. (1996). Distribution of alpha 2C-adrenergic receptor-like immunoreactivity in the rat central nervous system. *J. Comp. Neurol.* 372:135-165.

Ross, S.B. (1976). Long-term effects of N-2-chlorethyl-N-ethyl-2-bromobenzylamine hydrochloride on noradrenergic neurons in the rat brain and heart. *Br. J. Pharmacol.* 58:521–527.

Russo-Neustadt, A., Zomorodian, T.J. & Cotman, C.W. (1998). Preserved cerebellar tyrosine hydroxylase-immunoreactive neuronal fibers in a behaviorally aggressive subgroup of Alzheimer's disease patients. *Neuroscience* 87: 55–61.

Saper, C.B., Sorrentino, D.M., German, D.C. & de Lacalle, S. (1991). Medullary catecholaminergic neurons in the normal brain and in Parkinson's disease. *Ann. Neurol.* 29:577-584.

Savola, J.M., Hill, M., Engstrom, M., Merivuori, H., Wurster, S., McGuire, S.G., Fox, S.H., Crossman, A.R. & Brotchie, J.M. (2003). Fipamezole (JP-1730) is a potent α2 adrenergic receptor antagonist that reduces levodopa-induced dyskinesia in the MPTP-lesioned primate model of Parkinson's disease. *Mov. Disord.* 18:872-883.

Scatton, B., Dennis, T. & Curet, O. (1984). Increase in dopamine and DOPAC levels in noradrenergic terminals after electrical stimulation of the ascending noradrenergic pathways. *Brain Res.* 298, 193–196.

Scatton, B., Dennis, T., L'Heureux, R., Monfort, J.-C., Duyckaerts, C. & Javoy-Agid, F. (1986). Degeneration of noradrenergic and serotonergic but not dopaminergic neurons in the lumbar spinal cord of parkinsonian patients. *Brain Res.* 380:181-185.

Scheinin, M., Lomasney, J.W., Hayden-Hixson, D.M., Schambra, U.B., Caron, M.G., Lefkowitz, R.J. & Fremeau, R.T. (1994). Distribution of α_2-adrenergic receptor subtype gene expression in rat brain. *Mol. Brain Res.* 21:133-149.

Scheneck, C.H., Bundlie, S.R. & Mahowald, M.W. (2003). REM behavior disorder (RBD): Delayed emergence of parkinsonism and/or dementia in 65% of older men initially diagnosed with idiopathic RBD, and an analysis of the minimum and maximum tonic and/or phasic electromyographic abnormalities found during REM sleep. *Sleep* 26:A316.

Schroeder, J.P., Cooper, D.A., Schank, J.R., Lyle, M.A., Gaval-Cruz, M., Ogbonmwan, Y.E., Pozdeyev, N., Freeman, K.G., Iuvone, P.M., Edwards, G.L., Holmes, P.V. & Weinshenker, D. (2010). Disulfiram attenuates drug-primes reinstatement of cocaine seeking via inhibition of dopamine β-hydroxylase. *Neuropsychopharmacology* 35: 2440–2449.

Sethi, K. (2008). Levodopa unresponsive symptoms in Parkinson disease. *Mov. Disord.* 23: S521-S533.

Shannak, K., Rajput, A., Rozdilsky, B., Kish, S., Gilbert ,J. & Hornykiewicz, O. (1994). Noradrenaline, dopamine and serotonin levels and metabolism in the human hypothalamus: observations in Parkinson's disease and normal subjects. *Brain Res.* 639:33-41.

Singh, N., Pillay, V. & Choonara, Y.E. (2007). Advances in the treatment of Parkinson's disease. *Prog. Neurobiol.* 81:29-44.

Simon, H., Le Moal ,M. & Calas, A. (1979). Efferents and afferents of the ventral tegmental-A10 region studied after local injection of [^{3}H]leicine and horseradish peroxidase. Brain Res. 178:17-40.

Slaughter, J.R., Slaughter, K.A., Nichols, D., Holmes, S.E. & Martens, M.P. (2001). Prevalence, clinical manifestations, etiology, and treatment of depression in Parkinson's disease. *J. Neuropsychiatry Clin. Neurosci.* 13:187-196.

Srinivasan, J. & Schmidt, W.J. (2003). Potentiation of parkinsonian symptoms by depletion of locus coeruleus noradrenaline in 6-hydroxydopamine-induced partial degeneration of substantia nigra in rats. *Eur. J. Neurosci.* 17:2586-2592.

Srinivasan, J. & Schmidt, W.J. (2004a). Behavioral and neurochemical effects of noradrenergic depletions with N-(2-chloroethyl)-N-ethyl-2-bromobenzylamine in 6-hydroxydopamine-induced rat model of Parkinson's disease. *Behav. Brain Res.* 151:191-199

Srinivasan, J. & Schmidt, W.J. (2004b). The effect of the α_2-adrenoreceptor antagonist idazoxan against 6-hydroxydopamine-induced Parkinsonism in rats: multiple facets of action? *Naunyn-Schmiedeberg's Arch. Pharmacol.* 369:629-638.

Srinivasan, J. & Schmidt, W.J. (2004c). Treatment with α_2-adrenoceptor anatgonists, 2-methoxy idazoxan, protects 6-hydroxydopamine-induced Parkinsonian symptoms in rats: neurochemical and behavioral evidence. *Behav. Brain Res.* 154:353-363.

Strazielle, C., Lalonde, R., Hebert, C. & Reader, T.A. (1999). Regional brain distribution of noradrenaline uptake sites, and of α_1-,α_2- and β-adrenergic receptors in PCD mutant mice: a quatitative autoradiographic study. *Neuroscience* 94:287-304.

Swanson, L.W. & Hartman, B.K. (1975). The central adrenergic system. An immunofluorescence study of the location of cell bodies and their efferent connections in the rat utilizing dopamine-β-hydroxylase as a marker. *J. Comp. Neurol.* 163: 467-505.

Szot, P. (2006). Comparison of noradrenergic receptor distribution in the hippocampus of rodents and humans: Implications for differential drug response. *Lett. Drug Design Disc.* 3:645-652.

Szot, P., Leverenz, J., Peskind, E., Kiyasu, E., Rohde, K., Miller, M.A. & Raskind, M. (2000). Tyrosine hydroxylase and norepinephrine transporter mRNA expression in the locus coeruleus in Alzheimer's disease. *Mol. Brain Res.* 84: 135–140.

Szot, P., Miguelez, C., White, S.S., Franklin, A., Sikkema, C., Wilkinson, C.W., Ugedo, L. & Raskind, M.A. (2010). A comprehensive analysis of the effect of DSP4 on the locus coeruleus noradrenergic system in the rat. *Neuroscience* 166:279-291.

Szot, P., White, S.S., Greenup, J.L., Leverenz, J.B., Peskind, E.R. & Raskind, M.A. (2006). Compensatory changes in the noradrenergic nervous systemin the locus coeruleus and hippocampus of postmortem subjects with Alzheimer's disease and dementia with Lewy bodies. *J. Neurosci.* 26: 467–478.

Szot, P., White, S.S., Greenup, J.L., Leverenz, J.B., Peskind, E.R. & Raskind, M.A. (2007). Changes in adrenoreceptors in the prefrontal cortex of subjects with dementia: Evidence of compensatory changes. *Neuroscience* 146: 471–480.

Taylor, T.N., Caudle, W.M., Sheperd, K.R., Noorian, A., Jackson, C.R., Iuvone, P.M., Weinshenker, D., Greene, J.G. & Miller, G.W. (2009). Nonmotor symptoms of

Parkinson's disease revealed in an animal model with reduced monoamine storage capacity. *J. Neurosci.* 29:8103-8113.

Theron, C.N., de Villiers, A.S. & Taljaard, J.J. (1993). Effects of DSP-4 on monoamine and monoamine metabolites levels and on beta adrenoreceptor binding kinetics in rat brain at different times after administration. *Neurchem. Res.* 18:1321–1327.

Thomas, S.A., Matsumoto, A.M. & Palmiter, R.D. (1995). Noradrenaline is essential for mouse fetal development. *Nature* 374: 643–646.

Thomas, S.A., Marck, B.T., Palmiter, R.D. & Matsumoto, A.M. (1998). Restoration of norepinephrine and reversal of phenotypes in mice lacking dopamine β-hydroxylase. *J. Neurochem.* 70: 2468–2476.

Tohgi, H., Ueno, M., Abe, T., Takahashi, S. & Nozaki, Y. (1992). Concentrations of monoamines and their metabolites in the cerebral spinal fluid from patients with senile dementia of the Alzheimer's type and vascular dementia of the Binswanger's type. *J. Neurol. Transm. Park. Dis. Dement. Sect.* 4:69-77.

Tomlinson, B.E., Irving, D. & Blessed, G. (1981). Cell loss in the locus coeruleus in senile dementia of the Alzheimer's type. J. *Neurol. Sci.* 49, 419–428.

Turkka, J.T., Juujarvi, K.K. & Myllyla, V.V. (1987). Correlation of autonomic dysfunction to CSF concentrations of noradrenraline and 3-methoxy-4-hydroxyphenylglycol in Parkinson's disease. *Eur. Neurol.* 26:29-34.

Ungerstedt, U. (1971). Stereotaxic mapping of the monoamine pathways in the rat brain. *Acta. Physiol. Scand. Suppl.* 361:1-48.

Van Gaalen, M., Kawahara, H., Kawahara, Y. & Westernik, B.H.C. (1997). The locus coeruleus noradrenergic system in the rat brain studied by dual-probe microdilaysis. *Brain Res.* 763:56-62.

Villegier, A.-S., Drouin, C., Bizot, J.-C., Marien, M., Glowinski, J., Colpaert, F. & Tassin, J.-P. (2003). Stimulation of postsynaptic α_{1b}- and α_2-adrenrgic receptors amplifies dopamine-mediated locomotor activity in both rats and mice. *Synapse* 50:277-284.

Walsh, S., Finn, D.P. & Dowd, E. (2011). Time-course of nigrostriatal neurodegeneration and neuroinflammation in the 6-hydroxydopamine-induced axonal and terminal models of Parkinson's disease in the rat. *Neuroscience* 175:251-161.

Wang, Y., Zhang, Q.J., Liu, J., Ali, U., Gui, Z.H., Hui ,Y.P., Chen, L., Wu, Z.H. & Li, Q. (2010). Noradrenergic lesion of the locus coeruleus increases apomorphine-induced circling behavior and the firing activity of substantia nigra pars reticulate neurons in a rat model of Parkinson's disease. Brain Res. 1310:189-199.

Waterhouse, B.D., Lin, C.S., Burne, R.A. & Woodward, D.J. (1983). The distribution of neocortical projection neurons in the locus coeruleus. *J. Comp. Neurol.* 217:418-431.

Winkler, C., Kirik, D., Bjorklund, A. & Cenci, M.A. (2002). L-DOPA-induced dyskinesia in the intrastriatal 6-hydroxydopamine model of parkinson's disease: relation to motor and cellular parameters of nigrostriatal function. *Neurobiol Dis* 10:165-186.

Wolfman, C., Abo, V., Calvo, D., Medina, J., Dajas, F. & Silveiro, R. (1994). Recovery of central noradrenergic neurons one year after the administration of the neurotoxin DSP4. *Neurochem. Int.* 25:395- 400.

Yamada, H., Aimi, Y., Nagatsu, I., Taki, K., Kudo, M. & Arai, R. (2007). Immunohistochemical detection of L-DOPA-derived dopamine within serotonergic fibers in the striatum and the substantia nigra pars reticulata in Parkinsonian model rats. *Neurosci. Res.* 59:1-7.

Zarow, C., Lyness, S.A., Mortimer, J.A. & Chui, H.C. (2003). Neuronal loss is greater in the locus coeruleus than nucleus basalis and substantia nigra in Alzheimer' and Parkinson disease. *Arch. Neurol.* 60:337-341.

Zeng, D. & Lynch, K.R. (1991). Distribution of α_2-adrenergic receptor mRNAs in the rat CNS. *Mol. Brain Res.* 10:219-225.

Ziegler, M.G., Lake, C.R. & Kopin, I.J. (1977). The sympathetic-nervous-system defect in primary orthostatic hypotension. *N. Engl. J. Med.* 296:293-297.

Ziemssen, T. & Reichmann, H. (2007). Non-motor dysfunction in Parkinson's disease. *Parkinsonism Relat. Disord.* 13:323-332.

Zhou, Q.Y. & Palmiter, R.D. (1995). Dopamine-deficient mice are severely hypoactive, adipsic and aphagic. *Cell* 83:1197-1209

12

The Energy Crisis in Parkinson's Disease: A Therapeutic Target

Mhamad Abou-Hamdan, Emilie Cornille, Michel Khrestchatisky, Max de Reggi and Bouchra Gharib
NICN, UMR6184, CNRS, Aix-Marseille University, Marseille France

1. Introduction

The energy demand of the brain is very large: it accounts for 20% of the body's energy consumption, even though its weight is less than 2% of the total body mass. In the adult, brain energy comes primarily from glucose through oxidative glycolysis. The end product is acetyl-coenzyme A (acetyl-CoA), which enters the mitochondria and feeds into the tricarboxylic acid (TCA) cycle to produce energy in the form of reductants, such as NADH. The chemical energy of NADH is then used by the respiratory chain, or electron transport chain, to synthesize ATP (Fig. 1). Energy depletion is a major factor in the cascade of events culminating in dopaminergic neuronal death in Parkinson's disease (PD). There are two reasons for that. First, a frequent feature of the disease, as well as of other neurodegenerative diseases, is an alteration of glucose metabolism. Second, there is a decrease of mitochondrial respiratory chain activity due to, in particular, inhibition of the electron transport system complex I (NADH-ubiquinone oxidoreductase).

Complex I activity is redox-dependent and thiol-regulated; therefore its inhibition is associated with oxidative stress. Depletion of GSH, a major antioxidant and redox modulator, is observed in the substantia nigra of parkinsonian patients, as well as in the mouse MPTP model of the disease. Conversely, the restoration of GSH levels preserves complex I activity. Accordingly, the maintenance of cellular redox homeostasis by thiol agents protects against nigrostriatal toxicity.

In the case of the alteration of glucose metabolism, the brain has the ability to adapt its metabolism and to increase its reliance on lipids for energy production, through fatty acid β-oxidation. The process involves a mitochondrial oxido-reductase superfamily with broad substrate specificity. The penultimate step of the process is catalyzed by L-3-hydroxyacyl-CoA dehydrogenase (HADH II) (EC 1.1.1.35). HADH II overexpression protects against acute brain injury and chronic neurodegeneration. By-products of fatty acid β–oxidation are the ketone bodies β-hydroxybutyrate and acetoacetate. When injected into mice or rats, or administered in the form of a ketogenic diet, ketone bodies have a protective role in a broad spectrum of cerebral injuries and diseases.

In the present report, we examine the brain energy metabolism, its alterations associated with PD and how fatty acid β-oxidation can compensate such impairment. Energy store boosting agents have potential therapeutic properties. Pantethine, the precursor of vitamin

B5, is one of them, with the advantage of targeting multiple pathways involved in disease process. By itself or by its constituents (Fig. 2), pantethine regulates lipid metabolism, in addition to its anti-oxidant and anti-inflammatory properties, giving rise to the promise of an original therapeutic strategy against PD.

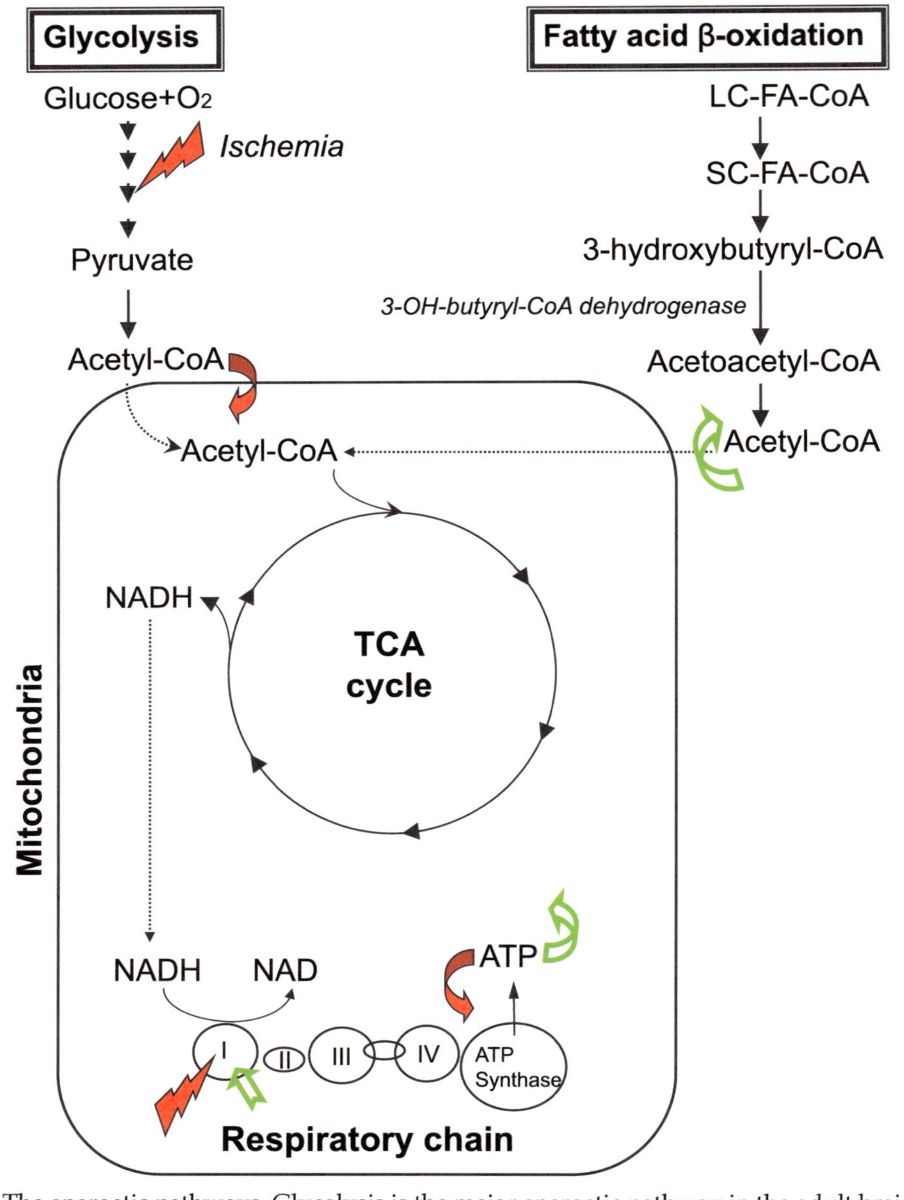

Fig. 1. The energetic pathways. Glycolysis is the major energetic pathway in the adult brain. It is impaired in Parkinson's disease, leading to an energy crisis, which is compensated by fatty acid-β–oxidation. Solid symbols (red) indicate the injuries and alterations occurring in the processes leading to the disease; open symbols (green) indicate the protective effects of pantethine.

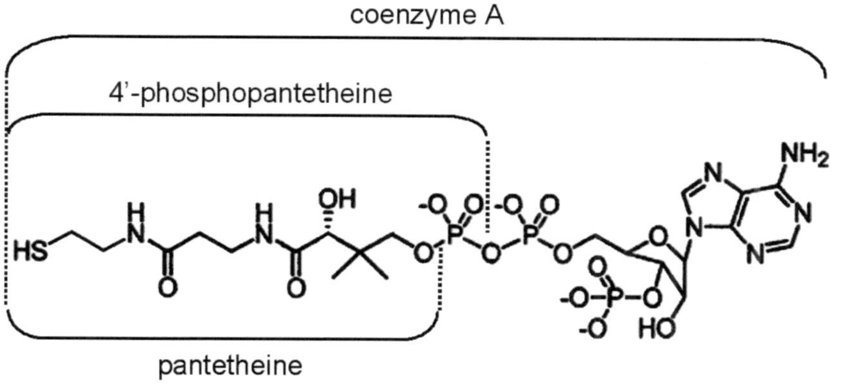

Fig. 2. Pantethine forms the active moiety of CoA. Pantetheine, the reduced form of pantethine, is first 4′-phosphorylated by pantothenate kinase and then adenylated by phosphopantetheine adenylyl transferase (CoaD) to form dephospho-CoA; finally, dephospho-CoA is phosphorylated to coenzyme A by the enzyme dephosphocoenzyme A kinase (CoaE). Lipids are metabolized as fatty acids linked to the SH group of pantetheine, in the form of acyl-CoA thioesters.

2. Brain energy metabolism

Although the brain represents only 2% of the body weight, it receives 15% of the cardiac output and accounts for 20% of total body oxygen consumption as well as 25% of total body glucose utilization. Under physiological conditions, glycolysis is, by far, the major energetic pathway in the adult brain. Glucose is broken down in the presence of oxygen, yielding pyruvate and lactate. Evidence accumulated during the past decade supports the notion that astrocytes play a pivotal role in the regulation of brain-glucose metabolism, via the so-called neuron-astrocyte lactate shuttle (Escartin et al., 2006; Hertz, 2004; Schurr, 2006). Owing to their strategic location surrounding cerebral blood capillaries, astrocytes form the first cellular barrier encountered by glucose entering the brain parenchyma, which makes them a prevalent site of glucose uptake. Blood-borne glucose crosses the vascular endothelial cells and enters brain cells through specific hexose transporters of the glucose transporter family (GLUT) (McEwen and Reagan, 2004; Vannucci et al., 1997). When the supply of oxygen therefore does not match precisely the demand, e.g. during neuronal activation or under pathological conditions, glucose may be broken down anaerobically, to produce lactate in order to supply energy faster. This process has, however, low energetic efficiency.
The following step of energy production is the conversion of pyruvate to acetyl-CoA which is used by mitochondria, the power house of living cells. Mitochondria produce the reductant NADH via the tricarboxilic acid cycle; then the chemical energy of NADH is used by the electron transport chain (ETC) to synthesize ATP. Mammalian ETC is composed of least 49 individual polypeptides which constitute a series of electron carriers organized in four enzymatic complexes plus the ATP synthase machinery. Complex I (NADH ubiquinone oxidoreductase) (EC1.6.5.3) is a very large enzymatic set catalyzing the first step of the ETC (Saraste, 1999; Schultz and Chan, 2001). The enzyme oxidizes NADH, transferring electrons to Ubiquinone (Coenzyme Q, CoQ), a lipid soluble electron carrier

embedded in the lipid bilayer of the inner mitochondrial membrane. Complex II (succinate-ubiquinone oxidoreductase) (EC1.3.5.1), bound to the inner mitochondrial membrane, catalyzes the oxidation of succinate to fumarate with the reduction of ubiquinone to ubiquinol. Complex III (ubiquinol-cytochrome C oxidoreductase; EC 1.10.2.2) is the oligomeric protein complex that transfers electrons from ubiquinol to cytochrome C and links proton translocation to this electron transfer by the proton motive Q cycle mechanism (Trumpower, 1990). Complex IV (cytochrome C oxidase (EC 1.9.3.1) is a transmembrane protein which receives electrons from cytochrome C and transfers them to one oxygen molecule, converting molecular oxygen to water. In the whole process, a transmembrane difference of proton electrochemical potential is established that the ATP synthase then uses to synthesize ATP. Mitochondrial dysfunction results in a dwindling supply of ATP, a failure in maintaining cellular homeostasis and activation of cell death pathways.

3. Energy crisis in Parkinson's disease

PD, Huntington's disease (HD) and Alzheimer's disease (AD) are age-related diseases of diverse etiologies, but energy crisis is a common factor. The link between PD and mitochondria was first established with the identification of a deficiency in the activity of complex I in the substantia nigra of PD patients (Schapira et al., 1989) and it has been then confirmed by several authors (see reviews in (Banerjee et al., 2009; Schapira, 2006)). Complex I deficiency was noticed not only in the brain but also in the peripheral tissues of PD patients (Krige et al., 1992; Wallace et al., 1992). Whether mitochondrial dysfunction is the cause or effect of PD pathogenesis is debatable. However, it is clear that dopaminergic neurons are especially susceptible to energy deficit, meaning that mitochondrial dysfunction may underlie selective dopaminergic neuro-degeneration in PD (Beal, 2005).

The seminal discovery that MPTP (1-methyl-4-phenyl-1,2,3,6-tetrahydropyridine) causes PD-like symptoms in humans (Langston et al., 1983) and the ensuing rapid unraveling of the molecular mechanism of its toxicity strongly stimulated the interest of the PD research community in the role of mitochondria in PD pathology. MPTP is metabolized to its toxic form MPP^+ (1-methyl-4-phenylpyridinium ion) by mitochondrial monoamine oxidase (MAO) (Chiba et al., 1984), specifically by MAO B (Heikkila et al., 1984) and is rapidly concentrated in the mitochondria (Ramsay et al., 1986b). Once accumulated, MPP^+ specifically inhibits the oxidation of NAD-linked substrates (Nicklas et al., 1985) by blocking the electron transfer through the ETC complex I (Ramsay et al., 1986a). It also inhibits the activity of a key TCA (tricarboxylic acid) enzyme KGDHC (α-ketoglutarate dehydrogenase complex) thereby impairing the ATP synthesis and inducing "**energy crisis**" *in vivo* (Mizuno et al., 1988b) and *in vitro* (Mizuno et al., 1988a). The rather selective toxicity of MPP+ to dopaminergic neurons in SN (substantia nigra) was explained by the fact that MPP+ is selectively accumulated by the dopamine uptake system involving the dopamine transporters (DAT) (Javitch et al., 1985). Platelets which also express DAT (Frankhauser et al., 2006) have been shown to accumulate MPP+ with high efficiency and suffer from mitochondrial failure as a result of MPP+ exposure (Buckman et al., 1988). Human platelets also contain high levels of MAO B and share a number of properties with aminergic neurons including receptors, uptake sites and storage granules for amine neurotransmitters. As platelets are more available for research than PD brain samples or muscle biopsy specimens, they were a natural choice for PD tissue samples in earlier studies on the status of complex I in PD. Low complex I activities have been reported in both PD platelet homogenates and mitochondria isolated from PD platelets, although the degree of its inhibition varied within a wide range. Other ETC complexes in PD platelets are also concerned: complex II (Yoshino et al., 1992), complex II + complex III (Haas et al., 1995), and complex IV (Benecke et al., 1993). Several studies showed impaired complex I, II+III, and IV activities in PD muscle (Bindoff et al., 1991; Blin et al., 1994; Cardellach et al., 1993); whereas no differences were observed in other studies (DiDonato et al., 1993; Mann et al., 1992; Reichmann et al., 1994). Similar conflicting results were reported in the ETC in PD lymphocytes (Martin et al., 1996; Yoshino et al., 1992). Such inconsistency in the experimental data may be explained by significant methodological differences in these studies, e.g. difficulties in obtaining the relevant tissue samples, individual variability of PD patients and many other factors, as was suggested (Parker et al., 2008).

Complex I activity is reduced in mitochondria isolated from PD frontal cortex (Keeney et al., 2006; Parker et al., 2008); it is believed to be an early pathogenic event in PD. Ample data strongly suggest that MPTP-induced ETC disruption per se is sufficient to trigger the death of nigrostriatal neurons and to cause PD-like symptoms in animals and humans. Thus, despite some conflicting results, systemic complex I deficiency might be a predominant feature in PD pathogenesis (Banerjee et al., 2009). Accordingly, ^{1}H and ^{31}P magnetic resonance spectrometry demonstrated mitochondrial dysfunction in the putamen and midbrain of both early and advanced PD subjects, with a bilateral reduction of high-energy phosphates; the changes were associated with abnormally elevated lactate levels. In contrast, low-energy metabolites such as adenosine diphophosphate and inorganic phosphate were within normal ranges. These results provide strong in vivo evidence that mitochondrial dysfunction of mesostriatal neurons is a central and persistent phenomenon in the pathogenesis cascade of PD which occurs early in the course of the disease (Hattingen et al., 2009; Henchcliffe et al., 2008).

Paraquat and rotenone are other neurotoxins that inhibit mitochondrial complex I activity, whereas there are substantial differences in their action (Richardson et al., 2005). Rotenone rat models of PD have been developed that reproduce essential biochemical and behavioral human PD features (Alam and Schmidt, 2002; Betarbet et al., 2000; Greenamyre et al., 2003; Sherer et al., 2003).

Complex I activity is redox-dependent and thiol-regulated (Annepu and Ravindranath, 2000; Sriram et al., 1998). Since PD pathogenesis consistently involve reactive oxygen and nitrogen species (Bove et al., 2005; Li et al., 2003; Przedborski, 2005; Przedborski and Ischiropoulos, 2005) this may explain, at least in part, complex I inhibition. Thus, depletion of GSH, an antioxidant and redox modulator, may be one of the early events leading to the inhibition of complex I activity and loss of mitochondrial function (Chinta and Andersen, 2006; Jha et al., 2000).

4. Mitochondrial dysfunction and the genetic causes of the disease

In the past decade, a rapidly expanding list of Mendelian-inherited gene mutations has provided great insight into the mechanisms leading to loss of the nigrostriatal dopaminergic neurons in familial PD which constitutes less than 10% of the total number of PD cases. In recent years, a plethora of studies of the multifunctional consequences of these mutations point towards the disruption of mitochondrial function culminating in neuronal dysfunction and death.

α-Synuclein was the first gene associated with familial PD. It was followed by four other genes linked conclusively to autosomal recessive (parkin, PINK-1, DJ-1) or dominant (LRRK2) Parkinsonism (Bogaerts et al., 2008; Henchcliffe and Beal, 2008).

PINK1. Mutations in phosphatase and tensin homologue (PTEN)-induced putative kinase (PINK1) cause a rare form of autosomal recessive, PD early onset Parkinsonism following the parkin mutations (Valente et al., 2004; Winklhofer and Haass, 2010). Loss of PINK1 function increases the propensity of cells to oxidative stress-induced cell death and imbalance of calcium homeostasis. The experiments suggest that the impairment of mitochondrial calcium efflux promotes ROS formation that inhibits glucose uptake, resulting in reduced substrate delivery and respiration (Gandhi et al., 2009).

Parkin is a multifaceted ubiquitin ligase (Moore, 2006). Mutations in the *parkin* gene serve as the most common cause of young onset PD (Farrer et al., 2001; Lucking et al., 2000). Loss of function of E3 ligase activity has been suggested to result in accumulation of toxic substrates leading to autosomal recessive form of PD (Dawson, 2006). *Parkin* gene expression is up-regulated in various stress examples and has a wide range of neuroprotective capacities, including protection against mitochondrial dysfunction, endoplasmatic reticulum stress, exitotoxicity, proteasome inhibition, and overexpression of α-synuclein, tau, and other proteins. Future studies of the biochemical interactions between PINK1 and parkin and identification of other components in this pathway are likely to provide insight into PD pathogenesis, and might identify new therapeutic targets (Henchcliffe and Beal, 2008).

DJ-1 and **LRRK2**. DJ-1 has structural similarities with the stress-inducible Escherichia coli chaperone Hsp31 and mutations in the *DJ-1* gene are associated with rare cases of early onset autosomal recessive PD (Andersen, 2004). The loss of DJ-1 function leads to a striking sensitivity to the herbicide paraquat and the insecticide rotenone; this suggests that DJ-1 may have a role in the protection from oxidative stress caused by environmental toxins. It has been clearly demonstrated that, while overexpression of DJ-1 protects neurons from oxidative stress-induced damage, conversely DJ-1 deficiency renders cells more susceptible to oxidative injury. Mutations in leucin-rich repeat kinase 2 (*LRRK2* gene) cause autosomal dominant PD (Paisan-Ruiz et al., 2004; Zimprich et al., 2004). The precise physiological role of this protein is unknown but the presence of multiple functional domains suggests involvement in a wide variety of functions. A possible mechanism of LRRK2 action is at the mitochondrial level.

5. Lipids as an alternative carbon source for energy production

The brain has the ability to use fatty acids as an alternative carbon source. Fatty acid β-oxidation parallels glycolysis (Fig. 1). This occurs normally during embryonic development and, in adults, under conditions of inadequate glucose supply or increased energy demand, as well as under pathological conditions, such as neurodegeneration, hypoxia/ischemia and traumatic brain injury (Prins, 2008).

5.1 Lipid metabolism and regulation of mitochondrial function

Peroxisome Proliferator-Activated Receptors (PPARs) regulate development, tissue differentiation, inflammation, wound healing, mitochondrial function, lipid and glucose metabolism (Reddy et al., 2006; Reddy, 2001). PPARs are expressed in CNS neurons and astrocytes, raising the possibility of exploring the neuroprotective efficacy of PPAR agonists in several neurodegenerative disorders (Bordet et al., 2006; Heneka and Landreth, 2007; Woods et al., 2003). Gene-knockout experiments have revealed that, consistent with their distinct expression patterns, each PPAR subtype performs a specific function in fatty acid homeostasis. PPAR-α targets genes function together to coordinate the complex metabolic changes necessary to conserve energy during fasting and feeding in cases where catabolic enzymes promote fatty acid β–oxidation.

It is now well established that damage to dopaminergic neurons involves oxidative stress, microglial activation-mediated inflammation and mitochondrial impairment, which ultimately culminate in activation of an apoptotic pathway. The PPAR-γ agonist pioglitazone was shown to exert protective effects in a mouse model of PD; it attenuated the MPTP intoxication-induced glial activation and prevented dopaminergic cell loss in the substantia nigra pars compacta (Breidert et al., 2002). These findings were paralleled by another study showing that the treatment with pioglitazone may offer an opportunity for treatment of PD to slow its progression (Dehmer et al., 2004).

PPAR-γ coactivator 1α (PGC-1α) is a master regulator of mitochondrial biogenesis and respiration (Lehman et al., 2000; Lin et al., 2002; Puigserver et al., 1998; Wu et al., 1999). It transduces many physiological stimuli into specific metabolic programs, often by stimulating mitochondrial activity. For example, PGC-1α regulates both β–oxidation of fatty acids and gluconeogenesis in liver (Herzig et al., 2001; Puigserver et al., 2003; Rhee et al., 2003; Yoon et al., 2001). The importance of PGC-1α in these metabolic programs was further revealed through the generation of PGC-1α null mice. These mice display a reduced basal expression of many mitochondrial genes in liver, brain, skeletal muscle and heart, compared with wild-type animals (Arany et al., 2005; Leone et al., 2005; Lin et al., 2004). Moreover, it has been shown that PGC-1α knockout (KO) mice displayed neurodegenerative lesions in the brain, particularly in the striatum; the animals also showed behavioral abnormalities (Leone et al., 2005; Lin et al., 2004). At present, the cause of the brain lesions is unclear, but the lesions observed in many genetic models with altered ROS levels raise the possibility that PGC-1α plays an important role in the control of ROS in vivo (St-Pierre et al., 2006). PGC-1α and PGC-1β are powerfully induced by ROS, and these coactivators, in turn, regulate a complex and multifaceted ROS defense system. In the MPTP model, PGC-1α KO mice have a greatly increased sensitivity to damage by oxidative stress in the dopaminergic cells of the substantia nigra and hippocampal neurons. Conversely, the overexpression of PGC-1α in cultured dopaminergic neurons from embryonic rat midbrain resulted in activation of electron transport genes and protection against neuronal damage induced by mutant α-synuclein (Zheng et al., 2010). The same authors found in postmortem brain tissue samples from PD patients that the gene sets with the strongest association with PD contained nuclear genes encoding subunits of the ETC proteins. These genes all showed decreased expression in substantia nigra dopaminergic neurons even in the earliest stages of PD. Furthermore, a second gene set associated with PD and also underexpressed in the earliest stages of PD encodes enzymes involved in glucose metabolism. These results are compelling because many studies have already implicated dysfunctional mitochondria and altered energy metabolism as well as defective glucose metabolism in PD. The authors realized that these gene sets had in common the master transcriptional regulator, PGC-1α and surmised that disruption of PGC-1α expression might be a root cause of PD.

5.2 Fatty acid β-oxidation

As in the case of glycolysis, the end product of fatty acid β-oxidation is acetyl-CoA (Fig. 1) which feeds into the TCA cycle to produce energy in the form of NADH and $FADH_2$. The enzymes involved in fatty acid β-oxidation all act on acyl-CoA, i.e. fatty acids linked to CoA as thioesters. They belong to an oxido-reductase superfamily with broad substrate specificity. The enzymes are subdivided into several groups, according to the substrate chain length. Each of the constituent steps of the pathway comprises three consecutive enzymatic reactions catalyzed by a trifunctional enzymatic complex: 2-enoyl-CoA hydratase, 3-hydroxyacyl-CoA dehydrogenase and 3-ketoacyl-CoA thiolase. The reactions yield acetyl-CoA plus a chain-shortened acyl-CoA (at each step, the fatty acid chain loses two carbons) (Eaton et al., 2000).

In the present review, we focus attention on the penultimate step of the process, i.e. acyl-CoA dehydrogenation. It involves four classes of enzymes: short-chain acyl-CoA dehydrogenase (SCAD, active with C_4 and C_6), medium-chain acyl-CoA dehydrogenase (MCAD, active with C_4 to C_{12}), long-chain acyl-CoA dehydrogenase (LCAD, active with C_8 to C_{20}) and very-long-chain acyl-CoA dehydrogenase (VLCAD, active with C_{12} to C_{24}). SCAD, MCAD and LCAD are homotetramers located in the mitochondrial matrix. VLCAD, however, is a homodimer and is located in the inner mitochondrial membrane. VLCAD is a constituent of the trifunctional protein described above.

Short chain 3-hydroxyacyl-CoA dehydrogenase (SCHAD) also known as L-3-hydroxyacyl-CoA dehydrogenase/amyloid-peptide binding alcohol dehydrogenase (HADH II/ABAD) is predominantly a mitochondrial enzyme (Furuta et al., 1997; Kobayashi et al., 1996) that belongs to the short-chain dehydrogenase/reductase superfamily (Jornvall et al., 1995). It acts on a wide spectrum of substrates, including steroids, cholic acids, and fatty acids, with a preference for short chain methyl-branched acyl-CoAs. Abnormally low or high levels of SCHAD in certain brain regions may contribute to the pathogenesis of some neural disorders. The human SCHAD gene and its protein product are therefore potential targets for intervention in conditions such as PD, AD and an X-linked mental retardation, which may arise from the impaired degradation of branched fatty acid chains and of isoleucine (Yang et al., 2005; Zschocke et al., 2000).

The levels of SCHAD/HADH II are significantly reduced in the ventral midbrain of both PD patients and of a PD mouse model generated by MPTP injection (Przedborski et al., 2004). Conversely, transgenic mice with increased expression of human HADH II/ABAD are significantly more resistant to MPTP; overexpression of the enzyme mitigates MPTP-induced impairment of oxidative phosphorylation and ATP production (Tieu et al., 2004). This observation suggests that a new way to prevent PD may be to increase expression of SCHAD/HADH II in the midbrain.

6. Therapeutic strategies to target the energy crisis

6.1 Potential therapeutic compounds

Coenzyme Q (CoQ) is a component of the electron transport chain where it accepts electrons from complexes I and II (Beal, 2004). Its administration increases mitochondrial uncoupling protein (UCP) expression in the nervous system of primates, and this is associated with marked neuroprotection in both *in vitro* and *in vivo* models of MPTP, paraquat and rotenone-induced mitochondrial dysfunction. CoQ_{10} exerts significant protection against MPTP-induced dopamine depletion and loss of tyrosine hydroxylase immunoreactive neurons in aged mice (Shults et al., 2002).

Creatine is a nitrogenous guanidine compound that helps to supply energy to muscle and nerve cells (Adhihetty and Beal, 2008). Chronic administration of creatine protects against MPTP-induced dopamine loss and improves the survival of neurons in the substantia nigra (Matthews et al., 1999).

α-Lipoic acid (ALA) is a disulfide compound found in mitochondria as a coenzyme for pyruvate dehydrogenase and α-ketoglutarate dehydrogenase. Dietary supplementation with α-lipoic acid in old rats improved ambulatory activity, decreased oxidative damage, and improved mitochondrial function (Hagen et al., 1999). *In vitro*, pre-treatment of PC12 cells with R-lipoic acid acts to prevent depletion of GSH content and preserves the mitochondrial complex I activity which normally is impaired as a consequence of GSH loss (Bharat et al., 2002).

Carnitine transports long-chain fatty acid into the mitochondrial matrix for subsequent β–oxidation (Di Lisa et al., 1985; Rosenthal et al., 1992). Carnitine also facilitates the removal of short-chain and medium chain fatty acids that accumulate in the mitochondria during normal and abnormal metabolism. Carnitine and acetyl-L-carnitine attenuate neuronal damage produced by 3-nitropropionic acid, rotenone, and MPTP *in vitro* (Snyder et al., 1990; Virmani et al., 1995).

Nicotinamide is a precursor of NADH, a substrate for Complex I (NADH-ubiquinone oxidoreductase). It is also an inhibitor of poly-ADP-ribose polymerase, which is activated by DNA damage and in turn depletes both NADH and ATP. Activation of poly-ADP-ribose polymerase plays a role in neuronal injury induced by both ischemia and MPTP (Eliasson et al., 1997; Mandir et al., 1999).

6.2 Ketone bodies

If the amounts of acetyl-CoA generated by fatty acid β-oxidation challenge the processing capacity of the TCA cycle or if activity in the TCA cycle is low, acetyl-CoA is used in the biosynthesis of ketone bodies via β–hydroxy-metylglutaryl-CoA (HMG-CoA) synthesis. The main ketone bodies are D-β-hydroxybutyrate (DβHB) and acetoacetate (ACA). They are produced by hepatocytes and are transported to the tissues, including the brain; astrocytes are also ketogenic, although to a lesser extent (Guzman and Blazquez, 2001).

DβHB and ACA have a protective role in a broad spectrum of cerebral injuries and diseases and they preserve neuronal cell integrity and stability *in vitro*. The experimental approaches used are intravenous infusion of mice or rats with DβHB (Prins, 2008) or administration of a ketogenic diet (Maalouf et al., 2009). Exogenous ketone bodies have been employed successfully in both rapidly developing pathologies (glutamate excitotoxicity, hypoxia/ischemia) and neurodegenerative conditions (PD, AD) [for review see(Prins, 2008)]. In vitro DβHB prevents neuronal damage induced by glucose deprivation (Izumi et al., 1998). Following MPP+ exposure, administration of 4 mmol/L of DβHB increased the survival of cultured neurons (Kashiwaya et al., 2000). In the rotenone *in vitro* model, application of 8 mmol/L of DβHB improved mitochondrial membrane potential and reduced cytochrome C release by mouse neuronal cultures (Imamura et al., 2006); under the same conditions, cell survival was increased by 60% in human neuroblastoma cell culture. *In vivo*, 24 h infusion of DβHB, using mini-osmotic pumps, protected SNpc dopaminergic neurons against MPTP in a dose-dependent and stereospecific manner and prevented the development of PD-like motor abnormalities in mice (Tieu et al., 2003). Tieu's studies provide *in vivo* and *in vitro* evidence that DβHB protects not by alleviating MPTP-related complex I inhibition, but by enhancing oxidative phosphorylation via a mechanism dependent on mitochondrial complex II (succinate-ubiquinone oxidoreductase).

Therefore, modulation of DβHB levels may be a neuroprotective strategy for the treatment of neurodegenerative diseases such as PD. However, the long-term effects of the chronic use of DβHB on the cellular metabolism, and especially on mitochondrial function, are not known. DβHB has been administered orally for several months to two 6-months-old infants with hyperinsulinemic hypoglycemia (Plecko et al., 2002). The high dosage (up to 32 g/d) seemed to be tolerated by these patients. In addition, ketogenic diets have been used in humans as a treatment for refractory epilepsy. In general, patients tolerate the ketogenic diet well with mild side effects (Freeman et al., 2006). However, long-term ketone therapy will have to take into consideration possible adverse effects.

6.3 Pantethine

A promising emerging therapeutic strategy involves fatty acids combined with pantethine. CoA is central in these fields, as illustrated by pantothenate kinase-associated neurodegeneration (PKAN). Pantothenate kinase catalyzes pantetheine phosphorylation to 4'-phosphopantetheine, the first step of CoA synthesis (Fig. 2). PKAN, due to insufficient kinase activity, occurs in early adulthood and its symptoms, such as dystonia, rigidity and tremor, recall PD and it may lead to PD in late adulthood. PKAN results in a decrease of CoA levels associated with mitochondrial dysfunction. These defects can be reversed by pantethine, the oxidized form of pantetheine. Dietary pantethine increased CoA synthesis, improved mitochondrial function, rescued brain degeneration, enhanced locomotor abilities, and increased lifespan in a Drosophila model of PKAN (Rana et al., 2010). Moreover, pantethine circumvented the impairment of fatty acid β-oxidation in rat liver mitochondria and microvessels of the brain (Morisaki et al., 1983). It has been shown recently that pantethine mitigated MPTP neurotoxicity in the mouse via the enhancement of fatty acid β–oxidation, leading to increased levels of circulating ketone bodies and improved mitochondrial function (Cornille et al., 2010). In addition, pantethine attenuates MPTP-induced neuroinflammation, as shown by reduced expression of macrophage antigen-1 (MAC-1), a critical trigger of microglial activation associated with neurodegeneration (Pei et al., 2007) (Fig. 3). Ultimately, pantethine protects from MPTP-induced blood-brain barrier (BBB) leakage (Fig. 4) and significantly attenuates the clinical scores (Fig. 5).

7. Concluding remarks and future perspectives

Deficits in mitochondrial activity in combination with increased oxidative stress, and aging-associated damage to mitochondrial DNA are key biochemical abnormalities associated with the pathogenesis of not only in sporadic PD but also in familial forms of the disease. Factors that trigger these mitochondrial abnormalities are still elusive, however one may speculate that strategies aimed at correcting these biochemical abnormalities might be useful in halting or slowing down the progression of PD. In this regard some of the candidate drugs which showed great efficacy in experimental models of PD have already made it to clinical trials. Preliminary clinical trial data on Coenzyme Q10 and creatine have shown some promise. There is also a great deal of enthusiasm following the recent identification of novel mitochondrial targets such as PGC-1α and the sirtuin family of enzymes that are known to modulate aging, mitochondrial biogenesis, metabolic homeostasis and mitochondria-dependent cell death. These observations hold promise for future development of neuroprotective strategies in PD by targeting mitochondrial dysfunction. However it is important to remember that PD is a multi-factorial disease and mitochondrial dysfunction may only be a part of this complex process. Future research should thus focus on developing neuroprotective strategies by targeting multiple pathways involved in the disease process. Therapeutic approaches targeting both mitochondrial dysfunction and oxidative damage in neurodegenerative diseases and aging have great promise (Beal, 2005). Pantethine provides an example of molecule able to restore mitochondrial function while displaying antioxidant and anti-inflammatory properties. Perhaps, this safe and effective compound of natural origin merits consideration for broader use against pathologies such as PD.

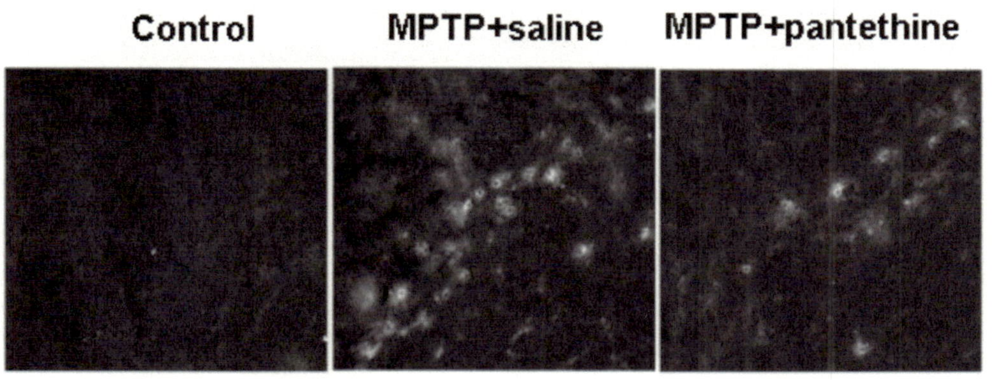

Fig. 3. Attenuation of microglial reaction by pantethine treatment in MPTP-injected mice.

The figure shows macrophage antigen-1 (Mac-1) immunostaining in SNpc, two days after MPTP injection. Microglial reaction was drastically reduced in pantethine-treated mice as compared to saline ones. No immunostaining was observed in control animals.

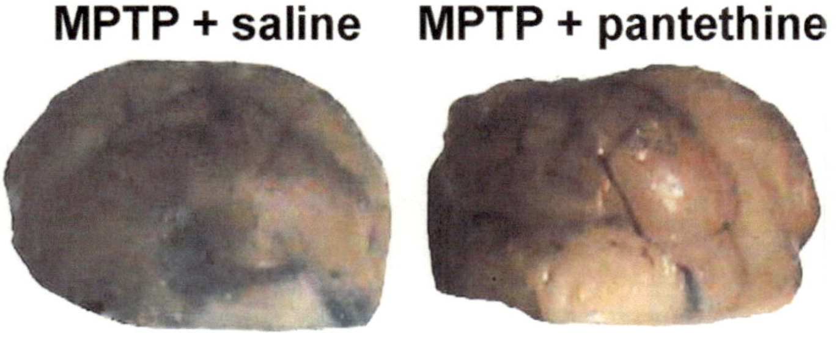

Fig. 4. Prevention of BBB leakage by pantethine treatment in MPTP-injected mice.

Evans blue was administered intravenously on day 16 after MPTP injection. The figure shows brains of saline mice with a diffuse dye leakage, and some intensively stained areas. In contrast, brains of pantethine-treated mice looked normal, with limited stained areas.

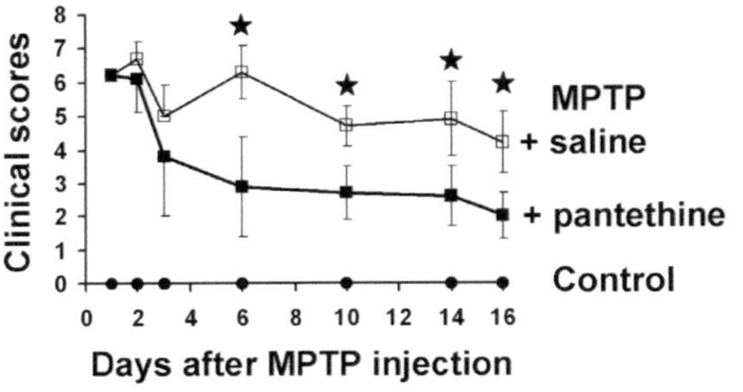

Fig. 5. Attenuation of the clinical scores by pantethine treatment in MPTP-injected mice.

Mice were injected with MPTP and then treated or not treated with pantethine. Under our experimental conditions, the scores were 6.2 in both groups 24 hours after MPTP injection and they decreased much more rapidly in the pantethine group. (*) Significant difference between the two groups, according to the Student t test ($p < 0.01$).

8. Acknowledgements

The authors thank Howard Rickenberg for the critical reading of the manuscript.

9. References

Adhihetty, P.J. & Beal, M.F. (2008). Creatine and its potential therapeutic value for targeting cellular energy impairment in neurodegenerative diseases. *Neuromolecular Medicine,* Vol.10, pp. 275-290

Alam, M. & Schmidt, W.J. (2002). Rotenone destroys dopaminergic neurons and induces parkinsonian symptoms in rats. *behavioural brain research,* Vol.136, pp. 317-324

Andersen, J.K. (2004). Oxidative stress in neurodegeneration: cause or consequence? *Nature Medicine,* Vol.10 Suppl, pp. S18-25

Annepu, J. & Ravindranath, V. (2000). 1-Methyl-4-phenyl-1,2,3,6-tetrahydropyridine-induced complex I inhibition is reversed by disulfide reductant, dithiothreitol in mouse brain. *Neuroscience Letters,* Vol.289, pp. 209-212

Arany, Z.; He, H.; Lin, J.; Hoyer, K.; Handschin, C.; Toka, O.; Ahmad, F.; Matsui, T.; Chin, S.; Wu, P.H.; Rybkin, II; Shelton, J.M.; Manieri, M.; Cinti, S.; Schoen, F.J.; Bassel-Duby, R.; Rosenzweig, A.; Ingwall, J.S.& Spiegelman, B.M. (2005). Transcriptional coactivator PGC-1 alpha controls the energy state and contractile function of cardiac muscle. *Cell Metabolism,* Vol.1, pp. 259-271

Banerjee, R.; Starkov, A.A.; Beal, M.F.& Thomas, B. (2009). Mitochondrial dysfunction in the limelight of Parkinson's disease pathogenesis. *Biochimica et Biophysica Acta,* Vol.1792, pp. 651-663

Beal, M.F. (2004). Therapeutic effects of coenzyme Q10 in neurodegenerative diseases. *Methods in Enzymology,* Vol.382, pp. 473-487

Beal, M.F. (2005). Mitochondria take center stage in aging and neurodegeneration. *Annals of Neurology,* Vol.58, pp. 495-505

Benecke, R.; Strumper, P.& Weiss, H. (1993). Electron transfer complexes I and IV of platelets are abnormal in Parkinson's disease but normal in Parkinson-plus syndromes. *Brain,* Vol.116 (Pt 6), pp. 1451-1463

Betarbet, R.; Sherer, T.B.; MacKenzie, G.; Garcia-Osuna, M.; Panov, A.V.& Greenamyre, J.T. (2000). Chronic systemic pesticide exposure reproduces features of Parkinson's disease. *Nature Neuroscience,* Vol.3, pp. 1301-1306

Bharat, S.; Cochran, B.C.; Hsu, M.; Liu, J.; Ames, B.N.& Andersen, J.K. (2002). Pre-treatment with R-lipoic acid alleviates the effects of GSH depletion in PC12 cells: implications for Parkinson's disease therapy. *Neurotoxicology,* Vol.23, pp. 479-486

Bindoff, L.A.; Birch-Machin, M.A.; Cartlidge, N.E.; Parker, W.D., Jr.& Turnbull, D.M. (1991). Respiratory chain abnormalities in skeletal muscle from patients with Parkinson's disease. *Journal of the Neurological Sciences,* Vol.104, pp. 203-208

Blin, O.; Desnuelle, C.; Rascol, O.; Borg, M.; Peyro Saint Paul, H.; Azulay, J.P.; Bille, F.; Figarella, D.; Coulom, F.; Pellissier, J.F.& et al. (1994). Mitochondrial respiratory failure in skeletal muscle from patients with Parkinson's disease and multiple system atrophy. *Journal of the Neurological Sciences,* Vol.125, pp. 95-101

Bogaerts, V.; Theuns, J.& van Broeckhoven, C. (2008). Genetic findings in Parkinson's disease and translation into treatment: a leading role for mitochondria? *Genes, Brain and behavior,* Vol.7, pp. 129-151

Bordet, R.; Gele, P.; Duriez, P.& Fruchart, J.C. (2006). PPARs: a new target for neuroprotection. *Journal of Neurology, Neurosurgery and Psychiatry,* Vol.77, pp. 285-287

Bove, J.; Prou, D.; Perier, C.& Przedborski, S. (2005). Toxin-induced models of Parkinson's disease. *NeuroRx,* Vol.2, pp. 484-494

Breidert, T.; Callebert, J.; Heneka, M.T.; Landreth, G.; Launay, J.M.& Hirsch, E.C. (2002). Protective action of the peroxisome proliferator-activated receptor-gamma agonist pioglitazone in a mouse model of Parkinson's disease. *Journal of Neurochemistry,* Vol.82, pp. 615-624

Buckman, T.D.; Chang, R.; Sutphin, M.S.& Eiduson, S. (1988). Interaction of 1-methyl-4-phenylpyridinium ion with human platelets. *Biochemical and Biophysical Research Communications,* Vol.151, pp. 897-904

Cardellach, F.; Marti, M.J.; Fernandez-Sola, J.; Marin, C.; Hoek, J.B.; Tolosa, E.& Urbano-Marquez, A. (1993). Mitochondrial respiratory chain activity in skeletal muscle from patients with Parkinson's disease. *Neurology,* Vol.43, pp. 2258-2262

Chiba, K.; Trevor, A.& Castagnoli, N., Jr. (1984). Metabolism of the neurotoxic tertiary amine, MPTP, by brain monoamine oxidase. *Biochemical and Biophysical Research Communications,* Vol.120, pp. 574-578

Chinta, S.J. & Andersen, J.K. (2006). Reversible inhibition of mitochondrial complex I activity following chronic dopaminergic glutathione depletion in vitro: implications for Parkinson's disease. *Free Radical Biology and Medicine,* Vol.41, pp. 1442-1448

Cornille, E.; Abou-Hamdan, M.; Khrestchatisky, M.; Nieoullon, A.; de Reggi, M.& Gharib, B. (2010). Enhancement of L-3-hydroxybutyryl-CoA dehydrogenase activity and circulating ketone body levels by pantethine. Relevance to dopaminergic injury. *BMC Neuroscience,* Vol.11, pp. 51

Dawson, T.M. (2006). Parkin and defective ubiquitination in Parkinson's disease. *Journal of Neural Transmission Supplementa,* pp. 209-213

Dehmer, T.; Heneka, M.T.; Sastre, M.; Dichgans, J.& Schulz, J.B. (2004). Protection by pioglitazone in the MPTP model of Parkinson's disease correlates with I kappa B alpha induction and block of NF kappa B and iNOS activation. *Journal of Neurochemistry*, Vol.88, pp. 494-501

Di Lisa, F.; Bobyleva-Guarriero, V.; Jocelyn, P.; Toninello, A.& Siliprandi, N. (1985). Stabilising action of carnitine on energy linked processes in rat liver mitochondria. *Biochemical and Biophysical Research Communications*, Vol.131, pp. 968-973

DiDonato, S.; Zeviani, M.; Giovannini, P.; Savarese, N.; Rimoldi, M.; Mariotti, C.; Girotti, F.& Caraceni, T. (1993). Respiratory chain and mitochondrial DNA in muscle and brain in Parkinson's disease patients. *Neurology*, Vol.43, pp. 2262-2268

Eaton, S.; Bursby, T.; Middleton, B.; Pourfarzam, M.; Mills, K.; Johnson, A.W.& Bartlett, K. (2000). The mitochondrial trifunctional protein: centre of a beta-oxidation metabolon? *Biochemical Society Transactions*, Vol.28, pp. 177-182

Eliasson, M.J.; Sampei, K.; Mandir, A.S.; Hurn, P.D.; Traystman, R.J.; Bao, J.; Pieper, A.; Wang, Z.Q.; Dawson, T.M.; Snyder, S.H.& Dawson, V.L. (1997). Poly(ADP-ribose) polymerase gene disruption renders mice resistant to cerebral ischemia. *Nature Medicine*, Vol.3, pp. 1089-1095

Escartin, C.; Valette, J.; Lebon, V.& Bonvento, G. (2006). Neuron-astrocyte interactions in the regulation of brain energy metabolism: a focus on NMR spectroscopy. *Journal of Neurochemistry*, Vol.99, pp. 393-401

Farrer, M.; Chan, P.; Chen, R.; Tan, L.; Lincoln, S.; Hernandez, D.; Forno, L.; Gwinn-Hardy, K.; Petrucelli, L.; Hussey, J.; Singleton, A.; Tanner, C.; Hardy, J.& Langston, J.W. (2001). Lewy bodies and parkinsonism in families with parkin mutations. *Annals of Neurology*, Vol.50, pp. 293-300

Frankhauser, P.; Grimmer, Y.; Bugert, P.; Deuschle, M.; Schmidt, M.& Schloss, P. (2006). Characterization of the neuronal dopamine transporter DAT in human blood platelets. *Neuroscience Letters*, Vol.399, pp. 197-201

Freeman, J.; Veggiotti, P.; Lanzi, G.; Tagliabue, A.& Perucca, E. (2006). The ketogenic diet: from molecular mechanisms to clinical effects. *Epilepsy Research*, Vol.68, pp. 145-180

Furuta, S.; Kobayashi, A.; Miyazawa, S.& Hashimoto, T. (1997). Cloning and expression of cDNA for a newly identified isozyme of bovine liver 3-hydroxyacyl-CoA dehydrogenase and its import into mitochondria. *Biochimica et Biophysica Acta*, Vol.1350, pp. 317-324

Gandhi, S.; Wood-Kaczmar, A.; Yao, Z.; Plun-Favreau, H.; Deas, E.; Klupsch, K.; Downward, J.; Latchman, D.S.; Tabrizi, S.J.; Wood, N.W.; Duchen, M.R.& Abramov, A.Y. (2009). PINK1-associated Parkinson's disease is caused by neuronal vulnerability to calcium-induced cell death. *Molecular Cell*, Vol.33, pp. 627-638

Greenamyre, J.T.; Betarbet, R.& Sherer, T.B. (2003). The rotenone model of Parkinson's disease: genes, environment and mitochondria. *Parkinsonism and Related Disorders*, Vol.9 Suppl 2, pp. S59-64

Guzman, M. & Blazquez, C. (2001). Is there an astrocyte-neuron ketone body shuttle? *Trends Endocrinol Metab*, Vol.12, pp. 169-173

Haas, R.H.; Nasirian, F.; Nakano, K.; Ward, D.; Pay, M.; Hill, R.& Shults, C.W. (1995). Low platelet mitochondrial complex I and complex II/III activity in early untreated Parkinson's disease. *Annals of Neurology*, Vol.37, pp. 714-722

Hagen, T.M.; Ingersoll, R.T.; Lykkesfeldt, J.; Liu, J.; Wehr, C.M.; Vinarsky, V.; Bartholomew, J.C.& Ames, A.B. (1999). (R)-alpha-lipoic acid-supplemented old rats have improved mitochondrial function, decreased oxidative damage, and increased metabolic rate. *Faseb Journal,* Vol.13, pp. 411-418

Hattingen, E.; Magerkurth, J.; Pilatus, U.; Mozer, A.; Seifried, C.; Steinmetz, H.; Zanella, F.& Hilker, R. (2009). Phosphorus and proton magnetic resonance spectroscopy demonstrates mitochondrial dysfunction in early and advanced Parkinson's disease. *Brain,* Vol.132, pp. 3285-3297

Heikkila, R.E.; Manzino, L.; Cabbat, F.S.& Duvoisin, R.C. (1984). Protection against the dopaminergic neurotoxicity of 1-methyl-4-phenyl-1,2,5,6-tetrahydropyridine by monoamine oxidase inhibitors. *Nature,* Vol.311, pp. 467-469

Henchcliffe, C. & Beal, M.F. (2008). Mitochondrial biology and oxidative stress in Parkinson disease pathogenesis. *Nature Clinical Practive Neurology,* Vol.4, pp. 600-609

Henchcliffe, C.; Shungu, D.C.; Mao, X.; Huang, C.; Nirenberg, M.J.; Jenkins, B.G.& Beal, M.F. (2008). Multinuclear magnetic resonance spectroscopy for in vivo assessment of mitochondrial dysfunction in Parkinson's disease. *Annals of the New York Academy of Sciences,* Vol.1147, pp. 206-220

Heneka, M.T. & Landreth, G.E. (2007). PPARs in the brain. *Biochimica et Biophysica Acta,* Vol.1771, pp. 1031-1045

Hertz, L. (2004). The astrocyte-neuron lactate shuttle: a challenge of a challenge. *Journal of Cerebral Blood Flow and Metabolism,* Vol.24, pp. 1241-1248

Herzig, S.; Long, F.; Jhala, U.S.; Hedrick, S.; Quinn, R.; Bauer, A.; Rudolph, D.; Schutz, G.; Yoon, C.; Puigserver, P.; Spiegelman, B.& Montminy, M. (2001). CREB regulates hepatic gluconeogenesis through the coactivator PGC-1. *Nature,* Vol.413, pp. 179-183

Imamura, K.; Takeshima, T.; Kashiwaya, Y.; Nakaso, K.& Nakashima, K. (2006). D-beta-hydroxybutyrate protects dopaminergic SH-SY5Y cells in a rotenone model of Parkinson's disease. *Journal of Neuroscience Research,* Vol.84, pp. 1376-1384

Izumi, Y.; Ishii, K.; Katsuki, H.; Benz, A.M.& Zorumski, C.F. (1998). beta-Hydroxybutyrate fuels synaptic function during development. Histological and physiological evidence in rat hippocampal slices. *Journal of Clinical Investigation,* Vol.101, pp. 1121-1132

Javitch, J.A.; D'Amato, R.J.; Strittmatter, S.M.& Snyder, S.H. (1985). Parkinsonism-inducing neurotoxin, N-methyl-4-phenyl-1,2,3,6 -tetrahydropyridine: uptake of the metabolite N-methyl-4-phenylpyridine by dopamine neurons explains selective toxicity. *Proceedings of the National Academy of Sciences of the U S A,* Vol.82, pp. 2173-2177

Jha, N.; Jurma, O.; Lalli, G.; Liu, Y.; Pettus, E.H.; Greenamyre, J.T.; Liu, R.M.; Forman, H.J.& Andersen, J.K. (2000). Glutathione depletion in PC12 results in selective inhibition of mitochondrial complex I activity. Implications for Parkinson's disease. *Journal of Biological Chemistry,* Vol.275, pp. 26096-26101

Jornvall, H.; Persson, B.; Krook, M.; Atrian, S.; Gonzalez-Duarte, R.; Jeffery, J.& Ghosh, D. (1995). Short-chain dehydrogenases/reductases (SDR). *Biochemistry,* Vol.34, pp. 6003-6013

Kashiwaya, Y.; Takeshima, T.; Mori, N.; Nakashima, K.; Clarke, K.& Veech, R.L. (2000). D-beta-hydroxybutyrate protects neurons in models of Alzheimer's and Parkinson's disease. *Proceedings of the National Academy of Sciences of the U S A,* Vol.97, pp. 5440-5444

Keeney, P.M.; Xie, J.; Capaldi, R.A.& Bennett, J.P., Jr. (2006). Parkinson's disease brain mitochondrial complex I has oxidatively damaged subunits and is functionally impaired and misassembled. *J Neurosci,* Vol.26, pp. 5256-5264

Kobayashi, A.; Jiang, L.L.& Hashimoto, T. (1996). Two mitochondrial 3-hydroxyacyl-CoA dehydrogenases in bovine liver. *J Biochem,* Vol.119, pp. 775-782

Krige, D.; Carroll, M.T.; Cooper, J.M.; Marsden, C.D.& Schapira, A.H. (1992). Platelet mitochondrial function in Parkinson's disease. The Royal Kings and Queens Parkinson Disease Research Group. *Annals of Neurology,* Vol.32, pp. 782-788

Langston, J.W.; Ballard, P.; Tetrud, J.W.& Irwin, I. (1983). Chronic Parkinsonism in humans due to a product of meperidine-analog synthesis. *Science,* Vol.219, pp. 979-980

Lehman, J.J.; Barger, P.M.; Kovacs, A.; Saffitz, J.E.; Medeiros, D.M.& Kelly, D.P. (2000). Peroxisome proliferator-activated receptor gamma coactivator-1 promotes cardiac mitochondrial biogenesis. *Journal of Clinical Investigation,* Vol.106, pp. 847-856

Leone, T.C.; Lehman, J.J.; Finck, B.N.; Schaeffer, P.J.; Wende, A.R.; Boudina, S.; Courtois, M.; Wozniak, D.F.; Sambandam, N.; Bernal-Mizrachi, C.; Chen, Z.; Holloszy, J.O.; Medeiros, D.M.; Schmidt, R.E.; Saffitz, J.E.; Abel, E.D.; Semenkovich, C.F.& Kelly, D.P. (2005). PGC-1alpha deficiency causes multi-system energy metabolic derangements: muscle dysfunction, abnormal weight control and hepatic steatosis. *PLoS Biolology,* Vol.3, pp. e101

Li, N.; Ragheb, K.; Lawler, G.; Sturgis, J.; Rajwa, B.; Melendez, J.A.& Robinson, J.P. (2003). Mitochondrial complex I inhibitor rotenone induces apoptosis through enhancing mitochondrial reactive oxygen species production. *Journal of Biological Chemistry,* Vol.278, pp. 8516-8525

Lin, J.; Wu, H.; Tarr, P.T.; Zhang, C.Y.; Wu, Z.; Boss, O.; Michael, L.F.; Puigserver, P.; Isotani, E.; Olson, E.N.; Lowell, B.B.; Bassel-Duby, R.& Spiegelman, B.M. (2002). Transcriptional co-activator PGC-1 alpha drives the formation of slow-twitch muscle fibres. *Nature,* Vol.418, pp. 797-801

Lin, J.; Wu, P.H.; Tarr, P.T.; Lindenberg, K.S.; St-Pierre, J.; Zhang, C.Y.; Mootha, V.K.; Jager, S.; Vianna, C.R.; Reznick, R.M.; Cui, L.; Manieri, M.; Donovan, M.X.; Wu, Z.; Cooper, M.P.; Fan, M.C.; Rohas, L.M.; Zavacki, A.M.; Cinti, S.; Shulman, G.I.; Lowell, B.B.; Krainc, D.& Spiegelman, B.M. (2004). Defects in adaptive energy metabolism with CNS-linked hyperactivity in PGC-1alpha null mice. *Cell,* Vol.119, pp. 121-135

Lucking, C.B.; Durr, A.; Bonifati, V.; Vaughan, J.; De Michele, G.; Gasser, T.; Harhangi, B.S.; Meco, G.; Denefle, P.; Wood, N.W.; Agid, Y.& Brice, A. (2000). Association between early-onset Parkinson's disease and mutations in the parkin gene. *New England Journal of Medicine,* Vol.342, pp. 1560-1567

Maalouf, M.; Rho, J.M.& Mattson, M.P. (2009). The neuroprotective properties of calorie restriction, the ketogenic diet, and ketone bodies. *Brain Research Reviews,* Vol.59, pp. 293-315

Mandir, A.S.; Przedborski, S.; Jackson-Lewis, V.; Wang, Z.Q.; Simbulan-Rosenthal, C.M.; Smulson, M.E.; Hoffman, B.E.; Guastella, D.B.; Dawson, V.L.& Dawson, T.M. (1999). Poly(ADP-ribose) polymerase activation mediates 1-methyl-4-phenyl-1,

2,3,6-tetrahydropyridine (MPTP)-induced parkinsonism. *Proceedings of the National Academy of Sciences of the U S A*, Vol.96, pp. 5774-5779

Mann, V.M.; Cooper, J.M.; Krige, D.; Daniel, S.E.; Schapira, A.H.& Marsden, C.D. (1992). Brain, skeletal muscle and platelet homogenate mitochondrial function in Parkinson's disease. *Brain*, Vol.115 (Pt 2), pp. 333-342

Martin, M.A.; Molina, J.A.; Jimenez-Jimenez, F.J.; Benito-Leon, J.; Orti-Pareja, M.; Campos, Y.& Arenas, J. (1996). Respiratory-chain enzyme activities in isolated mitochondria of lymphocytes from untreated Parkinson's disease patients. Grupo-Centro de Trastornos del Movimiento. *Neurology*, Vol.46, pp. 1343-1346

Matthews, R.T.; Ferrante, R.J.; Klivenyi, P.; Yang, L.; Klein, A.M.; Mueller, G.; Kaddurah-Daouk, R.& Beal, M.F. (1999). Creatine and cyclocreatine attenuate MPTP neurotoxicity. *Experimental Neurology*, Vol.157, pp. 142-149

McEwen, B.S. & Reagan, L.P. (2004). Glucose transporter expression in the central nervous system: relationship to synaptic function. *European Journal of Pharmacology*, Vol.490, pp. 13-24

Mizuno, Y.; Sone, N.; Suzuki, K.& Saitoh, T. (1988a). Studies on the toxicity of 1-methyl-4-phenylpyridinium ion (MPP+) against mitochondria of mouse brain. *Journal of the Neurological Sciences*, Vol.86, pp. 97-110

Mizuno, Y.; Suzuki, K.; Sone, N.& Saitoh, T. (1988b). Inhibition of mitochondrial respiration by 1-methyl-4-phenyl-1,2,3,6-tetrahydropyridine (MPTP) in mouse brain in vivo. *Neuroscience Letters*, Vol.91, pp. 349-353

Moore, D.J. (2006). Parkin: a multifaceted ubiquitin ligase. *Biochemical Society Transactions*, Vol.34, pp. 749-753

Morisaki, N.; Matsuoka, N.; Shirai, K.; Sasaki, N.; Saito, Y.& Kumagai, A. (1983). Effect of pantethine on fatty acid oxidation in microvessels of rat brain. *Tohoku Journal of Experimental Medicine*, Vol.141, pp. 41-45

Nicklas, W.J.; Vyas, I.& Heikkila, R.E. (1985). Inhibition of NADH-linked oxidation in brain mitochondria by 1-methyl-4-phenyl-pyridine, a metabolite of the neurotoxin, 1-methyl-4-phenyl-1,2,5,6-tetrahydropyridine. *Life Sciences*, Vol.36, pp. 2503-2508

Paisan-Ruiz, C.; Jain, S.; Evans, E.W.; Gilks, W.P.; Simon, J.; van der Brug, M.; Lopez de Munain, A.; Aparicio, S.; Gil, A.M.; Khan, N.; Johnson, J.; Martinez, J.R.; Nicholl, D.; Carrera, I.M.; Pena, A.S.; de Silva, R.; Lees, A.; Marti-Masso, J.F.; Perez-Tur, J.; Wood, N.W.& Singleton, A.B. (2004). Cloning of the gene containing mutations that cause PARK8-linked Parkinson's disease. *Neuron*, Vol.44, pp. 595-600

Parker, W.D., Jr.; Parks, J.K.& Swerdlow, R.H. (2008). Complex I deficiency in Parkinson's disease frontal cortex. *Brain Research*, Vol.1189, pp. 215-218

Pei, Z.; Pang, H.; Qian, L.; Yang, S.; Wang, T.; Zhang, W.; Wu, X.; Dallas, S.; Wilson, B.; Reece, J.M.; Miller, D.S.; Hong, J.S.& Block, M.L. (2007). MAC1 mediates LPS-induced production of superoxide by microglia: the role of pattern recognition receptors in dopaminergic neurotoxicity. *Glia*, Vol.55, pp. 1362-1373

Plecko, B.; Stoeckler-Ipsiroglu, S.; Schober, E.; Harrer, G.; Mlynarik, V.; Gruber, S.; Moser, E.; Moeslinger, D.; Silgoner, H.& Ipsiroglu, O. (2002). Oral beta-hydroxybutyrate supplementation in two patients with hyperinsulinemic hypoglycemia: monitoring of beta-hydroxybutyrate levels in blood and cerebrospinal fluid, and in the brain by in vivo magnetic resonance spectroscopy. *Pediatric Research*, Vol.52, pp. 301-306

Prins, M.L. (2008). Cerebral metabolic adaptation and ketone metabolism after brain injury. *Journal of Cerebral Blood Flow and Metabolism,* Vol.28, pp. 1-16

Przedborski, S. (2005). Pathogenesis of nigral cell death in Parkinson's disease. *Parkinsonism and Related Disorders,* Vol.11 Suppl 1, pp. S3-7

Przedborski, S. & Ischiropoulos, H. (2005). Reactive oxygen and nitrogen species: weapons of neuronal destruction in models of Parkinson's disease. *Antioxidants and Redox Signaling,* Vol.7, pp. 685-693

Przedborski, S.; Tieu, K.; Perier, C.& Vila, M. (2004). MPTP as a mitochondrial neurotoxic model of Parkinson's disease. *Journal of Bioenergetics and Biomembranes,* Vol.36, pp. 375-379

Puigserver, P.; Rhee, J.; Donovan, J.; Walkey, C.J.; Yoon, J.C.; Oriente, F.; Kitamura, Y.; Altomonte, J.; Dong, H.; Accili, D.& Spiegelman, B.M. (2003). Insulin-regulated hepatic gluconeogenesis through FOXO1-PGC-1alpha interaction. *Nature,* Vol.423, pp. 550-555

Puigserver, P.; Wu, Z.; Park, C.W.; Graves, R.; Wright, M.& Spiegelman, B.M. (1998). A cold-inducible coactivator of nuclear receptors linked to adaptive thermogenesis. *Cell,* Vol.92, pp. 829-839

Ramsay, R.R.; Salach, J.I.; Dadgar, J.& Singer, T.P. (1986a). Inhibition of mitochondrial NADH dehydrogenase by pyridine derivatives and its possible relation to experimental and idiopathic parkinsonism. *Biochemical and Biophysical Research Communications,* Vol.135, pp. 269-275

Ramsay, R.R.; Salach, J.I.& Singer, T.P. (1986b). Uptake of the neurotoxin 1-methyl-4-phenylpyridine (MPP+) by mitochondria and its relation to the inhibition of the mitochondrial oxidation of NAD+-linked substrates by MPP+. *Biochemical and Biophysical Research Communications,* Vol.134, pp. 743-748

Rana, A.; Seinen, E.; Siudeja, K.; Muntendam, R.; Srinivasan, B.; van der Want, J.J.; Hayflick, S.; Reijngoud, D.J.; Kayser, O.& Sibon, O.C. (2010). Pantethine rescues a Drosophila model for pantothenate kinase-associated neurodegeneration. *Proceedings of the National Academy of Sciences of the U S A,* Vol.107, pp. 6988-6993

Reddy, H.K.; Koshy, S.K.; Wasson, S.; Quan, E.E.; Pagni, S.; Roberts, A.M.; Joshua, I.G.& Tyagi, S.C. (2006). Adaptive-outward and maladaptive-inward arterial remodeling measured by intravascular ultrasound in hyperhomocysteinemia and diabetes. *Journal of Cardiovascular Pharmacology and Therapeutics,* Vol.11, pp. 65-76

Reddy, J.K. (2001). Nonalcoholic steatosis and steatohepatitis. III. Peroxisomal beta-oxidation, PPAR alpha, and steatohepatitis. *American Journal of Physiology. Gastrointestinal and Liver Physiology,* Vol.281, pp. G1333-1339

Reichmann, H.; Janetzky, B.; Bischof, F.; Seibel, P.; Schols, L.; Kuhn, W.& Przuntek, H. (1994). Unaltered respiratory chain enzyme activity and mitochondrial DNA in skeletal muscle from patients with idiopathic Parkinson's syndrome. *European Neurology,* Vol.34, pp. 263-267

Rhee, J.; Inoue, Y.; Yoon, J.C.; Puigserver, P.; Fan, M.; Gonzalez, F.J.& Spiegelman, B.M. (2003). Regulation of hepatic fasting response by PPARgamma coactivator-1alpha (PGC-1): requirement for hepatocyte nuclear factor 4alpha in gluconeogenesis. *Proceedings of the National Academy of Sciences of the U S A,* Vol.100, pp. 4012-4017

Richardson, J.R.; Quan, Y.; Sherer, T.B.; Greenamyre, J.T.& Miller, G.W. (2005). Paraquat neurotoxicity is distinct from that of MPTP and rotenone. *Toxicological Sciences,* Vol.88, pp. 193-201

Rosenthal, R.E.; Chanderbhan, R.; Marshall, G.& Fiskum, G. (1992). Prevention of post-ischemic brain lipid conjugated diene production and neurological injury by hydroxyethyl starch-conjugated deferoxamine. *Free Radical Biology and Medicine,* Vol.12, pp. 29-33

Saraste, M. (1999). Oxidative phosphorylation at the fin de siecle. *Science,* Vol.283, pp. 1488-1493

Schapira, A.H. (2006). Mitochondrial disease. *Lancet,* Vol.368, pp. 70-82

Schapira, A.H.; Cooper, J.M.; Dexter, D.; Jenner, P.; Clark, J.B.& Marsden, C.D. (1989). Mitochondrial complex I deficiency in Parkinson's disease. *Lancet,* Vol.1, pp. 1269

Schultz, B.E. & Chan, S.I. (2001). Structures and proton-pumping strategies of mitochondrial respiratory enzymes. *Annual Review of Biophysics and Biomolecular Structure,* Vol.30, pp. 23-65

Schurr, A. (2006). Lactate: the ultimate cerebral oxidative energy substrate? *Journal of Cerebral Blood Flow & Metabolism,* Vol.26, pp. 142-152

Sherer, T.B.; Betarbet, R.; Testa, C.M.; Seo, B.B.; Richardson, J.R.; Kim, J.H.; Miller, G.W.; Yagi, T.; Matsuno-Yagi, A.& Greenamyre, J.T. (2003). Mechanism of toxicity in rotenone models of Parkinson's disease. *J Neurosci,* Vol.23, pp. 10756-10764

Shults, C.W.; Oakes, D.; Kieburtz, K.; Beal, M.F.; Haas, R.; Plumb, S.; Juncos, J.L.; Nutt, J.; Shoulson, I.; Carter, J.; Kompoliti, K.; Perlmutter, J.S.; Reich, S.; Stern, M.; Watts, R.L.; Kurlan, R.; Molho, E.; Harrison, M.& Lew, M. (2002). Effects of coenzyme Q10 in early Parkinson disease: evidence of slowing of the functional decline. *Archives of Neurology,* Vol.59, pp. 1541-1550

Snyder, J.W.; Kyle, M.E.& Ferraro, T.N. (1990). L-carnitine delays the killing of cultured hepatocytes by 1-methyl-4-phenyl-1,2,3,6-tetrahydropyridine. *Archives of Biochemistry and Biophysics,* Vol.276, pp. 132-138

Sriram, K.; Shankar, S.K.; Boyd, M.R.& Ravindranath, V. (1998). Thiol oxidation and loss of mitochondrial complex I precede excitatory amino acid-mediated neurodegeneration. *J Neurosci,* Vol.18, pp. 10287-10296

St-Pierre, J.; Drori, S.; Uldry, M.; Silvaggi, J.M.; Rhee, J.; Jager, S.; Handschin, C.; Zheng, K.; Lin, J.; Yang, W.; Simon, D.K.; Bachoo, R.& Spiegelman, B.M. (2006). Suppression of reactive oxygen species and neurodegeneration by the PGC-1 transcriptional coactivators. *Cell,* Vol.127, pp. 397-408

Tieu, K.; Perier, C.; Caspersen, C.; Teismann, P.; Wu, D.C.; Yan, S.D.; Naini, A.; Vila, M.; Jackson-Lewis, V.; Ramasamy, R.& Przedborski, S. (2003). D-beta-hydroxybutyrate rescues mitochondrial respiration and mitigates features of Parkinson disease. *Journal of Clinical Investigation,* Vol.112, pp. 892-901

Tieu, K.; Perier, C.; Vila, M.; Caspersen, C.; Zhang, H.P.; Teismann, P.; Jackson-Lewis, V.; Stern, D.M.; Yan, S.D.& Przedborski, S. (2004). L-3-hydroxyacyl-CoA dehydrogenase II protects in a model of Parkinson's disease. *Annals of Neurology,* Vol.56, pp. 51-60

Trumpower, B.L. (1990). The protonmotive Q cycle. Energy transduction by coupling of proton translocation to electron transfer by the cytochrome bc1 complex. *Journal of Biological Chemistry,* Vol.265, pp. 11409-11412

Valente, E.M.; Abou-Sleiman, P.M.; Caputo, V.; Muqit, M.M.; Harvey, K.; Gispert, S.; Ali, Z.; Del Turco, D.; Bentivoglio, A.R.; Healy, D.G.; Albanese, A.; Nussbaum, R.; Gonzalez-Maldonado, R.; Deller, T.; Salvi, S.; Cortelli, P.; Gilks, W.P.; Latchman, D.S.; Harvey, R.J.; Dallapiccola, B.; Auburger, G.& Wood, N.W. (2004). Hereditary early-onset Parkinson's disease caused by mutations in PINK1. *Science,* Vol.304, pp. 1158-1160

Vannucci, S.J.; Maher, F.& Simpson, I.A. (1997). Glucose transporter proteins in brain: delivery of glucose to neurons and glia. *Glia,* Vol.21, pp. 2-21

Virmani, M.A.; Biselli, R.; Spadoni, A.; Rossi, S.; Corsico, N.; Calvani, M.; Fattorossi, A.; De Simone, C.& Arrigoni-Martelli, E. (1995). Protective actions of L-carnitine and acetyl-L-carnitine on the neurotoxicity evoked by mitochondrial uncoupling or inhibitors. *Pharmacological Research,* Vol.32, pp. 383-389

Wallace, D.C.; Shoffner, J.M.; Watts, R.L.; Juncos, J.L.& Torroni, A. (1992). Mitochondrial oxidative phosphorylation defects in Parkinson's disease. *Annals of Neurology,* Vol.32, pp. 113-114

Winklhofer, K.F. & Haass, C. (2010). Mitochondrial dysfunction in Parkinson's disease. *Biochimica et Biophysica Acta,* Vol.1802, pp. 29-44

Woods, J.W.; Tanen, M.; Figueroa, D.J.; Biswas, C.; Zycband, E.; Moller, D.E.; Austin, C.P.& Berger, J.P. (2003). Localization of PPARdelta in murine central nervous system: expression in oligodendrocytes and neurons. *Brain Research,* Vol.975, pp. 10-21

Wu, Z.; Puigserver, P.; Andersson, U.; Zhang, C.; Adelmant, G.; Mootha, V.; Troy, A.; Cinti, S.; Lowell, B.; Scarpulla, R.C.& Spiegelman, B.M. (1999). Mechanisms controlling mitochondrial biogenesis and respiration through the thermogenic coactivator PGC-1. *Cell,* Vol.98, pp. 115-124

Yang, S.Y.; He, X.Y.& Schulz, H. (2005). 3-Hydroxyacyl-CoA dehydrogenase and short chain 3-hydroxyacyl-CoA dehydrogenase in human health and disease. *FEBS Journal,* Vol.272, pp. 4874-4883

Yoon, J.C.; Puigserver, P.; Chen, G.; Donovan, J.; Wu, Z.; Rhee, J.; Adelmant, G.; Stafford, J.; Kahn, C.R.; Granner, D.K.; Newgard, C.B.& Spiegelman, B.M. (2001). Control of hepatic gluconeogenesis through the transcriptional coactivator PGC-1. *Nature,* Vol.413, pp. 131-138

Yoshino, H.; Nakagawa-Hattori, Y.; Kondo, T.& Mizuno, Y. (1992). Mitochondrial complex I and II activities of lymphocytes and platelets in Parkinson's disease. *Journal of Neural Transmission.Parkinson's disease and Dementia Section,* Vol.4, pp. 27-34

Zheng, B. et al. (2010). PGC-1alpha, a potential therapeutic target for early intervention in Parkinson's disease. *Science Translational Medicine,* Vol.2, pp. 52ra73

Zimprich, A. et al.(2004). Mutations in LRRK2 cause autosomal-dominant parkinsonism with pleomorphic pathology. *Neuron,* Vol.44, pp. 601-607

Zschocke, J.; Ruiter, J.P.; Brand, J.; Lindner, M.; Hoffmann, G.F.; Wanders, R.J.& Mayatepek, E. (2000). Progressive infantile neurodegeneration caused by 2-methyl-3-hydroxybutyryl-CoA dehydrogenase deficiency: a novel inborn error of branched-chain fatty acid and isoleucine metabolism. *Pediatric Research,* Vol.48, pp. 852-855

13

Analysis of Transcriptome Alterations in Parkinson's Disease

Elena Filatova, Maria Shadrina, Petr Slominsky and Svetlana Limborska
Institute of Molecular Genetics Russian Academy of Sciences, Russian Federation

1. Introduction

The information that stems from the primary structure of DNA lies within the basis of every sign formation, although the regulation of any process occurs in different levels of cellular processes including transcription. In this context analysis of gene transcription is of great importance to improve our understanding of the pathogenesis of diverse disorders, and Parkinson's disease (PD) is not an exception. However, each disease has its own unique etiopathogenesis within organs and tissues, which is caused by disease-specific processes in cells, as well as at the genetic level. Knowledge of the etiology and pathogenesis of diseases at a cellular level opens wide prospects for diagnosis and treatment, even for complex and incurable disorders such as PD. Therefore, it is necessary to study the pathogenesis of specific disease at the cellular and genetic levels. Accordingly, the expression profiles of large numbers of genes are being studied in different neurodegenerative disorders, including PD. Although the mechanisms that initiate neuronal pathology in sporadic PD remain largely obscure, in this chapter we have tried to summarize all current knowledge in the field of the PD transcriptomics.

2. Analysis of gene expression in PD

2.1 Analysis of gene expression in brain tissues

The general approach in studying gene expression in PD is the analysis of transcript levels in tissues of the brain (the main organ that is affected in PD), which exhibit lesions that result in symptoms of PD. Unfortunately, only post-mortem tissues can be used in such studies. In addition, DNA microarrays are actively used in this type of study and there is a tendency to combine these data with the results of genome-wide association studies (GWAS) of single nucleotide polymorphisms (SNPs) and point mutations in PD (Elstner, 2009). Combined analysis allows the identification of a number of candidate genes for further study; therefore, residual genes are more likely involved in the pathogenesis of PD (Horan, 2009, Noureddine, 2005).

Thus, several tens of genes implicated in different metabolic pathways that are disturbed in PD have been identified during the analysis of transcription profiles in the substantia nigra of patients with PD. Mitochondrial dysfunction, oxidative stress, ubiquitin-proteasomal degradation of proteins, differentiation and functioning of dopaminergic (DA) neurons, DA metabolism, inflammation, apoptosis, and several other processes are among such metabolic pathways.

During the development of PD, there is a common tendency toward a decrease in the expression of genes that are involved in the pathogenesis of this disease (Table 1). According to some studies, the data expression of genes associated with mitochondrial functioning and oxidative stress (*PARK7* and *PINK*) is downregulated. Although the levels of expression of genes involved in the ubiquitin-proteasomal system (UPS) were both increased and decreased in neurons of patients with PD, the downregulation of these genes is predominant especially regarding the expression of genes associated with monogenic forms of PD: *SNCA, UCHL1,* and *ATP13A2*. In addition, a lower number of transcripts were observed for lysosomal genes (mainly genes encoding proton-transporting ATP synthases) (Bossers, 2009, Duke, 2006, Elstner, 2009, Hauser, 2005, Simunovic, 2010, Simunovic, 2009).

The very interesting work of Grünblatt and co-workers (Grünblatt, 2004) showed, for the first time, the global changes in gene expression in the substantia nigra pars compacta (SNpc) of postmortem parkinsonian brains compared with aged-matched controls. It was shown that major gene downregulation was observed in the signal transduction, protein degradation, dopaminergic transmission and metabolism, ion transport, and protein modification/phosphorylation, as well as in the energy pathways/glycolysis functional classes, in PD. Regarding genes that are upregulated differentially in PD, these cluster mainly in biological processes involving cell adhesion/cytoskeleton, extracellular-matrix components, cell cycle, protein modification/phosphorylation, protein metabolism, transcription, and inflammation/stress.

Similar results were obtained later by Simunovic et al. (Simunovic, 2009), as one can see in the Table 1. Their data show a set of deregulated genes that are directly or indirectly involved in programmed cell death (PCD) confirming the current concept of the apoptotic death of the DA neuron. In addition, data show a dysfunction of both mitochondria and the UPS, which are major contributors to PCD and the pathogenesis of Parkinson's disease (Duke, 2006). It should be noted that the expression of *SNCA*, a component of Lewy bodies and the pathologic accumulation of which is caused by oxidative stress, mitochondrial dysfunction, and impairment of cellular proteolytic mechanisms (Lundvig, 2005, as cited in Simunovic, 2009), was also deregulated.

The expression of genes involved in the differentiation, survival, and functioning of DA neurons also changes. There is evidence of decreased expression of the *NR4A2* transcription factor gene and of the *ST13* chaperone gene. *NR4A2* encodes a transcriptional factor that is required for the differentiation of postmitotic DA neurons and for the control of the expression of genes with protein products that are associated with DA synthesis and storage, notably, the tyrosine hydroxilase gene *TH*, the dopamine-transporter gene *SLC6A3*, the vesicular monoamine transporter gene *VMAT2*, and the amino acid decarboxylase gene *AADC* (Chinta & Andersen, 2005). In turn, decreased levels of expression of the *ALDH*, *ARPP-21* and *VMAT2* genes are also possible markers of PD. The latter six genes are directly involved in the synthesis, metabolism and functioning of DA. A decrease in their expression may seriously disturb neurotransmitter storage and correlate with DA neurons dysfunction. The *PDXK* gene is also directly involved in the synthesis of DA. The increase of the expression of this gene in DA neurons can be explained by an adaptive mechanism of enhancement of DA metabolism in the residually functioning DA neurons of the substantia nigra, or by L-DOPA treatment (Tan, 2005). In PD, the expression of DA receptors also changes: the level of expression of D3 is reduced by 40-45% in the nucleus accumbens and in the tegmentum, and the level of D2 is increased by 15% in the tegmentum (Ryoo, 1998, Simunovic, 2010).

Decrease of expression	Increase of expression	Reference
Mitochondrial functioning, oxidative phosphorylation		
Cytochrome c subunits genes		(Grünblatt, 2004, Simunovic, 2010, Simunovic, 2009)
NADH dehydrogenase subunits genes and NADH dehydrogenase-affecting proteins genes		(Bossers, 2009, Hauser, 2005, Simunovic, 2010, Simunovic, 2009)
	MTND2 (subunit of NADH dehydrogenase)	(Elstner, 2009)
proton-transporting ATP-synthase complex genes,		(Simunovic, 2010, Simunovic, 2009)
other genes related with mitochondrial dysfunction		(Bossers, 2009, Elstner, 2009, Hauser, 2005, Simunovic, 2010, Simunovic, 2009)
Oxidative stress		
Genes of different subunits of PIK3	Genes of different subunits of PIK3	(Grünblatt, 2004, Simunovic, 2009)
PINK1 и PARK7		(Simunovic, 2010, Simunovic, 2009)
Ubiquitin-proteasomal system of protein degradation, proteolysis/peptidolysis, lysosomes		
HIP2		(Grünblatt, 2004, Moran, 2006, Simunovic, 2010, Simunovic, 2009)
ATP6V1E1		(Grünblatt, 2004, Simunovic, 2009)
ATP13A2, RIMS3	*RIMS1*	(Simunovic, 2010, Simunovic, 2009)
SNCA		(Dachsel, 2007, Simunovic, 2010, Simunovic, 2009)
UCHL1		(Hauser, 2005, Simunovic, 2010, Simunovic, 2009)
SKP1A		(Grünblatt, 2004)
proton-transporting ATP-synthase complex genes		(Grünblatt, 2004, Simunovic, 2010, Simunovic, 2009)
Other genes involved in protein degradation, proteasome subunits genes		(Bossers, 2009, Grünblatt, 2004, Hauser, 2005, Simunovic, 2010, Simunovic, 2009)

Table 1. Alterations in the transcription of genes involved in different pathways in brain tissues (substantia nigra) of patients with Parkinson's disease.

Decrease of expression	Increase of expression	Reference
Cytoskeleton, adhesion		
TUBB2 (tubulins), genes coding different proteins from kinesin family		(Grünblatt, 2004, Simunovic, 2009)
Cytoskeleton, cell adhesion proteins genes	Cytoskeleton, cell adhesion proteins genes	(Grünblatt, 2004, Simunovic, 2009)
MAPT		(Simunovic, 2010)
Transcription, translation, chaperones, protein modification		
ST13		(Simunovic, 2010)
NR4A2		(Bossers, 2009, Simunovic, 2009)
Other genes involved in these pathways	Other genes involved in these pathways	(Grünblatt, 2004, Noureddine, 2005, Simunovic, 2009)
Signal transduction, synaptic transmission, neurotransmitters and neurotransmitter metabolism		
GABARAPL2	Neurotrasmitters receptors genes	(Grünblatt, 2004, Noureddine, 2005, Simunovic, 2009)
RIMS3		(Moran, 2006, Simunovic, 2010, Simunovic, 2009)
ALDH1A1	*PENK*	(Grünblatt, 2004)
SEC22L1, *ARPP-21*		(Grünblatt, 2004, Zhang, 2005)
	PDXK (DA synthesis)	(Duke, 2007, Elstner, 2009)
	SRGPA3 (Signal transduction)	(Elstner, 2009)
Genes involved in synaptic transmission		(Bossers, 2009, Noureddine, 2005, Simunovic, 2009)
Ion-channels genes	Ion-channels genes	(Simunovic, 2010, Simunovic, 2009)
Transport		
solute carrier family genes	solute carrier family genes	(Grünblatt, 2004, Simunovic, 2009)
Other transport protein genes *VMAT*	Other transport protein genes	(Grünblatt, 2004)
TRAPPC4		(Elstner, 2009)

Table 1. Alterations in the transcription of genes involved in different pathways in brain tissues (substantia nigra) of patients with Parkinson's disease (continuation).

The expression of genes involved in synaptic transmission and signal transduction is also altered in PD. Over the past years, there has been emerging evidence that the survival of DA neurons depends on their unique properties of electrical activity involving Na^+, K^+, and Ca^{2+} channels; moreover, the association between mitochondrial dysfunction and reactive oxygen species (ROS) production and K^+ and Ca^{2+} channel activation has been suspected as a major contributor to the pathogenesis Parkinson's disease (Michel, 2007 and Surmeier, 2007, as cited in Simunovic, 2009). Many molecules related to these mechanisms were shown as being deregulated in the data set (Simunovic, 2009). In addition, the calcium channel subunit b3 (CACNB3), the ATPase type 13A2 (PARK9), and several subunits of Ca^{2+} transporting ATPases (ATP2A3, ATP2B2, and ATP2C1) were downregulated in PD further substantiating the involvement of a deficit in organelle function and of Ca^{2+} sequestering. A decrease in the level of the transcripts of the GABA receptor genes (*GABRB1, GABARAPL1/3,* and *GABARAPL2*) has also been discovered in PD, supporting the previous suggestion that GABAergic synapses are reduced in the substantia nigra of Parkinson's disease brains, resulting in a reduction of DA neuron inhibition and an increase in neurotransmission and function of the remaining functional DA neurons (Miller & Federoff, 2005, as cited in Simunovic, 2009). In contrast, the expression of genes encoding glutamatergic, cholinergic, somatostatinergic, and dopaminergic receptors was increased (Simunovic, 2009). The deregulation of several genes pointed to impairment of synaptic function and plasticity; some of these genes were also identified in other studies, such as *SYNGR3, NSF, SV2B, SYN1, SYT1,* and dynamin (Miller, 2006). The genes that were deregulated in the study of Simunovic mediate important mechanisms involved in the maintenance of synaptic function and integrity, such as those encoding a number of proteins from the SNARE complex (priming of the synaptic vesicle and synaptic vesicle surface proteins), which play a role in vesicle binding and fusion to the plasma membrane (Brunger, 2005).

However, the genes and mechanisms described above do not cover the whole spectrum of possible pathogenetic pathways underlying the sporadic form of PD. Several authors observed the upregulation of genes involved in cell adhesion and cytoskeleton (*MAPT, PARVA* (parvin, alpha), *LGALS9,* and selectin ligand P (*SELPLG*)), components of extracellular matrix (genes encoding structural proteins and phosphorylating proteins), cell cycle, inflammatory stress, and induced apoptosis (*TRAF3,* TNF receptor-associated factor 3) (Table 1). Simunovic et al. (Simunovic, 2009) detected deregulation of microtubulin-associated genes, such as *MAPT, MAPRE1, TCP1* (which participate in the unfolding of translated proteins in the cytosol, such as actin and tubulin (Stirling, 2007, as cited in Simunovic, 2009)) and of multiple subunits of tubulin, but not of the microtubule-affinity regulating kinase (MARK1) and microtubule-associated protein (MAP2), as described elsewhere (Miller, 2006, Moran, 2007). Recently, the underexpression of a set of genes that are expressed in response to the *PPARGC1A* gene has also been shown in patients with PD in a genome-wide expression study (Zheng, 2010). Activation of *PPARGC1A* results in increased expression of nuclear-encoded subunits of the mitochondrial respiratory chain (Zechner, 2010). Taken together, the results of Simunovic and co-workers are consistent with other observations that point to a functional disconnect of the striatonigral trophic signaling pathways (Miller, 2006).

Currently, much data has been obtained regarding altered gene expression in brain tissues of patients with PD, especially in the substantia nigra. However, as can be seen in the studies described above, previous observations are reproduced rarely. Each study reports on different spectra of transcripts. The study of Moran et al. (Moran, 2006) is an exception, as it partly reproduced the results of Zhang et al. (Zhang, 2005), which can be explained by the fact that these authors used the same methods. Bossers et al. also replicated some of the results of Grünblatt et al. and Zhang et al. (*ALDH1A1, SNCA, UCHL1, VMAT2, GBE1* and *NR4A2*) (Bossers, 2009). However, Moran et al. admit that they could not confirm the data of Grünblatt and Hauser, although they found similar changes in the expression of some genes ,including *ALDH1A1* and *NR4A2*. Such difference probably can be explained by the diverse approaches in experimental design (different populations, different methods, and diverse comparison groups), despite the fact that all studies were performed using post-mortem samples of substantia nigra obtained from patients with PD.

Given the apparent lack of concordance among published data sets, one might wonder about the relevance of these transcriptional approaches regarding PD pathogenesis. Certainly, the use of post-mortem brain tissues appears to represent the best opportunity for finding PD-specific changes in gene expression. Furthermore, such "benchmarks" facilitate the evaluation of clinical samples and model systems for their utility in PD research. However, the approaches used to generate and analyse microarray data are not standardized; therefore, they could account for much of the apparent discrepancy observed among reported gene lists (Sutherland, 2009).

Nevertheless, despite the differences in individual gene expression data, many researchers report alterations in the expression profiles of whole groups of genes involved in specific cellular processes. Thus, a tendency toward downregulation of genes related to mitochondrial function and the ubiquitin-proteasomal system is observed, as well as the alteration of the expression of genes involved in oxidative stress, DA metabolism, transport proteins, microtubule-associated proteins of movement, and cytoskeletal proteins, thereby approving supposed picture of PD pathogenesis (Table 1). However, it is important to understand that alterations of expression likely represent late stages of PD (post mortem tissues) and cannot fully represent the entire pathogenesis of PD.

Case-control expression analysis in a degenerative disease like PD raises difficult issues when attempting to uncover pathways contributing to disease initiation. It would be advantageous to target tissues that express the proteins that are fundamental to the disease process and that are different in individuals who are at risk for the disease. At the same time, we need to account for any influences of the pathological process on these profiles. Microarray data of predilection brain sites, such as the SN, illustrate the cytoarchitectural differences between cases and controls; however, to understand some of the early pathogenic processes, ideally we would want to assay a brain region that is very similar to the SN but that is only affected belatedly.

The ability of the pathway approach that was used in the analyses of Sutherland and co-workers (Sutherland, 2009) to provide adequate specificity for PD over other neurodegenerative conditions is an additional consideration. This issue remains unclarified and requires further investigation. It is important to recognize that there may be genetic expression patterns that are common among neurodegenerative diseases in general. These may reflect common pathological changes (such as cell death, markers of oxidative stress or neuroinflammation, and etc) or shared risk factors that influence neurodegeneration. Inherent difficulties remain regarding the generation of reproducible gene expression data from post mortem brain, even if an optimal region of the brain could be assayed. Furthermore, this information can only be used retrospectively, for the potential benefit of future PD patients. Therefore, there is considerable interest in developing strategies to obtain human RNA from sources that are more accessible, such as the blood or neuronal-like cell lines. However, there is a real concern that peripheral tissues, such as whole blood, may express few proteins that are fundamental for the disease process and, therefore, may have limited ability to demonstrate case-control differences that are relevant to disorders of the nervous system (Matigian, 2008). The lack of available gene expression data from multiple tissues of patients with PD at various stages of the disease precludes such an analysis, but highlights the need for ongoing research efforts in this area. At present, the search for expression markers of early stages of PD in tissues that are more available (e.g. blood and cerebrospinal fluid) is urgent.

2.2 Analysis of gene expression in the peripheral blood of patients with PD

Unfortunately, little is known currently about the expression of single genes and the expression profiles of groups of genes in the blood of patients with PD. Only a few studies report changes in the number of transcripts or protein concentration in blood cells or in plasma.

To date, there is only one report of a genome-wide expression study in the blood of patients with PD. It was shown that only 22 among 20000 genes are significantly downregulateded in PD (Scherzer, 2007). According to other data, a decreased number of transcripts has been shown for two of these genes, *HIP2* and *ST13,* in the substantia nigra of patients with PD (Table 1). However, Scherzer et al. noticed that one of the 22 genes that was most underexpressed in PD was the heat-shock protein-70-interacting protein ST13, which belongs to the ubiquitin–proteasome pathway. ST13 is a cofactor of the heat-shock protein 70 (HSP70) and stabilizes its chaperone activity (Shi, 2007). HSP70 modulates the folding of SNCA and suppresses its toxicity in cells, yeast, and flies (Auluck, 2002, Flower, 2005, and Klucken, 2004, as cited in Scherzer, 2007). ST13 stabilizes the ADP state of HSP70, which has a high affinity for substrate proteins. Via its own chaperone activity, *ST13* may contribute to the interaction of *HSP70* with various target proteins (Hohfeld, 1995) that may play a role in the pathogenesis of PD. However, it is necessary to mention that we have not found any alterations in the expression of the *ST13* gene in patients with PD in Russia (Shadrina, 2010).

There are only a few studies on expression changes of single genes as well. Increased expression of *SNCA* was shown in the peripheral blood of Korean patients with a sporadic form of PD (Kim, 2004). Another study showed a direct correlation between the levels of expression of cyto/chemokines (MCP-1, RANTES, MIP-1-α, IL-8, IFN-γ, IL-1β, TNF-α, and NF-κB(p65)) in peripheral white blood cells in patients with PD and stages of PD (Reale, 2009). These results reflect the deregulation of cytokines in the blood of patients with PD and possibly indicate the activation of inflammation. Recent data reported by Grünblatt et al., based on their previous study (Grünblatt, 2004), show that the expression levels of *HIST1H3E, PSMA2, LAMB2,* and *ALDH1A1* may be biomarkers for PD diagnosis, with an achieved sensitivity and specificity of more than 80% (Grünblatt, 2010). However, the sensitivity of the clinical diagnosis of PD in symptomatic patients remains higher, as it is estimated as 91% (Hughes, 2002).

Furthermore, some studies also described alterations of protein concentrations in the blood of patients with PD. Armentero et al. showed increased levels of glycogen synthase kinase 3 (GSK-3) in peripheral lymphocytes in patients with PD (Armentero, 2010). GSK-3 has been implicated in the regulation of axonal transport (Morfini, 2002 and Pigino, 2003, as cited in Armentero, 2010) and modulates the ubiquitylation of synphilin-1, as well as its degradation, which is promoted by SIAH (Avraham, 2005, as cited in Armentero, 2010). Caronti et al. demonstrated a reduction of dopamine transporter immunoreactivity in peripheral blood lymphocytes in the early clinical stages of PD (Caronti, 2001). Despite these promising results, we have shown that the expression of *GSK3B* gene was not altered in the peripheral blood of Russian patients with PD (Filatova, 2011).

Nevertheless, the study of gene expression in the blood opens broad prospects for the identification of biomarkers for diagnosis of PD. Expression-profile analysis in PD will possibly allow the elucidation of the pathogenesis of the early stages of PD, which, in turn, opens wide prospects for a more adequate treatment or preventive correction of this disease.

2.3 Analysis of gene expression in different models of PD

Since the discovery of PD as a single nosological form, researchers have been trying to identify the mechanisms underlying disease development and approaches to test drugs before clinical usage. However, human brain tissues are not sufficient for these purposes because of their inaccessibility during the lives of the patients. Under these circumstances, researches have had to develop various models of PD involving cell lines (including induced pluripotent stem cells) and animals (mice, rats, monkeys, and flies). Currently there is a great variety of such models, which can be divided into two large groups: genetic (endogenous) and nongenetic (exogenous). Genetic models are based on altered expression of genes involved in the pathogenesis of PD or on altered functioning of proteins encoded by these genes. Nongenetic models are based on the introduction of different inductors (e.g. neurotoxins and drugs) into model organisms or on surgery approaches that lead to parkinsonian syndrome.

Despite this variety of models of PD and their large impact on the elucidation of pathogenesis of this disease, the picture of the etiopathogenesis of the disorder remains approximate. Nevertheless, some reports describe changes in the whole transcriptome of model organisms.

A monkey model with MPTP-induced parkinsonism was used to show that the same pathways are altered in the substantia nigra and in the striatum, as described previously in paragraph 2.1 and in Table 1 (Ohnuki, 2010); among them are mitochondrial dysfunction, oxidative stress, signal transduction, synaptic transmission, neurotransmitters, and neurotransmitter metabolism. Genes coding for the DA phenotype, such as *DAT, AADC, TH, VMAT2,* and *ADLH1A1,* were significantly downregulated in the SN of this MPTP, which is in line with the loss of DA neuronal function that occurs in PD and MPTP model systems. Genes involved in synaptic function and cytoskeletal stability represented a major class of genes that exhibited decreased expression. It was observed that some genes were consistently downregulated across the studies of PD patients. These genes were *D4S234E, NSF, CADPS, SYNJ1, AMPH, MAP1B, MAPT,* dynein complex component, kinesin family members, tubulins and catenins. Interestingly, the downregulation of *D4S234E,* which is a neuronal endosomal gene, showed the highest concordance across PD studies. This gene is involved in the regulation of AMPA-receptor trafficking in spines and may participate in the control of synaptic strength (Alberi, 2005, as cited in Ohnuki, 2010). The downregulation of the AMPA receptor GRIA3 was also consistently observed in PD studies. These observations may provide further insight for the evaluation of the neuroprotective effects of AMPA-positive allosteric modulators for the treatment of PD (O'Neill, 2005, as cited in Ohnuki, 2010). Downregulation of these synaptic transcripts in both MPTP models and PD patients suggests a significant failure in the production of the proteins necessary for vesicle trafficking and neurotransmitter release and transmission. The downregulation of several microtubule-associated proteins was also consistent in cross-comparison study (Ohnuki, 2010). The downregulation of *ACTR1A,* which is a component of the dynein complex, and several kinesin family member genes (*KIF3A, KLC1, KIF2A,* and *KIFAP3*) was observed in both the SN and STR (striatum). As pointed out by Miller et al. (Miller, 2006), the dynein complex and the members of the kinesin family are particularly important for bidirectional axonal transport and for the understanding of the association between the SN and the STR. Together with the downregulation of cadherins (Miller, 2006) and the overrepresentation of the cell adhesion pathway in the STR, the deregulation of the cell adhesion process seems apparent (Ohnuki, 2010).

Multiple mechanisms have also been shown as involved in neuronal cell death in PD and model systems. Apoptotic cell death is one of the key mechanisms. Pathway enrichment of this category suggests its contribution to the cellular functions in PD and model systems. The observed upregulation of proapoptotic genes (*BCL10* and *TPD52L*) and the downregulation of the antiapoptotic gene *XIAP* support the current concept of apoptosis in PD. Interestingly, XIAP is an ubiquitin–protein ligase of the UPS and has been shown to promote proteasomal degradation of caspase-3 and enhances its antiapoptotic effect (Ohnuki, 2010).

The UPS is one of the most well studied contributors to neuronal cell death in PD and model systems. The UPS is involved in the protein disposal process in cells and exerts protective effects from toxic proteins (Duke, 2006). The consistent downregulation of *UCHL1* across studies implies the impairment of the ability to degrade toxic proteins. Notably, the downregulation of β-TrCP was found in the STR of the MPTP model (Ohnuki, 2010). β-TrCP is a component of the SCF ubiquitin-ligase complex, which comprises SKP1, cullin, and the F-box protein. β-TrCP functions as an F-box protein that recognizes specific targets for ubiquitination, thereby regulating the function of specific proteins, , including β-catenin and NF-κB, via protein degradation. Interestingly, SKP1, which is another component of the SCF complex, is downregulated in the SN of PD patients, as assessed using microarray data (Mandel, 2005). Furthermore, a knockdown model of SKP1 exhibited increased susceptibility to cell death (Mandel, 2009). Thus, the reduction of SCF ubiquitin-ligase activity may play an important role in neuronal cell death both in the MPTP model and in patients with PD. MPTP-induced neuronal cell death is thought to affect surrounding cells to produce signals that feed back on the remaining DA neurons (Pattarini, 2008). Genes involved in neuroinflammation likely participate in this process. In agreement with earlier studies, treatment with MPTP led to the upregulation of the astrocyte marker GFAP. Although none of the typical microglial markers, such as CD40 and CD68, was detected in the study (Ohnuki, 2010), the upregulation of complement component genes (C1S and C4B), IL-11, and proinflammatory cytokines (CXCL13 and CXCL4) suggests microglial activation (Ohnuki, 2010). These observations support the notion that microglia-derived proinflammatory factors play a role in the process of dopaminergic MPTP-induced neuronal toxicity (Whitton, 2007).

Neurotrophic support by neurotrophic and growth factors protects DA neurons (Evans & Barker, 2008). The observed downregulation of *BDNF, FGF1, FGF13,* and *PACAP* in the STR of the MPTP model is in agreement with previous evidence. Regarding BDNF, the PD patient study found a decrease in BDNF expression in nigrostriatal DA neurons (Nagatsu, 2000). Certain transcription factors involved in survival and differentiation of DA neurons may participate in the neuroprotective function, as the loss of Nurr1 (NR4A2) (Ohnuki, 2010). Therefore, the upregulation of factors such as Nurr1 and TCF7L2 may improve the protective effects against MPTP toxicity (Bassilana, 2005). Similar to this, the upregulation of TCF7L2 was observed in the SN of the MPTP model. In contrast, Ohnuki and co-workers found robust downregulation of TCF7L2 in the STR of the MPTP model. As activation of TCF7L2 by β-catenin leads to the transcriptional initiation of the Wnt target genes (Clevers, 2006), the downregulation of TCF7L2 may influence several genes associated with survival, differentiation, and cytoskeletal stability. However, there was low consistency across the data sets of patients with PD with the exception of the occipital cortex of patients with PD (Vogt, 2006). *SKP1* was also downregulated in the same region and in the BA9 region of patients with PD (Vogt, 2006, Zhang, 2005). As the pathological process of Lewy bodies

begins in the brainstem and olfactory bulb and extends gradually to the substantia nigra and, ultimately, to the cerebral cortex (Braak, 2006), the deregulation of these genes may be associated with disease stage, in particular, with the late stage of PD.
The mitochondrial dysfunction, oxidative stress, signal transduction, synaptic transmission, neurotransmitters, and neurotransmitter metabolism pathways were also altered in the mouse models described in two other reports (Chin, 2008, Smith, 2009). Similar results were obtained in the mice and cell models described by Chung et al. and Yacoubian et al. (Chung, 2005, Yacoubian, 2008), although the two latter groups discovered changes mostly in the number of transcripts of regulatory genes.
In addition, proof of the role of mitochondrial dysfunction in PD was obtained from a genetic (SNCA A30P) fly model of the disease (Xun, 2007). This finding additionally emphasizes the role of mitochondrial dysfunction in the pathogenesis of PD.
Therefore, analysis of gene expression revealed that a number of significant pathways, including mitochondrial dysfunction, oxidative stress response, various transport pathways, signal transduction, synaptic transmission, neurotransmitters, neurotransmitter metabolism, and apoptosis, are involved in the development of PD. Nevertheless, much remains to be discovered to obtain the full picture of the pathogenesis of this disease. For example, the recently discovered microRNAs may offer new insight into the cellular mechanisms that occur during neurodegeneration.

3. MicroRNA expression in Parkinson's disease

Currently, research on miRNAs in the context of neurodegeneration is accumulating rapidly; the goal of this review is to provide the most complete data on the expression of microRNAs in connection with the etiopathogenesis of Parkinson's disease. Studies published recently shed some light on the role of microRNAs in the differentiation of dopaminergic neurons and raises the question of whether microRNAs are involved in the etiology of PD. There are also various reviews in this field (Barbato, 2009, Bushati & Cohen, 2008, De Smaelea, 2010, Fiore, 2008, Hébert & De Strooper, 2007, Lau & de Strooper, 2010, Nelson & Keller, 2007, Nelson, 2008, Roshan, 2009, Saugstad, 2010, Weinberg & Wood, 2009).
Genome-encoded microRNAs (miRNAs) are known regulators of gene expression. The significance of miRNAs in various biological processes has been suggested by studies that showed an important role for these small RNAs in the regulation of cellular differentiation. However, the role of miRNAs in the regulation of the physiology of differentiated cells is not well established. Furthermore, the existence of neuron-specific miRNAs argues in favor of their important role in neuronal differentiation and/or specialized functions. The involvement of miRNAs in neuronal differentiation is strongly supported by dynamic changes in miRNA expression during brain development (Krichevsky, 2003, Miska, 2004, Smirnova, 2005). The significance of miRNAs in neuronal physiology is also suggested by data that show miRNA involvement in dendritic-spine formation and neurite outgrowth *in vitro* (Schratt, 2006, Vo, 2005). In summary, although there is mounting evidence of the importance of the roles of miRNAs in neuronal cell differentiation, their role in differentiated, postmitotic neurons has not been addressed fully (Schaefer, 2007).

3.1 What is a microRNA?

miRNAs are a class of small noncoding RNAs that induce translational repression or degradation of a target mRNA upon imperfect base pairing to its 3′ untranslated region

(3'UTR). The biogenesis and mechanism of action of miRNAs are covered in detail in a number of excellent reviews (Bartel, 2004, Bartel, 2009, Bushati & Cohen, 2007), therefore, it will be summarized briefly here. Structurally, mature miRNAs are single-stranded RNA molecules of about 21 nucleotides (nt) derived from a 70-100 nt hairpin precursor (pre-miRNA). miRNA genes are mostly transcribed by RNA polymerase II, with the exception of some human genes that are transcribed by RNA polymerase III (Borchert, 2006). The primary transcript, which can be up to hundreds of nt long, is then processed by the RNAse III enzyme Drosha in the nucleus, to yield a pre-miRNA. The pre-miRNA is subsequently translocated to the cytoplasm via an exportin-5-dependent mechanism. Once in the cytosol, pre-miRNAs are further processed by a second RNAse III enzyme, Dicer. Cleavage generates an imperfect, siRNA-like duplex that is unwound and whose strand with the weakest base pairing at the 5' end is preferentially loaded into the RNA-induced silencing complex (RISC). Binding of the miRNA to its target occurs within the RISC and target silencing requires the presence of proteins belonging to the Argonaute (AGO) family. Complementarity between the 5' end of the miRNA, the seed region, and the 3'UTR of the target mRNA appears to be critical for the binding, where more variability is tolerated in the base pairing at the 3' end of the miRNA (Bartel, 2004, Bushati & Cohen, 2007). However, the range of action of miRNAs remains under active debate, as others showed that miRNAs are only active onto 3'UTR (Gu, 2009). Moreover, the mechanisms of miRNA processing at the posttranscriptional level are only beginning to be elucidated (Lau & de Strooper, 2010).

miRNAs regulate approximately 30% of genes in the human genome (Rajewsky, 2006). The mechanism by which miRNAs silence gene expression remains an active and controversial field of investigation (Cannell, 2008, Filipowicz, 2008, Lau & de Strooper, 2010, Vasudevan, 2007). Single miRNAs are able to target up to a few hundreds of different mRNAs (cooperativity) (Brennecke, 2005, John, 2004, Krek, 2005, Lewis, 2005). It is hardly surprising that the number of roles assigned to miRNAs during all stages of central nervous system (CNS) development and function is rapidly expanding (Fiore, 2008). One of the main mechanisms appears to be the blocking of translational initiation, but other mechanisms are likely involved (Jackson & Standart, 2007, Pillai, 2007, Standart & Jackson, 2007). Processing bodies (Pbodies), which are cytoplasmic foci that were originally identified as sites of mRNA storage and degradation, are critical structure for miRNA-mediated deadenylation and degradation. In addition to Pbodies, neurons contain a variety of functionally related high-molecular-weight ribonucleoprotein particles (nRNP) that are involved in the storage, dendritic trafficking, and translational control of neuronal mRNAs (Barbee, 2006, Krichevsky & Kosik, 2001).

Elucidation of the precise biological functions of these miRNAs has been the subject of many studies. miRNAs are involved in cell differentiation, development, apoptosis, stress resistance, tumor formation, and in neurodegenerative disorders (Bushati & Cohen, 2008, Plasterk, 2006, Santosh, 2009). Earlier studies provide some evidence of the involvement of miRNAs in Parkinson's disease (Nelson, 2008), but do not offer a full, comprehensive view of the microRNA-dependent regulation of PD genes.

It is possible that simple computational prediction of microRNA targets will shed some light on the behavior of target genes involved in Parkinson's disease. In addition, the identification of mRNA targets currently relies on prediction software (Bartel, 2009). Prediction of miRNAs using computer-based methods exhibits many advantages and aids in recognizing the molecular hallmarks of the disease that can lead to the development of effective screening tools for miRNA targets. However, the prediction of microRNA targets may be hindered by numerous problems, including tissue-specific expression and lack of validation. Moreover, interpretation of results is often not as evident and is further complicated by the small overlap set of predictions when comparing different algorithms. Such weakness of *in silico* studies can be partially compensated by predicting targets using multiple programs. The outputs can be effectively used for the development of a molecular marker for diagnosis and prognosis. Computer-based prediction of microRNA target selection undoubtedly reduces the noise, but is not sufficient to estimate the efficiency of each microRNA on the multiple targets. Therefore, computational prediction may not guide optimized selection of any single microRNA for efficient knock down and level of action; further validation of these findings using experimental approaches is required. Additional analysis and experimental validation of these results is mandatory to resolve the complexity of the selection of microRNA targets in the future (Santosh, 2009).

3.2 MicroRNAs in Parkinson's disease

As stated earlier, some studies provide evidences of the involvement of miRNAs in Parkinson's disease (Nelson, 2008), but they do not offer a full, comprehensive view of the microRNA-dependent regulation of PD genes. However, a causal link between a specific miRNA and a disease has been established in just a few cases, and most of the mechanistic data originate from invertebrate model systems.

An important work regarding the role of miRNAs in PD performed in Asa Abeliovich's laboratory indicates that a particular miRNA plays a significant role in the pathogenesis of this disease (Kim, 2007). Kim et al. profiled a panel of 224 miRNA precursors from the brains of Parkinson's patients and found that several miRNAs were deregulated, including the downregulation of miR-133b, which is enriched in dopaminergic neurons of the midbrain and, if overexpressed, suppresses their maturation and function. The authors showed experimentally that miR-133b is relatively highly expressed at the tissue level in the midbrain under normal conditions, but not in PD. Furthermore, the general knockout of miRNAs *in vivo*, or of miR-133b by itself in cultures of dopaminergic neurons, cultures derived from ES cells, or midbrain cultures, dramatically decreases the levels of tyrosine hydroxylase and dopamine transporter in dopaminergic neurons. Mir-133 appears to act as a negative regulator of dopaminergic neuron maturation, as overexpression and inhibition of miR-133b resulted in the decrease and increase, respectively, of the number of DA neurons in these cultures. The data also support the hypothesis that miR-133b and the paired-like homeodomain transcription factor PITX3 regulate each other's expression. In homology with miR-124, miR-133b seems to be a component of a negative feedback loop. In this case, miR-133b targets the transcription factor and marker for DA neurons, PITX3, which in turn is a positive regulator of miR-133b. Thus, loss of Pitx3 leads to the loss of miR-133b in the PD model. Interestingly, aphakia mice are deficient in Pitx3, which is a homeobox transcription factor required for the survival of DA neurons and for motor activity (van den Munckhof, 2003, as cited in Fuchs, 2007). Polymorphisms in *PITX3* have also been associated with PD in humans (Bergman, 2008, Fuchs, 2007).

This study is important for a number of reasons. First, it indicates a discrete role for a particular miRNA in dopaminergic function. Second, no particular miRNA–mRNA pair had been strongly implicated previously in a prevalent neurodegenerative disease. In other words, these investigators provided plausible molecular neurobiological breakthroughs for both miRNA function and dysfunction. This study also demonstrates how miRNAs can be an important component of a "downward spiral" during neurodegeneration (Nelson, 2008).

Whether the loss of the miRNA contributes to the etiology of PD is an important, albeit unanswered, question. This has not been addressed directly in the mouse model because mutants lacking miR-133b are not available.

The relationship between miR-133b and the maturation of DA neurons is especially intriguing, for two reasons. Firstly, mice with a conditional deletion of Dicer in DA neurons display progressive loss of DA neurons (Kim, 2007). Importantly, this phenotype is also observed *in vitro* in a dopaminergic stem cell differentiation paradigm, and can be partially rescued by transfection of the cultures with a small RNA population isolated from wild type cells. Secondly, and puzzlingly, miR-133b is undetectable in the midbrain of patients with Parkinson's disease (Kim, 2007). This apparent contradiction awaits further validation; however, it strongly suggests additional functions of miR-133 in DA neurons.

Interestingly, neurodegeneration is also observed in mice that lack Dicer specifically in the cerebellum. In these animals, Purkinje neurons progressively degenerate and the animals develop ataxia (Schaefer, 2007). Authors demonstrated an essential role for Dicer and miRNAs in the regulation of postmitotic neuronal survival. Although Dicer deficiency had no immediate impact on Purkinje cell function, the long-term absence of Dicer resulted in a neurodegenerative process. This pattern of Purkinje cell degeneration in the absence of miRNAs bears obvious similarities to processes associated with the slow, progressive neurodegenerative diseases, such as Alzheimer's and Parkinson's diseases. Deletion of Dicer impairs the ability of embryonic stem cells to differentiate into DA neurons, by blocking miRNA biogenesis. As Dicer deletion was partially rescued by transfection of a small RNA derived from embryonic mouse midbrain, it is likely that microRNAs are involved in the differentiation and survival of DA neurons (Kim, 2007). In addition, specific deletion of Dicer *in vivo*, in mouse midbrain dopaminergic neurons, leads to cell death in the substantia nigra. Behavioral studies of these animals revealed reduced locomotion in an open-field assay, which was reminiscent of the phenotype of human patients with PD. Thus, although miR-133b is involved in the differentiation and function of DA neurons, additional microRNAs should be responsible for the Dicer deletion phenotype in DA neurons (Sethupathy & Collins, 2008).

Together, these observations raise the possibility that the loss of miRNAs is involved in the emergence and/or progression of PD. Although its expression is lost in PD samples, these findings indicate that miR-133b cannot be the miRNA species that is responsible for the embryonic stem cell Dicer phenotype or the progressive loss of mouse midbrain DA neurons in Dicer mutants. PD probably results from the loss of PITX3-dependent expression of genes other than miR-133b. The miRNA(s) carrying a protective potential against DA neuron neurodegeneration remain unidentified. This profound loss of DA neurons in the substantia nigra contrasts with results of a study in which Dicer was removed from the dopaminoceptive neurons of the striatum (Cuellar, 2008). A range of phenotypes was observed, including reduction of the size of the brain and of neurons, ataxia, wasting, and premature death; however, the dopaminoceptive neurons survived throughout the lives of the animals. Therefore, in general, Dicer does not seem to be required for the promotion of cell survival in all postmitotic neurons, as Dicer is also dispensable in mature olfactory neurons (Choi, 2008). Notably, dysfunction, but not necessarily extensive loss, of dopaminoceptive neurons has also been implicated in PD (Evans & Lees, 2004).

Another miRNA has also been associated with the development of PD. A linkage analysis in PD reported in 2001 for identified a linkage peak on chromosome 8 that harbored the fibroblast growth factor 20 (FGF20) gene (Scott, 2001), which is preferentially expressed in the substantia nigra and promotes the survival of dopaminergic neurons. A subsequent Comparative Genomic Analysis Study (CGAS) reported in 2004 identified rs1989754 within FGF20 as associated with PD (van der Walt, 2004). Therefore, Wang et al. (Wang, 2008) selected FGF20 for further association testing using a family-based design. The authors observed that the strongest association (P = 0.0001) occured with rs12720208 [C/T], a SNP that was demonstrated as mediating the allele-specific *in vitro* targeting of miR-433 to the 3'UTR of *FGF20*. The authors also showed that miR-433 is highly expressed in the brain. Unlike prior studies, these researches went even further by providing human *in vivo* validation and testing a molecular mechanism by which differential miR-433 targeting potentially leads to PD. In cell culture experiments and in PD brains, increased translation of FGF20 was correlated with increased expression of α-synuclein.

Two independent GWASs for PD did not test rs12720208 (Fung, 2006, Maraganore, 2005). However, one of these studies tested a nearby SNP (rs1989754) and found no signal for association (P = 0.40) (Fung, 2006). The other study also tested another SNP within FGF20 (rs17515020) and observed a modest signal for association with PD (P = 0.03) (Maraganore, 2005). However, this result was not significant after correction for multiple testing (Maraganore, 2005). According to the phased HapMap CEU genotype data, rs12720208 is not in strong LD with either rs1989754 (r2 = 0.1) or rs17515020 (r^2 = 0.029); therefore, this SNP may still be associated with PD independently. Given that this study was not confounded by population stratification because of the use of a family-based association study design, and given that there is compelling functional evidence for both allele-specific targeting and an underlying molecular mechanism for the role of miR-433–FGF20 in PD pathogenesis, rs12720208 is the most attractive human poly-miRTS for use in future replication studies (Sethupathy & Collins, 2008). However, there was no association between the *FGF20* SNP rs12720208 and Parkinson's disease in Spanish patients (de Mena, 2010).

Overexpression of SNCA appears to be a common feature in PD and other α-synucleinopathies. In addition, it was demonstrated recently that miR-7 interacts *in vitro* with the 3'UTR of *SNCA*, represses the expression α-synuclein and inhibits α-synuclein-mediated cell death (Junn, 2009). Of note, miR-7 inhibits the cellular susceptibility of neuroblastoma cells to oxidative stress induced by a mutant form of SNCA, providing evidence that miRNAs protect neuronal cells against cellular stress. The presence of miR-7 in the substantia nigra was also validated, thus supporting a physiological role for this molecule in DA neurons. However, miR-7 was initially reported as highly expressed in the mouse pituitary gland (Bak, 2008, as cited in Lau & de Strooper, 2010) and its expression was ~15-fold lower in the substantia nigra compared with the pituitary gland, leaving open the possibility that other miRNAs regulate dopaminergic neurons in amore dynamic and efficient manner (Lau & de Strooper, 2010).

One of the latest studies on this subject revealed a previously unknown mechanism of regulation of SNCA levels in the nervous system (Doxakis, 2010). Specifically, two brain-enriched miRNAs, miR-7 and miR-153, were shown to bind directly to the 3'UTR of the *SNCA* mRNA and reduce its levels significantly. RNA and protein expression analysis showed developmental and tissue coexpression among miR-7, miR-153, and SNCA. The results of the study indicate that miR-7 and miR-153 have synergistic effect, require the 3'UTR of *SNCA* mRNA to regulate SNCA protein expression, do not interact with the coding region of *SNCA* to regulate the expression of SNCA protein, and act at the pretranslational level. Taking into consideration the two types of miRNA function, these findings strongly suggest that miR-7 and miR-153 play a role in the modulation/buffering of SNCA protein levels in the nervous system.

As neither of the miRNAs is fully complementary to the *SNCA* mRNA – to allow endonucleolytic cleavage by Argonaute proteins – the degradation effect is likely to stem from the accelerated level of deadenylation and decapping of the *SNCA* mRNA, induced by the binding of miR-7 and miR-153 to its 3'UTR (Behm-Ansmant, 2006 and Eulalio, 2009, as cited in Doxakis, 2010). miR-7, miR-153, and the *SNCA* mRNA and protein show highest expression in neural tissues, such as the midbrain, hippocampus, and cortex (the levels of miR-7, miR-153, and *SNCA* mRNA are significantly higher in neurons compared with astrocytes), and lowest expression in nonneural tissues, such as the lung and heart. Interestingly, all three RNA species show highest expression in the midbrain, indicating that deregulation of their expression levels may be important in the pathogenesis of PD. The *SNCA* protein is also detected in the lung, as a result of the high amount of peripheral blood present in this tissue. Moreover, the expression profiles of the *SNCA* mRNA and protein are similar, indicating that, during development, a constant level of the miRNA-regulated *SNCA* mRNA is translated into protein. These results suggest that miR-7 and miR-153 are coexpressed with SNCA in neurons to regulate its levels via a transcriptional feed-forward loop that fine-tunes, rather than blocks, the expression and translation of the *SNCA* mRNA (Doxakis, 2010).

4. Conclusions

Most neurochemical and gene expression studies on the mechanism of DA neuron death in PD and its animal models, have been conducted at a time when the majority of dopamine neurons are dead. However, the detailed profile of the crucial initial neurochemical and gene expression changes in injured (but not dead) neurons is more important, as the early genetic and biochemical alterations differ from those that occur at the time of neuronal death.

It is also important to emphasize that mRNA data reveal information on the transcriptional activation of genes, but do not provide much information on the actual protein levels and function. In addition, array data cannot predict whether deregulated gene expression is a primary or a secondary effect of cell function. For example, a gene could be down- or upregulated by factors such as miRNAs or transcriptional activators (or inhibitors), independent of its protein function and/or as a consequence of positive and negative feedback loops. Moreover, protein function relies on the interaction of down- and upstream factors within a pathway, i.e. downstream factors are more dependent on upstream signaling compared with upstream factors, which may influence a cascade of downstream events that can include multiple pathways. Thus, the consequences of deregulated gene expression are exerted on multiple levels within a complex and dynamic interplay of factors and mechanisms. Laser-microscopy-based microarray studies can only provide a "snapshot" of these events. Nevertheless, several studies showed that many genes associated with the pathogenesis of Parkinson's disease are deregulated in single captured postmortem DA neurons. This could provide a "molecular fingerprint identity" of a late-stage DA neuron affected by sporadic Parkinson's disease. The striking downregulation of PARK genes is a key aspect. As their mutation-induced malfunction in the familial forms of Parkinson's disease rapidly accelerates DA neuron degeneration, the results from the studies reviewed may support the view that these genes are also involved in the pathogenesis of sporadic Parkinson's disease. Data also point to an imbalance in neuronal homeostasis and stress characterized by factors related to high metabolic rate, neurotransmission and ion-channel activity. This stress may be part of the normal homeostasis and aging of DA neurons, but could be exacerbated in the presence of an unfavorable imbalance. In addition, the array data suggest a disintegration of key cellular functions, such as mitochondria-associated energy metabolism, protein degradation, synaptic function, and cytoskeletal integrity, revealing a cellular state that is characterized by programmed cell death. However, despite this cellular demise, some genes linked to survival mechanisms were upregulated, indicating the activation of compensatory mechanisms. Finally, the lack or the relatively modest deregulation of genes important for the DA neuronal phenotype suggests that the DA neurotransmitter identity (including DA production) seems to be sustained even when the neurons are severely damaged. It appears that the gene expression profile of the DA neurons of late-stage Parkinson's disease is consistent with the view that Parkinson's disease is a complex disorder and that multiple factors and cellular pathways are involved in its pathogenesis.

To date, whether miRNAs are also actively involved in the etiology or progression of neurodegenerative disorders remains uncertain. These small regulators clearly seem to be required for the survival of specific types of mature neurons in some model organisms; however, whether the loss of individual miRNAs can account for the drastic disease phenotypes remains to be determined. As many different cellular processes have been implicated in neurodegenerative disorders, the miRNAs involved in these pathways will obviously be found as misregulated in disease tissues. However, the degree to which their misregulation is causative in the diseases remains a pressing, but unanswered, question. Identification of causal links opens prospects for therapeutic intervention, perhaps by replacing missing miRNAs or blocking the activity of miRNAs that are overexpressed. Similarly, some miRNAs seem to have a neuroprotective role; therefore, they could potentially be used to prevent, or at least decelerate, the progressive loss of neurons in the diseased brain. These are tantalizing prospects that remain far from our grasp (Bushati & Cohen, 2008). Studies of miRNA in neurodegenerative diseases are emerging. Currently, both changes in the expression profiles of several miRNA and polymorphisms affecting the interactions between miRNAs and their targets are being addressed in various studies on neurodegenerative disease. It is difficult to determine if the changes in miRNA expression detected in the brains or cerebrospinal fluid (CSF) of patients are primary or secondary events, or both. Nevertheless early or late in the evolution of the disease, they may contribute to the pathogenesis of the observed lesions and neuronal loss. Unique patterns of miRNA expression in the CSF of particular neurodegenerative diseases may be useful as molecular biomarkers for disease diagnosis and, eventually, for the prediction of therapeutic responses. The identification of miRNAs that cause a specific pathology could open new therapeutic perspectives to block endogenous miRNAs or deliver exogenous miRNAs. To date either antisense oligonucleotides that are chemically modified (Meister, 2004) or expressed sequences corresponding to multiple miRNA seed targets (miRNA sponge) (Ebert, 2007) have been used as microRNA inhibitors. Delivery of these molecules to the central nervous system, while avoiding toxicities, may be the challenge of future research in this area. Furthermore, as specific nuclear or cytoplasmic protein accumulation causes the neuropathological manifestation in several neurodegenerative disorders, the identification of microRNAs that regulate the translation of these targets may represent the first step toward therapeutic applications. The second step might be the evaluation of the quantitative effects of specific amounts of "therapeutic" microRNAs on the proteome (Barbato, 2009).

5. Acknowledgements

This work has been supported in part by grants of the Russian Basic Research Foundation (Grants 07-04-01511, 07-04-00027, 09-04-01237-a), State Contracts (02.740.11.0084, P419, P1055), Russian Academy of Sciences program "Molecular and Cellular Biology" Russian Academy of Sciences program "Basic Sciences for Medicine".

6. References

Armentero, M.T., Sinforiani, E., Ghezzi, C., Bazzini, E., Levandis, G., Ambrosi, G., Zangaglia, R., Pacchetti, C., Cereda, C., Covab, E., Basso, E., Celi, D., Martignoni, E., Nappi, G. & Blandini, F. (2010). Peripheral expression of key regulatory kinases in Alzheimer's disease and Parkinson's disease. *Neurobiology of Aging*, (January 2010), pp. ISSN 0197-4580

Barbato, C., Ruberti, F. & Cogoni, C. (2009). Searching for MIND: MicroRNAs in Neurodegenerative Diseases. *Journal of Biomedicine and Biotechnology*, Vol.2009, (August 2009), pp. 871313, ISSN 1110-7251

Barbee, S.A., Estes, P.S., Cziko, A.M., Hillebrand, J., Luedeman, R.A., Coller, J.M., Johnson, N., Howlett, I.C., Geng, C., Ueda, R., Brand, A.H., Newbury, S.F., Wilhelm, J.E., Levine, R.B., Nakamura, A., Parker, R. & Ramaswami, M. (2006). Staufen- and FMRP-containing neuronalRNPs are structurally and functionally related to somatic P bodies. *Neuron*, Vol.52, No.6, (December 2006), pp. 997-1009, ISSN 1097-4199

Bartel, D.P. (2004). MicroRNAs: Genomics, Biogenesis, Mechanism, and Function. *Cell*, Vol.116, (January 2004), pp. 281-297, ISSN 0092-8674

Bartel, D.P. (2009). MicroRNAs: target recognition and regulatory functions. *Cell*, Vol.136, No.2, (January 2009), pp. 215-233, ISSN 0092-8674

Bassilana, F., Mace, N., Li, Q., Stutzmann, J.M., Gross, C.E., Pradier, L., Benavides, J., Ménager, J. & Bezard, E. (2005). Unraveling substantia nigra sequential gene expression in a progressive MPTP-lesioned macaque model of Parkinson's disease. *Neurobiol Dis*, Vol.20, No.1, (October 2005), pp. 93-103, ISSN 0969-9961

Bergman, O., Hakansson, A., Westberg, L., Nordenström, K., Carmine Belin, A., Sydow, O., Olson, L., Holmberg, B., Eriksson, E. & Nissbrandt, H. (2008). PITX3 polymorphism is associated with early onset Parkinson's disease. *Neurobiol Aging*, Vol.31, No.1, (January 2010), pp. 554-565, ISSN 0197-4580

Borchert, G.M., Lanier, W. & Davidson, B.L. (2006). RNA polymerase III transcribes human microRNAs. *Nat Struct Mol Biol*, Vol.13, No.12, (December 2006), pp. 1097-1101, ISSN 1545-9985

Bossers, K., Meerhoff, G., Balesar, R., van Dongen, J.W., Kruse, C.G., Swaab, D.F. & Verhaagen, J. (2009). Analysis of Gene Expression in Parkinson's Disease: Possible Involvement of Neurotrophic Support and Axon Guidance in Dopaminergic Cell Death. *Brain Pathology*, Vol.19, No.1, (January 2009), pp. 91-107, ISSN 1015-6305

Braak, H., Müller, C.M., Rüb, U., Ackermann, H., Bratzke, H., de Vos, R.A. & Del Tredici, K. (2006). Pathology associated with sporadic Parkinson's disease--where does it end? *J Neural Transm Suppl*, Vol.2006, No.70, (2006), pp. 89-97, ISSN 0303-6995

Brennecke, J., Stark, A., Russell, R.B. & Cohen, S.M. (2005). Principles of MicroRNA–Target Recognition. *PLoS Biology*, Vol.3, No.3, (March 2005), pp. e85, ISSN 1545-7885

Brunger, A.T. (2005). Structure and function of SNARE and SNARE-interacting proteins. *Q Rev Biophys*, Vol.38, No.1, (February 2005), pp. 1-47, ISSN 1469-8994

Bushati, N. & Cohen, S.M. (2007). microRNA Functions. *Annu Rev Cell Dev Biol*, Vol.23, (May 2007), pp. 175-205, ISSN 1530-8995

Bushati, N. & Cohen, S.M. (2008). microRNAs in neurodegeneration. *Current Opinion in Neurobiology*, Vol.18, (June 2008), pp. 292-296, ISSN 1873-6882

Cannell, I.G., Kong, Y.W. & Bushell, M. (2008). How do microRNAs regulate gene expression? *Biochemical Society Transactions*, Vol.36, No.6, (December 2008), pp. 1224–1231, ISSN 1470-8752

Caronti, B., Antonini, G., Calderaro, C., Ruggieri, S., Palladini, G., Pontieri, F.E. & Colosimo, C. (2001). Dopamine transporter immunoreactivity in peripheral blood lymphocytes in Parkinson's disease. *J Neural Transm*, Vol.108, No.7, (July 2001), pp. 803–807, ISSN 1435-1463

Chin, M.H., Qian, W.-J., Wang, H., Petyuk, V.A., Bloom, J.S., Sforza, D.M., Lac´an, G., Liu, D., Khan, A.H., Cantor, R.M., Bigelow, D.J., Melega, W.P., Camp, D.G., Smith, R.D. & Smith, D.J. (2008). Mitochondrial Dysfunction, Oxidative Stress, and Apoptosis Revealed by Proteomic and Transcriptomic Analyses of the Striata in Two Mouse Models of Parkinson's Disease. *Journal of Proteome Research*, Vol.7, No.2, (January 2008), pp. 666-677, ISSN 1535-3907

Chinta, S.I. & Andersen, J.K. (2005). Dopaminergic neurons. *Intern J Biochem Cell Biol*, Vol.37, No.5, (May 2005), pp. 942-946, ISSN 1357-2725

Choi, P.S., Zakhary, L., Choi, W.Y., Caron, S., Alvarez-Saavedra, E., Miska, E.A., McManus, M., Harfe, B., Giraldez, A.J., Horvitz, R.H. & et al. (2008). Members of the miRNA-200 family regulate olfactory neurogenesis. *Neuron*, Vol.57, (January 2008), pp. 41-55, ISSN 1097-4199

Chung, C.Y., Seo, H., Sonntag, K.C., Brooks, A., Lin, L. & Isacson, O. (2005). Cell type-specific gene expression of midbrain dopaminergic neurons reveals molecules involved in their vulnerability and protection. *Hum Mol Genet*, Vol.14, No.13, (July 2005), pp. 1709-1725, ISSN 1460-2083

Clevers, H. (2006). Wnt/beta-catenin signaling in development and disease. *Cell*, Vol.127, No.3, (November 2006), pp. 469-480, ISSN 0092-8674

Cuellar, T.L., Davis, T.H., Nelson, P.T., Loeb, G.B., Harfe, B.D., Ullian, E. & McManus, M.T. (2008). Dicer loss in striatal neurons produces behavioral and neuroanatomical phenotypes in the absence of neurodegeneration. *Proc Natl Acad Sci U S A*, Vol.105, (April 2008), pp. 5614-5619, ISSN 1091-6490

Dachsel, J.C., Lincoln, S.J., Gonzalez, J., Ross, O.A., Dickson, D.W. & Farrer, M.J. (2007). The Ups and Downs of alpha-Synuclein mRNA Expression. *Movement Disorders*, Vol.22, No.2, (November 2006), pp. 293-295, ISSN 1531-8257

de Mena, L., Cardo, L.F., Coto, E., Miar, A., Díaz, M., Corao, A.I., Alonso, B., Ribacoba, R., Salvador, C., Menéndez, M., Moris, G. & Alvarez, V. (2010). FGF20 rs12720208 SNP and microRNA-433 variation: No association with Parkinson's disease in Spanish patients. *Neuroscience Letters*, Vol.479 (July 2010), pp. 22-25, ISSN 0304-3940

De Smaelea, E., Ferrettia, E. & Gulino, A. (2010). MicroRNAs as biomarkers for CNS cancer and other disorders. *Brain Research*, Vol.1338, (April 2010), pp. 100 - 111, ISSN 1872-6240

Doxakis, E. (2010). Post-transcriptional Regulation of α-Synuclein Expression by mir-7 and mir-153. *The Journal of Biological Chemistry*, Vol.285, (April 2010), pp. 12726-12734, ISSN 1083-351X

Duke, D.C., Moran, L.B., Pearce, R.K.B. & Graeber, M.B. (2007). The medial and lateral substantia nigra in Parkinson's disease: mRNA profiles associated with higher brain tissue vulnerability. *Neurogenetics* Vol.8, (January 2007), pp. 83-94, ISSN 1364-6753

Duke, D.C., Moran, L.B., Kalaitzakis, M.E., Deprez, M., Dexter, D.T., Pearce, R.K. & Graeber, M.B. (2006). Transcriptome analysis reveals link between proteasomal and mitochondrial pathways in Parkinson's disease. *Neurogenetics,* Vol.7, No.3, (July 2006), pp. 139-148, ISSN 1364-6753

Ebert, M.S., Neilson, J.R. & Sharp, P.A. (2007). MicroRNA sponges: competitive inhibitors of small RNAs in mammalian cells. *Nature Methods,* Vol.4, No.9, (August 2007), pp. 721 - 726, ISSN 1548-7105

Elstner, M., Morris, C.M., Heim, K., Lichtner, P., Bender, A., Mehta, D., Schulte, C., Sharma, M., Hudson, G., Goldwurm, S., Giovanetti, A., Zeviani, M., Burn, D.J., McKeith, I.G., Perry, R.H., Jaros, E., Kruger, R., Wichmann, H.-E., Schreiber, S., Campbell, H., Wilson, J.F., Wright, A.F., Dunlop, M., Pistis, G., Toniolo, D., Chinnery, P.F., Gasser, T., Klopstock, T., Meitinger, T., Prokisch, H. & Turnbull, D.M. (2009). Single-Cell Expression Profiling of Dopaminergic Neurons Combined with Association Analysis Identifies Pyridoxal Kinase as Parkinson's Disease Gene. *Ann Neurol,* Vol.66, (December 2009), pp. 792-798, ISSN 1531-8249

Evans, A.H. & Lees, A.J. (2004). Dopamine dysregulation syndrome in Parkinson's disease. *Curr Opin Neurol,* Vol.17, (August 2004), pp. 393-398, ISSN 1473-6551

Evans, J.R. & Barker, R.A. (2008). Neurotrophic factors as a therapeutic target for Parkinson's disease. *Expert Opin Ther Targets,* Vol.12, No.4, (April 2008), pp. 437-447, ISSN 1744-7631

Filatova, E.V., Shadrina, M.I., Karabanov, A.V., Slominsky, P.A., Illarioshkin, S.N., Ivanova-Smolenskaya, I.A. & Limborska, S.A. (2011). Expression of GSK3B gene in peripheral blood in patient with Parkinson's Disease. *Molekuliarnaia biologiia,* Vol.45, No.2, (March 2011), pp. 1-5, ISSN 0026-8984

Filipowicz, W., Bhattacharyya, S.N. & Sonenberg, N. (2008). Mechanisms of post-transcriptional regulation by microRNAs: are the answers in sight? *Nature Reviews. Genetics,* Vol.9, (February 2008), pp. 102-114, ISSN 1471-0064

Fiore, R., Siegel, G. & Schratt, G. (2008). MicroRNA function in neuronal development, plasticity and disease. *Biochimica et Biophysica Acta,* Vol.1779 No.8, (August 2008), pp. 471-478, ISSN 0006-3002

Fuchs, J., Mueller, J.C., Lichtner, P., Schulte, C., Munz, M., Berg, D., Wullner, U., Illig, T., Sharma, M. & Gasser, T. (2007). The transcription factor PITX3 is associated with sporadic Parkinson's disease. *Neurobiology of Aging,* Vol.30, No.5, (May 2009), pp. 731-738, ISSN 0197-4580

Fung, H.-C., Scholz, S., Matarin, M., Simón-Sánchez, J., Hernandez, D., Britton, A., Gibbs, J.R., Langefeld, C., Stiegert, M.L., Schymick, J., Okun, M.S., Mandel, R.J., Fernandez, H.H., Foote, K.D., Rodríguez, R.L., Peckham, E., De Vrieze, F.W., Gwinn-Hardy, K., Hardy, J.A. & Singleton, A. (2006). Genome-wide genotyping in Parkinson's disease and neurologically normal controls: first stage analysis and public release of data. *Lancet Neurol,* Vol.5, (November 2006), pp. 911-916, ISSN 1474-4465

Grünblatt, E., Zehetmayer, S., Jacob, C.P., Müller, T., Jost, W.H. & Riederer, P. (2010). Pilot study: peripheral biomarkers for diagnosing sporadic Parkinson's disease. *J Neural Transm,* Vol.117, No.12, (December 2010), pp. 1387-1393, ISSN 1435-1463

Grünblatt, E., Mandel, S., Jacob-Hirsch, J., Zeligson, S., Amariglo, N., Rechavi, G., Li, J., Ravid, R., Roggendorf, W., Riederer, P. & Youdim, M.B.H. (2004). Gene expression profiling of parkinsonian substantia nigra pars compacta; alterations in ubiquitin-proteasome, heat shock protein, iron and oxidative stress regulated proteins, cell adhesion/cellular matrix and vesicle trafficking genes. *J Neural Transm*, Vol.111, (September 2004), pp. 1543-1573, ISSN 1435-1463

Gu, S., Jin, L., Zhang, F., Sarnow, P. & Kay, M.A. (2009). Biological basis for restriction of microRNA targets to the 3' untranslated region in mammalian mRNAs. *Nature Structural & Molecular Biology*, Vol.16, No.2, (February 2009), pp. 144-150, ISSN 1545-9985

Hauser, M.A., Li, Y.-J., Xu, H., Noureddine, M.A., Shao, Y.S., Gullans, S.R., Scherzer, C.R., Jensen, R.V., McLaurin, A.C., Gibson, J.R., Scott, B.L., Jewett, R.M., Stenger, J.E., Schmechel, D.E., Hulette, C.M. & Vance, J.M. (2005). Expression Profiling of Substantia Nigra in Parkinson Disease, Progressive Supranuclear Palsy, and Frontotemporal Dementia With Parkinsonism. *Arch Neurol*, Vol.62, (June 2005), pp. 917-921, ISSN 1538-3687

Hébert, S.S. & De Strooper, B. (2007). miRNAs in Neurodegeneration. *Science*, Vol.317, (August 2007), pp. 1179-1180, ISSN 1095-9203

Hohfeld, J., Minami, Y. & Hartl, F.-U. (1995). Hip, a Novel Cochaperone Involved in the Eukaryotic Hsc70/Hsp40 Reaction Cycle. *Cell*, Vol.83, (November 1995), pp. 589-598, ISSN 0092-8674

Horan, M.P. (2009). Application of serial analysis of gene expression to the study of human genetic disease. *Hum Genet*, Vol.126, (July 2009), pp. 605-614, ISSN 1432-1203

Hughes, A.J., Daniel, S.E., Ben-Shlomo, Y. & Lees, A.J. (2002). The accuracy of diagnosis of parkinsonian syndromes in a specialist movement disorder service. *Brain*, Vol.125, No.4, (April 2002), pp. 861-870, ISSN 1460-2156

Jackson, R.J. & Standart, N. (2007). How Do MicroRNAs Regulate Gene Expression? *Sci. STKE 2007*, (January 2007), pp. re1, ISSN 1525-8882

John, B., Enright, A.J., Aravin, A., Tuschl, T., Sander, C. & Marks, D.S. (2004). Human MicroRNA Targets. *PLoS Biology*, Vol.2, No.11, (November 2004), pp. e363, ISSN 1545-7885

Junn, E., Lee, K.-W., Jeong, B.S., Chan, T.W., Im, J.-Y. & Mouradian, M.M. (2009). Repression of -synuclein expression and toxicity by microRNA-7. *Proc Natl Acad Sci U S A*, Vol.106 No.31 (August 2009), pp. 13052-13057 ISSN 1091-6490

Kim, J., Inoue, K., Ishii, J., Vanti, W.B., Voronov, S.V., Murchison, E., Hannon, G. & Abeliovich, A. (2007). A microRNA feedback circuit in midbrain dopamine neurons. *Science*, Vol.317, No.5842, (August 2007), pp. 1220-1224, ISSN 1095-9203

Kim, S., eon, B.S.J., Heo, C., Im, P.S., Ahn, T.-B., Seo, J.-H., Kim, H.-S., Park, C.H., Choi, S.H., Cho, S.-H., Lee, W.J. & Suh, Y.-H. (2004). α-Synuclein induces apoptosis by altered expression in human peripheral lymphocytes in Parkinson's disease. *FASEB J*, (August 2004), pp. ISSN 1530-6860

Krek, A., Grün, D., Poy, M.N., Wolf, R., Rosenberg, L., Epstein, E.J., MacMenamin, P., da Piedade, I., Gunsalus, K.C., Stoffel, M. & Rajewsky, N. (2005). Combinatorial microRNA target predictions. *Nature Genetics*, Vol.37, (April 2005), pp. 495 - 500, ISSN 1546-1718

Krichevsky, A.M. & Kosik, K.S. (2001). Neuronal RNA granules: a link between RNA localization and stimulation-dependent translation. *Neuron*, Vol.32, No.4, (November 2001), pp. 683-696, ISSN 1097-4199

Krichevsky, A.M., King, K.S., Donahue, C.P., Khrapko, K. & Kosik, K.S. (2003). A microRNA array reveals extensive regulation of microRNAs during brain development. *RNA*, Vol.9, No.10, (October 2003), pp. 1274-1281, ISSN 1469-9001

Lau, P. & de Strooper, B. (2010). Dysregulated microRNAs in neurodegenerative disorders. *Seminars in Cell & Developmental Biology*, Vol.21 (September 2010), pp. 768-773, ISSN 1096-3634

Lewis, B.P., Burge, C.B. & Bartel, D.P. (2005). Conserved Seed Pairing, Often Flanked by Adenosines, Indicates that Thousands of Human Genes are MicroRNA Targets. *Cell*, Vol.120, No.1, (January 2005), pp. 15-20, ISSN 0092-8674

Mandel, S., Grunblatt, E., Riederer, P., Amariglio, N., Jacob-Hirsch, J., Rechavi, G. & Youdim, M.B. (2005). Gene expression profiling of sporadic Parkinson's disease substantia nigra pars compacta reveals impairment of ubiquitin-proteasome subunits, SKP1A, aldehyde dehydrogenase, and chaperone HSC-70. *Ann N Y Acad Sci*, Vol.1053, (August 2005), pp. 356-375, ISSN 1749-6632

Mandel, S.A., Fishman-Jacob, T. & Youdim, M.B. (2009). Modeling sporadic Parkinson's disease by silencing the ubiquitin E3 ligase component, SKP1A. *Parkinsonism Relat Disord*, Vol.15, No.Suppl 3, (December 2009), pp. S148-151, ISSN 1873-5126

Maraganore, D.M., de Andrade, M., Lesnick, T.G., Strain, K.J., Farrer, M.J., Rocca, W.A., Pant, P.V.K., Frazer, K.A., Cox, D.R. & Ballinger, D.G. (2005). High-Resolution Whole-Genome Association Study of Parkinson Disease. *Am J Hum Genet*, Vol.77, (September 2005), pp. 685-693, ISSN 1537-6605

Matigian, N.A., McCurdy, R.D., Féron, F., Perry, C., Smith, H., Filippich, C., McLean, D., McGrath, J., Mackay-Sim, A., Mowry, B. & Hayward, N.K. (2008). Fibroblast and lymphoblast gene expression profiles in schizophrenia: are non-neural cells informative? *PLoS ONE*, Vol.3, No.6, (June 2008), pp. e2412, ISSN 1932-6203

Meister, G., Landthaler, M., Dorsett, Y. & Tuschl, T. (2004). Sequence-specific inhibition of microRNA- and siRNA-induced RNA silencing. *RNA*, Vol.10, No.3, (March 2004), pp. 544-550, ISSN 1469-9001

Miller, R.M., Kiser, G.L., Kaysser-Kranich, T.M., Lockner, R.J., Palaniappan, C. & Federoff, H.J. (2006). Robust dysregulation of gene expression in substantia nigra and striatum in Parkinson's disease. *Neurobiol Dis*, Vol.21, No.2, (February 2006), pp. 305-313, ISSN 0969-9961

Miska, E.A., Alvarez-Saavedra, E., Townsend, M., Yoshii, A., Sestan, N., Rakic, P., Constantine-Paton, M. & Horvitz, H.R. (2004). Microarray analysis of microRNA expression in the developing mammalian brain. *Genome Biol*, Vol.5, (August 2004), pp. R68, ISSN 1465-6914

Moran, L.B., Duke, D.C., Deprez, M., Dexter, D.T., Pearce, R.K.B. & Graeber, M.B. (2006). Whole genome expression profiling of the medial and lateral substantia nigra in Parkinson's disease. *Neurogenetics*, Vol.7, (March 2006), pp. 1-11, ISSN 1364-6753

Moran, L.B., Croisier, E., Duke, D.C., Kalaitzakis, M.E., Roncaroli, F., Deprez, M., Dexter, D.T., Pearce, R.K. & Graeber, M.B. (2007). Analysis of alpha-synuclein, dopamine and parkin pathways in neuropathologically confirmed parkinsonian nigra. *Acta Neuropathologica*, Vol.113, No.3, (March 2007), pp. 253-263, ISSN 1432-0533

Nagatsu, T., Mogi, M., Ichinose, H. & Togari, A. (2000). Changes in cytokines and neurotrophins in Parkinson's disease. *J Neural Transm Suppl*, Vol.2000, No.60, (2000), pp. 277-290, ISSN 0303-6995

Nelson, P.T. & Keller, J.N. (2007). RNA in brain disease: no longer just "the messenger in the middle". *J Neuropathol Exp Neurol*, Vol.66, No.6, (June 2007), pp. 461-468, ISSN 0022-3069

Nelson, P.T., Wang, W.-X. & Rajeev, B.W. (2008). MicroRNAs (miRNAs) in Neurodegenerative Diseases. *Brain Pathology*, Vol.18, (January 2008), pp. 130-138, ISSN 1750-3639

Noureddine, M.A., Li, Y.J., van der Walt, J.M., Walters, R., Jewett, R.M., Xu, H., Wang, T., Walter, J.W., Scott, B.L., Hulette, C., Schmechel, D., Stenger, J.E., Dietrich, F., Vance, J.M. & Hauser, M.A. (2005). Genomic convergence to identify candidate genes for Parkinson disease: SAGE analysis of the substantia nigra. *Mov Disord*, Vol.20, No.10, (October 2005), pp. 1299-1309, ISSN 1531-8257

Ohnuki, T., Nakamura, A., Okuyama, S. & Nakamura, S. (2010). Gene expression profiling in progressively MPTP-lesioned macaques reveals molecular pathways associated with sporadic Parkinson's disease. *Brain Research*, Vol.1346, (June 2010), pp. 26-42, ISSN 1872-6240

Pattarini, R., Rong, Y., Qu, C. & Morgan, J.I. (2008). Distinct mechanisms of 1-methyl-4-phenyl-1,2,3,6-tetrahydropyrimidine resistance revealed by transcriptome mapping in mouse striatum. *Neuroscience*, Vol.155, No.4, (September 2008), pp. 1174-1194, ISSN 1873-7544

Pillai, R.S., Bhattacharyya, S.N. & Filipowicz, W. (2007). Repression of protein synthesis by miRNAs: how many mechanisms? *TRENDS in Cell Biology*, Vol.17, No.3, (March 2007), pp. 118-126, ISSN 1879-3088

Plasterk, W.P.K.a.R.H.A. (2006). The Diverse Functions of MicroRNAs in Animal Development and Disease. *Dev Cell*, Vol.11, No.4, (October 2006), pp. 441-450, ISSN 1878-1551

Rajewsky, N. (2006). MicroRNA target predictions in animals. *Nature Genetics*, Vol.38, (May 2006), pp. S8 - S13, ISSN 1546-1718

Reale, M., Iarlori, C., Thomas, A., Gambi, D., Perfetti, B., Di Nicola, M. & Onofrj, M. (2009). Peripheral cytokines profile in Parkinson's disease. *Brain Behav Immun*, Vol.23, No.1, (July 2008), pp. 55-63, ISSN 1090-2139

Roshan, R., Ghosh, T., Scaria, V. & Pillai, B. (2009). MicroRNAs: novel therapeutic targets in neurodegenerative diseases. *Drug Discovery Today*, Vol.14, No.23/24, (December 2009), pp. 1123-1129, ISSN 1878-5832

Ryoo, H.L., Pierrotti, D. & Joyce, J.N. (1998). Dopamine D3 receptor is decreased and D2 receptor is elevated in the striatum of Parkinson's disease. *Mov Disord*, Vol.13, (September 1998), pp. 788-797, ISSN 0885-3185

Santosh, S., Arora, N., Sarma, P., Pal-Bhadra, M. & Bhadra, U. (2009). InteractionMap and Selection of microRNA Targets in Parkinson's Disease-Related Genes. *Journal of Biomedicine and Biotechnology*, (November 2009), pp. ID363145, ISSN 1110-7251

Saugstad, J.A. (2010). MicroRNAs as effectors of brain function with roles in ischemia and injury, neuroprotection, and neurodegeneration. *J Cereb Blood Flow Metab*, Vol.30, No.9, (September 2010), pp. 1564-1576, ISSN 1559-7016

Schaefer, A., O'Carroll, D., Tan, C.L., Hillman, D., Sugimori, M., Llinas, R. & Greengard, P. (2007). Cerebellar neurodegeneration in the absence of microRNAs. *JEM* Vol.204, No.7, (July 2007), pp. 1553-1558, ISSN 1540-9538

Scherzer, C.R., Eklund, A.C., Morse, L.J., Liao, Z., Locascio, J.J., Fefer, D., Schwarzschild, M.A., Schlossmacher, M.G., Hauser, M.A., Vance, J.M., Sudarsky, L.R., Standaert, D.G., Growdon, J.H., Jensen, R.V. & Gullans, S.R. (2007). Molecular markers of early Parkinson's disease based on gene expression in blood. *Proc Natl Acad Sci U S A*, Vol.104 No.3, (January 2007), pp. 955–960, ISSN 1091-6490

Schratt, G.M., Tuebing, F., Nigh, E.A., Kane, C.G., Sabatini, M.E., Kiebler, M. & Greenberg, M.E. (2006). A brain-specific microRNA regulates dendritic spine development. *Nature*, Vol.439, No.7074, (January 2006), pp. 283-289, ISSN 1476-4687

Scott, W.K., Nance, M.A., Watts, R.L., Hubble, J.P., Koller, W.C., Lyons, K., Pahwa, R., Stern, M.B., Colcher, A., Hiner, B.C., Jankovic, J., Ondo, W.G., Allen, F.H.J., Goetz, C.G.,

Small, G.W., Masterman, D., Mastaglia, F., Laing, N.G., Stajich, J.M., Slotterbeck, B., Booze, M.W., Ribble, R.C., Rampersaud, E., West, S.G., Gibson, R.A., Middleton, L.T., Roses, A.D., Haines, J.L., Scott, B.L., Vance, J.M. & Pericak-Vance, M.A. (2001). Complete genomic screen in Parkinson disease: evidence for multiple genes. *JAMA*, Vol.286, No.18, (November 2001), pp. 2239-2244, ISSN 1538-3598

Sethupathy, P. & Collins, F.S. (2008). MicroRNA target site polymorphisms and human disease. *Trends in Genetics*, Vol.24 No.10, (September 2008), pp. 489-497, ISSN 0168-9479

Shadrina, M.I., Filatova, E.V., Karabanov, A.V., Slominsky, P.A., Illarioshkin, S.N., Ivanova-Smolenskaya, I.A. & Limborska, S.A. (2010). Expression analysis of suppression of tumorigenicity 13 gene in patients with Parkinson's disease. *Neuroscience Letters*, Vol.473 (April 2010), pp. 257-259, ISSN 0304-3940

Shi, Z.-z., Zhang, J.-w. & Zheng, S. (2007). What we know about ST13, a co-factor of heat shock protein, or a tumor suppressor? *Journal of Zhejiang University SCIENCE B*, Vol.8, No.3, (March 2007), pp. 170-176, ISSN 1862-1783

Simunovic, F., Yi, M., Wang, Y., Stephens, R. & Sonntag, K.C. (2010). Evidence for Gender-Specific Transcriptional Profiles of Nigral Dopamine Neurons in Parkinson Disease. *PLoS ONE*, Vol.5, No.1, (January 2010), pp. e8856, ISSN 1932-6203

Simunovic, F., Yi, M., Wang, Y., Macey, L., Brown, L.T., Krichevsky, A.M., Andersen, S.L., Stephens, R.M., Benes, F.M. & Sonntag, K.C. (2009). Gene expression profiling of substantia nigra dopamine neurons: further insights into Parkinson's disease pathology. *Brain*, Vol.132, No.Pt 7, (December 2008), pp. 1795-1809, ISSN 1460-2156

Smirnova, L., Gräfe, A., Seiler, A., Schumacher, S., Nitsch, R. & Wulczyn, F.G. (2005). Regulation of miRNA expression during neural cell specification. *Eur J Neurosci*, Vol.21, No.6, (March 2005), pp. 1469-1477, ISSN 1460-9568

Smith, D.J. (2009). Mitochondrial dysfunction in mouse models of Parkinson's disease revealed by transcriptomics and proteomics. *J Bioenerg Biomembr*, Vol.41, No.6, (December 2009), pp. 487-491, ISSN

Standart, N. & Jackson, R.J. (2007). MicroRNAs repress translation of m7Gppp-capped target mRNAs in vitro by inhibiting initiation and promoting deadenylation. *Genes Dev*, Vol.21, (August 2007), pp. 1975-1982, ISSN 0890-9369/07

Sutherland, G.T., Halliday, G.M., Silburn, P.A., Mastaglia, F.L., Rowe, D.B., Boyle, R.S., O'Sullivan, J.D., Ly, T., Wilton, S.D. & Mellick, G.D. (2009). Do Polymorphisms in the Familial Parkinsonism Genes Contribute to Risk for Sporadic Parkinson's Disease? *Movement Disorders*, Vol.24, No.6, (February 2009), pp. 833-838, ISSN 1531-8257

Tan, E.K., Cheah, S.Y., Fook-Chong, S., Yew, K., Chandran, V.R., Lum, S.Y. & Yi, Z. (2005). Functional COMT variant predicts response to high dose pyridoxine in Parkinson's disease. *Am J Med Genet B Neuropsychiatr Genet*, Vol.137B, No.1, (August 2005), pp. 1-4, ISSN 1552-485X

van der Walt, J.M., Noureddine, M.A., Kittappa, R., Hauser, M.A., Scott, W.K., McKay, R., Zhang, F., Stajich, J.M., Fujiwara, K., Scott, B.L., Pericak-Vance, M.A., Vance, J.M. & Martin, E.R. (2004). Fibroblast Growth Factor 20 Polymorphisms and Haplotypes Strongly Influence Risk of Parkinson Disease. *The American Journal of Human Genetics*, Vol.74, No.6, (June 2004), pp. 1121-1127, ISSN 1537-6605

Vasudevan, S., Tong, Y. & Steitz, J.A. (2007). Switching from Repression to Activation: MicroRNAs Can Up-Regulate Translation. *Science*, Vol.318, (December 2007), pp. 1931-1934, ISSN 1095-9203

Vo, N., Klein, M.E., Varlamova, O., Keller, D.M., Yamamoto, T., Goodman, R.H. & Impey, S. (2005). A cAMP-response element binding protein-induced microRNA regulates neuronal morphogenesis. *Proc Natl Acad Sci U S A*, Vol.102, No.45, (November 2005), pp. 16426-16431, ISSN 1091-6490

Vogt, I.R., Lees, A.J., Evert, B.O., Klockgether, T., Bonin, M. & Wüllner, U. (2006). Transcriptional changes in multiple system atrophy and Parkinson's disease putamen. *Exp Neurol*, Vol.199, No.2, (June 2006), pp. 465-478, ISSN 1090-2430

Wang, G., van der Walt, J.M., Mayhew, G., Li, Y.-J., Zu¨chner, S., Scott, W.K., Martin, E.R. & Vance, J.M. (2008). Variation in the miRNA-433 Binding Site of FGF20 Confers Risk for Parkinson Disease by Overexpression of a-Synuclein. *The American Journal of Human Genetics*, Vol.82, (February 2008), pp. 283-289, ISSN 1537-6605

Weinberg, M.S. & Wood, M.J.A. (2009). Short non-coding RNA biology and neurodegenerative disorders: novel disease targets and therapeutics. *Human Molecular Genetics*, Vol.18, No.R1, (April 2009), pp. R27-R39, ISSN 1460-2083

Whitton, P.S. (2007). Inflammation as a causative factor in the aetiology of Parkinson's disease. *Br J Pharmacol*, Vol.150, No.8, (April 2007), pp. 963-976, ISSN 1476-5381

Xun, Z., Sowell, R.A., Kaufman, T.C. & Clemmer, D.E. (2007). Protein Expression in a Drosophila Model of Parkinson's Disease. *J Proteome Res*, Vol.6, No.1, (January 2007), pp. 348-357, ISSN 1535-3907

Yacoubian, T.A., Cantuti-Castelvetri, I., Bouzou, B., Asteris, G., McLean, P.J., Hyman, B.T. & Standaert, D.G. (2008). Transcriptional dysregulation in a transgenic model of Parkinson disease. *Neurobiology of Disease*, Vol.29, (November 2007), pp. 515-528, ISSN 1095-953X

Zechner, C., Lai, L., Zechner, J.F., Geng, T., Yan, Z., Rumsey, J.W., Collia, D., Chen, Z., Wozniak, D.F., Leone, T.C. & Kelly, D.P. (2010). Total Skeletal Muscle PGC-1 Deficiency Uncouples Mitochondrial Derangements from Fiber Type Determination and Insulin Sensitivity. *Cell Metabolism*, Vol.12, No.6, (December 2010), pp. 633-642, ISSN 1932-7420

Zhang, Y., James, M., Middleton, F.A. & Davis, R.L. (2005). Transcriptional Analysis of Multiple Brain Regions in Parkinson's Disease Supports the Involvement of Specific Protein Processing, Energy Metabolism, and Signaling Pathways, and Suggests Novel Disease Mechanisms. *American Journal of Medical Genetics Part B (Neuropsychiatric Genetics)*, Vol.137B, (August 2005), pp. 5-16, ISSN 1552-485X

Zheng, B., Liao, Z., Locascio, J.J., Lesniak, K.A., Roderick, S.S., Watt, M.L., Eklund, A.C., Zhang-James, Y., Kim, P.D., Hauser, M.A., Grünblatt, E., Moran, L.B., Mandel, S.A., Riederer, P., Miller, R.M., Federoff, H.J., Wüllner, U., Papapetropoulos, S., Youdim, M.B., Cantuti-Castelvetri, I., Young, A.B., Vance, J.M., Davis, R.L., Hedreen, J.C., Adler, C.H., Beach, T.G., Graeber, M.B., Middleton, F.A., Rochet, J.-C. & Scherzer, C.R. (2010). PGC-1a, A Potential Therapeutic Target for Early Intervention in Parkinson's Disease. *Sci Transl Med*, Vol.2, No.52, (October 2010), pp. 52ra73, ISSN 1946-6242

14

Brain Mitochondrial Dysfunction and Complex I Syndrome in Parkinson´s Disease

Laura B. Valdez[1], Manuel J. Bandez[2], Ana Navarro[2]† and Alberto Boveris[1]
[1]*Laboratory of Free Radical Biology, School of Pharmacy and Biochemistry, University of Buenos Aires,*
[2]*Department of Biochemistry and Molecular Biology, School of Medicine, University of Cádiz,*
[1]*Argentina*
[2]*Spain*

1. Introduction

1.1 Clinical characteristics of Parkinson's disease

Parkinson's disease (PD) is an old-age neurodegenerative disease with a small but significant genetic risk. The prevalence of PD is of 0.3% in the whole population, affecting more than 1% of the humans over 60 years of age (de Lau & Breteler, 2006). Parkinson´s disease is characterized by the progressive loss of dopamine due to degeneration of dopaminergic neurons in the *substancia nigra, striatum* body and brain cortex. In addition, α-synuclein-positive Lewy bodies in brainstem and neocortex are consistently found at autopsy (Forno, 1996; Jellinger & Mizuno, 2003). Therefore, in patients with PD, movements, sleep, autonomic functions and cognition become progressively impaired.

Complex factors contribute to the appearance of PD but with a constant mitochondrial involvement and a decreased capacity to produce energy (ATP) in the affected brain areas (Shapira, 1998; Shapira, 2008). Mitochondrial dysfunction in the human frontal cortex is to be considered a factor contributing to impaired cognition in PD.

2. Environmental aspects and experimental models

Both environmental chemicals and genetic susceptibility are thought to contribute to the etiology of sporadic PD (Nagatsu, 2002). Despite of familial PD was correlated with a series of genes mutations, the etiology of idiopathic PD, which accounts for more than 90% of PD, is still not fully understood. It is well documented that there is an epidemiological link between PD and individuals who lives and works in rural areas and who has been exposed to various herbicides and insecticides (Gorell et al. 1998; Ayala et al., 2007; Gomez et al., 2007).

Although the etiopathogenesis of PD is still elusive, *post mortem* studies support the involvement of oxidative stress in neurons with an increased production of superoxide

radical (O_2^-) and hydrogen peroxide (H_2O_2) and of mitochondrial dysfunction, especially of complex I of mitochondrial respiratory chain (Shapira et al., 1989; Shapira et al., 1990a, 1990b; Gomez et al., 2007; Navarro & Boveris, 2009; Navarro et al., 2009).
The early hints about the central role of mitochondria in the pathogenesis of PD resulted from the observation that human exposure to 1-methyl-4-phenyl-1,2,3,6-tetrahydropyridine (MPTP), a contaminant in synthetic opiates, triggered an acute and permanent parkinsonism with death of dopamine neurons (Langston et al., 1983). It was found that the MPTP active metabolite is the 1-methyl-4-phenilpyridinium ion (MPP^+). This compound is accumulated in mitochondria and produces their toxicity by inhibiting mitochondrial complex I, the proton pumping NADH:ubiquinone oxidoreductase.
As was mentioned above, epidemiological research indicates that exposure to pesticides and welding elevates the risk of PD (Chade et al., 2006; Dhillon et al., 2008). Most of pesticides are inhibitors of mitochondrial complex I, which is the first and the most vulnerable complex in the series of membrane H^+ pumps of the mitochondrial respiratory chain (Wallace et al., 1997). The pesticide rotenone ((2R,6aS,12aS)-1,2,6,6a,12,12a-hexahydro-2-isopropenyl-8,9-dimethoxychromeno [3,4-b]furo(2,3-h)chromen-6-one) is a powerful inhibitor of mitochondrial complex I: in isolated beef heart and liver mitochondria, rotenone median inhibitory concentration (IC_{50}) is 0.05 nmol/mg protein with a Ki of 4 nM (Degli, 1998). When neuron cultures are exposed to rotenone, the cells increase the O_2^- production rate leading them to death (Ahmadi et al., 2003; Moon et al., 2005). Furthermore, dopaminergic neuronal cells exposed to rotenone reproduce many of the features of PD including α-synuclein inclusions bodies in rats (Betarber et al., 2000; Sherer et al., 2003).
The above mentioned inhibitors of complex I, rotenone and MPTP, are typically used in the experimental model of PD in laboratory animals.

3. Genetic aspects

Although most PD cases are sporadic, the discovery of genes linked to familial form of disease due to mutations in the SNCA (α-synuclein), PARK2, DJ-1, PINK1, and LRRK2 genes has provided important clues about the disease progress (Henchcliffe & Beal., 2008; Zheng et al., 2010). In the sporadic disease, α-synuclein and degenerating mitochondria are the major components of Lewy bodies, the hall mark cytoplasmic inclusions found in PD brains. Biochemical complex I deficiency is found in PD patients not only in *substancia nigra* but also in platelets (Henchcliffe & Beal, 2008).
Recently, Zheng and coworkers (2010) reported that decreases in expression of 10 gene sets are associated with PD, even in probable subclinical disease and in tissues, outside *substancia nigra*. These 10 gene sets encode proteins responsible for interconnected cellular processes: nuclear-encoded mitochondrial electron transfer, mitochondrial biogenesis, glucose oxidation, and glucose sensing (Zheng et al., 2010). The authors showed that bioenergetics genes responsive to the master regulation of PGC-1α, including genes for nuclear-encoded electron transfer carriers are under expressed in patients with PD and in incipient Lewy body diseases. Furthermore, co-activation by PGC-1α up-regulates nuclear subunits of mitochondrial respiratory chain complexes I, II, III, IV, and V and blocks dopamine neuron loss in cellular models of PD-linked α-synocleinopathy and rotenone toxicity. Moreover, genetic ablation of PGC-1α in mice markedly enhanced MPTP-induced dopamine neuron loss in the *substancia nigra* (St-Pierre et al., 2006).

4. Pathophysiological aspects

Physiological, clinical and genetic studies support the relationship between PD and energy metabolism in neurons, including mitochondrial electron transport carriers and cytosolic glucose utilization. *In vivo* and *ex vivo* experimental results have shown that PD is primarily associated to two interdependent situations of brain mitochondria: (a) mitochondrial dysfunction; and (b) mitochondrial oxidative damage. In addition, defective oxidative phosphorylation was reported in muscle, and increased level of 8-hydroxydeoxyguanosine was found in PD patients plasma (Henchcliffe & Beal, 2008).

4.1 Mitochondrial complex I and physiological production of superoxide, nitric oxide and peroxynitrite

Mitochondrial complex I (NADH-UQ reductase) catalyzes electron transfer from NADH to ubiquinone and it is the main molecular pathway to link the tricarboxylic acid cycle, the coenzyme NADH and the mitochondrial respiratory chain. Complex I is a supra-molecular protein complex composed of about 40 polypeptide subunits and contains FMN and iron-sulphur centers (Walker, 1992; Walker et al., 1992). Two complex I-linked UQ-pools have been detected (Raha & Robinson, 2000). Non-covalent hydrophobic bonds are essential in keeping together the whole structure of complex I; low concentrations of detergents, natural and synthetic steroids (Boveris & Stoppani, 1970) and hydrophobic pesticides, such as rotenone and pyridaben (Gomez et al., 2007), are effective in disrupting intra-complex I polypeptide hydrophobic bonds and in inhibiting complex I electron transfer activity.

Complex I produces significant amounts of O_2^- in physiological conditions (0.80-0.90 nmol O_2^-/min.mg protein) through the auto-oxidation reaction of flavin-semiquinone ($FMNH^•$) with molecular oxygen. It is understood that the ubisemiquinone ($UQH^•$) auto-oxidation contribution, in complex I, is negligible (Boveris & Cadenas, 2000; Turrens & Boveris, 1980). Superoxide anion production yields an O_2^- steady state concentration of 0.1-0.2 nM in the mitochondrial matrix (Boveris & Cadenas, 2000; Boveris et al., 2006; Valdez et al., 2006). The O_2^- production rate by complex I is increased by inhibition of electron transfer with rotenone (Boveris & Chance, 1973) or by complex I dysfunction (Hensley et al., 2000; Navarro et al., 2009; Navarro et al., 2011).

Both, nitric oxide (NO) and peroxynitrite ($ONOO^-$) have been proposed as direct inhibitors of complex I. Mitochondrial NO production is carried out by the mitochondrial nitric oxide synthase (mtNOS), an isoenzyme of the NOS family located in mitochondrial inner membrane (Tatoyan & Giulivi, 1998; Giulivi et al., 1998). Nitric oxide is produced at a rate of 1.0-1.4 nmol NO/min.mg protein and kept at a steady state level of 200-350 nM in the mitochondrial matrix (Boveris et al., 2006; Valdez et al., 2006). Peroxynitrite is generated in the mitochondrial matrix through the diffusion controlled reaction ($k = 1.9 \times 10^{10}$ M^{-1} s^{-1}) between two free radicals: O_2^- and NO. This reaction contributes with 0.38 μM $ONOO^-$/sec in the mitochondrial matrix or 0.92 nmol/min. mg protein (Valdez et al., 2000). In this approximation the contribution of cytosolic NO has not been considered. Peroxynitrite is normally reduced by the mitochondrial reductants NADH, UQH_2 and GSH and kept at intramitochondrial steady state level of 2-5 nM (Valdez et al., 2000). When the steady state concentration of $ONOO^-$ is enhanced up to 25-40 nM, tyrosine nitration, protein oxidation and damage to iron sulfur centers might takes place, leading to a sustained complex I inhibition and increased generation of O_2^- by complex I.

4.2 Brain mitochondrial dysfunction: Complex I syndrome

Several studies have shown a mitochondrial dysfunction and a reduced activity of mitochondrial complex I in *substantia nigra* (Schapira et al., 1990a; Schapira et al., 1990b; Schapira, 2008b) and in frontal cortex (Navarro et al., 2009; Navarro & Boveris, 2009) in PD patients.

Gomez et al. (2007) and Navarro et al. (2009) have shown that the *in vitro* treatment of rat brain mitochondria with rotenone (1-10 μM) inhibits complex I activity without changes in complexes II, III and IV activities. In addition, coupled mitochondria isolated from rat brain incubated with rotenone showed a dose-dependent decrease in respiratory control with malate and glutamate as substrates, without modifications in the O_2 consumption when succinate was used as substrate (Gomez et al., 2007; Navarro et al., 2009).

Rats treated with rotenone (2 mg/kg weight, i.p. and daily, during 30 to 60 days) showed a selective nigrostriatal dopaminergic degeneration similar to the one observed in PD. Respiration rates were assessed in 1 mm^3 brain cortex cubes, a thickness that allows O_2 diffusion to the center of the cube avoiding anaerobic areas. Control samples had a respiratory rate of about 0.45 μmol O_2/min. g striatum (Table 1). Rotenone treated rats during 30 and 60 days decreased 17% and 35%, respectively, the striatal O_2 uptake.

Experimental condition	**O_2 consumption** (ng-at O/min.g striatum)
Control	896 ± 8
30 days rotenone	744 ± 8*
60 days rotenone	582 ± 5*#

Table 1. **Striatal O_2 consumption in rotenone-treated rats during 30 and 60 days.** Respiratory rates were determined in 1 mm^3 rat striatum cubes in air-saturated Krebs suspending medium at 30ºC. The values are means ± SEM: n = 3 per group (15 rats each group in pools of 5 rats). *p<0.05, rotenone treated rats *vs.* control rats; #p<0.05, 60 days-rotenone treated rats *vs.* 30 days-rotenone treated rats.

The same phenomenon was observed in isolated striatal mitochondria. Mitochondrial state 3 respiration decreased by about 13% and 30% after 30 and 60 days of rotenone treatment, with malate-glutamate as complex I substrate. Due to the fact that no changes were observed in state 4 respiration, the respiratory control also declined (Table 2). When succinate was used as complex II substrate, a slight impairment in state 3 respiration (20%) was observed after 60 days of rotenone administration.

The respiratory deficiency was further examined by assaying the activity of mitochondrial respiratory complexes. Table 3 shows that complex I activity decreased after 30 and 60 days of rotenone administration by 17% and 57%, respectively; complex IV activity declined 23% after 60 days of treatment; and complex II activity was not modified showing, once more, the highest and selective susceptibility of complex I to the oxidative, nitrosative and/or nitrative damage associated with rotenone treatment. The pattern observed for the decline of complex I activity in striatal mitochondria was also observed in the reduction of biochemical mtNOS (27% and 62%, in 30 and 60 days rotenone-treated rats) (Table 3) and functional mtNOS activities (29% and 71%), in accordance to the reported physical and functional interaction between complex I and mtNOS (Franco et al, 2006; Valdez & Boveris, 2007; Navarro et al., 2010).

Experimental conditions	Oxygen consumption (ng-at O/min. mg protein)		
	Control	Rotenone	
		30 days	60 days
Substrate: malate-glutamate			
State 4	42 ± 3	40 ± 3	38 ± 3
State 3	166 ± 9	144 ± 8*	116 ± 7*#
Respiratory control	3.9 ± 0.3	3.6 ± 0.3*	3.1 ± 0.4*
Substrate: succinate			
State 4	60 ± 4	58 ± 4	52 ± 4
State 3	240 ± 14	220 ± 11	192 ± 9*#
Respiratory control	4.0 ± 0.3	3.7 ± 0.3	3.7 ± 0.3

Table 2. **Striatum mitochondrial O_2 uptake of rotenone-treated rats during 30 and 60 days.** The values are means ± SEM: n = 3 per group (15 rats each in pools of 5 rats). *$p<0.05$, rotenone treated rats *vs.* control rats; # $p<0.05$, 60 days-rotenone treated rats *vs.* 30 days-rotenone treated rats.

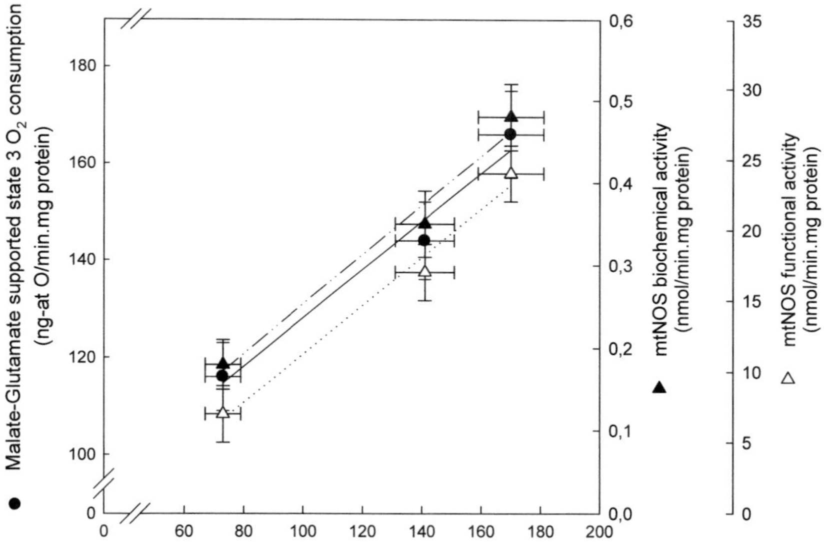

Fig. 1. Linear correlations between mitochondrial complex I activity and malate-glutamate supported state 3 respiration (•) ($r^2 = 0.97$) and between mitochondrial complex I activity and mtNOS biochemical (▲) ($r^2 = 0.98$) and functional activities (Δ) ($r^2 = 0.98$).

Linear correlations (Fig. 1) were obtained between mitochondrial complex I activity and either malate-glutamate supported state 3 O_2 uptake ($r^2 = 0.97$) or mtNOS biochemical ($r^2 = 0.98$) and functional activities ($r^2 = 0.98$), indicating that the pattern observed for the decline of complex I activity is associated to the reduction of mtNOS activity and to the impairment of striatum mitochondrial respiration.

Experimental condition	Complex I (nmol. min^{-1}. mg $protein^{-1}$)	Complex II (nmol. min^{-1}. mg $protein^{-1}$)	Complex IV (min^{-1}. mg $protein^{-1}$)	mtNOS (nmol. min^{-1}. mg $protein^{-1}$)
Control	170 ± 11	119 ± 9	75 ± 8	0.48 ± 0.04
30 days rotenone	141 ± 10*	117 ± 9	61 ± 5	0.35 ± 0.04*
60 days rotenone	73 ± 6*#	115 ± 9	58 ± 5*	0.18 ± 0.03*#

Table 3. **Striatum mitochondrial enzymatic activities of rotenone-treated rats during 30 and 60 days.** The values are means ± SEM: n = 3 per group (15 rats each in pools of 5 rats). *$p<0.05$, rotenone treated rats *vs.* control rats; #$p<0.05$, 60 days-rotenone treated rats *vs.* 30 days-rotenone treated rats.

The experimental quantitative evidence shows a range of 35% to 73% of a decline of complex I activity in brain mitochondria in aging and in neurodegenerative diseases. A value of about 50% is considered a limit of a tolerable functional impairment in terms of energy production that is compatible with the physiological function. For instance, complex I is inactivated by 36% in aged rat whole brain mitochondria (Navarro & Boveris, 2007), by 73% in aged rat hippocampal mitochondria (Navarro et al., 2008), by 57% in rat striatal mitochondria in experimental parkinsonism (Table 3 and Fig. 1), and by 43% in cortex mitochondria of human PD patients (Navarro et al., 2010). The data included in Tables 1 and 2 and in Fig. 1 allow to making some quantitative considerations respect to the basal respiration of striatal tissue under no neurological stimulus (in physiological conditions the striatal route is constantly activated). Taking into account the striatal O_2 consumption in control rats of 896 ng-at O/min. g tissue, a mitochondrial content of 12 mg protein/g striatum, and the mitochondrial respirations (in ng-at O/min. mg protein) in state 3 of 166 (malate-glutamate) and of 240 (succinate) and in state 4 of 42 and 60 (respectively), the fraction of mitochondria in state 3 and in state 4 can be calculated (Boveris & Boveris, 2007):

$$\text{Tissue } O_2 \text{ consumption (ng-at O/min x g tissue)} =$$
$$\text{mg protein/g tissue x [(a x state 3 } O_2 \text{ uptake) + (1 – a) x (state 4 } O_2 \text{ uptake)]}$$

The state 4 and state 3 mitochondrial O_2 consumption were calculated considering the detected O_2 uptake rates (Table 2) and the substrate supply in physiological conditions: [(3 x rate with malate-glutamate) + (rate with succinate)]/4. Therefore, striatal mitochondria are in the tissue about 20% in state 3 and about 80% in state 4. Under conditions of increased ATP demand, striatum mitochondria will be able to increase ATP synthesis up to 5 times by switching mitochondria from the resting state 4 to the active state 3. At variance, in experimental parkinsonism, after 60 days of rotenone treatment, mitochondria are 8% in state 3 and 92% in state 4, showing that in parkinsonism, striatal mitochondria are severely limited in their capacity to respond to ATP demands.

Moreover, similar mitochondrial complex I dysfunctions were reported in skeletal muscle and platelets of PD patients (Mann et al., 1992). This condition of complex I impairment is likely to be of pathogenic importance because intoxication of experimental animals with inhibitors of complex I (rotenone, MPTP, MPP^+) (Bougria et al., 1995; Gomez et al., 2007) reproduces the clinical symptoms of PD in human subjects.

4.3 Brain mitochondrial oxidative damage

The mtNOS and complex I functional association in brain has been linked to the development of neurodegenerative diseases (Navarro et al., 2010). As it has been early proposed (Hensley et al., 2000), changes in complex I proteins are certainly an explanation for the increase in O_2^- and H_2O_2 production rates. Rat treated with rotenone during 30 and 60 days increased the O_2^- production rates by about 13% and 37%, respectively (Table 4). This enhancement is in agreement with an increased generation of phospholipids oxidation and protein oxidation products in striatal mitochondria (Fig. 2 A and B).

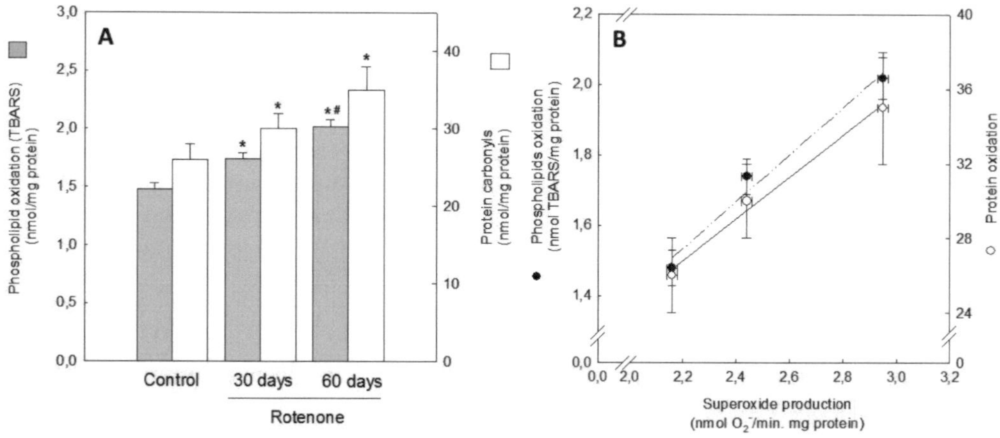

Fig. 2. **A**. Protein carbonyls and phospholipid oxidation products in striatal mitochondria of rotenone-treated rats. The values are means ± SEM: n=3 per group (15 rats each in pools of 5 rats). $^*p < 0.05$, rotenone treated rats *vs.* control rats; $\#p<0.05$, 60 days-rotenone treated rats *vs.* 30 days-rotenone treated rats. **B.** Linear correlations between O_2^- production rate and either phospholipid oxidation (•) ($r^2 = 0.98$) or protein oxidation (o) ($r^2 = 0.99$) products.

Navarro and co-workers (2009) have shown a marked impairments of tissue and malate-glutamate supported state 3 mitochondrial respiration and of complex I activity, associated with an oxidative damage, in frozen samples of frontal cortex (area 8) in PD patients in comparison to age-matched healthy controls (Navarro et al., 2009). Thus, human cortex mitochondrial dysfunction in PD is now added to the classical recognition of mitochondrial dysfunction in *substantia nigra,* which was early considered as specifically sensitive brain area in PD (Schapira et al., 1990a).

Experimental condition	O_2^- production (nmol/min. mg protein)
Control	2.16 ± 0.02
30 days rotenone	2.44 ± 0.02*
60 days rotenone	2.95 ± 0.02*#

Table 4. **Striatum mitochondrial superoxide anion production of rotenone-treated rats during 30 and 60 days.** The values are means ± SEM: n = 3 per group (15 rats each in pools of 5 rats). $^*p<0.05$, rotenone treated rats *vs.* control rats; $\#p<0.05$, 60 days-rotenone treated rats *vs.* 30 days-rotenone treated rats.

Mitochondrial complex I is particularly sensitive in terms of inhibition and inactivation to oxidants, oxygen free radicals and reactive nitrogen species. The mitochondrial dysfunction is currently described as "complex I syndrome", that includes decreased tissue O_2 uptake, decreased malate/glutamate-supported mitochondrial respiration, reduced complex I (NADH-dehydrogenase) activity, increased phospholipid and protein oxidation products, increased protein nitration products, and increased O_2^- and H_2O_2 production rates (Boveris et al., 2010). Interestingly, high doses of vitamin E are able to restore to normal the age-dependent complex I syndrome in hippocampus and brain cortex (Navarro et al., 2010).This "complex I syndrome" has been observed in PD and in other neurodegenerative diseases (Schapira et al., 1990a; Schapira et al., 1990b; Cooper et al., 1992; Schapira, 2008; Carreras et al., 2004; Navarro & Boveris, 2007; Navarro et al., 2009), as well as in aging (Boveris& Navarro, 2008) and in ischemia-reperfusion (Gonzalez-Flecha et al., 1993; Valdez et al., 2011).

The molecular mechanisms responsible for complex I syndrome are likely accounted for a series of processes and reactions that lead synergistically to complex I inactivation. The involved processes and reactions are, in the first place, the lipid peroxidation process and the reactions of the reactive free radical intermediates (mainly $ROO^\bullet$) with complex I. In the second place, the reactions of the aldehydes produced in the lipid peroxidation process (4-HO-nonenal and malonaldehyde) with amino groups of the polypeptide chain of the complex I proteins. In the third place, nitration of complex I proteins following to the increased formation of $ONOO^-$, the chemical species produced by the intramitochondrial reaction of NO and O_2^-at the vicinity of NADH-dehydrogenase active center (Turrens & Boveris, 1980). The three mentioned processes provide synergistically pathways leading to complex I inactivation. Interestingly, complex I inactivation is accompanied by increased auto-oxidation and O_2^- production rate and subsequently an enlarged generation of H_2O_2 (Hensley et al., 2000; Navarro et al., 2011). It is understood that the reactions that inactivate complex I, mediated by free radicals ($ROO^\bullet$), aldehydes and $ONOO^-$, change the native non-covalent intermolecular forces bonding and synergistically promote covalent cross linking with protein inactivation (Liu et al., 2003).

5. Conclusions

Parkinson's disease is characterized by persistent, coordinated, nuclear-encoded cellular energy defects to which nigral dopamine neurons are intrinsically more susceptible than others cells. Complex I dysfunction in PD may be a biochemically detectable "tip of the iceberg" of a deeper molecular defect comprising the entire nuclear-encoded electron transfer chain. Under expression of PGC-1α-controlled genes involved in cellular energetic might represent a common link for these diverse manifestations of defects in mitochondrial biogenesis, and abnormal glucose utilization. One of the basic postulates of the mitochondrial theory of aging and neurodegenerative diseases is that there is a significant reduction in the capacity for ATP production in the brain and other organs of old mammals. The concept of a decrease in the effectiveness of the mitochondrial process of energy transduction (or oxidative phosphorylation) is expressed as an under function of "the mitochondrial redox-energy axis" (Yap et al., 2010). Although mitochondrial complexes, complex I (Valdez et al., 2004; Boveris & Navarro, 2008; Navarro et al., 2009), complex IV (Valdez et al., 2004; Boveris & Navarro, 2008), and complex V (Lam et al., 2009), are considered the main targets in neurodegeneration and aging, there are also cytosolic enzymes whose activities are simultaneously decreased, such as succinyl-CoA-transferase (Lam et al. 2009) and as 6-phosphofructo-2-kinase (Herrero-Mendez et al., 2009). The cytosolic-mitochondrial interaction is certainly affected and there is recognition of a depressed glucose metabolism as the earliest and consistent abnormality in neurodegenerative diseases (Yap et al., 2009).

6. Acknowledgments

This work was supported by research grants from the University of Buenos Aires (B005), Agencia Nacional de Promoción Científica y Tecnológica (PICT 38326, PICT 1138), and Consejo Nacional de Investigaciones Científicas y Técnicas (PIP 688) in Argentina; and from Ministerio de Ciencia e Innovación (SAF2008-03690) and Plan Andaluz de Investigación 2007-2008 (CTS-194) in Spain.

7. References

Ahmadi, FA.,Linseman, DA., Grammatopoulos, TN., Jones, SM.,Bouchard, RJ., Freed, CR., Heidenreich, KA. &Zawada, WM. (2003). The pesticide rotenone induces caspase-3-mediatedapoptosis in ventral mesencephalic dopaminergic neurons. *J. Neurochem* 87: 914–921.

Ayala, A., Venero, JL., Cano, J. & Machado, A. (2007) Mitochondrial toxins and neurodegenerative diseases. *Front Biosci* 12: 986-1007

Betarbet, R., Sherer, TB., MacKenzie, G., Garcia-Osuna, M., Panov, AV. & Greenamyre, JT. (2000) Chronic systemic pesticide exposure reproduces features of Parkinson's disease. *Nat Neurosci* 3: 1301-1306

Bougria, M., Vitorica, J., Cano, J. & Machado, A. (1995) Implication of dopamine transporter system on 1-methyl-4-phenylpyridinium and rotenone effect in striatal synaptosomes. *Eur J Pharmacol* 291: 407-415

Boveris, A. & Cadenas, E. (2000) Mitochondrial production of hydrogen peroxide regulation by nitric oxide and the role of ubisemiquinone. *IUBMB Life* 50: 245-250.

Boveris, A. & Chance, B. (1973) The mitochondrial generation of hydrogen peroxide. *Biochem J.* 134: 617-630

Boveris, A. & Navarro, A. (2008) Brain mitochondrial dysfunction in aging. *IUBMB Life* 60: 308-314

Boveris, A. & Stoppani, AOM. (1970) Inhibition of electron and energy transfer in mitochondria by 19-nor-ethynyltestosterone acetate. *Arch Biochem Biophys* 141: 641-655

Boveris, A., Carreras, MC. & Poderoso, JJ. (2010) The regulation of cell energetics and mitochondrial signaling by nitric oxide. In: *Nitric oxide: Biology and Pathobiology*, Ignarro, L., pp. 441-482, Elsevier Academic Press Inc, London, UK.

Boveris, A., Valdez, LB., Zaobornyj, T. & Bustamante, J. (2006) Mitochondrial metabolic states regulate nitric oxide and hydrogen peroxide diffusion to the cytosol. *Biochim Biophys Acta* 1757: 535-542

Boveris, DL. & Boveris, A. (2007) Oxygen delivery to the tissues and mitochondrial respiration. *Front Biosci.* 12: 1014-1023

Carreras, MC., Franco, MC., Peralta, JG. & Poderoso, JJ. (2004) Nitric oxide, complex I, and the modulation of mitochondrial reactive species in biology and disease. *Mol Aspects Med* 25: 125-139

Chade, AR., Kasten, M. & Tanner, CM. (2006) Nongenetic causes of Parkinson's disease. *J Neural Transm Suppl* 70: 147-151

Cooper, JM., Mann, VM., Krige, D. & Schapira, AH. (1992) Human mitochondrial complex I dysfunction. *Biochim Biophys Acta* 1101: 198-120

de Lau, LM. & Breteler, MM. (2006) Epidemiology of Parkinson's disease. *Lancet Neurol* 5: 525-535

Degli, EM. (1998) Inhibitors of NADH-ubiquinone reductase: an overview. *Biochim Biophys Acta* 1364: 222-235

Dhillon, AS., Tarbutton, GL., Levin, JL., Plotkin, GM., Lowry, LK.,Nalbone, JT. & Shepherd, S. (2008) Pesticide/environmental exposures and Parkinson's disease in East Texas. *J Agromedicine* 13: 37-48

Forno, LS. (1996) Neuropathology of Parkinson's disease. *J Neuropathol Exp Neurol* 55: 259-272

Franco, MC., Arciuch, VG., Peralta, JG., Galli, S., Levisman, D., Lopez, LM., Romorini, L., Poderoso, JJ. & Carreras, MC. (2006) Hypothyroid Phenotype is contributed by mitochondrial complex I inactivation due to translocated neuronal nitric-oxide synthase. *J Biol Chem* 281: 4779-4786

Giulivi, C., Poderoso, JJ. & Boveris, A. (1998) Production of nitric oxide by mitochondria. *J. Biol Chem* 273: 11038-11043

Gomez, C., Bandez, MJ. & Navarro, A (2007) Pesticides and impairment of mitochondrial function in relation with the parkinsonian syndrome. *Front Biosci* 12: 1079-1093

González-Flecha, B., Cutrin, JC. & Boveris, A. (1993) Time course and mechanism of oxidative stress and tissue damage in rat liver subjected to in vivo ischemia-reperfusion. *J Clin Invest* 91: 456-464

Gorell, JM., Johnson, CC., Rybicki, BA., Peterson, EL. & Richardson, RJ. (1998) The risk of Parkinson's disease with exposure to pesticides, farming, well water, and rural living. *Neurology* 50: 1346-1350

Henchcliffe, C. & Beal, MF. (2008) Mitochondrial biology and oxidative stress in Parkinson disease pathogenesis. *Nat Clin Pract Neurol* 4: 600-609

Hensley, K., Kotake, Y., Sang, H., Pye, Q., Wallis, G., Kolker, L., Tabatabaie, T., Stewart, C., Konishi, Y., Nakae, D. & Floyd, R. (2000) Dietary choline restriction causes complex I dysfunction and increased H_2O_2 generation in liver mitochondria. *Carcinogenesis* 21: 983-989

Herrero-Mendez, A., Almeida, A., Fernández, E., Maestre, C., Moncada, S. & Bolaños, JP. (2009) The bioenergetic and antioxidant status of neurons is controlled by continuous degradation of a key glycolytic enzyme by APC/C-Cdh1. *Nat Cell Biol.* 11: 747-752

Jellinger, KA. & Mizuno, Y. (2003) Parkinson's disease. In: *Neurodegeneration: The molecular pathology of dementia and movement disorders*, Dickson, D., pp. 159-187, Neuropath Press

Lam, PY., Yin, F., Hamilton, RT., Boveris, A., Cadenas, E. (2009) Elevated neuronal nitric oxide synthase expression during ageing and mitochondrial energy production. *Free Radic Res* 43: 431-439

Langston, JW., Ballard, JW., Tetrud, JW. & Irwin, I. (1983) Chronic parkinsonism in human due to a product of meperidine-analog synthesis. *Science* 219: 979-980

Liu, Q., Raina, AK., Smith, MA., Sayre, LM. & Perry, G. (2003) Hydroxynonenal, toxic carbonyls, and Alzheimer disease. *Mol Aspects Med* 24: 305-313

Mann, VM., Cooper, JM., Krige, D., Daniel, SE., Schapira, AH. & Marsden, CD. (1992) Brain, skeletal muscle and platelet homogenate mitochondrial function in Parkinson's disease. *Brain* 115: 333-342

Mizuno, Y., Ohta, S., Tanaka, M., Takamiya, S., Suzuki, K., Sato, T., Oya, H., Ozawa, T. & Kagawa, Y. (1989) *Biochem Biophys Res Commun* 163: 1450-1455

Moon, Y., Lee, KH., Park, JH., Geum, D. & Kim, K. (2005). Mitochondrial membrane depolarization and the selective death of dopaminergic neurons by rotenone: protective effect of coenzyme Q10. *J. Neurochem*. 93: 1199–1208.

Nagatsu, T. (2002) Amine-related neurotoxins in Parkinson's disease: past, present, and future. *Neurotoxicol Teratol* 24: 565-569

Navarro, A. & Boveris, A. (2007) The mitochondrial energy transduction system and the aging process. *Am J Physiol Cell Physiol* 292: C670-686

Navarro, A. & Boveris, A. (2008) Mitochondrial nitric oxide synthase, mitochondrial brain dysfunction in aging, and mitochondria-targeted antioxidants. *Adv Drug Deliv Rev* 60: 1534-1544

Navarro, A. & Boveris, A. (2009) Brain mitochondrial dysfunction and oxidative damage in Parkinson's disease. *J Bioenerg Biomembr* 41: 517-521

Navarro, A., Bández, MJ., Gómez, C., Repetto, MG. &Boveris, A. (2010) Effects of rotenone and pyridaben on complex I electron transfer and on mitochondrial nitric oxide synthase functional activity. *J Bioenerg Biomembr* 42: 405-412

Navarro, A., Bandez, MJ., Lopez-Cepero, JM., Gómez, C. &Boveris, A. (2011) High doses of vitamin E improve mitochondrial dysfunction in rat hippocampus and frontal cortex upon aging. *Am J Physiol Regul Integr Comp Physiol* 300: R827-834

Navarro, A., Boveris, A., Bández, MJ., Sánchez-Pino, MJ., Gómez, C., Muntané, G. & Ferrer, I. (2009) Human brain cortex: mitochondrial oxidative damage and adaptive response in Parkinson disease and in dementia with Lewy bodies. *Free Rad Biol Med* 46: 1574-1580

Navarro, A., López-Cepero, JM., Bández, MJ., Sánchez-Pino, MJ., Gómez, C., Cadenas, E. & Boveris, A. (2008) Hippocampal mitochondrial dysfunction in rat aging. *Am J Physiol Regul Integr Comp Physiol* 294: R501-509

Persichini, T., Mazzone, V., Polticelli, F., Moreno, S., Venturini, G., Clementi, E. & Colasanti, M. (2005) Mitochondrial type I nitric oxide synthase physically interacts with cytochrome oxidase. *Neuroscience Lett* 384: 254-259

Raha, S. & Robinson, BH. (2000) Mitochondria, oxygen free radicals, disease and ageing. *Trends Biochem Sci* 25: 502-508.

Schapira, AH. (2008[a]) Mitochondria in the aetiology and pathogenesis of Parkinson's disease. *Lancet Neurol* 7: 97-109

Schapira, AH. (2008[b]) Mitochondrial dysfunction in neurodegenerative diseases. *Neurochem Res* 33: 2502-2509

Schapira, AH., Cooper, JM., Dexter, D., Clark, JB., Jenner, P. & Marsden, CD. (1990[a]) Mitochondrial complex I deficiency in Parkinson's disease. *J Neurochem* 54: 823-827

Schapira, AH., Cooper, JM., Dexter, D., Jenner, P., Clark, JB. & Marsden, CD. (1989) Mitochondrial complex I deficiency in Parkinson's disease. *Lancet* 1: 1269

Schapira, AH., Mann, VM., Cooper, JM., Dexter, D., Daniel, SE., Jenner, P., Clark, JB. & Marsden, CD. (1990[b]) Anatomic and disease specificity of NADH CoQ1 reductase (complex I) deficiency in Parkinson's disease. *J Neurochem* 55: 2142-2145.

Shapira, AH. (1998) Mitochondrial dysfunction in neurodegenerative disorders. *Biochim Biophys Acta* 1366: 225-233

Sherer, TB., Betarbet, R., Testa, CM., Seo, BB., Richardson, JR., Kim, JH., Miller, GW., Yagi, T., Matsuno-Yagi, A. & Greenamyre JT. (2003) Mechanism of toxicity in rotenone models of Parkinson's disease. *J Neurosci* 23: 10756-10764

St-Pierre, J., Drori, S., Uldry, M., Silvaggi, JM., Rhee, J., Jäger, S., Handschin, C., Zheng, K., Lin, J., Yang, W., Simon, DK., Bachoo, R., Spiegelman, BM. (2006) Suppression of reactive oxygen species and neurodegeneration by the PGC-1 transcriptional coactivators. *Cell* 127: 397-408.

Tatoyan, A. & Giulivi, G. (1998) Purification and characterization of a nitric-oxide synthase from rat liver mitochondria. *J Biol Chem* 273: 11044-11048

Turrens, JF. & Boveris, A. (1980) Generation of superoxide anion by the NADH dehydrogenase of bovine heart mitochondria. *Biochem J* 191: 421-427

Valdez, LB. & Boveris, A. (2007) Mitochondrial nitric oxide synthase, a voltage-dependent enzyme, is responsible for nitric oxide diffusion to cytosol. *Front Biosci* 12:1210-1219

Valdez, LB., Alvarez, S., LoresArnaiz, S., Schöpfer, F., Carreras, MC.,Poderoso, JJ. & Boveris A. (2000) Reactions of peroxynitrite in the mitochondrial matrix. *Free Rad Biol Med* 29: 349-356

Valdez, LB., Zaobornyj, T. & Boveris, A. (2006) Mitochondrial metabolic states and membrane potential modulate mtNOS activity. *Biochim Biophys Acta* 1757: 166-172

Valdez, LB., Zaobornyj, T., Alvarez, S., Bustamante, J., Costa, LE. & Boveris, A. (2004) Heart mitochondrial nitric oxide synthase. Effects of hypoxia and aging. *Mol Aspects Med* 25: 49-59

Valdez, LB., Zaobornyj, T., Bombicino, SS., Iglesias, DE. & Boveris, A. (2011) Regulation of heart mitochondrial nitric oxide synthase (mtNOS) by oxygen. In *Mitochondrial Pathophysiology,* Cadenas, S. & Palau, F. In press. Transworld Research Network, Kerala, India.

Walker, JE. (1992) The NADH:ubiquinoneoxidoreductase (complex I) of respiratory chains. *Q Rev Biophys* 25: 253-324

Walker, JE., Arizmendi, JM., Dupuis, A., Fearnley, IM., Finel, M., Medd, SM., Pilkington, SJ., Runswick, MJ. & Skehel, JM. (1992) Sequences of 20 subunits of NADH:ubiquinoneoxidoreductase from bovine heart mitochondria. Application of a novel strategy for sequencing proteins using the polymerase chain reaction. *J Mol Biol* 226: 1051-1072

Wallace, KB., Eells, JT., Madeira, VM., Cortopassi, G. & Jones, DP. (1997) Mitochondria-mediated cell injury. Symposium overview. *Fundam Appl Toxicol* 38: 23-37

Yap, LP., Garcia. JV., Han, DS. & Cadenas, E. (2011) Role of nitric oxide-mediated glutathionylation in neuronal function: potential regulation of energy utilization. *Biochem J* 428: 85–93

Zheng, B., Liao Z., Locascio, JJ., Lesniak, KA., Roderick, SS., Watt, ML., Eklund, AC., Zhang-James, Y., Kim, PD., Hauser, MA., Grünblatt, E., Moran, LB., Mandel, SA., Riederer, P., Mille,r RM., Federoff, HJ., Wüllner, U., Papapetropoulos, S., Youdim, MB., Cantuti-Castelvetri, I., Young, AB., Vance, JM., Davis, RL., Hedreen, JC., Adler, CH., Beach, TG., Graeber, MB., Middleton, FA., Rochet, JC., Scherzer, CR. (2010) Global PD Gene Expression (GPEX) Consortium. PGC-1α, a potential therapeutic target for early intervention in Parkinson's disease. *Sci Transl Med* 2: 52ra73

15

Role of Microglia in Inflammatory Process in Parkinson's Disease

Hirohide Sawada[1,2], Hiromi Suzuki[3], Kenji Ono[3], Kazuhiro Imamura[4], Toshiharu Nagatsu[2,3] and Makoto Sawada[3]
[1]*Department of Medical Technology, Kobe Tokiwa University,*
[2]*Department of Pharmacology, School of Medicine, Fujita Health University,*
[3]*Department of Brain Life Science, Research Institute of Environmental Medicine, Nagoya University,*
[4]*Department of Neurology, Okazaki City Hospital,*
Japan

1. Introduction

1.1 What is Parkinson's disease

Parkinson's disease (PD) is the second most common neurodegenerative disease after Alzheimer's disease (AD). PD is characterized by degeneration and cell death in dopaminergic neurons in the substantia nigra pars compacta (SNpc) and loss of their nerve terminals in the striatum (putamen and caudate nucleus), accompanied by the depletion of the neurotransmitter dopamine (DA) in the striatum. This depletion causes motor symptoms, i.e., resting tremor, muscle rigidity, and akinesia. The level of tyrosine hydroxylase (TH), the rate-limiting enzyme of catecholamine (DA, noradrenaline, and adrenaline) synthase in the nigro-striatal region of PD patients is decreased (Nagatsu and Sawada M., 2007).

A small percentage of PD is familial with a hereditary history. However, most cases of PD (approximately 90-95 %) are sporadic without any hereditary history. In 2009, 16 causative genes of familial PD have been identified (Satake et al., 2009), including PARK1 (*α-synuclein*), PARK2 (*parkin*), PARK4 (*α-synuclein*), PARK5 (*UCHL-1*), PARK6 (*PINK1*), PARK7 (*DJ-1*), PARK8 (*LRRK2*), and PARK9 (*ATP13A2*). Sporadic PD and some cases of familial PD are characterized by the presence of cytoplasmic inclusions named Lewy bodies, which consist mainly of α-synuclein protein, the product of the PARK1 gene. α-Synuclein is observed not only in PD but also in various neurodegenerative diseases, such as dementia with Lewy bodies (DLB).

Based on their investigation of the distribution of α-synuclein-positive Lewy bodies and Lewy neurites in PD patients, Braak et al. (2003) proposed a hypothesis that the pathological process of PD starts first from the lower brain stem and then spreads to the midbrain, limbic system, and cerebral cortex. α-Synuclein-positive inclusions are observed in the anterior olfactory nucleus, dorsal motor nucleus of vagus nerves, and also in peripheral autonomic neurons including those of the sympathetic ganglia, adrenal medulla, and intestinal Auerbach's plexus. Braak et al. (2003) proposed that symptoms of PD appears when Lewy bodies are formed in dopaminergic neurons in the substantia nigra (SN) .

The neuronal cells overexpressing α-synuclein were reported to directly transfer α-synuclein protein to neighboring normal neuronal stem cells both in cell culture and in transgenic mice; PD-like pathological changes occurred in such stem cells with development of inclusion bodies, lysosomal failure, and apoptotic changes (Desplats et al., 2009). This study could explain the findings that PD patients who had been treated more than ten years prior to death by implantation of human fetal mesencephalic dopaminergic neurons into their striatum had continued to develop PD pathology with loss of dopaminergic neurons and, importantly, the formation of Lewy bodies in the graft cells (Kordower et al. and Li et al., 2008). These findings indicating that α-synuclein pathology may spread throughout the nervous system from one cell to another, like a prion infection, would appear to fit the above hypothesis offered by Braak et al. (Olanow and Prusiner, 2009).

The animal models of PD are produced by several neurotoxins of dopaminergic neurons, e.g., 1-methyl-4-phenyl-1,2,3,6-tetrahydropyridine (MPTP), 6-hydroxydopamine (6-OHDA), paraquat, and rotenone (Miller et al., 2009; Nagatsu and Sawada M., 2006). Systemic administration of MPTP produces PD in humans, monkeys, and various animals. MPTP enters into the brain through the blood brain barrier (BBB), is metabolized to 1-methyl-4-phenyl-pyridium ion (MPP^+) by monoamine oxidase (MAO) B in astrocytes, and is specifically transported into dopaminergic neurons in the SN. In these dopaminergic neurons, MPP^+ inhibits mitochondrial complex I, depletes ATP, and causes the release of reactive oxygen species (ROS), and apoptotic cell death. Since 6-OHDA does not cross the BBB, direct stereotaxic injection into the nigro-striatum is used to produce hemiparkinsonian animal models. Rotenone and paraquat are non-selective dopaminergic neurotoxins, which are used as a pesticide. Both compounds cause degeneration of dopaminergic neurons, accompanied by mitochondrial dysfunction, when chronically administered to animals. These neurotoxins also inhibit mitochondrial complex I and cause the release of ROS and the depletion of ATP in dopaminergic neurons in the SN, thus triggering cell death.

The pathogenesis of sporadic PD is still uncertain, but it is speculated to be cause by combined effects of susceptibility genes like familial PD genes and unknown exogenous factors such as nutrition and toxic environmental substances. The following mechanisms are considered: mitochondrial dysfunction, endoplasmic reticulum (ER) stress due to production of misfolded proteins, abnormal degradation of toxic oligomers of misfolded proteins caused by dysfunction of intracellular protein degradation systems including the ubiquitin-proteasome system and autophagy-lysosome system, excitotoxicity, and oxidative stress. Mitochondrial dysfunction in sporadic PD is supported by the findings of mitochondrial complex I deficiency in the nigro-striatum of postmortem brains from sporadic PD patients and inhibition of complex I in the SN mitochondria of animal PD models produced by treatment with neurotoxins. Mitochondrial dysfunction causes the production of free radicals, ROS. Abnormal degradation of misfolded proteins due to dysfunction of the caspase-independent autophagy-lysosome system and/or caspase-dependent ubiquitin-proteasome system might cause the formation of toxic oligomers of α-synuclein to Lewy bodies and dopaminergic cell death in the SN.

Another remarkable pathological mechanism operating in PD and in most other neurodegenerative diseases is the neuroinflammation that accompanies the activation of microglia, which cells, once activated, release various pro-inflammatory cytokines such as tumor necrosis factor (TNF)-α, interleukin (IL)-1β, and IL-6 (Nagatsu and Sawada M., 2005). The significance of neuroinflammation in AD and PD was proposed for the first time by

McGeer et al. in 1988. The present review will discuss the pathological significance of neuroinflammation in neurodegenerative diseases, especially in PD.

2. Neuroinflammation in Parkinson's disease

One of the neurodegenerative mechanisms at work in PD is the neuroinflammatory process. McGeer et al. (1988) were the first to report that the number of major histocompatibility complex (MHC) class II of human leukocyte antigen (HLA-DR)-positive activated microglia are observed in the SN along with the appearance of Lewy bodies and free melanin in sporadic PD brains. Various dopaminergic neurotoxins including MPTP, 6-OHDA, paraquat, and rotenone used to produce animal models of PD also cause the neuroinflammation that accompanies microglial activation.

Changes in the levels of cytokines, apoptosis-related proteins, and neurotrophins, detected by use of the enzyme-linked immunosolvent assay (ELISA), were reported to have occurred in the postmortem brain (striatum or SN) and/or cerebrospinal fluid (CSF) in sporadic PD patients (Mogi et al., 1994a, 1994b, 1996, 2000; Nagatsu, 2002; Nagatsu and Sawada M., 2005, 2006; Sawada M. et al., 2006); increased levels of cytokines and apoptosis-related proteins, such as TNF-α, IL-1β, IL-2, IL-4, IL-6, epidermal growth factor (EGF), transforming growth factor (TGF)-α, TGF-β, soluble FAS, TNF-α receptor 1 (p55), Bcl-2, caspase 1, and caspase 3; decreased levels of neurotrophins nerve growth factor (NGF) and brain-derived neurotrophic factor (BDNF). An increased level of IL-1β and decreased level of NGF in the striatum were also reported in MPTP-administered mice (Mogi et al., 1998).

Imamura et al. (2003) reported, based on their immunohistochemical study on PD brains, that MHC class II-positive activated microglia produced TNF-α and IL-6 in the putamen and SN, where damaged TH-positive dopaminergic neurons and neurites were associated with the pathology. In normal brain, there were few MHC class II-positive microglia in the putamen and SN. MHC class II-positive microglia became increased in number with the progression of neurodegeneration in these regions of PD patients. However, such microglia were also associated with non-degenerated dopaminergic neurites, and serotonergic or other neurites without neurodegeneration in PD brains. Moreover, significantly higher number of MHC class II-positive microglia were also observed in the hippocampus and cerebral cortex, where no cell death occurs in the examined PD brains. These immunohistochemical results suggest that activated microglia in the hippocampus and cerebral cortex in PD may be non-toxic or even neuroprotective in contrast to their neurotoxic role in the putamen and SN.

Imamura et al. (2005) further observed activated microglia both in the movement-regulating nigro-striatum and memory-regulating hippocampus in the brains from patients with DLB. In these patients, the levels of BDNF mRNA and immunochemically detected BDNF protein were significantly decreased in the hippocampus, where cell death occurs in DLB; but they were not decreased in the PD hippocampus. The mRNA level of IL-6 was greatly increased in the hippocampus of both PD and DLB patients compared with that for the normal controls. These results suggest that activated microglia in the hippocampus in PD might be non-toxic, or even neuroprotective in contrast to their neurotoxic effect in DLB.

Some systemic viral infections may also cause PD with neuroinflammation. Recently, C57BL/6J mice infected with H5N1 influenza virus were found to display acute neurological signs of mild encephalitis to coma (Jang et al., 2009). In this study, H5N1 virus had invaded from the peripheral nervous system (PNS) into the central nervous system

(CNS) spreading to higher levels of the neuroaxis. They observed activation of microglia, α-synuclein phosphorylation and aggregation, and dopaminergic neuron loss in the SN after long-term progression of the viral infection.

3. Neuroinflammation and microglia

Microglia are derived from myeloid cells having the property of high affinity for the brain and comprise about 10% of the total cells in CNS parenchyma (Ono et al., 1999; Sawada M. et al., 1998). Microglia play important physiological roles in the development, differentiation, and maintenance of neural cells in the brain. They also have immunological functions in the brain and serve to remove dead cells by phagocytic activity after brain injury or neurodegeneration. Microglia are normally in the resting stage, but are activated by some brain lesions in neurodegenerative diseases such as PD.

Activated microglia may play neurotoxic roles by producing pro-inflammatory cytokines such as TNF-α, IL-1, and IL-6, as well as, nitric oxide (NO) and ROS (Cassarino et al., 1997; Chao et al., 1992; Hunot et al., 1996; Kim et al., 2000; Koutsilieri et al., 2002; Liu et al., 1998; McGuire et al., 2001). On the other hand, activated microglia may also function neuroprotectively by producing neurotrophic components such as IL-10, TGF-β, plasminogen, glial cell line-derived neurotrophic factor (GDNF), BDNF, and NGF (Batchelor et al., 1999; Elkabes et al., 1996; Miwa et al., 1997; Nagata et al., 1993b; Nakajima et al., 2001; Sawada M. et al., 1995, 1999; Suzumura et al., 1993).

Pro-inflammatory cytokines such as TNF-α, IL-1β, and IL-6 are pleiotropic, and may produce either neurotoxic or neuroprotective effects (Arai et al., 2004; Barger et al., 1995; Bolin et al., 2002; Fisher et al., 2001; Liu et al., 1998; Mason et al., 2001; McGuire et al., 2001). TNF-α produced by microglia or astrocytes in the CNS is generally considered to be neurotoxic (Sawada M. et al., 1989; Suzumura et al., 1999). Microglial production of TNF-α is increased when the cells are stimulated with lipopolysaccharide (LPS; Sawada M. et al., 1989, 1995). Neurotoxin-mediated damage to dopaminergic neurons is attenuated in mice deficient in TNF-α or TNF receptors compared with the damage seen in wild-type mice (Ferger et al., 2004; Sriram et al., 2002). A recent study demonstrated that inhibition of TNF reduce the delayed and progressive neurodegeneration in the SN in PD rats (Harms et al., 2011). Two weeks after having received intrastriatal administration of 6-OHDA, PD model rats were injected in their SN with lentivirus encoding a dominant-negative TNF gene. The effects of this abnormal TNF included inhibition of the progressive loss of nigral dopaminergic neurons, when the rats were examined 5 weeks after the initial 6-OHDA administration. The lentivirus dominant-negative TNF therapy also attenuated microglial activation in PD rats. However, some other reports suggest opposite neuroprotective effects of TNF-α. For example, auto-immune-mediated demyelination model mice of multiple sclerosis with deficient TNF-α developed more severe neurological impairment than the normal multiple sclerosis model mice (Liu et al., 1998). Two different subtypes of the TNF receptors may act for neuronal death or survival by different signal transduction pathways (Yang et al., 2002).

LPS is a gram-negative bacterial endotoxin and is a microglial activator substance. LPS treatment causes neurotoxic effects on dopaminergic neurons in various cell culture systems (Gao et al., 2003; Gayle et al., 2002; Kim et al., 2000) or by direct injection into the SN (Arai et al., 2004; Castano et al., 2002; Iravani et al., 2005). LPS is recognized as an initiator of dopaminergic neuronal loss, and the degree of neuronal damage may depend on the concentration of LPS used for treatment. The neurotoxicity of microglia is increased by the production of TNF-α in response to LPS stimulation (Sawada M. et al., 1989, 1995). On the other hand, the neurotrophic effects of microglial activation induced by LPS have also been found in several cell culture studies (Elkabes et al., 1998; Kramer et al., 2002; Mallat et al., 1989; Miwa et al., 1997; Nakajima et al., 2001). The neurotrophic effects of LPS may be explained by the fact that LPS induces the secretion of not only pro-inflammatory cytokines but also neurotrophic compounds. Stimulation by LPS increases the microglial secretion of NT-3, NT-4/5, NGF, and BDNF (Elkabes et al., 1998; Miwa et al., 1997; Nakajima et al., 2001). A rat model of spinal cord injury showed improvement in locomotor function by an LPS-elicited increase in the level of neuroprotective GDNF (Hashimoto et al., 2005). Plasminogen produced by LPS-treated microglia was reported to promote the development of dopaminergic neurons (Nagata et al., 1993b; Nakajima et al., 1992).

Several studies indicate that damaged dopaminergic neurons release various factors that can active microglia. These factors are α-synuclein, matrix metalloproteinase 3 (MMP-3), and neuromelanin, all of which are released from damaged dopaminergic neurons and induce ROS production. α-Synuclein, which is a synaptic vesicle protein and a main component of Lewy bodies, the pathological hallmark of PD, may have an important role in both the onset and progression of PD. Extracellular aggregated α-synuclein induced microglial activation that enhanced neurotoxicity toward dopaminergic neurons, whereas low concentrations of α-synuclein failed to be neurotoxic (Zhang et al., 2005). Microglial enhancement of α-synuclein-mediated neurotoxicity depended on the phagocytosis of α-synuclein and production of ROS by microglia. Nitrated/oxidized α-synuclein was detected in nigral cytoplasmic inclusions, and inhibition of microglial-derived NO and superoxide provided significant neuroprotection to dopaminergic neurons (Gao et al., 2008). MMP3 is a zinc-dependent proteolytic enzyme that degrades the extracellular matrix; and it is released from damaged neurons, thereby inducing microglial activation with production of inflammatory cytokines such as TNF-α (Kim et al., 2005). MMP-3-deficient mice show reduced MMP-3-induced microglial production of NADPH oxidase-derived superoxide and dopaminergic cell death (Kim et al., 2007).

Microglial activation accompanied by the degeneration of dopaminergic neurons is an early event of neuroinflammation in PD. Purisai et al. (2007) reported that activation of microglia accompanied by the induction of NADPH oxidase was a priming event in paraquat-administered mice, which activation occurred at least 1 or 3 days after the administration. An *in vivo* positron emission tomography (PET) study imaging, microglial activation in nigro-striatal regions indicated that the activation was likely to occur early in the disease process and paralleled the loss of terminals in dopaminergic neurons, as revealed by use of [11C](R)-PK11195, a peripheral benzodiazepine receptor-binding ligand (Gerhard et al., 2006). However, microglial activation by chronic LPS infusion into the SN or single systemic injection in animals caused delayed and progressive neurodegeneration of nigral dopaminergic neurons (Gao et al., 2002; Qin et al., 2007). Using conditional amyotrophic lateral sclerosis (ALS) transgenic mice, Boillée et al. (2006) demonstrated that microglia had a great effect on the later phase of disease progression but little effect on the early phase of the disease.

4. Nuroprotective role of microgliae

Neurotrophic effects of microglial activation were reported in cell-culture studies (Elkabes et al., 1996, 1998; Miwa et al., 1997; Nagata et al., 1993a; Nakajima et al., 2001) and in studies using animal models of neurodegeneration (Hashimoto et al., 2005; Imai et al., 1999, 2007; Rabchevsky and Streit, 1997; Suzuki et al., 2001).

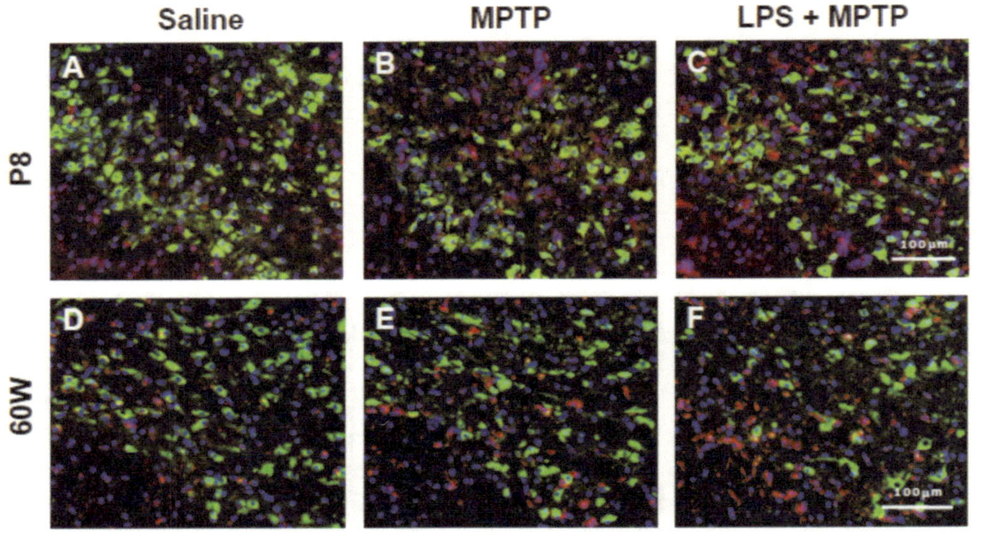

Fig. 1. Morphological changes due to MPTP administration in the SN. Immunostaining for tyrosine hydroxylase (TH)-positive dopaminergic (A9) neurons (green) and CD 11b-positive activated microglia (red) in the SN from mice treated with saline, MPTP, and LPS-MPTP are shown. In neonatal (P8) mice (**A**-**C**), dopaminergic (A9) neurons in the SN were decreased in MPTP-treated mice, whereas these neurons in the LPS-MPTP-treated mice were recovered, compared from MPTP-treated mice. The activated microglia had increased in number in the entire SN in mice treated with LPS-MPTP, as compared with saline- or MPTP-treated mice. In aged (60w) mice (**D**-**F**), numbers of the dopaminergic (A9) neurons were decreased in the order of saline, MPTP, and LPS-MPTP treatments. In the MPTP- and LPS-MPTP-treated mice, numbers of the activated microglia were increased with their accumulation in the SNc. P8 refers to postnatal day 8; and 60w, to 60-day-old mice (Sawada H. et al., 2007, J Neurosci Res, Vol. 85, No. 8, pp. 1752-1761, With permission of John Wiley and Sons).

Neonatal microglia are activated macrophage colony-stimulating factor (M-CSF)-dependently from late gestation up to two weeks after birth, and are very proliferative and easily activated under normal circumstances (Sawada M. et al., 1990; Thery et al., 1990). Sawada H. et al. (2007) showed that in MPTP-administered neonatal mice their microglia activated by treatment with systemic LPS showed neurotrophic potential toward dopaminergic neurons. Neonatal (postnatal day 7) mice treated with MPTP showed decreases in the number of dopaminergic (A9) neurons in the SN (Fig. 1 and 2), TH activity, and the levels of DA and the metabolite 3,4-dihydroxyphenylacetic acid in the midbrain. However, cell viability of dopaminergic (A9) neurons and these markers increased in mice treated with MPTP and LPS, along with marked LPS-induced activation of microglia (Fig. 1 and 2). A modest activation of microglia and a significant decrease in the number of dopaminergic (A9) neurons were observed in the MPTP-treated mice, whereas mice treated with the MPTP and LPS demonstrated marked microglial activation and a tendency toward recovery against cell toxicity, as compared with the MPTP-treated mice (Fig. 3A). These MPTP-LPS-treated mice showed increased levels of pro-inflammatory cytokines of IL-1β and IL-6. LPS-activated microglia in neonatal and aged mice had different phenotypic effects on dopaminergic neurons exposed to MPTP. In contrast, the number of dopaminergic neurons in the SN in aged mice (60 weeks) treated with MPTP was significantly decreased, and an increase in the number of microglia treated with MPTP and LPS produced a further decrease in the number of dopaminergic neurons (Fig. 1 and 2). The relationship between microglial activation and viability of dopaminergic (A9) neurons for the three groups (saline control, MPTP treated, and MPTP-LPS treated mice) of aged mice showed an inverse correlation (Fig. 3B). These results suggest that LPS-activated microglia in aged mice may be neurotoxic, whereas in neonatal mice they may have neurotrophic potential.

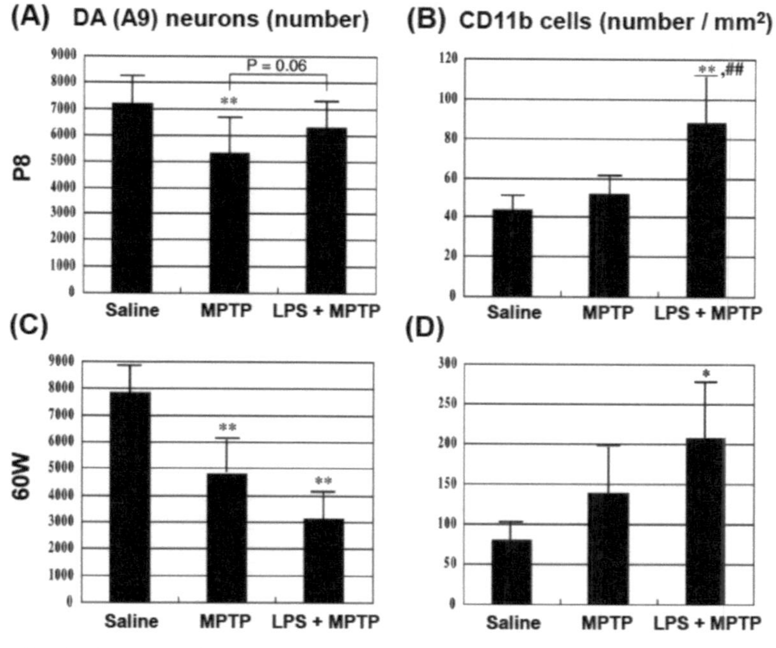

Fig. 2. Analysis of effects of LPS treatment on numbers of dopaminergic (A9) neurons and CD 11b-positive activated microglia in MPTP-treated neonatal and aged mice. **A**: Number of dopaminergic (A9) neurons of the SN for the saline, MPTP, and LPS-MPTP groups in P8 mice. The number of dopaminergic (A9) neurons in the MPTP group was significantly decreased, whereas that for the LPS-MPTP group was recovered. **B**: Number of CD11b-immunopositive microglial cells in the SN in P8 mice. The LPS-MPTP group demonstrated marked microglial activation. **C**: Number of dopaminergic (A9) neurons of the three groups in the SN of 60w mice. The number in the MPTP and LPS-MPTP groups was significantly decreased. **D**: Number of CD11b-immunopositive microglia for the three groups in the SN of 60w mice. Severe microglial activation was observed in the LPS-MPTP group. Values represent the mean±SD. $^{*}p < 0.05$; $^{**}p < 0.01$ versus saline group, $^{\#\#}p < 0.01$ versus MPTP group, by the use of the unpaired Student's *t* test (Sawada H. et al., 2007, J Neurosci Res, Vol. 85, No. 8, pp. 1752-1761, With permission of John Wiley and Sons).

Using an ischemic gerbil model, Imai et al. (2007) also showed neuroprotective effects of exogenously administered microglia. Microglia cells were isolated from neonatal gerbils by labeling with a fluorescent dye. When the isolated microglia were systemically injected into the subclavian artery in experimental ischemic gerbils, the cells migrated to ischemic hippocampal regions (CA1 pyramidal neurons); and the number of surviving hippocampal neurons was greater in the host gerbils than in the control ischemic animals. This neuroprotective effect was enhanced when the isolated microglia were stimulated by interferon-γ. Administration of exogenous microglia to the ischemic gerbils improved the performance of the animals in a passive-avoidance learning task. The ischemic animals revealed increased expression of neurotrophic factors BDNF and GDNF in their hippocampal regions. Thus, administration of isolated neonatal microglia may potentially have neurotrophic effects on injured brain regions.
Recently, Saijo et al. (2009) reported that an orphan nuclear receptor, Nurr1, protected dopaminergic neurons against impairment by inhibiting the expression of pro-inflammatory mediators produced by microglia and astrocytes, such as TNF-α, IL-1β, and inducible NO-synthesizing (iNOS) enzyme. Nurr1 is known to play an essential role in the generation and maintenance of dopaminergic neurons. When Nurr1 expression was reduced by shRNA, inflammatory substances were increased in microglia; and with further amplification by astrocytes, these substances caused dopaminergic neuron death in the SN.

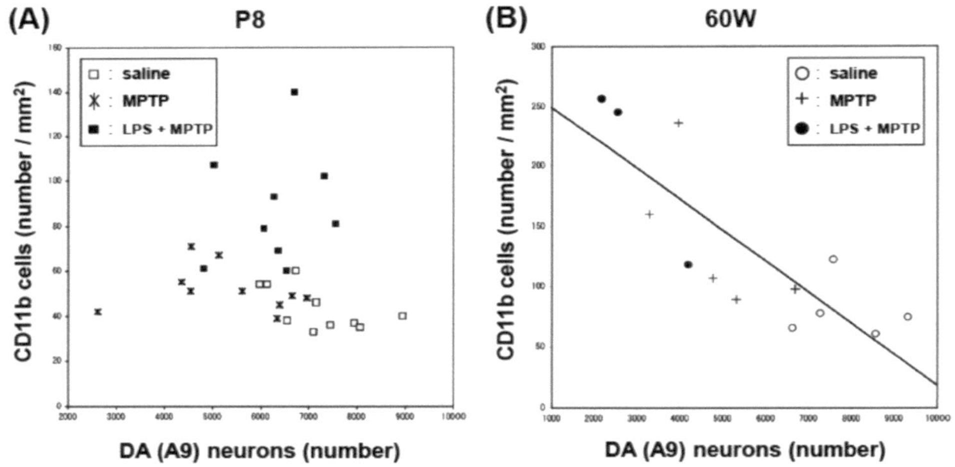

Fig. 3. Relationship between activated microglia and dopaminergic (A9) neurons in saline, MPTP, and LPS-MPTP groups of individual neonatal or aged mice. **A**: In P8 mice, only slight activation of microglia and decrease in number of dopaminergic (A9) neurons were found for the MPTP group, whereas the LPS-MPTP group demonstrated marked microglial activation and a tendency toward protection against loss of dopaminergic (A9) neurons compared with the MPTP group. **B**: In 60w mice, an inverse correlation (R=0.81) was observed between the 2 parameters when data for all 3 groups was plotted (Sawada H. et al., 2007, J Neurosci Res, Vol. 85, No. 8, pp. 1752-1761, With permission of John Wiley and Sons).

The question as to whether or not peripheral macrophages or lymphocytes can cross the BBB into the PD brain remains still controversial. However, peripheral T lymphocytes have been reported to be relevant to the pathogenesis of PD in relation to microglia. The infiltration of peripheral immune cells into the brain and its relevance to PD have been reported. Infiltrates of $CD4^+$ T cells were found in the SN of PD patients, and $CD4^+$ T cells were neurotoxic in MPTP-treated mice (Brochard et al., 2009). In contrast, mice lacking $CD4^+$ T cells showed attenuated nigro-striatal degeneration induced by MPTP. Another report indicated that nitrated α-synuclein, which is abundant in Lewy bodies, was detected in peripheral lymphocytes in cervical lymph nodes from MPTP-treated mice (Benner et al., 2008). The transfer of T cells from mice immunized with nitrated α-synuclein into MPTP-treated mice caused significant infiltration into the brain and a neuroinflammatory response with accelerated dopaminergic neuron loss (Benner et al., 2008). The consequence of two subsets of $CD4^+$ lymphocytes that acted on microglia was reported to be different (Reynolds et al., 2009). In the presence of nitrated α-synuclein, one subset, i.e., $CD4^+$ $CD25^-$ (effector) T cells, enhanced the microglial activation and neurotoxic responses by secreting TNF-α and IFN-γ; and the other, $CD4^+$ $CD25^+$ (regulatory) T cells, suppressed the microglia activation and induced microglia apoptosis by secreting IL-10 and TGF-β. On the other hand, the Th1 and Th17 cells, other subsets of $CD4^+$ T cells, increased the production of NO, superoxide, TNF-α and IL-1β from microglia, and decreased the production of neurotrophic factors such as insulin-like growth factor (IGF)-1 (Appel, 2009). Consequently, neuronal injury, which may trigger the release of increased levels of nitrated α-synuclein, may enhance the microglia-mediated neurotoxicity. $CD4^+$ $CD25^+$ T cells suppressed the inflammatory effects of Th17 cells. Another subset of $CD4^+$ T cells, Th2 cells, produced IL-4, increased the release of IGF-1 from microglia, and decreased the release of free radicals, resulting in enhanced neuronal protection.

5. Neurotoxic role of microglia

Many reports on postmortem PD brains and PD animal models indicate that activated microglia have neurotoxic effects and may play a significant role in progression of the disease (Block et al., 2007). Microglial activation was also reported to be neurotoxic in experimental PD models produced by MPTP (Furuya et al., 2004; Wu et al., 2002, 2003).

ROS production from microglia adversely affects the neurons. Previous studies demonstrated that NADPH oxidase-mediated microglial superoxide production is important to MPTP- or rotenone-induced dopaminergic toxicity (Gao et al., 2003; Wu et al., 2002, 2003). NADPH oxidase subunit (gp91)-deficient mice showed attenuated microglial production of superoxide and dopaminergic cell death (Wu et al., 2003).

There have been many reports indicating the neurotoxic effects of activated microglia, especially in aged animals (Sawada H. et al., 2007; Sawada M. et al., 2008; Sugama et al., 2003). Aging is thought to be an important factor in idiopathic PD. Aging is speculated to promote a change from the protective to the toxic phenotype of activated microglia, as in the toxic change in microglia hypothesized by Sawada M. et al. (2006). Cultures of amyloid β-peptide (Aβ)-stimulated microglia from aged rats were reported to show more evidence of toxicity than those from middle-aged or embryonic mice (Viel et al., 2001). Furthermore, MPTP neurotoxicity is greater in aged mice than in young mice, and is accompanied by age-related microglial activation (Sugama et al., 2003).

As described above, activated microglia acted in neuroprotection in MPTP-treated neonatal mice. However, microglia in neonatal or young animals might also act as neurotoxicity, depending on the condition of microglial activation. Sawada H. et al. (2010) reported that

LPS-activated neonatal microglia showed the neurotoxic phenotype in an ethanol-induced brain injury model produced by the stereotaxic injection of ethanol into the mouse striatum (Takeuchi et al., 1998; Toyama et al., 2008; Fig. 4). In this ethanol-injected model produced a large and round or oval shaped brain lesion without hemorrhage, infection or other unexpected effects that might affect the cytokine networks in the brain. Neonatal mice were pretreated with systemic LPS or saline injection (i.p.) daily for 5 days from postnatal day 3 (P3) to P7. Local injection of 100% ethanol (2.0 μl) produced more severe neuronal damage than seen in the MPTP-induced PD model. A large lesion with a necrotic core was observed in the ethanol-injected striatum; and activated microglia had migrated to the outside of this necrotic mass, where Fluoro-Jade B (FJB)-positive degenerative neurons were observed (Fig. 4). After the ethanol-induced damage, activated microglia accumulated in the FJB-positive regions and eliminated damaged neurons by causing delayed neuronal death (Fig. 4). By previous treatment with systemic LPS or saline treatment as a control, the volumes of necrotic and degenerative areas in the striatum were further increased along with an increase in the number of activated microglia by LPS (Table 1). The number of iNOS-positive microglia also tended to be increased by the LPS treatment.

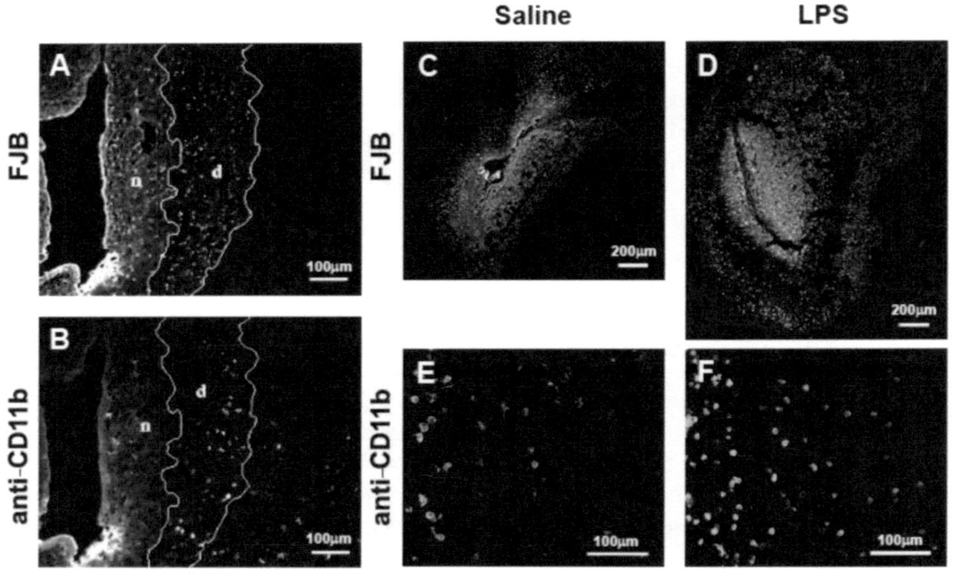

Fig. 4. Morphological changes due to ethanol injection into the striatum of neonatal (P8) mice; detection of neuronal injury by Fluoro-Jade B (FJB) staining and activated microglia by CD11b immunostaining. A large diameter of lesion was observed in ethanol-injected striatum 24 hr after the injection with the core of necrotic mass. Degenerative cells were observed outside the necrotic mass. **A:** In FJB staining, many FJB-positive cells were seen in the degenerative region. **B:** In CD11b immunostaining, the large number of activated microglia was found in the degenerative region. n; necrotic region, d; degenerative region. FJB-positive degenerative neurons are shown in saline-treated (**C**), and LPS-treated (**D**) mice. The number of FJB-positive degenerative cells was increased in LPS-treated mice. CD11b-positive microglia in ethanol-injected ipsilateral striatum are shown in saline-treated (**E**), and LPS-treated (**F**) mice. Increase in the number of activated microglia was observed most markedly in LPS-treated mice.

	Necrotic volumes (mm^3)	FJB (+) volumes (mm^3)	CD11b (+) cells (number/ mm^2)
Saline-treated	0.297±0.137	0.529±0.336	104.5±17.7
LPS-treated	0.696±0.281 *	1.443±1.136	210.6±51.7 **

Table 1. Volumes of the necrotic or FJB positive areas and number of the CD11b positive microglia in ethanol-injured striatum. These data are obtained from 4-5 of neonatal P8 mice. Values represent the mean±SD. ★ $p < 0.05$; ★★ $p < 0.01$, by use of the unpaired Student's *t* test.

6. Toxic change in microglia

Sawada M. et al. (1998, 1999, 2006) proposed a hypothesis of toxic change of microglia. He with collaborators separated two subsets of microglia with neuroprotective or neurotoxic phenotypes from mouse brain by cell sorting and established a cell line for each. The 6-3 cell line of one subset produced a greater amount of ROS stimulated by phorbol myristate acetate (PMA) than did the other, the Ra2 cell line. Both clones were dependent on granulocyte macrophage colony-stimulating factor (GM-CSF). When both microglia cell lines were co-cultured with N18 neuronal cells, which are sensitive to oxidative stress by hydrogen peroxide to produce dose-dependent cell death, and are stimulated with PMA, the viability of the N18 cells was increased when the cell were co-cultured with Ra2 cells and decreased in the presence of 6-3 cells. These results indicate that 6-3 cells were of the neurotoxic phenotype, and that Ra2 cells were of neuroprotective one.
A toxic change in microglia phenotypes from neuroprotection to neurotoxicity was observed by transfecting the cells with cDNA encoding HIV-1 Nef protein, indicating the conversion of microglia from a neurotrophic to a neurotoxic subtype (Vilhardt et al., 2002). When Ra2 cells were transfected with Nef protein by using lenti virus, these normally neuroprotective cells produced ROS with activation of NADPH oxidase, in contrast to the non-transfected Ra2 cells, which did not produce ROS. When Nef-Ra2 cells were co-cultured with N-18 neuronal cells, the viability of N-18 cells was decreased; whereas that of N-18 cells co-cultured with Ra2 cells was not lowered. These results suggest a toxic change in nef-transfected microglia accompanied by ROS production.
According to a report on conditional ALS transgenic mice, the disease progression was determined by the expression of mutant superoxide dismutase (SOD)1 protein not in motor neurons but in microglia (Boillée et al., 2006). Microglial activation was observed from the disease onset to the progression in the spinal cord in these animals. The disease progression accelerated in the transgenic mice that expressed mutant SOD1 in all systemic cells including microglia, whereas the viability was improved in the transgenic mice that expressed normal SOD1 only in their microglia. However, the early phase of disease progression showed no difference between above the two types of transgenic mice. This report concluded that microglia had little effect on the early disease phase but participated on the later disease progression in ALS. According to the hypothesis of toxic change in microglia by Sawada M., microglial toxic changes might appear during the progression phase of ALS.

Lai and Todd (2008) examined the effect of microglia by changing the severity of hypoxia-induced neuronal injury in a culture study. After exposing neuronal cells to various degrees of hypoxia, i.e., mild, moderate, or severe, the media from the neuronal cell culture were added to microglial cell culture. Neuroprotective phenotype of microglia was observed with the media from neurons with moderate hypoxia, but not with those from the cultured cells under mild or severe hypoxia.

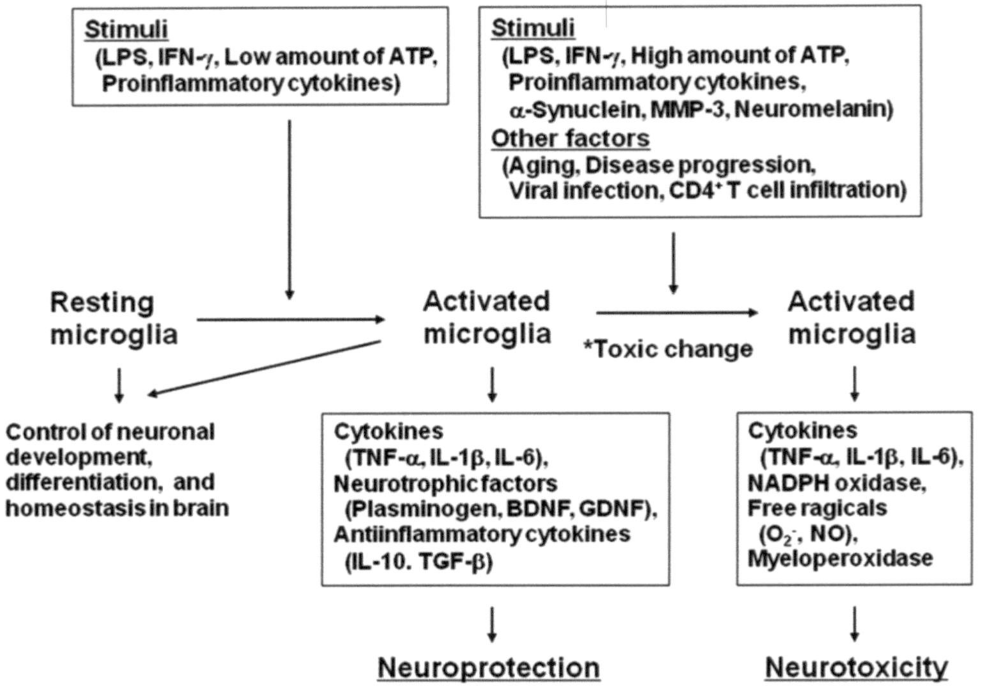

Fig. 5. This scheme shows a hypothesis of toxic change of microglia by two step activation of microglia proposed by Sawada M. et al. At the first step, activated microglia by the first stimulation probably by signaling molecules from injured neurons produce such as neurotrophins, neurotrophic cytokines, antioxidant, and may act for neuroprotection. At the secondary step, activated microglia, which are further stimulated by other factors such as a large amount of cytotoxic factors, may produce toxic change of microglia, which converts neuroprotective phenotypes to neurotoxic ones.

Inoue (2002) hypothesized that the fate of damaged neurons may be regulated in part by ATP through the activation of microglia. Microglia possess the functional P2 receptors, P2X and P2Y, which bind to purines and pyrimidines. Microglial activation is triggered by extracellular ATP or ADP, which is released from damaged neurons under pathological situations. Microglia showed membrane ruffling and enhanced chemotaxis in response to extracellular ATP or ADP produced by neuronal injuries (Honda et al., 2001). A low concentration of extracellular ATP (10-100 μM) stimulated microglial secretion of a neurotrophic substance plasminogen, with a peak response at 5-10 min after the stimulation. This secretion was ATP-concentration dependent (Inoue et al., 1998).

Thereafter, ATP at low-to-moderate concentrations (maximal secretion at 1 mM) stimulated TNF-α secretion from microglia, beginning at 2-3 hr after the stimulation (Hide et al., 2000). About 6 hr after the stimulation with ATP, the microglia showed increased release of IL-6, which secretion was ATP concentration dependent (10-1,000 μM; Shigemoto-Mogami et al., 2001). ATP also induced an increase in Ca^{2+} influx in a concentration-dependent manner. Furthermore, after the stimulation at high concentrations of ATP (10-1,000 μM) about 12 hr later microglial iNOS synthesis was induced; and this iNOS produced NO, then killed neuronal cells (Ohtani et al., 2000). Therefore, initial weaker and shorter stimulation of microglia by extracellular ATP may lead to neuroprotection by secretion of plasminogen, TNF-α, and IL-6; whereas stronger and longer exposures to ATP may be neurotoxic due to NO production. A recent report demonstrated that delayed neural damage was induced by iNOS expression by microglia in brain injured mouse model (Ono et al., 2010). Microglia themselves also release ATP depending on the LPS concentration (Ferrari et al., 1997).

As described above, Sawada M. et al. (2006) hypothesized that the microglial activation may occur in two steps in the PD brain (Fig. 5). At the first step, microglia activated by the first stimulation probably by signaling molecules from injured neurons produce neuroprotectants such as neurotrophins, neurotrophic cytokines, and antioxidant. At the secondary step, activated microglia, which are further stimulated by other factors such as a large amount of cytotoxic factors, may undergo toxic changes, thus converting them from the neuroprotective phenotype to the neurotoxic one, with the result being neuronal cell death in PD.

7. Conclusions

Neuroinflammation with activated microglia may play important roles in the pathogenesis of various neurodegenerative diseases including PD. Activation of microglia may be produced by some chemical signaling molecules released from the injured neurons such as dopaminergic neurons in the SN of the PD brain. Activated microglia may be neuroprotective, at least in the early phase, but may become neurotoxic later to contribute to the progression of the disease. Sawada M. et al. proposed a hypothesis of a toxic change in activated microglia from the neuroprotective phenotype to the neurotoxic one. Development of drugs to regulate activated microglia could be a promising approach for drug development for neurodegenerative diseases such as PD.

8. Acknowledgments

We thank Dr. R. Hishida, Dr. S. Muramatsu, and Dr. I. Nakano (Jichi Medical University, Department of Medicine, Division of Neurology), Dr. Y. Hirata (Gifu University, Faculty of Engineering, Department of Biomolecular Science), Dr. F. Imai (Fujita Health University, School of Medicine, Department of Neurosurgery), and Dr. M. Mogi (Aichi-Gakuin University, School of Pharmacy, Department of Medical Biochemistry) for their helpful advice and support of this work. Many of our studies described in this review were supported by grants-in-aid from the Ministry of Health, Labor, and Welfare of Japan (MS); Ministry of Education, Culture, Sports, Science, and Technology of Japan (MS); and Japan Health Sciences Foundation (MS).

9. References

Appel, S.H. (2009). CD4+ T cells mediate cytotoxicity in neurodegenerative diseases. *J Clin Invest*, Vol.119, No.1, pp.13-15.

Arai, H., Furuya, T., Yasuda, T., Miura, M., Mizuno, Y. and Mochizuki, H. (2004). Neurotoxic effects of lipopolysaccharide on nigral dopaminergic neurons are mediated by microglial activation, interleukin-1β, and expression of caspase-11 in mice. *J Biol Chem*, Vol. 279, No. 49, pp. 51647-51653.

Batchelor, P.E., Liberatore, G.T., Wong, J.Y.F., Porritt, M.J., Frerichs, F., Donnan, G.A. and Howells, D.W. (1999). Activated macrophages and microglia induce dopaminergic sptouting in the injured striatum and express brain-derived neurotrophic factor and glial cell line-derived neurotrophic factor. *J Neurosci*, Vol. 19, No. 5, pp. 1708-1716.

Barger, S.W., Hörster, D., Furukawa, K., Goodman, Y., Krieglstein, J. and Mattson, M.P. (1995). Tumor necrosis factors α and β protect neurons against amyloid β-peptide toxicity: evidence for involvement of a κB-binding factor and attenuation of peroxide and Ca^{2+} accumulation. *Proc Natl Acad Sci USA*, Vol. 92, No. 20, pp. 9328-9332.

Benner, E.J., Banerjee, R., Reynolds, A.D., Sherman, S., Pisarev, V.M., Tsiperson, V., Nemachek, C., Ciborowski, P., Przedborski, S., Mosley, R.L. and Gendelman, H.E. (2008). Nitrated α-synuclein immunity accelerates degeneration of nigral dopaminergic neurons. *PLoS ONE*, Vol. 3, No. 1, e1376.

Block, M.L., Zecca, L. and Hong, J.S. (2007). Microglia-mediated neurotoxicity: uncovering the molecular mechanisms. *Nat Rev Neurosci*, Vol. 8, No. 1, pp.57-70.

Boillée, S., Yamanaka, K., Lobsiger, C.S., Copeland, N.G., Jenkins, N.A., Kassiotis, G., Kollias, G. and Cleveland, D.W. (2006). Onset and progression in inherited ALS determined by motor neurons and microglia, *Science*, Vol. 312, No. 5778, pp. 1389-1392.

Bolin, L.M., Strycharska-Orczyk, I., Murray, R., Langston, J.W. and Monte, D.D. (2002). Increased vulnerability of dopaminergic neurons in MPTP-lesioned interleukin-6 deficient mice. *J Neurochem*, Vol. 83, No. 1, pp. 167-175.

Braak, H., Del Tredici, K., Rüb, U., de Vos, R.A.I., Steur, E.N.H.J. and Braak, E. (2003). Starting of brain pathology related to sporadic Parkinson's disease. *Neurobiol Aging*, Vol. 24, No. 2, pp. 197-211.

Brochard, V., Combadiére, B., Prigent, A., Laouar, Y., Perrin, A., Beray-Berthat, V., Bonduelle, O., Alvarez-Fischer, D., Callebert, J., Launay, J.M., Duyckaerts, C., Flavell, R.A., Hirsch, E.C. and Hunot, S. (2009). Infiltration of CD4+ lymphocytes into the brain contributes to neurodegeneration in a mouse model of Parkinson's disease. *J Clin Invest*, Vol. 119, No. 1, pp. 182-192.

Cassarino, D.S., Fall, C.P., Swerdlow, R.H., Smith, T.S., Halvorsen, E.M., Miller, S.W., Parks, J.P., Parker, W.D. Jr. and Bennett, J.P. Jr. (1997). Elevated reactive oxygen species and antioxidant enzyme activities in animal and cellular models of Parkinson's disease. *Biochem Biophys Acta*, Vol. 1362, No. 1, pp. 77-86.

Castano, A., Herrera, A. J., Cano, J. and Machado, A. (2002). The degenerative effect of a single intranigral injection of LPS on the dopaminergic system is prevented by dexamethasone, and not mimicked by rh-TNF-α, IL-1β and IFN-γ. *J Neurochem*, Vol. 81, No. 1, pp. 150-157.

Chao, C.C., Hu, S., Molitor, T.W., Shaskan, E.G. and Peterson, P.K. (1992). Activated microglia mediate neuronal cell injury via a nitric oxide mechanism. *J Immunol*, Vol. 149, No. 8, pp. 2736-2741.

Desplats, P., Lee, H.J., Bae, E.J., Patrick, C., Rockenstein, E., Crews, L., Spencer, B., Masliah, E. and Lee, S.J. (2009). Inclusion formation and neuronal cell death through neuron-to-neuron transmission of α-synuclein. *Proc Natl Acad Sci USA*, Vol. 106, No. 31, pp. 13010-13015.

Elkabes, S., DiCicco-Bloom, E.M. and Black, I.B. (1996). Brain microglia/macrophages express neurotrophins that selectively regulate microglial proliferation and function. *J Neurosci*, Vol. 16, No. 8, pp. 2508-2521.

Elkabes, S., Peng, L. and Black, I. B. (1998). Lipopolysaccharide differentially regulates microglial trk receptor and neurotrophin expression. *J Neurosci Res*, Vol. 54, No. 1, pp. 117-122.

Ferger, B., Leng, A., Mura, A., Hengerer, B. and Feldon, J. (2004). Genetic ablation of tumor necrosis factor-alpha (*TNF-α*) and pharmacological inhibition of TNF-synthesis attenuates MPTP toxicity in mouse striatum. *J Neurochem*, Vol. 89, No. 4, pp. 822-833.

Ferrari, D., Chiozzi, P., Falzoni, S., Hanau, S. and Di Virgilio, F. (1997). Purinergic modulation of interleukin-1β release from microglial cells stimulated with bacterial endotoxin. *J Exp Med*, Vol. 185, No. 3, pp. 579-582.

Fisher, J., Mizrahi, T., Schori, H., Yoles, E., Levkovitch-Verbin, H., Haggiag, S., Revel, M. and Schwartz, M. (2001). Increased post-traumatic survival of neurons in IL-6-knockout mice on a background of EAE susceptibility. *J Neuroimmunol*, Vol. 119, No. 1, pp. 1-9.

Furuya, T., Hayakawa, H., Yamada, M., Yoshimi, K., Hisahara, S., Miura, M., Mizuno, Y. and Mochizuki, H. (2004). Caspase-11 mediates inflammatory dopaminergic cell death in the 1-methyl-4-phenyl-1,2,3,6-tetrahydropyridine mouse model of Parkinson's disease. *J Neurosci*, Vol. 24, No. 8, pp. 1865-1872.

Gao, H.M., Jiang, J., Wilson, B., Zhang, W., Hong, J.S. and Liu, B. (2002). Microglial activation-mediated delayed and progressive degeneration of rat nigral dopaminergic neurons: relevance to Parkinson's disease, *J Neurochem*, Vol. 81, No. 6, pp. 1285-1297.

Gao, H.M., Hong, J.S., Zhang, W. and Liu, B. (2003). Synergistic dopaminergic neurotoxicity of the pesticide rotenone and inflammogen lipopolysaccharide: relevance to the etiology of Parkinson's disease. *J Neurosci*, Vol. 23, No. 4, pp. 1228-1236.

Gao, H.M., Kotzbauer, P.T., Uryu, K., Leight, S., Trojanowski, J.Q. and Lee, V.M. (2008). Neuroinflammation and oxidation/nitration of alpha-synuclein linked to dopaminergic neurodegeneration. *J Neurosci*, Vol. 28, No. 30, pp. 7687-7698.

Gayle, D. A., Ling, Z., Tong, C., Landers, T., Lipton, J. W. and Carvey, P. M. (2002). Lipopolysaccharide (LPS)-induced dopamine cell loss in culture: roles of tumor necrosis factor-alpha, interleukin-1beta, and nitric oxide. *Brain Res Dev Brain Res*, Vol. 133, No. 1, pp. 27-35.

Gerhard, A., Pavese, N., Hotton, G., Turkheimer, F., Es, M., Hammers, A., Eggert, K., Oertel, W., Banati, R.B. and Brooks, D.J. (2006). In vivo imaging of microglial with [^{11}C](R)-PK11195 PET in idiopathic Parkinson's disease. *Neurobiol Dis*, Vol. 21, No. 2, pp. 404-412.

Harms, A.S., Barnum, C.J., Ruhn, K.A., Varghese, S., Trevino, I., Blesch, A. and Tansey, M.G. (2011). Delayed dominant-negative TNF gene therapy halts progressive loss of nigral dopaminergic neurons in a rat model of Parkinson's disease. *Mol Ther*, Vol. 19, No. 1, pp. 46-52.

Hashimoto, M., Nitta, A., Fukumitsu, H., Nomoto, H., Shen, L. and Furukawa, S. (2005). Inflammation-induced GDNF improves locomotor function after spinal cord injury. *Neurorepot,* Vol. 16, No. 2, pp. 99-102.

Hide, I., Tanaka, M., Inoue, A., Nakajima, K., Kohsaka, S., Inoue, K. and Nakata, Y. (2000). Extracellular ATP triggers tumor necrosis factor-a release from rat microglia. *J Neurochem,* Vol. 75, No. 3, pp. 965-972.

Honda, S., Sasaki, Y., Ohsawa, K., Imai, Y., Nakamura, Y., Inoue, K. and Kohsaka, S. (2001). Extracellular ATP or ADP induce chemotaxis of cultured microglia through $G_{i/o}$-coupled P2Y receptors. *J Neurocsi,* Vol. 21, No. 6, pp. 1975-1982.

Hunot, S., Boissiere, F., Faucheux, B., Brugg, B., Mouatt-Prigent, A., Agid, Y. and Hirsch, E.C. (1996). Nitric oxide synthase and neuronal vulnerability in Parkinson's disease. *Neuroscience,* Vol. 72, No. 2, pp. 355-363.

Imai, F., Sawada, M., Suzuki, H., Zlokovic, B.V., Kojima, J., Kuno, S., Nagatsu, T., Nitatori, T., Uchiyama, Y. and Kanno, T. (1999). Exogenous microglia enter the brain and migrate into ischemic hippocampal lesions. *Neurosci Lett,* Vol. 272, No. 2, pp. 127-130.

Imai, F., Suzuki, H., Oda, J., Ninomiya, T., Ono, K., Sano, H. and Sawada, M. (2007). Neuroprotective effects of exogenous microglia in global brain ischemia. *J Cereb Blood Flow Metab,* Vol. 27, No. 3, pp. 488-500.

Imamura, K., Hishikawa, N., Sawada, M., Nagatsu, T., Yoshida, M. and Hashizume, Y. (2003). Distribution of major histocompatibility complex class II-positive microglia and cytokine profile of Parkinson's disease brains. *Acta Neuropathol,* Vol. 106, No. 6, pp. 518-526.

Imamura, K., Hishikawa, N., Ono, K., Suzuki, H., Sawada, M., Nagatsu, T., Yoshida, M. and Hashizume, Y. (2005). Cytokine production of activated microglia and decrease in neurotrophic factors of neurons in the hippocampus of Lewy body disease brains. *Acta Neuropathol,* Vol. 109, No. 2, pp. 141-150.

Inoue, K., Nakajima, K. Morimoto, T., Kikuchi, Y., Koizumi, S., Illes, P. and Kohsaka, S. (1998). ATP stimulation of Ca^{2+}-dependent plasminogen release from cultured microglia. *Br J Pharmacol,* Vol. 123, No. 7, pp. 1304-1310.

Inoue, K. (2002). Microglial activation by purines and pyrimidines. *Glia,* Vol. 40, No. 2, pp. 156-163.

Iravani, M.M., Leung, C.C.M., Sadeghian, M., Haddon, C.O., Rose, S. and Jenner, P. (2005). The acute and the long-term effects of nigral lipopolysaccharide administration on dopaminergic dysfunction and glial cell activation. *Eur J Neurosci,* Vol. 22, No. 2, pp. 317-330.

Jang, H., Boltz, D., Sturm-Ramirez, K., Shepherd, K.R., Jiao, Y., Webster, R. and Smeyne, R.J. (2009). Highly pathogenic H5N1 influenza virus can enter the central nervous system and induce neuroinflammation and neurodegeneration. *Proc Natl Acad Sci USA,* Vol. 106, No. 33, pp. 14063-14068.

Kim, W.G., Mohney, R.P., Wilson, B., Jeohn, G.H., Liu, B. and Hong, J.S. (2000). Regional difference in susceptibility to lipopolysaccharide-induced neurotoxicity in the rat brain: role of microglia. *J Neurocsi,* Vol. 20, No. 16, pp. 6309-6316.

Kim, Y.S., Kim, S.S., Cho, J.J., Choi, D.H., Hwang, O., Shin, D.H., Chun, H.S., Beal, M.F. and Joh, T.H. (2005). Matrix metalloproteinase-3: a novel signaling proteinase from apoptotic neuronal cells that activates microglia. *J Neurosci,* Vol. 25, No. 14, pp. 3701–3711.

Kim, Y.S., Choi, D.H., Block, M.L., Lorenzl, S., Yang, L., Kim, Y.J., Sugama, S., Cho, B.P., Hwang, O., Browne, S.E., Kim, S.Y., Hong, J.S., Beal, M.F. and Joh, T.H. (2007). A pivotal role of matrix metalloproteinase-3 activity in dopaminergic neuronal degeneration via microglial activation. *FASEB J*, Vol. 21, No. 1, pp. 179–187.

Kordower, J.H., Chu, Y., Hauser, R.A., Freeman, T.B. and Olanow, C.W. (2008). Lewy body-like pathology in long-term embryonic nigral transplants in Parkinson's disease. *Nat Med*, Vol. 14, No. 5, pp. 504-506.

Koutsilieri, E., Scheller, C., Grünblatt, E., Nara, K., Li, J., and Riederer, P. (2002). Free radicals in Parkinson's disease. *J Neurol*, Vol. 249, Suppl 2, II/1-II/5.

Kramer, B. C., Yabut, J. A., Cheong, J., Jnobaptiste, R., Robakis, T., Olanow C. W. and Mytilineou, C. (2002). Lipopolysaccharide prevents cell death caused by glutathione depletion: possible mechanisms of protection. *Neuroscience*, Vol. 114, No. 2, pp. 361-372.

Lai, A.Y. and Todd, K.G. (2008). Differential regulation of trophic and proinflammatory microglia effectors is dependent on severity of neuronal injury. *Glia*, Vol. 56, No. 3, pp. 259-270.

Li, J.Y., Englund, E., Holton, J.L., Soulet, D., Hagell, P., Lees, A.J., Lashley, T., Quinn, N.P., Rehncrona, S., Björklund, A., Winder, H., Revesz, T., Lindvall, O. and Brundin, P. (2008). Lewy bodies in grafted neurons in subjects with Parkinson's disease suggest host-to-graft disease propagation. *Nat Med*, Vol. 14, No. 5, pp. 501-503.

Liu, J., Marino, M.W., Wong, G., Grail, D., Dunn, A., Bettadapura, J., Slavin, A.J., Old, L. and Bernard, C.A. (1998). TNF is a potent anti-inflammatory cytokine in autoimmune-mediated demyelination. *Nat Med*, Vol. 4, No. 1, pp. 78-83.

Mallat, M., Houlgatte, R., Brachet, P. and Prochiantz, A. (1989). Lipopolysaccharide-stimulated rat brain macrophages release NGF in vitro. *Dev Biol*, Vol. 133, No. 1, pp. 309-311.

Mason, J. L., Suzuki, K., Chaplin, D.D. and Matsushima G.K. (2001). Interleukin-1β promotes repair of the CNS. *J Neorosci*, Vol. 21, No. 18, pp. 7046-7052.

McGeer, P.L., Itagaki, S., Boyes, B.E. and McGeer, E.G. (1988). Reactive microglia are positive for HLA-DR in the substantia nigra of Parkinson's and Alzheimer's disease brain. *Neurology*, Vol. 38, No. 8, pp. 1285-1291.

McGuire, S.O., Ling, Z.D., Lipton, J.W., Sortwell, C.E., Collier, T.J. and Carvey, P.M. (2001). Tumor necrosis factor α is toxic to embryonic mesencephalic dopamine neurons. *Exp Neurol*, Vol. 169, No. 2, pp. 219-230.

Miller, R.L., James-Kracke, M., Sun, G.Y. and Sun, A.Y. (2009). Oxidative and inflammatory pathway in Parkinson's disease. *Neurochem Res*, Vol. 34, No. 1, pp. 55-65.

Miwa, T., Furukawa, S., Nakajima, K., Furukawa, Y. and Kohsaka, S. (1997). Lipopolysaccharide enhances synthesis of brain-derived neurotrophic factor in cultured rat microglia. *J Neurosci Res*, Vol. 50, No. 6, pp. 1023-1029.

Mogi, M., Harada, M., Riederer, P., Narabayashi, H., Fujita, K. and Nagatsu, T. (1994a). Tumor necrosis factor-alpha (TNF-alpha) increases both in the brain and in the cerebrospinal fluid from parkinsonian patients. *Neurosci Lett*, Vol. 165, Nos. 1-2, pp. 208-210.

Mogi, M., Harada, M., Kondo, T., Riederer, P., Inagaki, H., Minami, M. and Nagatsu, T. (1994b). Interleukin-1 beta, interleukin-6, epidermal growth factor and transforming growth factor-alpha are elevated in the brain from parkinsonian patients. *Neurosci, Lett*, Vol. 180, No. 2, pp. 147-150.

Mogi, M., Harada, M., Kondo, T., Mizuno, Y., Narabayashi, H., Riederer, P. and Nagatsu T. (1996). Bcl-2 protein is increased in the brain from parkinsonian patients. *Neurosci Lett*, Vol. 215, No. 2, pp. 137-139.

Mogi, M., Togari, A., Ogawa, M., Ikeguchi, K., Shizuma, N., Fan, D.S., Nakano, I. and Nagatsu T. (1998). Effects of repeated administration of 1-methyl-4-phenyl-1,2,3,6-tetrahydropyridine (MPTP) to mice on interleukin-1 beta and nerve growth factor in the striatum. *Neurosci Lett,* Vol. 250, No. 1, pp. 25-28.

Mogi, M., Togari, A., Kondo, T., Mizuno, Y., Komure, O., Kuno, S., Ichinose, H. and Nagatsu T. (2000). Caspase activities and tumor necrosis factor receptor R1 level are elevated in the substantia nigra in Parkinson's disease. *J Neural Transm,* Vol. 107, No. 3, pp. 355-341.

Nagata, K., Takei, N., Nakajima, K., Saito, H. and Kohsaka, S. (1993a). Microglial conditioned medium promotes survival and development of cultured mesencephalic neurons from embryonic rat brain. *J Neorosci Res,* Vol. 34, No. 3, pp. 357-363.

Nagata, K., Nakajima, K. and Kohsaka, S. (1993b). Plasminogen promotes the development of rat mesencephalic dopaminergic neurons in vitro. *Brain Res Dev Brain Res,* Vol. 75, No. 1, pp. 31-37.

Nagatsu, T. (2002). Parkinson's disease: changes in apoptosis-related factors suggesting possible gene therapy. *J Neural Transm,* Vol. 109, Nos. 5-6, pp. 731-745.

Nagatsu, T. and Sawada, M. (2005). Inflammatory process in Parkinson's disease: role for cytokines. *Curr Pharm Design,* Vol. 11, No. 8, pp. 999-1016.

Nagatsu, T. and Sawada, M. (2006). Cellular and molecular mechanisms of Parkinson's disease: neurotoxins, causative genes, and inflammatory cytokines. *Cell Mol Neurobiol,* Vol. 26, Nos. 4-6, pp. 781-802.

Nagatsu, T. and Sawada, M. (2007). Biochenistry of postmortem brains in Parkinson's disease: historical overview and future prospects. *J Neural Transm, Suppl,* Vol. 72, pp. 113-120.

Nakajima, K., Tsuzaki, N., Nagata, K., Takemoto, N. and Kohsaka S. (1992). Production and secretion of plasminogen in cultured rat brain microglia. *FEBS Lett,* Vol. 308, No. 2, pp. 179-182.

Nakajima, K., Honda, S., Tohyama, Y., Imai, Y., Kohsaka, S. and Kurihara, T. (2001). Neurotrophin secretion from cultured microglia. *J Neurosci Res,* Vol. 65, No. 4, pp. 322-331.

Ohtani, Y., Minami, M. and Satoh, M. (2000). Expression of inducible nitric oxide synthase mRNA and production of nitric oxide are induced by adenosine triphosphate in cultured rat microglia. *Neurosci Lett,* Vol. 293, No. 1, pp. 72-74.

Olanow, C.W. and Prusiner, S.B. (2009). Is Parkinson's disease a prion disorder. *Proc Natl Acad Sci USA,* Vol. 106, No. 31, pp. 12571-12572.

Ono, K., Takii, T., Onozaki, K., Ikawa, M., Okabe, M. and Sawada, M. (1999). Migration of exogenous immature hematopoietic cells into adult mouse brain parenchyma under GFP-expressing bone marrow chimera. *Biochem Biophys Res Commun,* Vol. 262, No. 3, pp. 610-614.

Ono, K., Suzuki, H. and Sawada, M. (2010). Delayed neural damage is induced by iNOS-expressing microglia in a brain injury model. *Neurosci Lett,* Vol. 473, No. 2, pp.146-150.

Purisai, M.G., McCormack, A.L., Cumine, S., Li, J., Isla, M.Z. and Di Monte, D.A. (2007). Microglial activations as a priming event leading to paraquat-induced dopaminergic cell degeneration. *Neurobiol Dis,* Vol. 25, No. 2, pp. 392-400.

Qin, L., Wu, X., Block, M.L., Liu, Y., Breese, G.R., Hong, J.S., Knapp, D.J. and Crews, F.T. (2007). Systemic LPS causes chronic neuroinflammation and progressive neurodegeneration. *Glia,* Vol. 55, No. 5, pp. 453-462.

Reynolds, A.D., Stone, D.K., Mosley, R.L. and Gendelman, H.E. (2009). Nitrated α-synuclein-induced alterations in microglial immunity are regulated by CD4+ T cell Subsets. *J Immunol,* Vol. 182, No. 7, pp. 4137-4149.

Rabchevsky A. G. and Streit W. J. (1997). Grafting of cultured microglial cells into the lesioned spinal cord of adult rats enhances neurite outgrowth. *J Neorosci Res,* Vol. 47, No. 1, pp. 34-48.

Saijo, K., Winner, B., Carson, C.T., Collier, J.G., Boyer, L., Rosenfeld, M.G., Gage, F.H. and Glass, C.K. (2009). A Nurr1/CoREST pathway in microglia and astrocytes protects dopaminergic neurons from inflammation-induced death. *Cell,* Vol. 137, No. 1, pp. 47-59.

Satake, W., Nakabayashi, Y., Mizuta, I., Hirota, Y., Ito, C., Kubo, M., Kawaguchi, T., Tsunoda, T., Watanabe, M., Takeda, A., Tomiyama, H., Nakashima, K., Hasegawa, K., Obata, F., Yoshikawa, T., Kawakami, H., Sakoda, S., Yamamoto, M., Hattori, N., Murata, M., Nakamura, Y. and Toda, T. (2009). Genomic-wide association study identifies common variants at four loci as genetic risk factors for Parkinson's disease. *Nat Genet,* Vol. 41, No. 12, pp. 1303-1307.

Sawada, H., Hishida, R., Hirata, Y., Ono, K., Suzuki, H., Muramatsu, S., Nakano, I., Nagatsu, T. and Sawada, M. (2007). Activated microglia affect the nigro-striatal dopamine neurons differently in neonatal and aged mice treated with 1-methyl-4-phenyl-1,2,3,6-tetrahydropyridine. *J Neurosci Res,* Vol. 85, No. 8, pp. 1752-1761.

Sawada, H., Suzuki, H., Nagatsu, T. and Sawada, M. (2010). Neuroprotective and neurotoxic phenotypes of activated microglia in neonatal mice with respective MPTP- and ethanol-induced brain injury. *Neurodegenerative Dis,* Vol. 7, Nos. 1-3, pp. 64-67.

Sawada, M., Kondo, N., Suzumura, A. and Marunouchi T. (1989). Production of tumor necrosis factor-alpha by microglia and astrocytes in culture. *Brain Res,* Vol. 491, No. 2, pp. 394-397.

Sawada, M., Suzumura, A., Yamamoto, H. and Marunouchi T. (1990). Activation and proliferation of the isolated microglia by colony stimulating factor-1 and possible involvement of protein kinase C. *Brain Res,* Vol. 509, No. 1, pp. 119-124.

Sawada, M., Suzumura, A. and Marunouchi, T. (1995). Cytokine network in the central nervous system and its roles in growth and differentiation of glial and neuronal cells. *Int J Dev Neurosci,* Vol. 13, Nos. 3-4, pp. 253-264.

Sawada, M., Imai, F., Suzuki, H., Hayakawa, M., Kanno, T. and Nagatsu, T. (1998). Brain-specific gene expression by immortalized microglial cell-mediated gene transfer in the mammalian brain. *FEBS Lett,* Vol. 433, Nos. 1-2, pp. 37-40.

Sawada, M., Suzumura, A., Hosoya, H., Marunouch,i T. and Nagatsu T. (1999). Interleukin-10 inhibits both production of cytokines and expression of cytokine receptors in microglia. *J Neurochem,* Vol. 72, No. 4, pp. 1466-1471.

Sawada, M., Imamura, K. and Nagatsu, T. (2006). Role of cytokines in inflammatory process in Parkinson's disease. *J Neural Transm, Suppl,* Vol. 70, pp. 373-381.

Sawada, M., Sawada, H. and Nagatsu, T. (2008). Effects of aging on neuroprotective and neurotoxic properties of microglia in neurodegenerative diseases. *Neurodegenerative Dis,* Vol. 5, Nos. 3-4, pp. 254-256.

Shigemoto-Mogami, Y., Koizumi, S., Tsuda, M., Ohsawa, K., Kohsaka, S. and Inoue K. (2001). Mechanisms underlying extracellular ATP-evoked interleukin-6 release in mouse microglial cell line, MG-5. *J Neurochem,* Vol. 78, No. 6, pp. 1339-1349.

Sriram, K., Matheson, J.M., Benkovic, S.A., Miller, D.B., Luster, M.I. and O'Callaghan J.P. (2002). Mice deficient in TNF receptors are protected against dopaminergic neurotoxicity: implications for Parkinson's disease. *FASEB J,* Vol. 16, No. 11, pp. 1474-1476.

Sugama, S., Yang, L., Cho, B.P., DeGiorgio, L.A., Lorenzl, S., Albers, D.S., Beal, M.F., Volpe, B.T. and Joh, T.H. (2003). Age-related microglial activation in 1-methyl-4-phenyl-1,2,3,6-tetrahydropyridine (MPTP)-induced dopaminergic neurodegeneration in C57BL/6 mice. *Brain Res,* Vol. 964, No. 2, pp. 288-294.

Suzuki, H., Imai, F., Kanno, T. and Sawada, M. (2001). Preservation of neurotrophin expression in microglia that migrate into the gerbil's brain across the blood-brain barrier. *Neurosci Lett,* Vol. 312, No. 2, pp. 95-98.

Suzumura, A., Sawada, M., Yamamoto, H. and Marunouchi, T. (1993). Transforming growth factor-β suppresses activation and proliferation of microglia in vitro. *J Immunol,* Vol. 151, No. 4, pp. 2150-2158.

Suzumura, A., Ito, A., Yoshikawa, M. and Sawada, M. (1999). Ibudilast suppresses TNF alpha production by glial cells functioning mainly as type III phosphodiesterase inhibitor in the CNS. *Brain Res,* Vol. 837, Nos. 1-2, pp. 203-212.

Takeuchi, A., Isobe, K., Miyaishi, O., Sawada, M., Fan, Z.H., Nakashima, I. and Kiuchi K. (1998). Microglial NO induces delayed neuronal death following acute injury in the striatum. *Eur J Neurosci,* Vol. 10, No. 5, pp. 1613-1620.

Toyama, H., Hatano, K., Suzuki, H., Ichise, M., Momosaki, M., Kudo, G., Ito, F., Kato, T., Yamaguchi, H., Katada, K., Sawada, M. and Ito, K. (2008). In vivo imaging of microglial activation using a peripheral benzodiazepine receptor ligand: [11C]PK-11195 and animal PET following ethanol injury in rat striatum. *Ann Nucl Med,* Vol. 22, No. 5, pp. 417-424.

Thery, C., Hetier, E., Evrard, C. and Mallat, M. (1990). Expression of macrophage colony-stimulating factor gene in the mouse brain during development. *J Neorosci Res,* Vol. 26, No. 1, pp. 129-133.

Viel, J.J., McManus, D.Q., Smith, S.S. and Brewer, G.J. (2001). Age- and concentration-dependent neuroprotection and toxicity by TNF in cortical neurons from β-amyloid. *J Neurosci Res,* Vol. 64, No. 5, pp. 454-465.

Vilhardt, F., Plastre, O., Sawada, M., Suzuki, K., Wiznerowicz, M., Kiyokawa, E., Trono, D. and Krause, K.H. (2002). The HIV-1 Nef protein and phagocyte NADPH oxidase activation. *J Biol Chem,* Vol. 277, No. 44, pp. 42136-42143.

Wu, D.C., Jackson-Lewis, V., Vila, M., Tieu, K., Teismann, P., Vadseth, C., Choi, D-K., Ischiropoulos, H. and Przedborski, S. (2002). Blockade of microglial activation is neuroprotective in the 1-methyl-4-phenyl-1,2,3,6-tetrahydropyridine mouse model of Parkinson disease. *J Neurosci,* Vol. 22, No. 5, pp. 1763-1771.

Wu, D.C., Teismann, P., Tieu, K., Vila, M., Jackson-Lewis, V., Ischiropoulos, H. and Przedborski S. (2003). NADPH oxidase mediates oxidative stress in the 1-methyl-4-phenyl-1,2,3,6-tetrahydropyridine model of Parkinson disease. *Proc Natl Acad Sci USA,* Vol. 100, No. 10, pp. 6145-6150.

Yang, L., Lindholm, K., Konishi, Y., Li, R. and Shen, Y. (2002). Target depletion of distinct tumor necrosis factor receptor subtypes reveals hippocampal neuron death and survival through different signal transduction pathways. *J Neorosci,* Vol. 22, No. 8, pp. 3025-3032.

Zhang, W., Wang, T., Pei, Z., Miller D.S., Wu, X., Block, M.L., Wilson, B., Zhang, W., Zhou, Y., Hong, J.S. and Zhang, J. (2005). Aggregated alpha-synuclein activates microglia: a process leading to disease progression in Parkinson's disease. *FASEB J,* Vol. 19, No. 6, pp. 533-542.

16

Oxidative DNA Damage and the Level of Biothiols, and L-Dopa Therapy in Parkinson's Disease

Dorszewska Jolanta and Kozubski Wojciech
Poznan University of Medical Sciences, Laboratory of Neurobiology Department of Neurology, Chair and Department of Neurology, Poland

1. Introduction

Parkinson's disease (PD) is a chronic and progressive neurological disorder characterized by resting tremor, rigidity, and bradykinesia, affecting at least 1% of individuals above the age of 65 years. Parkinson's disease is a result of degeneration of the dopamine-producing neurons of the *substantia nigra*. Available therapies in PD will only improve the symptoms but not halt progression of disease. The most effective treatment for PD patients is therapy with L-3,4-dihydroxy-phenylalanine (L-dopa) (Olanow, 2008). As indicated in literature reports, L-dopa therapy leads to motor fluctuations and disabling involuntary movements called L-dopa-induced dyskinesia (Carta et al., 2006; Obeso et al., 2008). Literature reports indicate also that long-term administration of L-dopa in PD patients may not only alter arginine (Arg) levels but may also lead to increased concentrations of homocysteine (Hcy), the factor responsible for development of atherosclerosis and dysfunction of nigral endothelial cells (Muller et al., 1999).
Methylenetetrahydrofolate reductase (MTHFR) represents enzyme involved in remethylation of Hcy to methionine (Met). The C667T transition in *MTHFR* results in Ala>Val substitution in position 226 and, as a consequence, in 50 % decrease in the enzyme activity, and thus in an increased concentration of Hcy (Frosst et al., 1995). The study of Yasui et al. (2000) indicated that the TT genotype might be linked to pathogenesis of PD, particularly when the level of folates is low. Moreover, L-dopa metabolism via O-methylation by catechol-O-methyl-transferase (COMT) using S-adenosyl-L-methionine (SAM) leads to increase Hcy levels, hyper-Hcy (O'Suilleabhain et al., 2004a). A percentage 10-30% of PD patients exhibits hyper-Hcy. Hyper-Hcy in PD has been associated with affective and cognitive impairment, dementia, dyskinesia, and vascular disease (O'Suilleabhain et al., 2004b; Rogers et al., 2003; Zoccolella et al., 2006, 2009).
The exact mechanism of development and progression of PD pathology is not clear. It is known, that a complex interplay of multiple environmental and genetic factors has been involved in pathogenesis of PD and it is possibly that PD represents rather a syndrome but not a single disorder. Moreover, is likely that in pathogenesis of PD there are several mechanisms involved, such as: oxidative stress, mitochondrial dysfunction, DNA damage, protein aggregation, neuroinflammation, excitotoxicity, apoptosis and loss of trophic factors. The most probably is that all factors are represented targets for PD therapy.

2. 8-Oxo-2'-deoxyguanosine and L-dopa treatment in Parkinson's disease

Oxidative stress and excitotoxicity seems to play a pivotal role in pathogenesis of few major neurodegenerative diseases e.g. Alzheimer's disease (AD) and PD. The study of Jenner (2003) indicates that oxidative stress in the brain of PD patients may leads to formed reactive forms of oxygen (RFO). In the course of PD, RFO activate processes leading to the damage of DNA, proteins and lipids, and to a low level of antioxidants (Blake et al., 1997; Kikuchi et al., 2002). Moreover, in the patients suffering from PD, dopamine level-controlled deposition of ubiquitin- and α-synuclein-positive inclusion bodies (Lewy's bodies) takes place in the cytoplasm of dopaminergic neurons (Spillantini et al., 1997). Deposition of pathological proteins in brains of patients affected by the neurodegenerative diseases, result in pronounced neurotoxic effects on the central nervous system (CNS). In PD, augmented expression of α-synuclein may intensify oxidative stress (Hsu et al., 2000). Bergman et al. (1998) demonstrated that in the PD patients, dopaminergic neurons undergo oxidative damage of the compact portion of *substantia nigra* and dopamine levels decrease in putamen, a region of caudate nucleus. Moreover, ferrous ions released from damaged *substantia nigra* may provide an important substrate for oxidative reactions and for production of RFO (Jenner, 2003).

In PD, oxidative stress follows accumulation of the degradation products in the gray matter compact part of mesencephalon, and is accompanied not only by a high level of ferrous ions, and by decreased level of glutathione, malfunction of the respiratory chain complex I (Jenner, 2003; Schapira et al., 1990; Sian et al., 1994), and excessive oxidation processes, especially in patients treated with L-dopa (Spencer et al., 1994).

L-Dopa after oral intake undergoes metabolism, including oxidative metabolism of dopamine, and auto-oxidation, and is transported across the blood-brain barrier. Only less than 5% of an oral dose of L-dopa after took delivered to the brain. Remain plasmatic levels of L-dopa undergoes peripheral oxidative metabolism and may generate ROS. Likely peripheral oxidation status in PD might be affected by L-dopa therapy (Cornetta et al., 2009).

Some studies (e.g. Cornetta et al., 2009) suggest a toxic effect of L-dopa on neuronal cell *in vitro*, while *in vivo* studies in animal models are contradictory. However, in patients with PD some authors indicated on positive correlation between oxidative stress and L-dopa therapy (Florczak et al., 2008; Migliore at al., 2002), but there are also negative correlation between oxidative stress and L-dopa dosage in peripheral blood lymphocytes (in nine patients with PD et paper of Cornetta et al., 2009; Prigione et al., 2006).

As indicated by literature reports, interaction of reactive oxygen with nucleic acids leads to oxidation of guanine and formation of 8-oxo-2'-deoxyguanosine (8-oxo2dG). Oxidative modification of guanine at C8 position may take place either in nucleic acids or free cellular nucleosides and nucleotides, ready to be incorporated to newly synthesized DNA chains. Incorporation of the modified nucleotide to DNA may results in mutations due to pairing of 8-oxoguanosine with cytosine and adenosine. In the course of pairing with adenosine, 8-oxoguanosine induces GC→AT transversions (Hirano, 2008). 8-Oxoguanina or its nucleoside, 8-oxo2dG there are though to represent markers of oxidative DNA damage.

Augmented levels of 8-oxo2dG were demonstrated in brain and in lymphocytes of patients with PD (Alam et al., 1997; Dorszewska et al., 2007; Florczak et al., 2008; Kikuchi et al., 2002; Zhang et al., 1999). This indicates a gradual increase of nucleic acid damage during development of this disease, and high level of oxidized guanine in DNA is considered a risk factor for senescence and neurodegenerative diseases (e.g. PD).

The contribution of L-dopa therapy to oxidative damage and apoptosis in peripheral cells in PD patients is not clear, and is still debated.

2.1 Influence of L-dopa treatment on the level of 8-oxo-2dG in peripheral blood lymphocytes of Parkinson's disease patients

The aim of the study was to estimate the degree of oxidative damage to DNA (marker: 8-oxo2dG) in PD patients before and during treatment with L-Dopa, and in controls.

2.1.1 Patients

The studies were conducted on 98 patients with PD, including 37 women and 61 men aging 34-81 years (mean age: 60.8±10.7 years). Among the patients with PD, 27 patients (9 women and 18 men) awaited L-dopa treatment (patients' age: 34-79 years) and the remaining 71 individuals, 28 women and 43 men (patients' age: 35-81 years) were treated with L-dopa preparations in daily doses (up to 5 years treatment to 500 mg/day, 5-10 year treatment 500-800 mg/day, and over 10 year treatment 800-1500 mg/day).
Control group included 50 individuals, 34 women and 16 men, 22-76 years of age (mean age: 44.6±16.2 years).
Patients with PD were diagnosed using the criteria of UK Parkinson's Disease Society Brain Bank (Litvan et al., 2003), however stage of disease according to the scale of Hoehn and Yahr.
None of the control subjects had verifiable symptoms of dementia or any other neurological disorders and smoking, and drinking habits.
A Local Ethical Committee approved the study and the written consent of all patients or their caregivers was obtained.

2.1.2 Determination of 8-oxo2dG

Isolation of DNA. DNA was isolated from peripheral blood lymphocytes by fivefold centrifugation in a lytic buffer, containing 155 mM NH_4Cl, 10 mM $KHCO_3$, 0.1 mM Na_2EDTA, pH 7.4, in the presence of buffer containing 75 mM NaCl, 9 mM Na_2EDTA , pH 8.0, and sodium dodecyl sulfate and proteinase K (Sigma, St. Louis, MO). Subsequently, NaCl was added, the lysate was centrifuged, and DNA present in the upper layer was precipitated with 98% ethanol.
Enzymatic hydrolysis of DNA to nucleosides. DNA was hydrolyzed to nucleosides using P_1 nuclease (Sigma), for 2 h at 37°C in 10 mM NaOAc, pH 4.5. The solution was buffered with 100 mM Tris-HCl, pH 7.5. Subsequently, the DNA was hydrolyzed with alkaline phosphatase (1U/µl; Roche, Germany) for 1 h at 37 °C and the obtained nucleosides mixture was applied to high-pressure liquid chromatography system with both electrochemical and UV detection (HPLC/EC/UV).
Estimation of 8-oxo2dG. To determine 8-oxo2dG level, the nucleosides mixture was applied to the HPLC/UV system (P580A; Dionex, Germany) coupled to an electrochemical detector (CoulArray 5600; ESA, USA). Nucleosides were separated in a Termo Hypersil BDS C18 (250 x 4.6 x 5µm) column (Germany). The system was controlled, and the data were collected and processed using Chromeleon software (Dionex, Germany). The results were expressed as a ratio of oxidized nucleosides in the form of 8-oxo2dG to unmodified 2'dG (Olsen et al., 1999).

2.1.3 Results

In the patients with PD (Table 1), the levels of 8-oxo2dG in peripheral blood lymphocytes were significantly increased ($p<0.05$), as compared to the controls.

Parameter	Controls (22-76 years)	Patients with PD (34-81 years)
8-oxo2dG	13.7 ± 7.6	21.8 ± 17.8*

Table 1. Levels of DNA oxidative damage (8-oxo2dG/dG x 10^{-5}) in the PD patients and in control group. Results are expressed as a means ± SD. The nonparametric of Mann-Whitney test for unlinked variables was used. Differences significant at *$p<0.05$, as compared to the controls.

In the PD patients (Table 2) disease progress from stage I to IV (according to the scale of Hoehn and Yahr) resulted in higher level of 8-oxo2dG in DNA ($p<0.05$) also observed between stages I and III, and a tendency to further decrease in stage IV.

Parameter	Stage I (35-79 years)	Stage II (34-81 years)	Stage III (46-81 years)	Stage IV (56-78 years)
8-oxo2dG	17.4 ± 16.9	20.5 ± 14.2	25.2 ± 22.7	23.2 ± 12.8*

Table 2. Levels of oxidative DNA damage (8-oxo2dG/dG x 10^{-5}), as related to the stage of the PD according to the scale of Hoehn and Yahr. Results are expressed as means ± SD. The nonparametric of Mann-Whitney test for unlinked variables was used. Differences significant at *$p<0.05$, between stages I and IV of PD.

Pharmacotherapy with L-dopa (Table 3) affected the level of 8-oxo2dG ($p<0.01$), as compared to the healthy controls.

Parameter	Controls (22-76 years)	Patients with PD L-dopa (-) (34-79 years)	Patients with PD L-dopa (+) (35-81 years)
8-oxo2dG	13.7 ± 7.6	19.3 ± 17.3	22.6 ± 18.0**

Table 3. Levels of oxidative DNA damage (8-oxo2dG/dG x 10^{-5}), as related to pharmacotherapy with L-dopa (+) in the patients with PD. Results are expressed as means ± SD. The nonparametric of Mann-Whitney test for unlinked variables was used. Differences significant at **$p<0.01$, as compared to the controls.

Our results indicated that, L-dopa can modify the level of oxidative DNA damage (8-oxo2dG) in the peripheral blood cells of PD patients. On the other hand, it is interesting that in PD a significant increase in DNA damage has been observed in the IVth stage of the disease development (according to Hoehn and Yahr), even so 8-oxo2dG levels are increased between the stages I and III of the disease evolution. It seems that in PD the reason for increasing levels of oxidative process altered nucleic acids is thought to involve overproduction of free radicals as well as decreased levels of enzymatic and non-enzymatic antioxidants and less effective repair mechanisms. In AD patients have been found to contain lowered activity of specific 8-oxoguanine glycosylase 1, OGG1, and more oxidative DNA damage which might induce of apoptosis (Dorszewska et al., 2005, 2009a, 2010).

It seems that analysis of the level of oxidative stress (8-oxo2dG) may be represented targets for diagnosis of PD and therapy in future.

2.2 Influence of L-dopa treatment on the level of apoptotic factors in peripheral blood lymphocytes of Parkinson's disease patients

At the neuropathological studies, PD is mainly characterized by neuronal intracellular inclusions named Lewy's bodies with α-synuclein. These inclusions are now known to be comprised of filamentous polymers of α-synuclein, which may generate oxidative stress in the brain of PD patients. It could results from several mechanisms, such as depletion of antioxidants, defects in mitochondrial electron transport, neurotoxin exposure, and excessive oxidation of dopamine in the patients given L-dopa. Conway et al. (2001) showed that dopamine or L-dopa inhibits the fibrillization of α-synuclein filaments by stabilization of their structure.

However Alves Da Costa et al. (2002) showed that α-synuclein drastically lowered caspase-3 activity and p53 protein expression, and transcriptional activity, proteins controlled the apoptotic cascade. Blandini et al. (2004), Dorszewska et al. (2009b) and Iwashita (2004) showed that, apoptotic proteins such as: Bcl-2 family proteins and PARP are involved in the pathogenesis of PD as well.

The aim of the study was to estimate the levels of p53, and PARP proteins, and 85 kDa fragment, and two Bcl-2 family proteins: Bcl-2 and Bax in peripheral lymphocytes of patients with PD and in control group. The attention was also paid to L-dopa pharmacotherapy in PD.

2.2.1 Patients

The studies were conducted on 45 patients with PD, among their 22 patients, including 9 women and 13 men, aging 41-79 years (mean age: 58.0±10.7 years) awaited L-dopa treatment and 23 patients, including 11 women and 12 men aging 45-81 years (mean age: 68.0±8.6 years) were treated with L-dopa preparations in daily doses (up to 5 years treatment to 500 mg/day, 5-10 year treatment 500-800 mg/day, and over 10 year treatment 800-1500 mg/day).

The control group included 27 individuals, 19 women and 8 men, 35-73 years of age (mean age: 54.0±10.7 years).

Patients with PD were diagnosed using the criteria of UK Parkinson's Disease Society Brain Bank (Litvan et al., 2003), however stage of disease according to the scale of Hoehn and Yahr.

None of the control subjects had verifiable symptoms of dementia or any other neurological disorders and smoking, and drinking habits.

A Local Ethical Committee approved the study and the written consent of all patients or their caregivers was obtained.

2.2.2 Estimation of p53, Bax, Bcl-2, PARP proteins and 85-kDa subunit

Isolation of proteins. Blood was gradiated onto gradisol L at a 1:1 ratio and centrifuged, followed by collection of the interphase which was then rinsed in PBS buffer (0.9% NaCl in phosphate buffer) and centrifuged. The obtained lymphocyte precipitate was rinsed with radioimmunoprotein assay (RIPA) buffer (50 mM Tris-HCl, pH 7.2, 150 mM NaCl, 1% IGEPAL CA-630, 0.05% SDS, and 1% sodium deoxycholate), supplemented with a protease inhibitor cocktail (Sigma) and homogenized in a mixture of RIPA with protease inhibitor cocktail (16:1) and 0.5 μl PSMF (Sigma) in isopropanol (10 mg/100 μl), centrifuged, and the obtained supernatant underwent further analysis (Ohnishi et al., 1996).

Western Blot. The Bax and Bcl-2 proteins were analyzed in 12% and p53, and PARP proteins were analyzed in 7.5% polyacrylamide gel. Equivalent amounts of protein (30 μg protein/lane) were loaded to the wells. The gel-separated proteins were electrotransferred to nitrocellulose filter in a semidry Western Blot analysis apparatus (Apelex, France). To estimate the levels of the PARP protein, the filters were exposed first to an anti-PARP monoclonal antibody (G-2-10, IgG, 0.05 ml, Sigma, USA), diluted 1:2000, while the p53, Bax, Bcl-2 proteins were identified using anti-p53 (IgG-2a, 200 μg/1.0 ml; Santa Cruz, USA), anti-Bax (IgG-2b, 200 μg/1.0 ml; Santa Cruz, USA) and anti-Bcl-2 (IgG-1, 200 μg/1.0 ml; Santa Cruz, USA) mouse monoclonal antibody, respectively, diluted 1:500.

Subsequently, individual sheets of nitrocellulose filter were incubated with the second antibody, goad antimouse IgG-HRP (200 μg/0.5 ml; Santa Cruz, USA) at a dilution of 1:2000. To stain immunoreactive bands, peroxidase BMB was added (BM blue POD substrate precipitation; Roche, Germany). The surface area of the immunoreactive bands was registered using a densitometer (GS-710; Bio-Rad, Hercules, CA) in the Quantity One System.

2.2.3 Results

The studies disclosed significant decreased levels of apoptotic proteins (p53, Bax:Bcl-2, PARP, $p<0.01$; Bax, Bcl-2, $p<0.001$) in PD as compared to the controls (Table 4). Decreased level of apoptotic proteins in PD patients probably was result influence of α–synuclein on lower p53 protein expression and caspase-3 activity.

Parameter	Controls 35-73 years of age	PD patients 41-81 years of age
p53	0.52 ± 0.37	0.25 ± 0.14**
Bax	0.60 ± 0.50	0.13 ± 0.07***
Bcl-2	1.20 ± 0.77	0.15 ± 0.08***
Bax/Bcl-2	1.46 ± 3.77	1.13 ± 0.83**
PARP	2.12 ± 0.83	1.61 ± 1.12**
85-kDa	0.42 ± 0.80	0.41 ± 0.31

Table 4. Level of p53, Bax, Bcl-2, PARP proteins and of 85-kDa protein subunit in peripheral blood lymphocytes in PD patients and in the control group. Apoptotic proteins represent % of area of immunoreactivity bonds. Results are expressed as a means ± SD. The nonparametric test of Mann-Whitney was used. Differences significant at **$p<0.01$; ***$p<0.001$ as compared to the controls.

Simultaneously, in PD patients treated with L-dopa preparations (Table 5) levels of p53, Bax, Bcl-2 proteins increased unsignificant as compared with untreatment patients. In the PD patients treated with L-dopa significant increased only the levels of PARP protein ($p<0.001$ as compared to patients not treated with L-dopa) and 85-kDa fragment ($p<0.01$ as compared to patients untreated with L-dopa).

Parameter	Controls 35-73 years of age	PD patients L-dopa (-) 41-79 years of age	PD patients L-dopa (+) 45-81 years of age
p53	0.52 ± 0.37	0.19 ± 0.11**	0.30 ± 0.15
Bax	0.60 ± 0.50	0.12 ± 0.06***	0.14 ± 0.08***
Bcl-2	1.20 ± 0.77	0.15 ± 0.06***	0.16 ± 0.10***
Bax/Bcl-2	1.46 ± 3.77	1.00 ± 0.64	1.26 ± 0.97*
PARP	2.12 ± 0.83	0.82 ± 0.36***	2.36 ± 1.08(***)
85-kDa	0.42 ± 0.80	0.22 ± 0.13	0.58 ± 0.32***(**)

Table 5. Level of p53, Bax, Bcl-2, PARP proteins and of 85-kDa protein subunit in peripheral blood lymphocytes in PD patients untreatment L-dopa (-) and treatment L-dopa (+), and in the control group. Apoptotic proteins represent % of area of immunoreactivity bonds. Results are expressed as a means ± SD. The nonparametric test of Kruskal-Wallis was used. Differences significant at *$p<0.05$; **$p<0.01$; ***$p<0.001$ as compared to the controls, and (**)$p<0.01$; (***)$p<0.001$ between PD patients untreatment L-dopa (-) and treatment L-dopa (+).

However, (Table 6) long-term (more than 5 years) therapy of L-dopa in PD patients probably leads to apoptosis, because elevated levels of Bax:Bcl-2 ratio ($p<0.05$ as compared to the controls) and 85-kDa fragment ($p<0.05$ as compared to the controls).

Parameter	Controls	PD patients L-dopa < 5 years	PD patients L-dopa > 5 years
p53	0.52 ± 0.37	0.30 ± 0.13	0.30 ± 0.16
Bax	0.60 ± 0.50	0.14 ± 0.09**	0.15 ± 0.08***
Bcl-2	1.20 ± 0.77	0.19 ± 0.08*	0.15 ± 0.11***
Bax/Bcl-2	1.46 ± 3.77	0.85 ± 0.69	1.40 ± 1.03*
PARP	2.12 ± 0.83	2.03 ± 1.00	2.48± 1.12
85-kDa	0.42 ± 0.80	0.44 ± 0.20	0.64 ± 0.35**

Table 6. Level of p53, Bax, Bcl-2, PARP proteins and of 85-kDa protein subunit in peripheral blood lymphocytes in PD patients treatment L-dopa less and more than 5 years, and in the control group. Apoptotic proteins represent % of area of immunoreactivity bonds. Results are expressed as a means ± SD. The nonparametric test of Kruskal-Wallis was used. Differences significant at *$p<0.05$; **$p<0.01$; ***$p<0.001$ as compared to the controls.

It seems that pharmacological treatment of PD patients with L-dopa has a major role in modulating of levels in lymphocytes of some apoptotic proteins, important for this process. Further investigation is thus requisite to analysis expression and mutations of genes encoding proteins important for effective repair and/or apoptosis in PD patients treatment with L-dopa.

3. Homocysteine and asymmetric dimethylarginine and L-dopa treatment in Parkinson's disease

Elevated Hcy level is a risk factor for vascular diseases, cognitive impairment and dementia, and neurodegenerative diseases (e.g. PD). It is also known that vascular dementia and cognitive impairment worsen the prognosis of PD patients, and it is important to minimize the risk of their occurrence as much as possible. Gorell et al. (1994) indicated that patients with PD have shown an increased risk for cardiovascular disease and stroke. In PD not only Hcy, but also cysteine (Cys), product of Hcy metabolism may promote pathological alterations such as: atherosclerosis and thrombogenesis (Muller, 2008).

3.1 Metabolism of biothiols

In the body, Hcy is a point of intersection of two main metabolic pathways: transsulfuration and remethylation. Under physiological conditions, around 50% of Hcy is catabolized by transsulfuration and undergoes transformation to cystathionine and then to Cys. The remaining 50% of Hcy undergoes methylation to Met (Fig. 1).

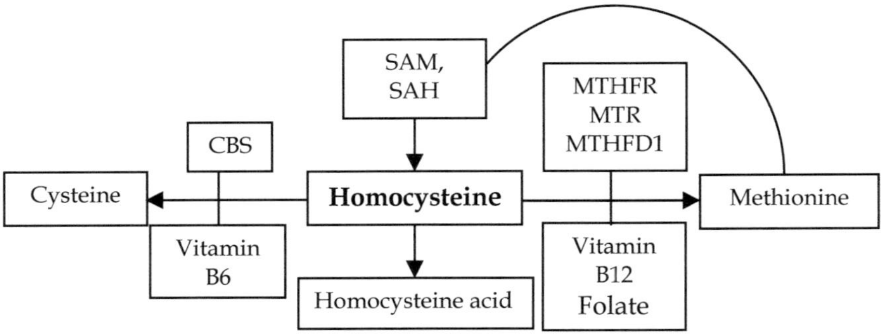

Fig. 1. Synthesis and metabolic pathways of homocysteine, CBS- cystationine β-synthase, MTHFR- 5,10-methylenetetrahydrofolate reductase, MTR- methionine synthase, MTHFD1- methylenetetrahydrofolate dehydrogenase/ methenyltetrahydrofolate cyclohydrolase/formyltetrahydrofolate synthetase, SAH- S-adenosylhomocysteine, SAM- S-adenosylmethionine.

Methionine is supplied with food and its transformation to Hcy involves several steps. At the first step, Met is transformed to SAM and is then demethylated to SAH (S-adenosylhomocysteine) and hydrolyzed to Hcy. SAM is the main donor of methyl groups in many reactions. A decreased content of SAM was demonstrated in the course of PD (Cheng et al., 1997).

The level of Hcy undergoes control, depending upon concentration of its metabolites: Cys and Met. In the case of Met deficit and low concentration of SAM, most Hcy undergoes remethylation to Met, catalyzed by methionine synthase (MTR). MTR is a vitamin B12-dependent enzyme responsible for transfer of methyl groups from N-methyltetrahydrofolate to Hcy, leading to formation of Met (Jarrett et al., 1996). Mutations in the MTR gene are responsible for decreased methylcobalamine level, and result in homocysteinuria, hyperhomocysteinemia and hypomethioninemia (Watkins et al., 2002). The tri-functional enzyme, methylenetetrahydrofolate dehydrogenase/ methenyltetrahydrofolate cyclohydrolase/formyltetrahydrofolate synthetase (MTHFD1) represents another enzyme linked to transformation of Hcy to Met. Homozygotes of both *MTHFR* and *MTHFD1* are at risk of cardiovascular diseases connected with elevated levels of Hcy, or folate level-related hypoplasia of neural tube (Hol et al., 1998). However, in the literature, less numerous data are available on the involvement of MTHFD1 in the pathogenesis of degenerative diseases (Dorszewska et al., 2007).

Under normal conditions, in the presence of a positive Met balance, most of Hcy undergoes transsulfuration catalyzed by cystathionine β-synthetase (CBS), which requires derivative of vitamin B6, pyridoxal phosphate.

Homocysteine or it oxidative product, homocysteine acid are thought to exhibit its pro-oxidative activity most probably through its direct interaction with NMDA receptors (it represents an agonist of NMDA receptor). Agnati et al. (2005) have shown that Hcy may pass the blood/brain barrier and that level of plasma Hcy corresponds to Hcy concentration in the brain.

3.2 Influence of L-dopa treatment on the plasma level of biothiols in Parkinson's disease

In PD, the high Hcy concentration may augment risk of the disease through its direct toxic effect on dopaminergic neurons. Studies *in vitro* on human dopaminergic neurons have documented a significant increase in neurotoxicity accompanying high Hcy levels (Duan et al., 2002). In parallel, elevated Hcy levels in PD have been shown to carry potential for deterioration of cognitive and motoric functions, for depression and elevated risk to develop vascular diseases (Kuhn et al., 1998).

Reports of the literature (Florczak et al., 2008; Miller et al., 2003) indicate that plasma Hcy levels in PD have been affected also by pharmacotherapy with L-dopa. It is indicated that in PD patients who are initiating L-dopa therapy, Hcy elevates within six weeks to a few months after L-dopa initiation (O'Suilleabhain et al., 2004a). Study Florczak et al., 2008 indicated that the sulfuric amino acids were also affected by duration of the L-dopa pharmacotherapy. The most exposed to neurotoxic effects of Hcy have seemed to be the patients during the first 5 years L-dopa treatment while its continued administration has resulted in stably elevated Hcy level. The study of Miller et al. (1997) indicates that L-dopa may induce elevated levels of Hcy during its methylation to 3-O-methyldopa (3-OMD) with involvement of COMT (catechol O-methyltransferase) both in peripheral blood leukocytes and in nigrostriatal neurons. In the course of the reaction, COMT in presence of magnesium ions induces in parallel transition of SAM to SAH and further hydrolysis of SAH to Hcy (Fig. 2).

Elevated level of Hcy in *substantia nigra* of PD patients has been demonstrated already after 3 months of L-dopa treatment (Yasui et al., 2003). Long-term administration of L-dopa is thought to promote benign vascular lesions in patients with PD and may result in the patients in cognitive disturbances or dementia, particular at late stages of treatment with the preparation (Muller et al., 1999). On the other hand, COMT has a broad detoxification potential in human. Two compounds are currently available, entacapone peripheral and tolcapone central blocking of COMT. COMT inhibition is also under suspicion to prevent motor complications and seems that has beneficial effect on the L-dopa-related hyper-Hcy as well (Muller, 2009a; Nevrly et al., 2010). Some animal studies shown that COMT inhibition can eliminate L-dopa-induced hyper-Hcy but not all previous studies confirm it.

Study Dorszewska et al. (2007) have shown that augmented plasma levels of Hcy in PD possibly could have developed due to altered processes of Hcy remethylation to Met and transsulfuration to Cys. Simultaneuosly, in the PD patients a decreased concentration of Met has been observed, paralleled by elevated levels of Cys and lowered ratio of Met and Cys to Hcy. The demonstrated at present decrease in Met to Hcy ratio may be linked to transformation of Hcy to thiolactone in endothelial cells. According to one of more recent hypothesis, sulfonic sulfur of thiol compounds may be involved in development of Hcy-induced arteriosclerotic lesions (Toohey, 2001). At the same time, the demonstrated at present increased plasma Cys level in PD may result from intensified release of the amino acid from proteins, due to substitution by the circulating Hcy or due to diminished transformation of Cys to glutathione, important for maintenance of redox homeostasis in the body.

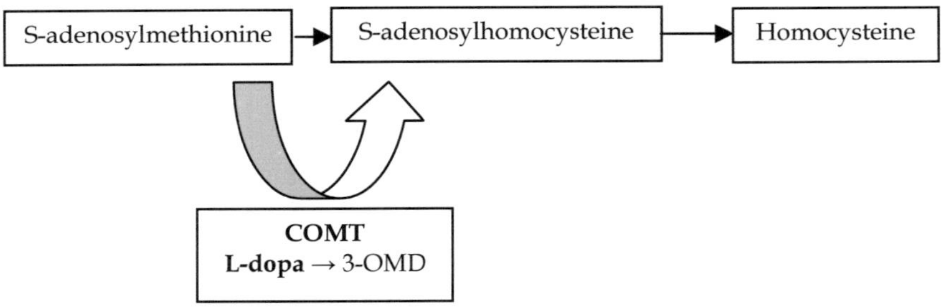

Fig. 2. COMT-mediated O-methylation of L-dopa, which results in formation of 3-methyldopa product, COMT- catecholamine-O-methyltrasferase, 3-OMD- 3-O-methyldopa.

In the literature there are studies of plasma Cys concentrations in PD patients (Dorszewska et al., 2007; Muller & Kuhn, 2009b) but there are no reported about relation between L-dope treatment and Cys status.

3.2.1 Patients

The studies were conducted on 98 patients with PD, including 37 women and 61 men aging 34-81 years (mean age: 60.8±10.7 years). Among the patients with PD, 27 patients (9 women and 18 men) awaited L-dopa treatment (patients' age: 34-79 years) and the remaining 71 individuals, 28 women and 43 men (patients' age: 35-81 years) were treated with L-dopa preparations in daily doses (up to 5 years treatment to 500 mg/day, 5-10 year treatment 500-800 mg/day, and over 10 year treatment 800-1500 mg/day).
Control group included 50 individuals, 34 women and 16 men, 22-76 years of age (mean age: 44.6±16.2 years).
Patients with PD were diagnosed using the criteria of UK Parkinson's Disease Society Brain Bank (Litvan et al., 2003), however stage of disease according to the scale of Hoehn and Yahr.
None of the control subjects had verifiable symptoms of dementia or any other neurological disorders and smoking, and drinking habits.
A Local Ethical Committee approved the study and the written consent of all patients or their caregivers was obtained.

3.2.2 Analysis of Cys concentrations

Preparation of samples. The analyzed plasma thiol compounds (Cys, Sigma, USA) were diluted with water at 2:1 ratio and reduced using 1% TCEP (Tris-(2-carboxyethyl)-phosphin-hydrochloride; Applichem, Germany) at 1:9 ratio. Subsequently, the sample was deproteinized using 1M $HClO_4$ (at 2:1 ratio) and applied to the HPLC/EC system.
Determination of thiol concentration. The samples were fed to the HPLC system (P580A; Dionex, Germany) coupled to an electrochemical detector (CoulArray 5600; ESA, USA). The analysis was performed in Termo Hypersil BDS C18 column (250 x 4.6 x 5µm) (Germany) in isocratic conditions, using the mobile phase of 0.15 M phosphate buffer, pH 2.8 supplemented with 8-10% acetonitrile for estimation of Cys (Accinni et al., 2000).

The system was controlled, and the data were collected and processed using Chromeleon software (Dionex, Germany).

3.2.3 Results

Pharmacotherapy with L-dopa of PD patients (Tables 7 and 8) leads to increase of the concentrations of metabolic product of Hcy, Cys ($p<0.01$) as compared to the controls, in the patients treated ($p<0.05$) as well as untreated ($p<0.01$) with L-dopa. Consequently, the ratio of Cys/Hcy in PD patients decreased, as compared to the controls ($p<0.05$) and to the untreated patients ($p<0.01$) as compared to treated PD patients with L-dopa.

Parameter	Controls (22-76 years)	Patients with PD (34-81 years)
Cys	220.7 ± 46.6	250.6 ± 49.6**
Cys/Hcy	19.3 ± 6.7	16.3 ± 6.5*

Table 7. Cysteine (μM) concentrations in the patients with PD and in control group. Results are expressed as a means ± SD. The nonparametric test of Mann-Whitney was used. Differences significant at *$p<0.05$, **$p<0.01$ as compared to the controls.

Parameter	Controls (22-76 years)	Patients with PD L-dopa (-) (34-79 years)	Patients with PD L-dopa (+) (35-81 years)
Cys	220.7 ± 46.6	263.6 ± 42.9**	244.7 ± 51.9*
Cys/Hcy	19.3 ± 6.7	20.7 ± 6.9	14.4 ± 5.4**(**)

Table 8. Cysteine (μM) concentrations as related to pharmacotherapy with L-dopa (+) in the patients with PD. Results are expressed as means ± SD. The nonparametric test of Mann-Whitney was used. Differences significant at *$p<0.05$, **$p<0.01$ as compared to the controls. Differences significant at (**)$p<0.01$, as compared to patients not treated with L-dopa (-).

Muller & Kohn (2009) indicated that only PD patients with an elevated level of Hcy above 15 μM showed an increase of Cys plasma level and elevated concentration of both risk factors (Hcy, Cys) may intervene in the neurodegenerative process. Present study indication that especially PD patients before L-dopa treatment showed increased level of Cys and L-dopa treatment only little decreased higher level of Cys. Increased plasma Cys level in PD may result from intensified release of the amino acid from proteins, due to substitution by the circulating Hcy or due to diminished transformation of Cys to glutathione, important for maintenance of redox homeostasis in the body. In culture of human hepatocytes 50% Cys has been demonstrated to transform into GSH (Mosharov et al., 2000). It seems also that intensity of dementive disease in particular disturbs transsulfuration of Hcy and leads to decreased levels of the agent (Cys), which provides the natural antioxidant, GSH. Homocysteine as well as Cys may serve as biomarkers for severity or progression of PD.

3.3 Influence of L-dopa treatment on the plasma level of Hcy and ADMA in Parkinson's disease patients

In the body Hcy is metabolized along two metabolic pathways, by the way of trassulfution and remethylation, involvement of SAM and SAH (Fig. 1). SAM is thought to provide the principal donor of methyl groups in numerous metabolic reactions, leading to formation of

methyl derivatives. One of the products of SAM methylation is thought to be asymmetric dimethylarginine (ADMA) (Gary & Clarke, 1998).
ADMA is an endogenous inhibitor of nitrogen oxide synthase (NOS) (Vallace et al., 1992). It arises from Arg contained in body proteins and may undergo hydrolysis to L-citruline and dimethylamine with involvement of dimethylaminohydrolase (DDAH). Homocysteine is thought to inhibit activity of DDAH (Stuhlinger et al., 2001) and might promote accumulation of ADMA that leads to a decreased production of nitrogen oxide (NO) and L-citruline from Arg with participation of NOS (Fig. 3).
NO plays an important role in control of vascular tone, in neurotransmission and in body protective mechanisms as well as in memory processes. Literature reports indicate that in PD the augmented activity of glia results in increased production of NO (McGeer et al., 1988).
ADMA is regarded to act as a risk factor for vascular diseases (Yoo & Lee, 2001). Its elevated levels were demonstrated in patients with hypercholesterolemia, hypertension, chronic heart failure and in atherosclerotic processes and during physiological aging (Kielstein et al., 2003). Role of ADMA in pathogenesis of PD is less known. Until now, in PD the levels on non-methylated substrate in biosynthesis of ADMA were examined only, and the elevated levels of Arg in cerebrospinal fluid were shown in PD patients with the decrease after L-dopa administration (Qureshi et al., 1995). Literature reports indicate also that long-term administration of L-dopa in PD patients may not only lead to increased concentrations of Hcy but may also alter Arg levels (Muller et al., 1999).

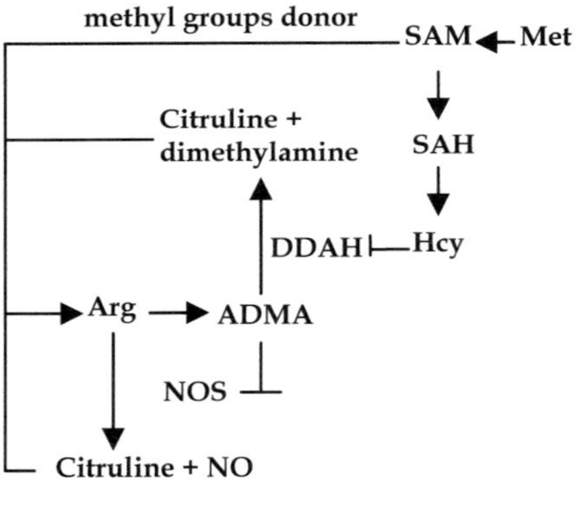

Fig. 3. The roles of methionine, homocysteine and arginine in metabolism of asymmetric dimethylarginine, Hcy- homocysteine, Met- methionine, ADMA- asymmetric dimethylarginine, Arg- arginine, NO- nitric oxide, NOS- NO synthase, DDAH- dimethylarginine dimethylaminohydrolase, SAM- S-adenosylmethionine, SAH- S-adenosylhomocysteine.

The present study was aimed at the estimation of plasma levels of Hcy and ADMA together with Met and Arg in patients with PD. The attention was also paid to developmental stages of the analyzed degenerative diseases and to L-dopa pharmacotherapy in PD.

3.3.1 Patients

The studies were conducted on 47 patients with PD, including 21 women and 26 men aging 41-86 years (mean age: 63.0±11.1 years). Among the patients with PD, 13 patients (3 women and 10 men) awaited L-dopa treatment (patients' age: 41-78 years) and the remaining 34 individuals, 18 women and 16 men (patients' age: 46-86 years) were treated with L-dopa preparations in daily doses (up to 5 years treatment to 500 mg/day, 5-10 year treatment 500-800 mg/day, and over 10 year treatment 800-1500 mg/day).

The control group included 35 individuals, 20 women and 15 men, 22-76 years of age (mean age: 45.1±16.0 years).

Patients with PD, on the other hand, were diagnosed using the criteria of UK Parkinson's Disease Society Brain Bank (Litvan et al., 2003). The stage of evolution of Parkinson's disease was defined according to the scale of Hoehn and Yahr. The tested patients represented stages I to IV of the disease evolution.

None of the control subjects had verifiable symptoms of dementia or any other neurological disorders.

A Local Ethical Committee approved the study and the written consent of all patients or their caregivers was obtained.

3.3.2 Analysis of Hcy and Met concentrations

Preparation of samples. The analyzed plasma thiol compounds (Hcy, Fluka Germany; Met, Sigma, USA) were diluted with water at 2:1 ratio and reduced using 1% TCEP (Tris-(2-carboxyethyl)-phosphin-hydrochloride; Applichem, Germany) at 1:9 ratio. Subsequently, the sample was deproteinized using 1M $HClO_4$ (at 2:1 ratio) and applied to the HPLC/EC system.

Determination of thiol concentration. The samples were fed to the HPLC system (P580A; Dionex, Germany) coupled to an electrochemical detector (CoulArray 5600; ESA, USA). The analysis was performed in Termo Hypersil BDS C18 column (250 x 4.6 x 5μm) (Germany) in isocratic conditions, using the mobile phase of 0.15 M phosphate buffer, pH 2.9, supplemented with 12.5-17% acetonitrile for estimation of Hcy and Met and 0.15 M phosphate buffer (Accinni et al., 2000).

The system was controlled and the data were collected and processed using Chromeleon software (Dionex, Germany).

3.3.3 Analysis of Arg and ADMA concentrations

Preparation of samples and derivatization. Plasma and the standard, containing solution of Arg and ADMA (Sigma, USA) were diluted with water at the ratio of 1.5:1.0 and, then, they were deproteinised using 8M $HCLO_4$ at the ratio of 5:1. Directly before HPLC analysis the samples were subjected to derivatization in a solution containing 10 mg OPA per 100 μl methanol supplemented with 900 μl 0.4 M borate buffer (pH 8.5) and 5μl 2-mercaptoethanol at the ratio of 1:1 (Pi et al., 2000).

Analysis of Arg and ADMA. The samples were fed to the HPLC system (P580A; Dionex, Germany) coupled to a fluorescence detector (RF2000; Dionex, Germany). The analysis was performed in a Termo Hypersil BDS C18 column (250 x 4.6 x 5μm) (Germany) in an isocratic conditions using 0.1 M phosphate buffer, pH 6.75 with 25 % methanol as the mobile phase. Arg and its methylated metabolites were measured fluorimetrically at excitation and emission wavelengths of 340 nm and 455nm, respectively.

The system was controlled and the data were collected and processed using Chromeleon software (Dionex, Germany).

3.3.4 Results

The study indicated that in patients with the diagnosed PD (Table 9) the augmented export of Hcy to plasma, ($p<0.001$ as compared to the controls), was accompanied by increased levels of circulating ADMA in analyzed neurodegenerative disease ($p<0.001$ as compared to the controls). In parallel, in the patients lower levels were observed of both Met ($p<0.01$ as compared to the controls), and Arg ($p<0.05$ as compared to the controls) expressed also by the lowered Met/Hcy and Arg/ADMA ratio ($p<0.001$ as compared to the controls).

Parameter	Controls (22-76 years)	Patients with PD (41-86 years)
Hcy	13.0 ± 4.3	20.1 ± 14.1***
Met	24.0 ± 6.9	18.7 ± 8.6**
Met/Hcy	2.1 ± 0.9	1.2 ± 0.8***
Arg	79.7 ± 24.4	68.4 ± 21.9*
ADMA	2.0 ± 1.0	3.8 ± 1.9***
Arg/ADMA	55.3 ± 40.5	25.8 ± 20.9***

Table 9. Homocysteine (μM), methionine (μM), asymmetric dimethylarginine (μM) and arginine (μM) concentrations in the patients with PD and in control group. Results are expressed as a means ± SD. The nonparametric test of Mann-Whitney was used. Differences significant at *$p<0.05$, **$p<0.01$, ***$p<0.001$, as compared to the controls.

Moreover, in the patients with PD (Fig. 4) development of the degenerative disease resulted in increased levels the risk factor for vascular diseases (Hcy), particularly pronounced in IVth stage of PD development ($p<0.05$ between Ist and IVth stage and between IInd and IVth stage of PD evolution). On the other hand, the Hcy remethylation product demonstrated a decreasing tendency only in the stage III of the disease, as compared to stage I of PD. In parallel, levels of the other analyzed risk factor of vascular diseases (ADMA) manifested higher correlation with concentration of its precursor. In parallel to the development of PD from stage I to stage IV of the disease evolution augmented levels of ADMA were accompanied by a decrease in the level of Arg (as compared to the Ist stage of PD). Also at the IInd stage of the degenerative disease evolution the highest levels of Met and ADMA and practically unaltered levels of Arg were accompanied by the lowest value of Arg/ADMA ratio ($p<0.01$ between stages I and II of PD evolution). In the IVth stage of PD development, however, both Met/Hcy ratio and Arg/ADMA ratio behaved in a similar manner demonstrating practically the lowest level ($p<0.05$, as compared to the Ist stage of the disease development).

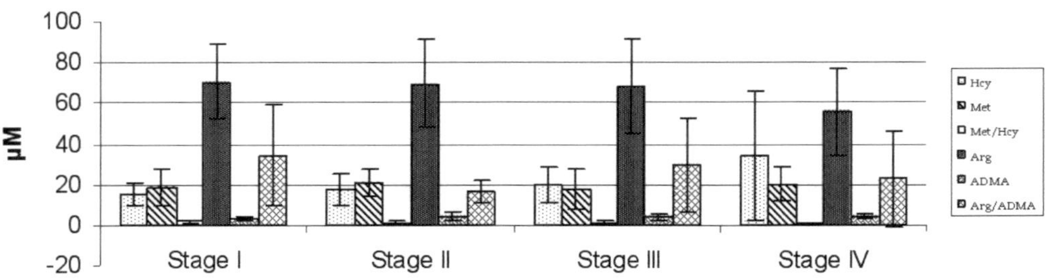

Mean ±SD; Hcy, Arg/ADMA, p<0.05 between stages I and IV of PD, and Hcy, Met/Hcy, p<0.05 between stages II and IV of PD; Arg/ADMA, p<0.01 between stages I and II of PD

Fig. 4. Hcy, Met, Arg and ADMA concentrations as related to the stage of the PD according to the scale of Hoehn and Yahr.

Pharmacotherapy with L-dopa preparations was demonstrated also to increase levels of both factors of vascular disease risk (Table 10), Hcy ($p<0.001$ as compared to the controls and $p<0.05$ as compared to patients not treated with L-dopa) and ADMA ($p<0.001$ as compared to the controls), although levels of ADMA increased also as a result of development of the degenerative disease ($p<0.01$ as compared to the controls). In parallel, in patients treated with L-dopa preparations levels of Met decreased ($p<0.001$ as compared to the controls) and so did concentrations of Arg ($p<0.05$ as compared to the controls and to L-dopa untreated patients), Met/Hcy ratios ($p<0.001$ as compared to the controls and $p<0.05$ as compared to patients not treated with L-dopa) and Arg/ADMA ratios ($p<0.001$, only as compared to the controls).

Parameter	Controls (22-76 years)	Patients with PD L-dopa (-) (41-78 years)	Patients with PD L-dopa (+) (46-86 years)
Hcy	13.0 ± 4.3	15.1 ± 5.1	22.0 ± 15.9$^{***(*)}$
Met	24.0 ± 6.9	21.0 ± 7.8	17.8 ± 8.8***
Met/Hcy	2.1 ± 0.9	1.6 ± 1.0*	1.0 ± 0.6$^{***(*)}$
Arg	79.7 ± 24.4	77.5 ± 19.7	64.4 ± 22.0$^{*(*)}$
ADMA	2.0 ± 1.0	3.3 ± 1.1**	4.1 ± 2.1***
Arg/ADMA	55.3 ± 40.5	22.8 ± 7.8***	26.7 ± 23.6***

Table 10. Homocysteine (μM), methionine (μM), asymmetric dimethylarginine (μM) and arginine (μM) concentrations as related to pharmacotherapy with L-dopa (+) in the patients with PD. The nonparametric test of Mann-Whitney was used. Results are expressed as means ± SD. Differences significant at $^{*}p<0.05$, $^{**}p<0.01$, $^{***}p<0.001$, as compared to the controls. Differences significant at $^{(*)}p<0.05$, as compared to patients not treated with L-dopa (-).

Present study indicated that ADMA may be involved in pathogenesis of PD. In development of PD the principal role is thought to be played by peroxinitrates (Padovan-Neto et al., 2009). This seems consistent with the demonstrated in present study ADMA level not elevated till the IInd stage of the disease development and the lower level of Arg, particularly accentuated in the IVth stage of PD evolution. Thus, a probability exists for involvement of reactive NO derivatives in induction of toxic damage to *substantia nigra* in PD.

In present study we have observed particularly in PD patients an evident decrease in Arg/ADMA ratio. The lowered ratio in blood is thought (Matsuoka et al., 1997) to be linked to development of hypercholesterolemia, congestive heart failure, arterial occlusive disease, heart failure and hypertension.

The levels of ADMA in PD have probably been affected also by pharmacotherapy with L-dopa. Both in the studies of Qureshi et al. (1995), and in present study decreased levels of Arg have been shown in patients treated with the drug. In the study of Qureshi et al. (1995) pharmacotherapy with L-dopa has been shown to generate nitrites, agents of neurotoxic activity, but in present studies seem that ADMA has not been shown to participate in their generation. Increased NO levels in PD have seemed to result rather from elevated activity of the glutaminergic system and altered neuronal metabolism.

It seems that ADMA may be regarded to represent a risk factor for PD and may be involved in pathogenesis of this neurodegenerative disease. Present results indicate also that developing neurodegenerative diseases are accompanied by disturbed metabolism of Hcy and ADMA and administration of L-arginine, in line with vitamins B6, B12 and folates, to PD patients may offer a modern therapy in this neurodegenerative disease.

4. Polymorphisms of *MTHFR, MTR, MTHFD1* and the level of biothiols in Parkinson's disease

The enzyme MTHFR plays a key role in regulating of Hcy metabolism. The study of Yasui et al. (2000) indicated that the TT *MTHFR* C677T genotype might also be linked to pathogenesis of PD, particularly when the level of folates is low. However, Fong et al. (2011) indicated on synergistic effects of polymorphisms in the folate metabolic pathway genes in PD not only C677T *MTHFR*, but also A2756G of *MTR* and A1049G, C1783T of *MTRR* (methionine synthase reductase). Yuan et al. (2009) showed on synergism between Hcy elevation after L-dopa administration in PD patients and *MTHFR*, CT and TT (C677T) genotypes. The study of Dorszewska et al. (2007) indicated that the genotypes TT (C677T), CC (A1298C) and AA (G1793A) of *MTHFR* have been the least frequent in patients with neurodegenerative disorders and their incidence has been slightly increased in the degenerative diseases (e.g. PD). In study of Dorszewska et al. (2007) also indicated that in PD patients Hcy has reached higher levels only in patients with CT genotype of *MTHFR* C677T. It seems that, particularly in persons with CT genotype of the C677T polymorphism of *MTHFR*, processes of Hcy transsulfuration to Cys become disturbed. Moreover, in PD the most pronounced alterations in Hcy levels in cases of A1298C polymorphism of *MTHFR* have been manifested in both genotypes AA and AC, even if this has not been expressed by the increased in parallel levels of oxidized guanine in DNA.
The enzyme of MTR is responsible for transfer of methyl groups from methyltetrahyrofolate to Hcy with involvement of methylcobalamin as the cofactor. The AG genetype of the A2756G polymorphism of *MTR* is probably linked to augmented levels of Hcy (Dorszewska et al., 2007). The increase of Hcy concentrations most probably results from lowered activity of MTR, induced by excessive oxidation of cobalamin (McCaddon et al. 2002) due to a more pronounced oxidative stress in degenerative syndromes. In parallel, the studies of Matsuo et al. (2001) indicate that *MTR* AG leads also to hypomethylation of DNA and to inactivation of several genes (low levels of SAM).
It seems also that the polymorphism G1958A of the gene coding for MTHFD1 enzyme may be involved in pathogenesis of PD, and heterozygote as well as homozygote (GA, AA) are thought to be responsible for increased levels of Hcy (Dorszewska et al., 2007). MTHFD1 represents another folate-dependent enzyme, which catalyzes transformation of tetrahydrofolate to 10-formyl, 5,10-methenyl and 5,10-methylene derivatives. 10-Formyltetrahydrofolate and 5,10-methylenetetrahydrofolate are regarded to serve as donors of methyl groups in DNA biosynthesis. The study of Dorszewska et al. (2007) also indicated that significant differences of the levels of Cys/Hcy, *MTHFD1* GA (G1958) were between AD and PD groups. The results indicate that only polymorphisms of folate-dependent enzyme *MTHFD1* have pointed to significant differences in intensity of turnover of circulating thiols between both neurodegenerative diseases, AD and PD.
Some studies confirmed that the C677T *MTHFR* polymorphism should consider as a genetic risk factor in patients who are going to take L-dopa preparations and folates and vitamins B (6, 12) supplementation may be given to the treated PD patients.

5. Influence of L-dopa treatment duration on the level of oxidative damage to DNA and thiols compounds concentration in patients with Parkinson's disease

The discussion about value of the L-dopa treatment in PD concerning on: toxicity, biochemical effects, clinical motor complications, especially after long-term its administrations (Belcastro et al., 2010; Muller, 2009a). Long-term treatment with L-dopa in PD patients may be promotes Hcy levels increase. Moreover, only PD patients with hyper-Hcy (Hcy above 15 μM) may have disturbed metabolism Hcy to Cys. As showed, hyper-Hcy in PD patients has been correlated with duration of disease and L-dopa dose.

5.1 Patients (see point 2.1.1)

5.2 Analysis of Hcy and Met (see point 3.3.2), and Cys (see point 3.2.2) concentrations, and 8-oxo2dG level (see point 2.1.2)

5.3 Results

During the initial five years and within the following 10 years of treatment with L-dopa (Table 11), the levels of 8-oxo2dG were augmented ($p<0.05$, as compared to the controls). Similarly to 8-oxo2dG, the levels of Hcy were highest after the initial five years of L-dopa administration ($p<0.05$, as compared to the controls). Subsequent treatment for another five to ten years resulted in the elevated levels of Hcy ($p<0.01$, as compared to the controls) which were even more significant if the treatment was extended over ten years ($p<0.001$, as compared to the controls). Moreover, the initial five years of L-dopa treatment were accompanied by relatively low levels of Met ($p<0.05$, as compared to the controls) and a slight increase in concentration of Cys. After ten years of treatment, similar levels of Hcy and Met were detected (Met, $p<0.01$), as compared to the controls, and Cys, ($p<0.05$), as compared to the group treated for five to ten years.

Parameter	Controls (22-76 years)	Patients with PD		
		up to 5 year treatment (34-78 years)	5-10 year treatment (46-81 years)	over 10 year treatment (46-81 years)
8-oxo2dG	13.7 ± 7.6	21.5 ± 15.1*	17.5 ± 11.1	27.8 ± 23.0*
Hcy	12.6 ± 4.3	28.5 ± 33.6*	19.7 ± 9.0**	18.3 ± 6.9***
Met	24.2 ± 6.7	19.2 ± 6.2*	20.4 ± 9.1	18.2 ± 8.2**
Met/Hcy	2.2 ± 0.9	1.1 ± 0.5**	1.2 ± 0.6**	1.1 ± 0.5***
Cys	220.7 ± 46.6	232.3 ± 52.5	267.9 ± 47.1**	238.2 ± 53.3(*)
Cys/Hcy	19.3 ± 6.7	12.8 ± 5.3*	15.4 ± 5.1	14.4 ± 5.8**

Table 11. Levels of oxidative DNA damage (8-oxo2dG/dG x 10^{-5}), and homocysteine (μM), methionine (μM) and cysteine (μM) concentrations as related to duration of L-dopa administration to patients with PD. Results are expressed as means ± SD. Differences significant at *$p<0.05$, **$p<0.01$, ***$p<0.001$, as compared to the controls. Differences significant at (*)$p<0.05$ between patients treated with L-dopa for 5-10 year and those treated for over 10 year.

As shown by the literature (Spencer et al., 1995) and by our studies, the elevated level of oxidized guanine in DNA (8-oxo2dG) in PD reflects also pharmacotherapy with L-dopa preparations. In present study, levels of 8-oxo2dG in the patients treated with L-dopa

preparations have reflected duration of administration of the drug. Patients have seemed most exposed to oxidative stress, resulting from L-dopa administration, during the first 5 years of treatment with the preparation and following long-term (over 10 years) its administration. According to Spencer et al. (1995), the augmented oxidative stress in patients treated with L-dopa might have resulted from lowered levels of antioxidants (GSH), disturbed mitochondrial transport and from excessive oxidation of dopamine.
Reports of the literature (Miller et al., 2003) and present results indicate that plasma Hcy levels in PD have been affected also by pharmacotherapy with L-dopa. In present study levels of the sulfuric amino acid were also affected by duration of the pharmacotherapy. The most exposed to neurotoxic effects of Hcy have seemed to be the patients during the first 5 years L-dopa treatment while its continued administration has resulted in stably elevated Hcy level, it seems that all time are disturbed metabolism of Hcy to Met and Cys.
Treatment with L-dopa preparations seems to be a potential risk factor for vascular diseases in PD patients. According to Lamberti et al. (2005), administration of vitamin B12 and of folates decreases plasma level of Hcy particularly in patients with PD during treatment with L-dopa preparations and in this way prevents against intensification of vascular lesions and dementia in the patients.

6. Conclusion

In conclusion, L-dopa metabolism after administration in PD patients is an important component for Hcy elevation and for increase toxicity in peripheral blood lymphocytes. Therapy of L-dopa leads to increases of the level factors inducing in oxidative stress and apoptosis as well as changes concentrations of risk factors of vascular diseases such as: Hcy, Cys and ADMA especially after long-term therapy. Analysis of the level of 8-oxo2dG, Hcy, Cys and ADMA may be a new biomarkers of severity and progression of PD.
It seems that for elevated levels of biothiols in PD, is not only important genotype *MTHFR,* TT (C677T) but also CC (A1298C), AA (G1793A), and *MTHFD1,* AA (G1958A) and *MTR,* GG (A2756G), which have a tendency for increased frequency in PD patients. In PD, there are more significant differences of the levels of biothiols in patients with one of genotype: Hcy [*MTHFR*: CT (C677T) and GG (G1793A); *MTR,* AG (A2756G)], Met [*MTR,* AA (A2756G)], Cys [*MTR,* AG (A2756G)], and Met/Hcy [*MTHFR*: CC, CT (C677T) and AA (A1298C), and GG (G1793A); *MTHFD1* AA (G1958A); *MTR* AA (A2756G)]. Moreover only polymorphisms of folate-dependent enzyme *MTHFD1* have pointed to significant differences in intensity of turnover of circulating biothiols between both neurodegenerative diseases: AD, and PD, which differ in the localization of neurotoxic lesions in the CNS.
Therefore in PD, monitoring of thiols compound levels in particular Hcy, is recommended. In the patients with PD administration of vitamins B6, B12, folates may cause a decrease in Hcy level, due to increased efficiency of remethylation and transsulfuration processes.

7. References

Accinni, R., Bartesaghi, S., De Leo, G., Cursano, C.F., Achilli, G., Loaldi, A., Cellerino, C., & Parodi, O. (2000). Screening of homocysteine from newborn blood spots by high-performance liquid chromatography with coulometric array detection. *Journal of Chromatography A*, Vol.896, No.1-2, (Obctober 2000), pp. 183-189, ISSN 0021-9673

Agnati, L.F., Genedani, S., Rasio, G., Galantucci, M., Saltini, S., Filaferro, M., Franco, R., Mora, F., Ferre, S., & Fuxe, K. (2005). Studies on homocysteine plasma levels in Alzheimer's patients. Relevance for neurodegeneration. *Journal of Neural Transmission*, Vol.112, No.1, (January 2005), pp. 163-169, ISSN 0300-9564

Alam, Z.I., Jenner, A., Daniel, S.E., Lees, A.J., Cairns, N., Marsden, C.D., Jenner, P., & Halliwell, B. (1997). Oxidative DNA damage in the parkinsonian brain: an apparent selective increase in 8-hydroxyguanine levels in substantia nigra. *Journal of Neurochemistry*, Vol.69, No.3, (September 1997), pp. 1196-1203, ISSN 0022-3042

Alves Da Costa, C.A., Paitel, E., Vincent, B., & Checler, F. (2002). α-Synuclein lowers p53-dependent apoptotic response of neural cells. Abolishment by 6-hydroxydopamine and implication for Parkinson's disease. *Journal of Biological Chemistry*, Vol.277, No.52, (December 2002), pp. 50980-50984, ISSN 0021-9258

Belcastro, V., Pierguidi, L., Castrioto A., Menichetti, C., Gorgone, G., Ientile, F., Pisani F., Rossi, A. Calabresi P., & Tambasco N. (2010). Hyperhomocysteinemia recurrence in levodopa-treated Parkinson's disease patients. *European Journal of Neurology*, Vol.17, No.5, (May 2010), pp. 661-665, ISSN 1351-5101

Blake, C.I., Spitz, E., Leehey, M., Hoffer, B.J., & Boyson, S.J. (1997). Platelet mitochondrial respiratory chain function in Parkinson's disease. *Movement Disorders*, Vol.12, No.1, (January 1997), pp. 3-8, ISSN 0885-3185

Blandini, F., Cosentino, M., Mangiagalli, A., Marino, F., Samuele, A., Rasini, E., Fancellu, R., Tassorelli, C., Pacchetti, C., Martignoni, E., Riboldazzi, G., Calandrella, D., Lecchini, S., Frigo, G., & Nappi, G. (2004). Modifications of apoptosis-related protein levels in lymphocytes of patients with Parkinson's disease. The effect of dopaminergic treatment. *Journal of Neural Transmission*, Vol.111, No.8, (August 2004), pp. 1017-1030, ISSN 0300-9564

Bergman, H., Feingold, A., Nini, A., Raz, A., Slovin, H., Abeles, M., & Vaadia, E. (1998). Physiological aspects of information processing in the basal ganglia of normal and parkinsonian primates. *Trends in Neurosciences*, Vol.21, No.1, (January 1998), pp. 32-38, ISSN 0166-2236

Carta, M., Lindgren, H.S., Lundblad, M., Stancampiano, R., Fadda, F., & Cenci, M.A. (2006). Role of striatal L-DOPA in the production of dyskinesia in 6-hydroxydopamine lesioned rats. *Journal of Neurochemistry*, Vol.96, No.6, (March 2006), pp. 1718-1727, ISSN 0022-3042

Cheng, H., Gomes-Trolin, C., Aquilonius, S.M., Steinberg, A., Lofberg, C., Ekblom, J., & Oreland, L. (1997). Levels of L-methionine S-adenosyltransferase activity in erythrocytes and concentrations of S-adenosylmethionine and S-adenosylhomocysteine in whole blood of patients with Parkinson's disease. *Experimental Neurology*, Vol.145, No.2 Pt 1, (January 1997), pp. 580-585, ISSN 0014-4886

Conway, K.A., Rochet, J.C., Bieganski, R.M., & Lansbury, P.T.Jr. (2001). Kinetic stabilization of the alpha-synuclein protofibril by a dopamine-alpha-synuclein adduct. *Science*, Vol.249, No.5545, (November 2001), pp. 1346-1349, ISSN 0036-8075

Cornetta, T., Palma, S., Aprile, I., Padua, L., Tonali, P., Testa, A., & Cozzi, R. (2009). Levodopa therapy reduces DNA damage in peripheral blood cells of patients with Parkinson's disease. *Cell Biology & Toxicology*, Vol.25, No.4, (August 2009), pp. 321-330, ISSN 0742-2091

Dorszewska, J., Florczak, J., Rózycka, A., Jaroszewska-Kolecka, J., Trzeciak, W.H., & Kozubski, W. (2005). Polymorphisms of the CHRNA4 gene encoding the alpha4 subunit of nicotinic acetylcholine receptor as related to the oxidative DNA damage and the level of apoptotic proteins in lymphocytes of the patients with Alzheimer's disease. *DNA & Cell Biology*, Vol.24, No.12, (December 2005), pp. 786-794, ISDN 1044-5498

Dorszewska, J., Florczak, J., Rozycka, A., Kempisty B., Jaroszewska-Kolecka, J., Chojnicka K., Trzeciak,W.H., & Kozubski, W. (2007). Oxidative DNA damage and level of thiols as related to polymorphisms of MTHFR, MTR, MTHFD1 in Alzheimer's and Parkinson's diseases. *Acta Neurobiologiae Experimentalis,* Vol.67, No.2, (2007), pp. 113-129, ISSN 0065-1400

Dorszewska, J., Kempisty, B., Jaroszewska-Kolecka, J., Rozycka, A., Florczak, J., Lianeri, M., Jagodzinski, P.P., & Kozubski, W. (2009a). Expression and polymorphisms of gene 8-oxoguanine glycosylase 1 and the level of oxidative DNA damage in peripheral blood lymphocytes of patients with Alzheimer's disease. *DNA & Cell Biology,* Vol.28, No.11, (November 2009), pp. 579-588, ISSN 1044-5498

Dorszewska, J., Florczak, J., & Kozubski, W. (2009b). Level of oxidative DNA damage and expression of apoptotic proteins in patients with Parkinson's disease treatment with L-dopa. *Parkinsonism & Related Disorders, 15, Suppl. 2,* 111, ISSN 1353-8020, Abstracts of the XVIII WFN World Congress on Parkinson's Disease and Related Disorders. Miami Beach, FL, USA, December 13-16, 2009

Dorszewska, J., Dezor, M., Florczak, J., Kozubski, W. (2010). Expression of 8-oxoguanine DNA glycosylase 1 (OGG1) and the level of p53 and TNF-alpha proteins in peripheral lymphocytes in patients with Alzheimer's disease. *Alzheimer's Dementia, 6, 4,* P3186, Supp. 1, ISSN 1552-5260, Alzheimer's Association International Conference on Alzheimer's disease. Honolulu, Hawaii, USA, July 10-15, 2010

Duan, W., Ladenheim, B., Cutler, R.G., Kruman, I.I., Cadet, J.L., & Mattson, M.P. (2002). Dietary folate deficiency and elevated homocysteine levels endanger dopaminergic neurons in models of Parkinson's disease. *Journal of Neurochemistry,* Vol.80, No.1, (January 2002), pp. 101-110, ISSN 0022-3042

Florczak, J., Dorszewska, J., & Kozubski, W. (2008). Influence of L-dopa treatment duration on the level of oxidative damage to DNA and thiol compound concentration in patients with Parkinson's disease. *Neurologia i Neurochirurgia Polska,* Vol.42, No.1, Suppl. 1, (in Polish), pp. S36-S44, ISSN 0028-3843

Fong, C.S., Shyu, H.Y., Shieh, J.C., Fu, Y.P., Chin, T.Y., Wang, H.W., & Cheng C.W. (2011). Association of MTHFR, MTR, and MTRR polymorphisms with Parkinson's disease among ethnic Chinese in Taiwan. *Clinica Chimica Acta,* Vol.412, No.3-4, (January 2011), pp. 332-338, ISSN 0009-8981

Frosst, P., Blom, H.J., Milos, R., Goyette, P., Sheppard, C.A., Matthews, R.G., Boers, G.J., den Heijer, M., Kluijtmans, L.A., van den Heuvel, L.P., & Rozen, R. (1995). A candidate genetic risk factor for vascular disease: a common mutation in methylenetetrahydrofolate reductase. *Nature Genetics,* Vol.10, No.1, (May 1995), pp. 111-113, ISSN 1061-4036

Gary, J.D., & Clarke, S. (1998). RNA and protein interactions modulated by protein arginine methylation. *Progress in Nucleic Acid Research & Molecular Biology,* Vol.61, pp. 65-131, ISSN 0079-6603

Gorell, J.M., Johnson, C.C., & Rybicki, B.A. (1994). Parkinson's disease and its comorbid disorders: an analysis of Michigan mortality data, 1970 to 1990. *Neurology,* Vol.44, No.10, (October 1994), pp. 1865-1868, ISSN 0028-3878

Hirano, T. (2008). Repair system of 7, 8-dihydro-8-oxoguanine as a defense line against carcinogenesis. *Journal of Radiation Research,* Vol.49, No.4, (July 2008), pp. 329-340, ISSN 0449-3060

Hol, F.A., van der Put, N.M., Geurds, M.P., Heil, S.G., Trijbels, F.J., Hamel, B.C., Mariman, E.C., & Blom, H.J. (1998). Molecular genetic analysis of the gene encoding the trifunctional enzyme MTHFD (methylenetetrahydrofolate-dehydrogenase, ethenyltetrahydrofolate-cyclohydrolase, formyltetrahydrofolate synthetase) in patients with neural tube defects. *Clinical Genetics*, Vol.53, No.2, (February 1998), pp. 119-125, ISSN 1178-704X

Hsu, L.J., Sagara, Y., Arroyo, A., Rockenstein, E., Sisk, A., Mallory, M., Wong, J., Takenouchi, T., Hashimoto, M., & Masliah, E. (2000). alpha-synuclein promotes mitochondrial deficit and oxidative stress. *American Journal of Pathology*, Vol.157, No.2, (August 2000), pp. 401-410, ISSN 0002-9440

Iwashita, A., Yamazaki, S., Mihara, K., Hattori, K., Yamamoto, H., Ishida, J., Matsuoka, N., & Mutoh, S. (2004). Neuroprotective effects of a novel poly(ADP-ribose) polymerase-1 inhibitor, 2-{3-[4-(4-chlorophenyl)-1-piperazinyl]propyl}-4(3H)-quinazolinone (FR255595), in an in vitro model of cell death and in mouse 1-methyl-4-phenyl-1,2,3,6-tetrahydropyridine model of Parkinson's disease. *Journal of Pharmacology and Experimental Therapeutics*, Vol.309, No.3, (June 2004), pp. 1067-1078, ISSN 0022-3565

Jarrett, J.T., Amaratunga, M., Drennan, C.L., Scholten, J.D., Sands, R.H., Ludwig, M.L., & Matthews, R.G. (1996). Mutations in the B12-binding region of methionine synthase: how the protein controls methylcobalamin reactivity. *Biochemistry*, Vol.35, No.7, (February 1996), pp. 2464-2475, ISSN 0006-2979

Jenner, P. (2003). Oxidative stress in Parkinson's disease. *Annals Neurology*, Vol.53, pp. S26-S38, ISSN 0364-5134

Kielstein, J.T., Bode-Boger, S.M., Frolich, J.C., Ritz, E., Haller, & H., Fliser, D. (2003). Asymmetric dimethylarginine, blood pressure, and renal perfusion in elderly subjects. *Circulation*, Vol.107, No.14, (April 2003), pp. 1891-1895, ISSN 0009-7322

Kikuchi, A., Takeda, A., Onodera, H., Kimpara, T., Hisanaga, K., Sato, N., Nunomura, A., Castellani, R.J., Perry, G., Smith, M.A., & Itoyama, Y. (2002). Systemic increase of oxidative nucleic acid damage in Parkinson's disease and multiple system atrophy. *Neurobiology of Disease*, Vol.9, No.2, (March 2002), pp. 244-248, ISSN 0969-9961

Kuhn, W., Roebroek, R., Blom, H., van Oppenraaij, D., Przuntek, H., Kretschmer, A., Buttner, T., Woitalla, D., & Muller, T. 1998). Elevated plasma levels of homocysteine in Parkinson's disease. *European Neurology*, Vol.40, No.4, (November 1998), pp. 225-227, ISSN 0014-3022

Lamberti, P., Zoccolella, S., Armenise, E., Lamberti, S.V., Fraddosio, A., de Mari, M., Iliceto, G., & Livrea, P. (2005). Hyperhomocysteinamia in L-dopa treated Parkinson's disease patients: effect of cobalamin and folate dministration. *European Journal of Neurology*, Vol.12, No.5, (May 2005), pp. 365-368, ISSN 1351-5101

Litvan, I., Bhatia, K.P., Burn, D.J., Goetz, C.G., Lang, A.E., McKeith, I., Quinn, N., Sethi, K.D., Shults, C., & Wenning, G.K. (2003). Movement Disorders Society Scientific Issues Committee report: SIC Task Force appraisal of clinical diagnostic criteria for Parkinsonian disorders. *Movement Disorders*, Vol.18, No.5, (May 2003), pp. 467-486, ISSN 0885-3185

Matsuo, K., Suzuki, R., Hamajima, N., Ogura, M., Kagami, Y., Taji, H., Kondoh, E., Maeda, S., Asakura, S., Kaba, S., Nakamura, S., Seto, M., Morishima, Y., & Tajima, K. (2001). Association between polymorphisms of folate- and methionine-metabolizing enzymes and susceptibility to malignant lymphoma. *Blood*, Vol.97, No.10, (May 2001), pp. 3205-3209, ISSN 0006-4971

Matsuoka, H., Itoh, S., Kimoto, M., Kohno, K., Tamai, O., Wada, Y., Yasukawa, H., Iwami, G., Okuda, S., & Imaizumi, T. (1997). Asymmetric dimetylarginine, an endogenous nitric oxide synthase inhibitor, in experimental hypertension. *Hypertension*, Vol.29, No.1 Pt 2, (January 1997), pp. 242-247, ISSN 0914-911X

McCaddon, A., Regland, B., Hudson, P., & Davies, G. (2002). Functional vitamin B(12) deficiency and Alzheimer disease. *Neurology*, Vol.58, No.9, (May 2002), pp. 1395-1399, ISSN 0028-3878

McGeer, P.L., Itagaki, S., Boyes, B.E., & McGeer, E.G. (1988). Reactive microglia are positive for HLA-DR in the substantia nigra of Parkinson's and Alzheimer's disease brains. *Neurology*, Vol.38, No.8, (August 1988), pp. 1285-1291, ISSN 0028-3878

Migliore, L., Petrozzi, L., Lucetti, C., Gambaccini, G., Bernardini, S., Scarpato, R., Trippi, F., Barale, R., Frenzilli, G., Rodilla, V., & Bonuccelli, U. (2002). Oxidative damage and cytogenetic analysis in leukocytes of Parkinson's disease patients. *Neurology*, Vol.58, No.12, (June 2002), pp. 1809-1815, ISSN 0028-3878

Miller, J.W., Shukitt-Hale, B., Villalobos-Molina, R., Nadeau, M.R., Selhub. J., & Joseph, J.A. (1997). Effect of L-Dopa and the catechol-O-methyltransferase inhibitor Ro 41-0960 on sulfur amino acid metabolites in rats. *Clinical Neuropharmacology*, Vol.20, No.1, (February 1997), pp. 55-66, ISSN 0362-5664

Miller, J.W., Selhub, J., Nadeau, M.R., Thomas, C.A., Feldman, R.G., & Wolf, P.A. (2003). Effect of L-dopa on plasma homocysteine in PD patients: relationship to B-vitamin status. *Neurology*, Vol.60, No.7, (April 2003), pp. 1125-1129, ISSN 0028-3878

Mosharov, E., Cranford, M.R., & Banerjee, R. (2000). The quantitatively important relation ship between homocysteine metabolism and glutathione synthesis by the transsulfuration pathway and its regulation by redox changes. *Biochemistry*, Vol.39, No.42, (October 2000), pp. 13005-13011, ISSN 0006-2979

Muller, T., Werne, B., Fowler, B., & Kuhn, W. (1999). Nigral endothelial dysfunction, homocysteine, and Parkinson's disease. *Lancet*, Vol.354, No.9173, (July 1999), pp. 126-127, ISSN 0140-6736

Muller, T. (2008). Role of homocysteine in the treatment of Parkinson's disease. *Expert Review of Neurotherapeutics*, Vol.8, No.6, (June 2008), pp. 957-967, ISSN 1473-7175

Muller, T. (2009a). Possible treatment concept for the levodopa-related hyperhomocystenemia. *Cardiovascular Psychiatry & Neurology*, (September 2009), pp. 1-5, ISSN 2090-0163

Muller, T. & Kuhn, W. (2009b). Cysteine elevation in levodopa-treated patients with Parkinson's disease. *Movement Disorders*, Vol.24, No.6, (April 2009), pp. 929-932, ISSN 0885-3185

Nevrly, M., Kanovsky, P., Vranova, H., Langova, K., & Hlustik, P. (2010). Effect of entacapone on plasma homocysteine levels in Parkinson's disease patients. *Neurological Sciences*, Vol.31, No.5, (October 2010), pp. 565-569, ISSN 1590-1874

Obeso, J.A., Rodriguez-Oroz, M.C., Benitez-Temino, B. Blesa, F.J., Guridi, J., Marin, C., & Rodriguez, M. (2008). Functional organization of the basal ganglia: therapeutic implications for Parkinson's disease. *Movement Disorders*, Vol.23, Suppl. 3, pp. S548-S559, ISSN 0885-3185

Ohnishi, T., Inoue, N., Matsumoto, H., Omatsu, T., Ohira, Y., & Nagaoko, S. (1996). Cellular content of p53 protein in rat skin after exposure to the space environment. *Journal of Applied Physics*, Vol.81, No.1, (July 1996), pp. 183-185, ISSN 0021-8979

Olanow, C.W. (2008). Levodopa/dopamine replacement strategies in Parkinson's disease: future directions. *Movement Disorders*, Vol.23, Suppl. 3, pp. S613-S622, ISSN 0885-3185

Olsen, A., Siboska, G.E., Clark, B.F., & Rattan, S.I. (1999). N^6-Furfuryladenosine, kinetin, protects against Fenton reaction-mediated oxidative damage to DNA. *Biochemical Biophysical Research Communications*, Vol.265, No.2, (November 1999), pp. 499-502, ISSN 0006-291X

O'Suilleabhain, P.E., Bottiglieri, T., Dewey, R.B., Sharma, S., & Diaz-Arrastia, R. (2004a). Modest increase in plasma homocysteine follows levodopa initiation in Parkinson's disease. *Movement Disorders*, Vol.19, No.12, (December 2004), pp. 1403-1408, ISSN 0885-3185

O'Suilleabhain, P.E., Sung, V., Hernandez, C., Lacritz, L., Dewey, R.B.Jr., Bottiglieri, T., & Diaz-Arrastia, R. (2004b). Elevated plasma homocysteine level in patients with Parkinson disease: motor, affective, and cognitive associations. *Archives of Neurology*, Vol.61, No.6, (June 2004), pp. 865-868, ISSN 0003-9942

Padovan-Neto, F.E., Echeverry, M.B., Tumas, V., & Del-Bel, E.A. (2009). Nitric oxide synthase inhibition attenuates L-DOPA-induced dyskinesias in a rodent model of Parkinson's disease. *Neuroscience*, Vol.159, No.3, (March 2009), pp. 927-935, ISSN 0306-4522

Pi, J., Kumagai, Y., Sun, G., & Shimojo, N. (2000). Improved method for simultaneous determination of L-arginine and its mono- and dimethylated metabolites in biological samples by high-performance liquid chromatography. *Journal of Chromatography B: Biomedical Sciences & Applications*, Vol.742, No.1, (May 2000), pp. 199-203, ISSN 0378-4347

Prigione, A., Begni, B., Galbussera, A., Beretta, S., Brighina, L., Garofalo, R., Andreoni, S., Piolti, R., & Ferrarese C. (2006). Oxidative stress in peripheral blood mononuclear cells from patients with Parkinson's disease: negative correlation with levodopa dosage. *Neurobiology of Disease*, Vol.23, No.1, (July 2006), pp. 36-43, ISSN 0969-9961

Qureshi, G.A., Baig, S., Bednar, I., Sodersten, P., Forsberg, G., & Siden, A. (1995). Increased cerebrospinal fluid concentration of nitrite in Parkinson's disease. *Neuroreport*, Vol.6, No.12, (August 1995), pp. 1642-1644, ISSN 0959-4965

Rogers, J.D., Sanchez-Saffon, A., Frol, A.B., & Diaz-Arrastia, R. (2003). Elevated plasma homocysteine levels in patients treated with levodopa: association with vascular disease. *Archives of Neurology*, Vol.60, No.1, (January 2003), pp. 59-64, ISSN 0003-9942

Schapira, A.H., Cooper, J.M., Dexter, D., Clark, J.B., Jenner, P., & Marsden, C.D. (1990). Mitochondrial complex I deficiency in Parkinson's disease. *Journal of Neurochemistry*, Vol.53, No.3, (March 1990), pp. 823-827, ISSN 0022-3042

Sian, J., Dexter, D.T., Lees, A.J., Daniel, S., Agid, Y., Javoy-Agid, F., Jenner, P., & Marsden, C.D. (1994). Alterations in glutathione levels in Parkinson's disease and other neurodegenerative disorders affecting basal ganglia. *Annals of Neurology*, Vol.36, No.3, (September 1994), pp. 384-355, ISSN 0364-5134

Spencer, J.P., Jenner, A., Aruoma, O.I., Evans, P.J., Kaur, H., Dexter, D.T., Jenner, P., Lees, A.J., Marsden, D.C., & Halliwell, B. (1994). Intense oxidative DNA damage promoted by L-dopa and its metabolites. Implications for neurodegenerative disease. *FEBS Letters*, Vol.353, No.3, (October 1994), pp. 246-250, ISSN 0014-5793

Spencer, J.P., Jenner, P., & Halliwell, B. (1995). Superoxide-dependent depletion of reduced glutathione by L-DOPA and dopamine. Relevance to Parkinson's disease. *Neuroreport*, Vol.6, No.11, (July 1995), pp. 1480-1484, ISSN 0959-4965

Spillantini, M.G., Schmidt, M.L., Lee, V.M., Trojanowski, J.Q., Jakes, R., & Goedert, M. (1997). α-synuclein in Lewy bodies. *Nature*, Vol.388, No.6645, (August 1997), pp. 839-840, ISSN 0028-0836

Stuhlinger, M.C., Tsao, P.S., Her, J.H., Kimoto, M., Balint, R.F., & Cooke, J.P. (2001). Homocysteine impairs the nitric oxide synthase pathway: role of asymmetric dimethylarginine. *Circulation*, Vol.104, No.21, (November 20001), pp. 2569-2575, ISSN 0009-7322

Toohey, J.I. (2001). Possible involvement of sulfane sulfur in homocysteine-induced atherosclerosis. *Medical Hypotheses*, Vol.56, No.2, (February 2001), pp. 259-261, ISSN 0306-9877

Yasui, K., Kowa, H., Nakaso, K., Takeshima, T., & Nakashima, K. (2000). Plasma homocysteine and MTHFR C677T genotype in levodopa-treated patients with PD. *Neurology*, Vol.55, No.3, (August 2000), pp. 437-440, ISSN 0028-3878

Vallance, P., Leone, A., Calver, A., Collier, J., & Moncada, S. (1992). Accumulation of an endogenous inhibitor of nitric oxide synthesis in chronic renal failure. *Lancet*, Vol.339, No.8793, (March 1992), pp. 572-575, ISSN 0140-6736

Watkins, D., Ru, M., Hwang, H.Y., Kim, C.D., Murray, A., Philip, N.S., Kim, W., Legakis, H., Wai, T., Hilton, J.F., Ge, B., Dore, C., Hosack, A., Wilson, A., Gravel, R.A., Shane, B., Hudson, T.J., & Rosenblatt, D.S. (2002). Hyperhomocysteinemia due to methionine synthase deficiency, cblG: structure of the MTR gene, genotype diversity, and recognition of a common mutation, P1173L. *American Journal of Human Genetics*, Vol.71, No.1, (July 2003), pp. 143-153, ISSN 0002-9297

Yasui, K., Kowa, H., Nakaso, K., Takeshima, T., & Nakashima, K. (2000). Plasma homocysteine and MTHFR C677T genotype in levodopa-treated patients with PD. *Neurology*, Vol.55, No.3, (August 2000), pp. 437-440, ISSN 0028-3878

Yasui, K., Nakaso, K., Kowa, H., Takeshima, T., & Nakashima, K. (2003). Levodopa-induced hyperhomocysteinaemia in Parkinson's disease. *Acta Neurologica Scandinavica*, Vol.108, No.1, (July 2003), pp. 66-67, ISSN 0001-6314

Yoo, J.H. & Lee, S.C. (2001). Elevated levels of plasma homocysteine and asymmetric dimethylarginine in elderly patients with stroke. *Atherosclerosis*, Vol.158, No.2, (October 2001), pp. 425-430, ISSN 0021-9150

Yuan, R.Y., Sheu, J.J., Yu, J.M., Hu, C.J., Tseng, I.J., Ho, C.S., Yeh, C.Y., Hung, Y.L., & Chiang, T.R. (2009). Methylenetetrahydrofolate reductase polymorphisms and plasma homocysteine in levodopa-treated and non-treated Parkinson's disease patients. *Journal of Neurological Sciences*, Vol.287, No.1-2, (December 2009), pp. 64-68, ISSN 0022-510X

Zhang, J., Perry, G., Smith, M.A., Robertson, D., Olson, S.J., Graham, D.G., & Montine, T.J. (1999). Parkinson's disease is associated with oxidative damage to cytoplasmic DNA and RNA in substantia nigra neurons. *American Journal of Pathology*, Vol.154, No.5, (May 1999), pp. 1423-1429, ISSN 0002-9440

Zoccolella, S., Lamberti, P., Iliceto, G., Dell'Aquila, C., Diroma, C., Fraddosio, A., Lamberti, S.V., Armenise, E., Defazio, G., de Mari,.M., & Livrea, P. (2006). Elevated plasma homocysteine levels in L-dopa-treated Parkinson's disease patients with dyskinesias. *Clinical Chemistry and Laboratory Medicine*, Vol.44, No.7, pp. 863-866, ISSN 1434-6621

Zoccolella, S., Dell'Aquila, C., Abruzzese, G., Antonini, A., Bonuccelli, U., Canesi, M., Cristina, S., Marchese, R., Pacchetti, C., Zagaglia, R., Logroscino, G., Defazio, G., Lamberti, P., & Livrea, P. (2009). Hyperhomocysteinemia in levodopa-treated patients with Parkinson's disease dementia. *Movement Disorders*, Vol.24, No.7, (May 2009), pp. 1028-1033, ISSN 0885-3185

17

Inflammatory Responses and Regulation in Parkinson's Disease

Lynda J. Peterson and Patrick M. Flood
The University of North Carolina at Chapel Hill, U.S.A.

1. Introduction

Parkinson's disease (PD) is a slow, progressive neurodegenerative disorder affecting an estimated 6 million people worldwide (Litteljohn, Mangano et al. 2011). The etiology of the disease is characterized by increasing loss over time of dopaminergic neurons (DA-neurons) in the substantia nigra (SN) as well as the depletion of dopamine in the striatum, which eventually leads to pathological and clinical symptoms (Jenner and Olanow 2006). PET imaging and post-mortem analyses of the brains of PD patients indicate that the appearance of symptoms, including tremor, bradykinesia, rigidity, slowness of movement, and postural instability (Jellinger 2001), generally are manifest once 60% of DA-neurons have died and a 70% threshold decrease in normal DA activity has been reached (Klockgether 2004; Litteljohn, Mangano et al. 2011). Epidemiological studies indicate that only about 10% of PD cases are early onset , i.e. prior to the age of 50 and occur mainly in familial clusters (Mizuno, Hattori et al. 2001). These cases have established genetic bases due to mutations in several recently identified genes, including parkin, leucine-rich repeat kinase 2 (LRRK2), α-synuclein, PINK-1, or DJ-1 (Polymeropoulos, Lavedan et al. 1997; Lucking, Durr et al. 2000; Abou-Sleiman, Healy et al. 2003; Farrer, Haugarvoll et al. 2006; Sun, Latourelle et al. 2006; Jiang, Wu et al. 2007; Weng, Chou et al. 2007; Bonifati, Wu-Chou et al. 2008). The majority of PD cases (approximately 90%) are late onset and idiopathic (Tanner 2003). Although the etiology of idiopathic PD is uncertain, this form of PD particularly affects the elderly, with average onset of clinical symptoms between 60 and 65 years of age (Litteljohn, Mangano et al. 2011). Idiopathic PD is thus age-associated, with approximately 1% of the population being affected by 65-70 year of age, increasing to 4-5% at 85 years (Fahn 2003; Tansey, McCoy et al. 2007). However, the causes of idiopathic non-familial PD are probably multifactorial, with some form of genetic predisposition, environmental insults and/or aging all likely to be important factors in disease initiation and progression (Nagatsu and Sawada 2006; Dickson 2007; Vilar, Coelho et al. 2007; Singh, Singh et al. 2008).

While the exact cause of chronic neurodegeneration of PD is not known, increasing evidence suggests that chronic inflammation is the fundamental process mediating the progressive nature of the neurodegeneration characteristic of PD (McGeer, Yasojima et al. 2001; Hirsch and Hunot 2009). In animal PD models, long-term inflammation induces progressive loss of DA neurons within the SN brain region (Gao, Jiang et al. 2002; Dauer and Przedborski 2003; Bartels and Leenders 2007). Neuroinflammation, which is characterized by activation of both the innate and adaptive immune response, has been demonstrated in PD patients by the preponderance of activated microglia within the SN, and the increased production in the CNS of inflammatory mediators, such as cytokines, chemokines, reactive oxygen species (ROS) and reactive nitrites (Cicchetti, Lapointe et al. 2005; Loeffler, Camp et al. 2006; Ghosh, Roy et al. 2007; Cicchetti, Drouin-Ouellet et al. 2009). Post mortem analyses of brains from PD patients provide clear evidence of large numbers of human leukocyte antigen (HLA-DR) and CD11b-positive microglia in the SN, the brain region in which the degeneration of DA neurons is most prominent (McGeer, Itagaki et al. 1988). Expression of the inflammatory markers MHC II, TNFα and cyclooxygenase (COX-2) is also higher in SN tissue of patients with PD than in comparable tissue from unaffected controls (McGeer, Itagaki et al. 1988; Boka, Anglade et al. 1994; Knott, Stern et al. 2000). Additionally, levels of proinflammatory mediators, including TNFα, IL-1β, IL-6, (ROS), and eicosanoids, are all elevated in the SN, striatum, cerebrospinal fluid (CSF) and/or peripheral blood mononuclear cells (PBMC) of PD patients (McGeer, Itagaki et al. 1988; Qureshi, Baig et al. 1995; Mogi, Harada et al. 1996; Nagatsu, Mogi et al. 2000; Imamura, Hishikawa et al. 2003; Teismann and Schulz 2004; Nagatsu and Sawada 2006; Sawada, Imamura et al. 2006; Hirsch and Hunot 2009; Pisani, Moschella et al. 2010). Nitric oxide (NO) free radicals are also elevated in PD as indicated by increased nitrite (an indicator for NO) present in the CSF, as well as increased expression of inducible nitric oxide synthase (iNOS) within the SN of PD patients (Qureshi, Baig et al. 1995). Oxidative damage measured by the presence of nucleoside oxidation product 8-hydroxyguanosine, is approximately 16-fold higher in SN of PD patients and post-mortem analysis of the brains of PD patients also show evidence of the oxidation of lipids, DNA and proteins (Owen, Schapira et al. 1996; Spencer, Jenner et al. 1998; Halliwell 2006). Reduced levels of antioxidant glutathione (GSH) concomitant with increased concentrations of oxidized GSH, are found in the surviving SN neurons of PD patients compared to normal controls, indicating these neurons were undergoing increased oxidative stress (OS) at the time of death (Sofic, Lange et al. 1992; Pearce, Owen et al. 1997).

In addition to direct evidence for increased inflammatory activity within the CNS of patients with PD, other aspects of the etiology of PD suggest this is primarily an inflammatory disorder. For example, PD patients display decreased activity in mitochondrial complexes I and I/III (Krige, Carroll et al. 1992), and the inhibition of mitochondria respiratory complex-I after exposure to MPTP gives rise to PD-like pathologies in humans (Tetrud, Langston et al. 1989; Langston, Forno et al. 1999), primates, mice and rats (Yazdani, German et al. 2006; Jackson-Lewis and Przedborski 2007). This is because DA neurons appear to have an intrinsic sensitivity to complex I defects based on studies that demonstrate the selective neurotoxic effects of the pesticide rotenone on DA neurons only, despite the fact that rotenone inhibits complex I throughout the brain (Sherer, Betarbet et al. 2002). However, even direct inhibition of complex-I by MPTP in DA neurons results in neurodegeneration that is primarily inflammatory in nature (Ghosh, Roy et al. 2007; Qian, Gao et al. 2007; Qian and Flood 2008). Further evidence of the key role of inflammation in PD is seen in other features of the disease. For example, blood-brain-barrier (BBB) leakage has been found in positron-emission tomography (PET) images of the brains of PD patients (Kortekaas, Leenders et al. 2005), and is likely caused by increased inflammation in PD. In addition, increased angiogenesis also occurs in PD patients (Faucheux, Bonnet et al. 1999) , and in the SN of a monkey-model of PD (Barcia, Bautista et al. 2005). Increased expression of the angiogenic-stimulant vascular endothelial growth factor (VEGF) and its major receptor

VEGFR1, have been found post mortem in the SN of PD patients (Wada, Arai et al. 2006), and this is consistent with increased angiogenesis found in PD brains (Faucheux, Bonnet et al. 1999). Excess VEGF induces increased macrophage migration mediated by VEGFR1 (Huusko, Merentie et al. 2009) and VEGF also induces BBB disruption in animal models after brain injury (Zhang, Zhang et al. 2000; Nguyen, Julien et al. 2002; Rite, Machado et al. 2007; Argaw, Gurfein et al. 2009) as well as in a rat model of PD (Rite, Machado et al. 2007). The VEGFR antagonist, Cyclo-VEGI, reduces inflammation and vascular leakiness, and is neuroprotective against excitotoxin-induced neurodegeneration in rats (Ryu and McLarnon 2008). This suggests dysregulated VEGF expression in the PD brain is also a key part of the neuroinflammatory response and increased edema in PD (Kirk and Karlik 2003; Suidan, Dickerson et al. 2010) (Nguyen, Julien et al. 2002; Nguyen, Tatlipinar et al. 2006; Zhang, Wang et al. 2006).

It is also worth noting that the innate immune cells of the brain, including microglia, become more reactive with age and that this might contribute to increased neuroinflammation in the elderly at some time point after activation of the peripheral immune response (Godbout and Johnson 2009). It has been suggested that prolonged exposure over a lifetime to inflammatory cytokines in the brain might eventually lead to various neurologic disorders (Godbout and Johnson 2009). This increased susceptibility to chronic inflammation in the elderly could contribute to the increased risk of PD associated with age. With growing elderly populations in many countries, PD is potentially an expanding public health problem. It is therefore critical that therapeutic interventions be identified and developed, that can halt and eventually reverse the neurodegeneration characteristic in PD. Treatments that focus on reducing chronic inflammation and pro-inflammatory microglial cell activation offer great promise for this sort of therapy. Therapies that foster microglia phenotypes which are non-inflammatory and supportive of neuroregeneration, could also prove beneficial in treating PD in the future.

In this chapter, we will discuss inflammatory mechanisms that play a crucial role in the progression of PD, and the therapeutic efficacy of using several anti-inflammatory compounds to treat progressive PD. We will also discuss the biology of microglial cells, including the cellular and molecular mechanisms that activate and regulate their inflammatory response, the evidence that implicates their different inflammatory mediators in the destruction of DA-neurons, and the efficacy of using different anti-inflammatory cytokines such as IL-10 and 1β, natural anti-inflammatory compounds such as *sinomenine*, *luteolin*, and *curcumin*, and the anti-inflammatory drugs morphinans and cyclosporine A, cell-based treatments such as Treg therapy, and specific anti-inflammatory therapies such as NF-κB inhibitors and β2-Adrenergic Receptor (β2AR) agonists. in halting or reversing the degenerative effects of inflammation within the SN. Finally, we will propose a model for PD as it relates to chronic inflammation, and discuss some possible future directions for the therapeutic treatment of PD.

2. Neuroinflammation in Parkinson's Disease

2.1 Microglia and chronic inflammation in neurodegeneration

Over two decades ago, high levels of activated microglia were discovered in the SN of PD patients (McGeer, Itagaki et al. 1988), first suggesting a connection between inflammation and PD. Since then, a wide range of inflammatory mediators produced by active microglia have been identified post mortem in PD tissue samples (Hirsch 2000; Orr, Rowe et al. 2002). The presence of activated microglia has also been verified in the SN of PD animal models (rodents and primates) (Akiyama and McGeer 1989; Barcia, Sanchez Bahillo et al. 2004; Gao, Miao et al. 2011). Studies using animal models of PD have begun to elucidate the inflammatory mechanisms that underlie the neurodegeneration of DA neurons and loss of DA production which are hallmarks of the disease. It has been found that intranigral injection of the pathogen product lipopolysaccharide (LPS) induces increased levels of CD11b+ and microglia and neutrophils in the SN of rats when compared to levels found in the cortex (Ji, Kronenberg et al. 2009). This same study also observed pronounced damage to endothelial cells and BBB permeability within the SN of the LPS-injected rats (Ji, Kronenberg et al. 2009). In this model, direct intranigral injection LPS or administration of the neurotoxin 1-methyl-4-phenyl-1,2,3,6-tetrahydropyridine (MPTP) induced PD-like symptoms accompanied by increased activation of microglia in the SN. Of particular significance is another finding that activated microglia and elevated levels of pro-inflammatory TNFα could be detected in the SN of monkeys from 1 to 14 years after an initial brief administration of MPTP (McGeer, Schwab et al. 2003; Barcia, Sanchez Bahillo et al. 2004; Barcia, de Pablos et al. 2005). These observations suggested that a brief insult to the brain by toxins could induce a chronic inflammatory state with concomitant progressive neurodegeneration. Additional support for sustained inflammation after insult is provided by an unfortunate human example of accidental exposure to MPTP in contaminated illegal street-drugs. Post-mortem evidence of activated microglia and degeneration in the SN of these human patients remained evident from 3 to 16 years after intravenous injection of the toxin (Langston, Forno et al. 1999).

Among the many inflammatory factors produced by microglia, superoxide is one of the major mediators of neurodegeneration. DA neurons are especially vulnerable to oxidative insults and this strongly supports the association of microglia activation with progressive PD (Block and Hong 2007). It is known that the normal midbrain region encompassing the SN contains nearly five times more microglia than other areas of the brain (Kim, Mohney et al. 2000). Understanding the progressive nature of microglia-mediated neurotoxicity, and the common mechanism of microglia activation by various diverse toxins or insults, thus has prime therapeutic importance for treating PD (Nguyen, Julien et al. 2002).

2.2 Inflammatory mechanisms and dopaminergic-neuron death

Several different animal models of PD have found that both systemic inflammation and direct dopaminergic neurotoxicity can initiate or exacerbate the neuroinflammation and neurodegeneration that are hallmarks of the disease. Injection of MPTP results in chronic neuroinflammation and progressive neurotoxicity in humans (Langston, Forno et al. 1999) and other primates (McGeer, Schwab et al. 2003). In the former case, an accidental intravenous injection of MPTP-contaminated street-drugs left several patients ill with progressive motor-dysfunction which was shown in post mortem analysis to be mediated by DA-neuron loss in the SN, very similar to what is observed following MPTP injection in both rodent and primate models of neurodegeneration (Langston, Forno et al. 1999; Qin, Wu et al. 2007). Similarly a single systemic injection of LPS in an rodent model results in significant loss (23%) of DA neurons in the SN beginning at 7-months post treatment, increasing to a 47% loss at 10-months post injection (Qin, Wu et al. 2007). This delayed, progressive loss of DA neurons in the SN recapitulates some of the hallmark characteristics of PD. This model is further supported as a model for PD by a clinical case report that a patient displayed PD-related symptoms after accidental peripheral exposure to LPS (Niehaus and Lange 2003). However, the underlying mechanism that advances the progressive nature of the disease remains unclear. It is known that systemically injected LPS cannot readily cross the blood-brain barrier, and studies have shown that pro-inflammatory cytokines, actually mediate the mechanism of systemic LPS-induced DA neurotoxicity (Qin, Wu et al. 2007). Interestingly, systemic administration of LPS enhances motor neuron degeneration in animal models of another neurodegenerative disease, amyotrophic lateral sclerosis (ALS), 6 months after LPS injection (Nguyen, D'Aigle et al. 2004), suggesting this may be a common etiology for a number of chronic neurodegenerative conditions. In addition, systemic exposure to LPS was also shown to significantly exacerbate neuronal-cell death associated with ischemic insult in neonatal rats (Lehnardt, Massillon et al. 2003). The effects of systemic inflammation on neuronal survival may depend upon several factors such as brain region affected, length of time to allow cumulative effects, age of exposure to the inflammagen, presence of systemic TNFα, and severity of the inflammatory stimulation.

It now appears that it is the inflammatory cytokines TNFα, IL-1β and IL-6 which play major roles in the etiology of PD both systemically and within the CNS. First, TNFα produced in the periphery after systemic LPS injection is transported across BBB to enter the brain through a TNFα-receptor dependent mechanism (Gutierrez, Banks et al. 1993; Pan and Kastin 2002; Qin, Wu et al. 2007). TNFα then initiates an inflammatory cascade by interacting with TNFα receptors on the microglia, leading to the activation of transcription factor NF-κB within microglial cells, and resulting in the production of additional TNFα and other pro-inflammatory factors, and thus creating a persistent and self-perpetuating neuroinflammatory response that drives delayed and progressive loss of DA neurons in the SN (Park and Bowers 2010). In addition, TNFα is one of the primary pro-inflammatory cytokines that promote overproduction of ROS (Fernandez-Checa, Kaplowitz et al. 1997), a key player in DA-neurodegeneration (Gao and Hong 2008) (Qian, Flood et al. 2011). Another pro-inflammatory cytokine, IL-1β, is also under transcriptional control of NF-κB and is consequently up-regulated in neuroinflammation. Direct injection of recombinant IL-1β into the brains of rats induces astrocytic expression of hypoxia inducible factor (HIF-1α) which contributes to the induction of oxidative stress (Argaw, Zhang et al. 2006). IL-1β also induces the HIF-1α-VEGF pathway that results in increased BBB permeability and increased angiogenesis (Argaw, Zhang et al. 2006; Argaw, Gurfein et al. 2009), which are all found to be increased in PD patients (Kortekaas, Leenders et al. 2005). Similarly, IL-6 expression is controlled by NF-κB (Lappas, Permezel et al. 2002) and is increased under a variety of inflammatory conditions (Van Snick 1990; Dendorfer 1996), including an MPTP-induced mouse model of PD (Kohutnicka, Lewandowska et al. 1998). IL-6 expression from activated microglia coincides in the SN with loss of TH+ DA neurons after MPTP injection but is absent from the SN in uninjected controls (Kohutnicka, Lewandowska et al. 1998). Neuronal levels of IL-6 are also increased by oxidative stress which is another mediator of microglia activation, neuroinflammation and degeneration (Lee, Cho et al. 2010; Naik and Dixit 2011; Negi, Kumar et al. 2011).

In addition to inflammatory cytokines, oxidative stress appears to play a crucial role in the DA-neurodegeneration seen in PD. Oxidative stress occurs because of intracellular accumulation of reactive oxygen and nitrogen species (ROS & RNS) and, along with mitochondrial dysfunction and inflammation, has been identified as central in the mechanism underlying the inflammatory pathogenesis of PD (Bartels and Leenders 2007; Monahan, Warren et al. 2008). Impaired mitochondrial function has been observed in PD (Schapira, Cooper et al. 1989; Schapira 1994; Jenner and Olanow 1996; Sherer, Betarbet et al. 2002; Keeney, Xie et al. 2006; Schapira 2006), in which mitochondria generate ROS as by-products of molecular oxygen consumption in the electron transport chain. Oxidative stress is hypothesized to initiate DA neuron loss in the SN (Jenner and Olanow 1998; Lin and Beal 2006). The brain is hypersensitive to oxidative damage in part due to the fact that oxygen consumption by brain cells constitutes 20% of total oxygen consumption in body. Brain tissue is also enriched in peroxidizable fatty acids and has low levels anti-oxidant defenses (catalase, SOD, glutathione, glutathione peroxidase) (Floyd 1999; Floyd 1999). Within the brain, the SN is amongst regions most vulnerable to oxidative insult. The SN is characterized by a pro-oxidative state, and has a high metabolic rate with high levels of the oxidizable species DA, DA-derived ROS, neuromelanin and other molecules that render the SN vulnerable to the possible effects of peroxynitrite and sulfite (Marshall, Reist et al. 1999). Oxidative stress is part of the pro-inflammatory response of microglia within the CNS, and it has been found that NADPH oxidase (PHOX), is the major superoxide-producing enzyme of microglia. It is a molecular complex of membrane-associated cytochrome b558 (composed of 2 subunits: gp91phox and p22phox) and the cytosolic components: p47phox, p67phox, p40phox, and a small GTPase rac2 (Groemping and Rittinger 2005). Upon activation, the cytosolic subunits translocate to the membrane and form a functional enzyme to generate superoxide. Therapy directed against the oxidative stress response has proved beneficial in treatment for PD (Smith and Zigmond 2003; Jackson-Lewis and Smeyne 2005). Anti-inflammatory agents that inhibit NADPH oxidase activity are neuroprotective (Liu and Hong 2003; Qian, Block et al. 2006; Qian, Gao et al. 2007), and reduced DA neurotoxicity induced by LPS or MPTP has been demonstrated in PHOX-/- compared to wild-type mice (Gao, Liu et al. 2003; Qin, Liu et al. 2004). Pharmacological inhibition of PHOX by the specific inhibitor diphenyliodonium (DPI), also shows potent DA-neuroprotection *in vitro* (Qian, Gao et al. 2007). PHOX activity also regulates production of pro-inflammatory cytokines, such as TNFα, by activated microglia *in vitro* following LPS stimulation (Qin, Liu et al. 2004). This suggests that PHOX not only mediates superoxide production, but also controls the levels of other pro-inflammatory neurotoxic factors produced by activated microglia. Cell signaling pathways that regulate PHOX activity are still being elucidated but it has been shown that a microglial adhesion molecule, the integrin MAC1 (macrophage antigen complex 1), is closely linked with PHOX and plays an important role in microglia-mediated neuroinflammation and neurotoxicity (Hu, Zhang et al. 2008). Microglial- cell expressed MAC1 is indispensable for the enhanced neurotoxicity induced by LPS, a-synuclein, or MPTP in neuron-glia mixed cell cultures (Pei, Pang et al. 2007; Zhang, Dallas et al. 2007; Hu, Zhang et al. 2008). Furthermore, MAC1-deficient mice show resistance to MPTP-induced DA neurotoxicity *in vivo*. NADPH oxidase-generated oxygen free radicals are also required for MAC1-mediated phagocytosis in neutrophils (Coxon, Rieu et al. 1996). Therefore, the dual activity between MAC1 and NADPH oxidase might be a central mechanism underlying the reactive microgliosis that mediates oxidative damage and consequent progressive neurodegeneration after microglia activation.

2.3 Peripheral inflammation, microglial-cell activation and neurodegeneration

Neuroinflammation is an important defense mechanism against pathogens and environmental toxins damaging the brain. Under normal conditions, the central nervous system (CNS) and the brain especially are considered to be immune privileged (Neuwelt and Clark 1978; Smith, DeGirolami et al. 1992; Lotan and Schwartz 1994). Any immune response is very highly regulated with a finely balanced anti-inflammatory environment within the CNS combined with vigilant immune surveillance by circulating immune cells and those that are resident in the CNS. Under pathological conditions, the brain mounts an aggressive, acute inflammatory response to invading pathogens, infection, trauma, stroke or any other threat to homeostasis. These perturbations trigger the activation of microglia, the brain resident macrophages (Ransohoff and Perry 2009), as well as local invasions of circulating immune cells and the production of ROS and RNS (Mosley, Benner et al. 2006; Tansey, McCoy et al. 2007; Whitton 2007). The resident microglia aid in functional regulation of other immune cells particularly the helper T-cells and dendritic cells (DC) which also play critical roles in the initiation and maintenance of any neuroinflammatory response to pathological threats. However, inflammation in the brain is a 'two-edged sword' (Wyss-Coray and Mucke 2002) because if the tight regulation of the inflammatory process breaks down in any manner, the inflammatory response can switch from being beneficial to highly detrimental to brain function. In acute situations short-lived inflammatory mechanisms limit injury and promote healing (Wyss-Coray and Mucke 2002; McGeer and McGeer 2004). Microglia are the critical elements in an acute neuroinflammatory response that minimize tissue damage, restore tissue to homeostasis and promote would healing processes. Conversely, when inflammation is chronically sustained at high levels, this can lead to brain-tissue damage with concomitant initiation and progression of neuroinflammatory diseases such as PD.

While microglial cells are the major immunocompetent cells in the CNS and are important mediators in the pathogenesis of PD (Herrera, Tomas-Camardiel et al. 2005; Smeyne, Jiao et al. 2005; Zhou, Wang et al. 2005), up-regulation of humoral response and other peripheral immune components has been identified in both idiopathic and genetic cases of PD (Orr, Rowe et al. 2005). Elevated levels of IL-1β, TNFα, IL-6 have been described in post mortem tissue from PD patients (Mogi, Harada et al. 1994; Mogi, Harada et al. 1994; Mogi, Harada et al. 1996), and PD patients show higher levels of IL-1β, TNFα, Il-1, CD4+ and CD8+ cells in serum and CSF (Dobbs, Charlett et al. 1999; Bas, Calopa et al. 2001; Hisanaga, Asagi et al. 2001; Reale, Greig et al. 2009). CD8+ T cells have also been found associated with degenerating SN neurons (McGeer, Itagaki et al. 1988), and classical complement components have been isolated in the Lewy bodies that form in the SN of PD patients (Yamada, McGeer et al. 1992). Significantly, compromised BBB integrity has also been observed in PD patients (Kortekaas, Leenders et al. 2005), indicating that factors in peripheral inflammation have ready access to the brain and may also be involved in the neurodegenerative process probably via an effect on the activation of microglia. Complement proteins normally circulate in the blood in an inactive state, but in response to pathogenic threat, these proteins become activated in cascades of events that precipitate destruction and removal of the threat. Importantly for PD, studies have shown that complement factors C1q and mannose-binding lectins (MBL), participate in microglial cell activation and could be important in pathogenesis of neurodegeneration (Yamada, McGeer et al. 1992; Webster, Galvan et al. 2001; Whitton 2007). The importance of the classical complement pathway in PD has been established (Yamada, McGeer et al. 1992; Yamada, Chong et al. 1993), and MBL infiltration into the brain accompanies degeneration of TH+ neurons in MPTP-injected mice up to 28 days post MPTP administration in an animal model of PD (Chao, He et al. 2009). In the latter study, clear evidence of BBB breakdown was also documented, providing further evidence that peripheral immunity probably participates in the activation of microglia and consequent DA-neuron destruction.

Normally, immune surveillance protects the healthy brain from pathogen assault and damage. Memory T-cell surveillance of the CNS is first regulated via migration from the blood into the cerebral spinal fluid (CSF) through the choroid plexus barrier (Engelhardt and Ransohoff 2005), while the recruitment and infiltration of immune cells into brain tissue occurs through the post-capillary venules into the perivascular space that surrounds microvascular endothelial cells (MVEC) which are joined together by tight-junctions that form the blood-brain-barrier (Carrithers, Visintin et al. 2000; Pachter, de Vries et al. 2003). MVEC in the brain closely interact with astrocytes, pericytes, perivascular microglia and neuronal cells such as DA-producing neurons to form the neurovascular unit. Thus, at these crucial checkpoints the specific microenvironment within the CNS tissues determines whether the immune cells survive to mount antigen-specific inflammatory response or if they will be eliminated. CD4+ T cells play a critical role in the initiation and maintenance of any immune response in the CNS including the brain, but to survive in this normally anti-inflammatory environment, they need additional stimulatory signals. Generally, CD4+ must be activated in the peripheral lymphoid system prior to migration into the CNS. Activated CD4+Th cells differentiate into distinct effector subsets that express unique suites of cytokines that perform different immunoregulatory functions. For example Th1 and Th2 produce predominantly INF-γ and IL-4 respectively which have differential effects on the activation state of microglia amongst other disparate outcomes (Appel, Beers et al. 2009)

T cells express many sensor receptors with which they assess the microenvironment milieu. CD+4 interact with other immune cells such as antigen presenting cells (APC) that take-up, process and present antigens via the major histocompatibility complex molecules (MHC). MHCII is expressed mainly in cells of the lymphoid system such as T cells, B cells, macrophages, and DC (Matarese, De Rosa et al. 2008). Under non-inflammatory conditions, cells of the CNS express low levels of MCH and in the absence of histocompatibility molecules the survival or further differentiation of activated T cells is low. Constitutively expressed mediators also help prevent differentiation of Th cells, and conversely promote development of Tregs. For example, the neuropeptide Vasoactive Intestinal Peptide (VIP) up-regulates Treg function which has an inhibitory effect on microglia and macrophages (Delgado, Chorny et al. 2005; Fernandez-Martin, Gonzalez-Rey et al. 2006). Additionally, anti-inflammatory cytokines secreted by astrocytes and glial cells, such as IL-10 and TGFβ1, induce differentiation of Tregs (Chen and Wahl 2003). However, during inflammation TGFβ1 works with IL-6 or IL-21 to induce differentiation of pro-inflammatory IL-17-producing T cells (Th17) indicating the distinction between anti-inflammatory and pro-inflammatory is not always straight forward. In an animal model of PD, the DA-neuron neurodegenerative effects of MPTP administration were Th17-cell mediated, and the induction of Tregs by VIP attenuated this effect (Reynolds, Banerjee et al. 2007; Reynolds, Stone et al. 2010). However, as it has also been shown that TGFβ1/IL-6 increases production of IL-10 as well as IL-17, this IL-10 is then capable of suppressing the degenerative effects mediated by Th17 cells (McGeachy, Bak-Jensen et al. 2007).

3. Efficacy of anti-inflammatory agents halting or reversing degeneration

Mounting evidence indicates that numerous types of inflammatory mediators such as TNFα, prostaglandin (PGE2), NO, free radicals, and other products of activated immune cells can also play a role in the DA-neuron degeneration in several models of PD (Gao, Jiang et al. 2002; Dauer and Przedborski 2003; Bartels and Leenders 2007). Treatment using anti-inflammatory agents directed at a number of different pro-inflammatory targets could potentially halt, slow or even reverse PD disease progression. For example, steroidal anti-inflammatory drugs (SAIDS) such as dexamethasone have been used to stimulate neuroprotection against MPTP or LPS-induced toxicity (Kurkowska-Jastrzebska, Wronska et al. 1999; Castano, Herrera et al. 2002; Kurkowska-Jastrzebska, Litwin et al. 2004). In addition, non-steroidal anti-inflammatory drugs (NSAIDS), e.g. aspirin and ibuprofen, can reduce inflammation by inhibition of COX activity (Sairam, Saravanan et al. 2003)(Sairam et al. 2003). A prospective study found a significantly lower risk of developing PD in users of ibuprofen compared to non-users, and that the efficacy of taking ibuprofen was dose-dependently related to the number of weekly tablets of the drug taken (Gao, Chen et al. 2011). Microglial cell inhibitors such as minocycline have also shown neuroprotective characteristics in PD animal models (Du, Ma et al. 2001; Wu, Jackson-Lewis et al. 2002). Recently, strategies that directly inactivate the activation of the pro-inflammatory transcription factor NF-κB (Ghosh, Roy et al. 2007; Zhang, Qian et al. 2010), and/or activate the peroxisome proliferator-activated receptor-c (PPARc) (Bernardo, Ajmone-Cat et al. 2005), have produced beneficial modulation of inflammatory responses. Other strategies, including inhibition of ion channels in microglial cells (Thomas, Chartrand et al. 2007) can also be effective treatments aimed at halting progressive PD in an animal model of the disease. We will focus on five relatively new approaches in anti-inflammatory therapy for PD: (1) the use of exogenous anti-inflammatory cytokines IL-10 or TGFβ1, (2) the use of cell-based therapies such as regulatory T cells (Tregs), which are the major source of IL-10 or TGFβ1 in the resolution of neuroinflammation; (3) the use of morphinan-related compounds; (4) the targeting of NF-κB, the major transcriptional regulator of inflammation, and (5) the administration of beta2-adrenergic receptor (β2AR) agonists.

3.1 Therapies using anti-inflammatory cytokines: IL-10 and TGFβ

When acute inflammation is not resolved, i.e. the agent or event that originated the inflammatory response has not been eliminated, chronic inflammation can become entrenched and lead to neuroinflammation and degeneration. Normally, endogenous anti-inflammatory cytokines provide a negative-feedback mechanism which controls the continued activation of immune cells from potentially pathological effects (Moore, Lahiri et al. 2001; Strle, Zhou et al. 2001). Therefore, replacing or elevating the level of these anti-inflammatory regulators could be a therapeutic means to halt the chronic, pathological aspects of inflammation. IL10 and TGFβ1 are two major anti-inflammatory cytokines that are normally produced by Treg cells. Studies using exogenously supplied IL10 and TGFβ1 have shown potent effects in reducing neurotoxicity induced by either LPS or MPTP in PD models. In an *in vitro* model of PD, application of IL-10 to a mixed glial cell-neuron cell culture abrogated the degeneration of the neuron cells induced by either LPS or MPTP (Qian, Block et al. 2006). This inhibitory effect of IL10 was mediated through its inhibition of the production of TNFα, nitric oxide, and extracellular superoxide in the microglia cells within the mixed cell culture (Qian, Block et al. 2006). These *in vitro* effects of IL-10 are confirmed by *in vivo* results from a 6-OHDA rat model of PD. In this model, sustained administration of IL10 via a viral-vector, significantly protected DA-neuron from death and ameliorated behavioral deficits induced by intra-striatal delivery of 6-OHDA (Johnston, Su et al. 2008).

Several *in vitro* studies have shown that TGFβ1 can also protect neurons from cell death induced by oxidative stress (Prehn and Krieglstein 1994), glutamate excitotoxicity (Zhu, Yang et al. 2002), or chemical-induced hypoxia (Ruocco, Nicole et al. 1999). TGFβ1 suppresses the progression of neurodegeneration *in vivo* in an EAE model of MS (Szczepanik, Tutaj et al. 2005). Additionally, recombinant TGFβ1, intracerebrally delivered by a viral-vector, protects against brain injury induced by ischemia (Unsicker and Krieglstein 2002), excitotoxic-induced death (Ruocco, Nicole et al. 1999), and oxidative stress (Henrich-Noack, Prehn et al. 1996). Although exogenous TGFβ1 has thus been strongly suggested as a neuroprotective treatment, the molecular mechanisms underlying its neuroprotection have not been clearly elucidated. Recent evidence indicates that the neuroprotective effects of both IL10 and TGFβ1 are mainly due to their inhibition of ROS production in microglia during initial activation or in reactive microgliosis (Qian, Block et al. 2006; Qian, Wei et al. 2008). In mixed glial cell-neuronal cell cultures, application of TGFβ1 blocked neuron cell death through the inhibition of PHOX activity in cultures exposed to either LPS or MPTP. TGFβ1 prevented the ERK-dependent phosphorylation on p47phox in the microglial cells and blocked translocation and assembly of the PHOX molecular complex to the plasma membrane. Inhibition of PHOX activation consequently reduced oxidase activities induced by LPS (Qian, Wei et al. 2008). While the complete *in vivo* roles of IL10 and TGFβ1 in the regulation of chronic CNS inflammation in PD remain to be determined, both may provide promising basis for therapeutic use in PD treatments.

3.2 Morphinan-based anti-inflammatory therapeutics

Dextromethorphan (DM) is a well established drug that is used as the active ingredient in many cough suppressants. Over twenty years ago, it was recognized that DM and the metabolite dextrorphan (DX) could have anti-seizure effects in models of convulsive disorders such as epilepsy (Tortella, Ferkany et al. 1988). Dextrorphan was also shown to antagonize the *in vitro* excitation of spinal neurons by application of N-methyl-D-aspartate (NMDA), a glutamate receptor ligand (Church, Lodge et al. 1985). In addition, DX was found to block cortical neuron injury induced by NMDA or by glutamate (Choi 1987; Choi, Maulucci-Gedde et al. 1987; Choi, Peters et al. 1987; Koh and Choi 1987). Because NMDA receptors were known to mediate hypoxic injury in neuronal cell cultures, it was suggested that morphinan drugs, especially DX and DM, might be potential therapeutic treatments for brain injury from hypoxia of ischemia (Goldberg, Weiss et al. 1987). Additionally, since the loss of DA-neuron in PD leads to the secondary effect of hyperactive glutamatergic function, it was postulated that DM and DX might also be useful as adjunct therapies in treating PD (Albin, Young et al. 1989; Greenamyre and O'Brien 1991).

Several studies using PD animal models or *in vitro* cell cultures have shown that dextromethorphan and its metabolites are neuroprotective due to their anti-inflammatory properties and inhibitory function towards microglia activation (Liu, Qin et al. 2003; Zhang, Wang et al. 2004; Zhang, Qin et al. 2005). In the first of these studies, DM treatment protected DA-neurons from LPS-induced neuron death in mixed glial-neuronal cell cultures (Liu, Qin et al. 2003). Furthermore, the neuroprotective effects of DM were mediated through inhibiting microglial cell activation (Liu, Qin et al. 2003). Similarly, DM inhibited microglia activation and was neuroprotective when administered daily to mice that had been injected with MPTP (Zhang, Wang et al. 2004). Another metabolite of DM, 3-hydroxymorphinan (3-HM), was shown to have the greatest potency (of several tested methorphinans) for attenuating the loss of DA-neurons in the SN, as well as restoring motor functions in an MPTP-injection mouse-model of PD (Zhang, Qin et al. 2005). 3-HM also protected neuronal cells in mixed glial-neuronal cells cultures by reducing MPTP-induced microgliosis and decreasing the production of ROS. In addition to this neuroprotective property, 3-HM was also found to have neurotrophic effects. The neurotrophic effects of 3-HM were mediated by induction of increased expression of neurotrophic factors, including GDNF, EGF, NTF and TGFβ1, by astroglial cells in mixed cultures with neuronal cells (Zhang, Wang et al. 2004; Zhang, Shin et al. 2006). In another study using mixed neuron-glia cultures, both l-morphine and it synthetic steroenantiomer, d-morphine, reduced LPS or MPTP-induced DA-neuron death with similar efficacy (Qian, Tan et al. 2007). These results indicated that morphine exerts anti-inflammatory effects either by inhibition of direct microglial cell activation via LPS or through attenuating reactive microgliosis induced by MPTP. A naturally occurring d-morphinan, sinomenine, also has neuroprotective effects and will be discussed below (Qian, Xu et al. 2007).

While DM and other morphinan compounds appear to have strong neuroprotective properties in animal model systems of PD, early human trials using DM to treat PD patients were contradictory. While one study found daily high doses of DM could improve some motor-behavioral deficits in PD patients (Bonuccelli, Del Dotto et al. 1992), another similar trial using the same dose regimen reported no beneficial effects on PD motor-associated symptoms (Montastruc, Fabre et al. 1994). Significantly, more recent double-blind trials have confirmed that DM can improve motor function in PD patients, especially the dyskinesia associated with long-term levadopa treatment (Verhagen Metman, Blanchet et al. 1998; Verhagen Metman, Del Dotto et al. 1998). It has been suggested that the uncertainty over the true effects of DM might be due to the relatively rapid metabolism of DM *in vivo* (Werling, Lauterbach et al. 2007). Although, DX and other DM metabolites have shown similar neuroprotective properties in preclinical studies, only DM seems to function through multiple mechanisms rather than simply blocking activity of the NMDA-receptor (Werling, Lauterbach et al. 2007). In situ DM concentrations can be increased if given in conjunction with a low dose of the drug quinidine which retards metabolism of DM and leads to increased DM concentrations in plasma, resulting in greater bioavailability (Pope, Khalil et al. 2004). Clearly, DM presents an attractive potential for use in combinatorial treatment for at least ameliorating the motor deficits characteristic of PD and possibly for attenuating the activation of microglia and chronic inflammation also prominent in PD.

3.3 Sinomenine, luteolin and curcumin as treatments for Parkinson's disease

Several natural compounds isolated from plants, including sinomenine, luteolin and curcumin, are also being investigated for their ability to attenuate inflammation and provide neuroprotection against the loss of DA neurons. Although these three agents belong to different families of organic compounds, they have all shown anti-oxidant, anti-inflammatory and neuroprotective qualities *in vitro* cell-culture models of neurodegenerative diseases including PD. The first of these is sinomenine, a morphinan related alkaloid compound purified from a medicinal plant (Sinomenine acutum) that has been traditionally used to treat inflammatory disorders (Liu, Resch et al. 1994; Liu, Buchner et al. 1996). In a study using rat midbrain mixed glial cell-neuron cell cultures, sinomenine protected the neuronal cells from both LPS and MPP+ induced cell death (Qian, Xu et al. 2007). Sinomenine protected neurons by reducing release of extracelluar ROS and inhibiting PHOX/p47 from translocation to the plasma membrane where the complex becomes activated. These effects were mediated by inhibition of microglial cells since sinomenine failed to protect neuronal-cell enriched cultures which lacked microglia from MPP+ induced damage and death (Qian, Xu et al. 2007).

Another plant extract, the flavonoid luteolin, has also been used for its anti-oxidant and anti-inflammatory properties. Luteolin was demonstrated to have neuroprotective effects by inhibiting oxidative stress-induced cell death in the DA-producing SH-SY5Y cell line (Kang, Lee et al. 2004). In mixed glial-neuron midbrain cell cultures from rats, luteolin attenuated the loss of TH+ DA-neurons after addition of increasing concentrations of LPS. The protective effect of luteolin in these experiments was shown to be mediated through the inhibition of microglial cell activation, and reduced production of TNFα, NO and ROS (Chen, Jin et al. 2008). Similarly, curcumin, the active anti-inflammatory isolate from turmeric (Curcuma longa), is known to have anti-inflammatory neuroprotective effects in CNS disorders. In an experimental allergic encephalomyelitis (EAE) mouse model of MS, curcumin inhibited EAE development by attenuating microglia activation and IL-12 production as well as Th1 cell differentiation (Natarajan and Bright 2002). Curcumin also has shown protective effects against LPS-induced DA neuron cell death in mixed rat neuron-glial cell cultures which were mediated by inhibition of the production of proinflammatory factors in microglia (Yang, Zhang et al. 2008). Taken together, the neuroprotective results from these three natural plant products suggest an interesting possibility for PD therapeutics. Since these and other similar plant-based isolates can cross the BBB and have anti-inflammatory as well as anti-oxidant properties, they may provide new directions for adjunct therapy.

4. Anti-inflammatory cell-based strategy for Parkinson's disease therapy: Regulatory T-cells

An anti-inflammatory strategy currently being studied as a cell-based therapy in PD involves the therapeutic introduction of Treg cells. It is now believed that Tregs suppress immune reactivity through multiple mechanisms, such as release of IL-10 and TGFβ, induction of apoptotic tolerance, and suppression of metabolic functions in effector immune cells such as microglia and effector T-cells. As the primary source IL10 and TGF1β *in vivo*, Tregs have been shown to be the major cells which regulate the inflammatory response in a number of disorders through their effects on the innate and adaptive immune responses that have escaped normal pathways of control. Recent studies using models of neurodegeneration demonstrated that induction of an anti-inflammatory Treg response inhibited microglial activation, and promoted neuronal survival (Reynolds, Banerjee et al. 2007; Liu, Gong et al. 2009; Reynolds, Stone et al. 2009). In another report, adoptively transferred Treg cells attenuated a Th17-mediated inflammatory response in mice that had been injected with MPTP and concomitantly vaccinated with nitrated (N) α-synuclein. In this model, injection of N-α-synuclein elicited an adaptive immune response in conjunction with the MPTP-induced neurotoxicity both of which were ameliorated by the transfer of natural or VIP-induced Treg cells in these mice (Reynolds, Stone et al. 2010). Tregs have also been shown to promote neurotrophic factor production from astrocytes (Reynolds, Banerjee et al. 2007; Reynolds, Stone et al. 2010), indicating their potential for neuroregeneration of DA neurons.

Strategies that use Th2 cells are also being employed. Th2 cells inhibit microglial cell activation through the production of IL4 and IL10, and stimulate the production of GDNF by astrocytes, thereby providing neuroprotection against MPTP-induced neuronal death (Benner, Mosley et al. 2004). Copaxone, a peptide-based therapy approved for patients with MS, is thought to promote the development of Th2 cells which function to decrease CNS inflammation through the release of anti-inflammatory cytokines and neurotrophic factors (Kipnis and Schwartz 2002; Angelov, Waibel et al. 2003; Benner, Mosley et al. 2004; Schwartz 2004). Copaxone-induced T-cells also have neuroprotective effects in animal models of ALS and PD (Angelov, Waibel et al. 2003; Benner, Mosley et al. 2004). However, because the interactions amongst regulatory T cells, glial cells, neurons and other infiltrating leukocytes within the SN is incredibly complex and not well understood, further studies to elucidate the regulatory pathways involved are necessary to develop Th2-cell based therapies for PD patients.

5. Specific anti-inflammatory therapies

5.1 Therapies targeting pro-inflammatory transcription factor NF-κB

Many of the inflammatory mediators involved in inflammation and DA-neurodegeneration in PD are expressed in microglial cells and their regulation is primarily mediated by the transcription factor NF-κB. NF-κB was first described in 1986 as a transcription factor which is essential for the expression of mouse kappa light chain genes (Sen and Baltimore 1986; Sen and Baltimore 1986). It has since been shown that NF-κB functions to control gene expression of many of pro-inflammatory mediators (Tsoulfas and Geller 2001). Inflammatory cytokines such as TNFα and IL-1α and β, bacterial products such as lipopolysaccharide (LPS), and products of cellular damage strongly activate inflammatory responses through the activation of NF-κB. NF-κB subsequently plays an essential positive-feedback role in the inflammatory response through regulation of genes encoding inflammatory cytokines IL-1β, TNFα, and IL-12/23, as well as chemokines IL-8, MIP-1α, and MCP-1(Xia, Pauza et al. 1997; Roebuck 1999; Roebuck, Carpenter et al. 1999). NF-κB also mediates nitric oxide production (iNOS), expression of NADPH oxidase subunits p47 and p67 (Gauss, Nelson-Overton et al. 2007; Lawrence 2009), and adhesion molecules ICAM-1, VCAM, and E-selectin (Chen and Manning 1995; Tak and Firestein 2001). Activation of NF-κB is a key event in many chronic inflammatory diseases such as cardiovascular disease (Van der Heiden, Cuhlmann et al.), tissue reperfusion injury (Latanich and Toledo-Pereyra 2009), experimental autoimmune encephalomyelitis (EAE) (Vandenbroeck, Alloza et al. 2004), rheumatoid arthritis (Criswell 2010), and inflammatory bowel disease (IBD) (Atreya, Atreya et al. 2008). A large number of the therapeutic agents for treating human inflammatory conditions, including sulfasalazine, 5-aminosalicylates, and corticosteroids, as well as some natural anti-inflammatory compounds such as IL-10, TGFβ1, β2AR agonists, glutamate, and curcumin, may owe their anti-inflammatory effects to inhibition of NF-κB (Lawrence and Fong ; Wang, Boddapati et al. ; Pereira and Oakley 2008; Lawrence 2009). These anti-inflammatory agents are potent inhibitors of microglial activation, and are neuroprotective to DA neurons *in vitro* and *in vivo*. Clearly, NF-κB activity presents a key target to ameliorate chronic inflammation in humans. Therapeutic strategies to inhibit NF-κB activity in microglial cells may lead to more effective treatments for PD (Zhang, Qian et al. 2010; Flood, Qian et al. 2011).

The NF-κB family consists of dimeric transcription factors which include five members: c-Rel, RelA (p65), RelB, NF-κB1 (p50/p105), and NF-κB2 (p52/p100) (Flood, Qian et al. 2011). There are two major activation pathways: (1) the classical or canonical pathway, and (2) the alternate or noncanonical pathway. While the non-canonical pathway does not appear to play a major role in the activation of inflammation, the classical pathway is thought to regulate the production of most pro-inflammatory mediators and is characterized by activation of a dimer of Rel proteins p50 and p65. In the inactive state this Rel dimer is complexed within the cytosol to the inhibitory protein IκBα complex (Lawrence 2009). The classical NF-κB pathway is initiated upon phosphorylation, ubiquitination, and subsequent proteasome-dependent degradation of IκBα. The phosphorylation of IκBα on serine residues is mediated by IκB kinase (IKK), which is a molecular complex of three proteins consisting of a heterodimer of the two catalytic subunits IKKα and IKKβ, along with IKKγ (the NF-κB essential modulator, NEMO) (May, Marienfeld et al. 2002; Huxford and Ghosh 2009; Oeckinghaus and Ghosh 2009). Embryonic cells derived from genetic knock-out mice lacking IKKβ, IKKγ, or p65 are unresponsive to classical NF-κB inducers such as TNFα and IL-1β (Reuther-Madrid, Kashatus et al. 2002; Sizemore, Lerner et al. 2002; Sizemore, Agarwal et al. 2004). Activation of IKK in response to inflammatory mediators such as TNFα, IL-1β, and LPS, depends critically on the presence of the IKKγ (NEMO) subunit of the IKK complex (Rudolph, Yeh et al. 2000; May, Marienfeld et al. 2002), which results in the phosphorylation of the IκB by the kinase activity of IKKβ (Huxford and Ghosh 2009; Oeckinghaus and Ghosh 2009). An N-terminal region of NEMO associates with a hexapeptide sequence within the C-terminus of both IKKα and IKKβ (NEMO binding domain or NBD), and disruption or mutation of this NEMO-NBD interaction site on either IKKβ or IKKγ results in a loss of responsiveness of cells to pro-inflammatory signaling (Flood, Qian et al. 2011). Agents that block the activation of NF-κB are capable of inhibiting the two major inflammatory pathways in microglia—activation of oxidative stress and production of inflammatory mediators, including cytokines TNFα, IL-1β, IL-6, as well as chemokines associated with inflammation (Qian, Flood et al. 2010).

Selective IKKβ and IKKγ inhibitors that do not target IKKα or the non-canonical P100/p52 pathway, should be promising therapeutic agents for treating chronic inflammatory disorders including PD. Such specific NF-κB inhibitors have recently been used in murine models of PD to halt the progression of neurodegeneration induced by the neurotoxin MPTP (Ghosh, Roy et al. 2007), or by activation of CNS inflammation by the intracranial injection of LPS (Zhang, Qian et al. 2010). Pretreatment of animals with a peptide against the NEMO-binding domain (NBD peptide) prior to injection of MPTP into mice, significantly inhibits the activation of NF-κB within the midbrain region. This inhibition of NF-κB activation is accompanied by a concomitant reduction in inflammatory mediator mRNA expression within the SN, as well as the expression of microglial cell activation marker CD11b. Mice receiving the NBD peptide prior to MPTP injection also showed highly significant protection of the nigrostriatum from MPTP-induced neurodegeneration of the TH+ neurons and the loss of dopamine production, as well as improvement in their locomotor function compared with MPTP-injected mice given mutant peptide. More importantly, administration of NBD peptide 2 days after injection of MPTP showed substantial protection of TH+ neurons, suggesting that NBD peptide can be used therapeutically to slow down or halt the progression of DA-neurodegeneration in MPTP-treated animals (Ghosh, Roy et al. 2007). In addition, infrared analysis of the brains of NBD-treated animals determined that significant levels of the NBD peptide localized within the brain tissue, suggesting that the NBD peptide could cross the BBB and reach sites of neuroinflammation. The nature of the mechanism of NF-κB inhibition within the SN remains to be determined, but these data suggest NF-κB is a viable target for therapy for PD patients (Ghosh, Roy et al. 2007).

A second approach to inhibit inflammation has been to use small molecule inhibitors that specifically block function of IKKβ. One such specific inhibitor, called Compound A, is a small molecule inhibitor of the kinase activity of IKKβ but not IKKα. Compound A, also known as BAY-65-1942 (7-[2-(cyclopropylmethoxy)-6-hydroxyphenyl]-5-[(3S)-3-piperidinyl]-1,4-dihydro-2Hpyrido [2,3- d] [1,3]-oxazin-2-one hydrochloride), has been shown to specifically and effectively block the catalytic activity of IKKβ, inhibiting its ability to phosphorylate IκB and activate the cytosolic p50/p65 NF-κB heterodimers (Moss, Stansfield et al. 2007; Zhang, Qian et al. 2010). In one recent study, Zhang and colleagues (2010) used Compound A in an LPS-induced neurodegeneration model to inhibit the canonical NF-κB pathway and halt inflammation-induced DA-neurodegeneration. In this model, LPS was injected directly into one side of the midbrain of rats, leading to inflammation-induced degeneration of DA-neurons (Zhang, Qian et al. 2010). It was found that Compound A strongly inhibited the activation of NF-κB *in vitro* and *in vivo*, as well as the mRNA expression and subsequent release of pro-inflammatory mediators. Compound A also significantly inhibited LPS- and MPTP-induced DA-neurotoxicity *in vitro*, and this neuroprotective activity required the presence of microglial cells. Most importantly, administration of Compound A to animals injected intranigrally with LPS, attenuated LPS-induced DA neuronal loss and microglia activation within the SN ((Zhang, Qian et al. ; Zhang, Qian et al. 2010). These data provide strong evidence that NF-κB offers a promising potential therapeutic target to halt DA-neurodegeneration, and that much additional work needs to be performed to determine the optimal approach and agent best suited for the treatment of PD.

5.2 β2-AR agonists as PD therapeutics

A family of compounds that have recently been shown to potentially reduce inflammation and DA-neurodegeneration in animal models are the β2 adrenergic receptor agonists. The β2 adrenergic receptor (β2AR) is a G-protein coupled receptor (GPCR) which is known to regulate of smooth muscle function in the airway and vasculature. Interestingly, β2AR expression has also been identified on immune cells such as macrophages, microglia, T cells, and B cells, and signaling through this receptor can inhibit the inflammatory response of these cells (Koff, Fann et al. 1986; Severn, Rapson et al. 1992; van der Poll, Jansen et al. 1994; Sekut, Champion et al. 1995; Panina-Bordignon, Mazzeo et al. 1997; Farmer and Pugin 2000; Kin and Sanders 2006). Both short-acting and long-acting β2AR agonists have been used for pharmacological studies and clinical therapy, and results have indicated that they possess the ability to inhibit the inflammatory responses by immune cells. Several of these long-acting agonists such as salmeterol (Advair®) and formoterol (Symbicort®) are currently being used as anti-inflammatory therapeutics to treat asthma and chronic obstructive pulmonary disease (COPD) (Koto, Mak et al. 1996; Tashkin and Cooper 2004; McKeage and Keam 2009). However, potential use of β2AR agonists in neurodegenerative diseases in the CNS has not been well studied. Since most long-acting β2AR agonists are highly lipophilic and should readily cross the BBB, it is likely that these compounds could have an immunomodulatory effect on the progression of inflammation in PD patients by inhibiting the activation of microglia that normally express high levels of β2AR (Tanaka, Kashima et al. 2002).

When long-acting β2AR agonists were tested for DA-neuroprotective properties, it was found that the compounds can inhibit DA-neurodegeneration *in vitro*, even if used at extremely low doses. Furthermore, administration of the long-acting β2AR agonist salmeterol significantly protects DA neurons against LPS- and MPTP-induced cytotoxicity *in vivo* (Qian, Wu et al. 2011). Mechanistic studies using primary midbrain neuron-glia cultures demonstrated that salmeterol, as well as several other long-acting β2AR agonists, have potent neuroprotective effects through their inhibition of microglial inflammatory mediator production. These anti-inflammatory effects of salmeterol require the presence of β2AR, are mediated through the inhibition of both MAPK and NF-κB signaling pathways in activated microglia, and function independently of the canonical GPCR/cAMP/PKA signaling pathway. It was further determined that this inhibition is dependent on the expression of β-arrestin 2, which suggests a novel mechanism for the long-acting β2AR agonists in regulating CNS inflammatory conditions (Qian, Wu et al. 2011). Therefore, the high specific activity and effectiveness of β2AR agonists such as salmeterol at inhibiting inflammation and DA-neurodegeneration within the CNS in these animal models suggests they have potential for the treatment of chronic inflammatory disorders and in particular, Parkinson's disease.

6. Proposed model of neuroinflammation in PD

Inflammation associated with PD can be initiated in the brain by internal factors such as a brain injury, a genetic mutation or some other brain insult or dysfunction (Nagatsu and Sawada 2006; Tansey, McCoy et al. 2007; Hirsch and Hunot 2009; Qian, Flood et al. 2010)(Figure 1). These sorts of intracerebral inflammatory stimuli activate the microglia which then up-regulate production of inflammatory factors including inflammatory cytokines such as TNFα, IL-1β or IL-6, as well as NO and ROS (Nagatsu, Mogi et al. 2000; Nagatsu and Sawada 2006; Tansey, McCoy et al. 2007). These in turn stimulate a further inflammatory response which results in a self-perpetuating chronic inflammatory condition (Qian and Flood 2008; Qian, Flood et al. 2010). Alternatively, inflammation in the periphery might induce the initial inflammatory response within the brain. Normally, the microvascular endothelial cells that line the blood vessels in the brain are tightly joined to each other through cell-cell tight junctions, and thus form the blood-brain-barrier which excludes most substances or cells from entry into the brain (Zlokovic 2008). A chronic peripheral inflammatory response can work to disrupt the cell-cell junctions and the blood-brain barrier, allowing access of inflammatory factors and cells into the brain (Stamatovic, Keep et al. 2008; Zlokovic 2008). These can then activate microglia and initiate the perpetual round of pro-inflammatory factor production leading to chronic neuroinflammation. Once microglia are activated, from whatever the source of initial inflammatory stimulus, the microglial response increases secretion of inflammatory cytokines and release of NO (Qian and Flood 2008). Microglial activation also precipitates an enhanced respiratory burst and release of ROS (Colton and Gilbert 1987). These various inflammatory mediators can trigger cell death in neurons (Chao, Hu et al. 1992; Colton and Gilbert 1993; Taylor, Jones et al. 2005), including DA neurons which seem to be especially vulnerable. Dying neurons then stimulate an intensified inflammatory response as the brain attempts to restore stasis (Qian, Flood et al. 2010). Therapies aimed at halting neurodegeneration are increasingly based on intervention to top the chronic inflammatory response, including introduction of anti-inflammatory drugs, compounds, cytokines and Treg cells, which inherently release anti-inflammatory cytokines such as TGFβ1 and IL-10.

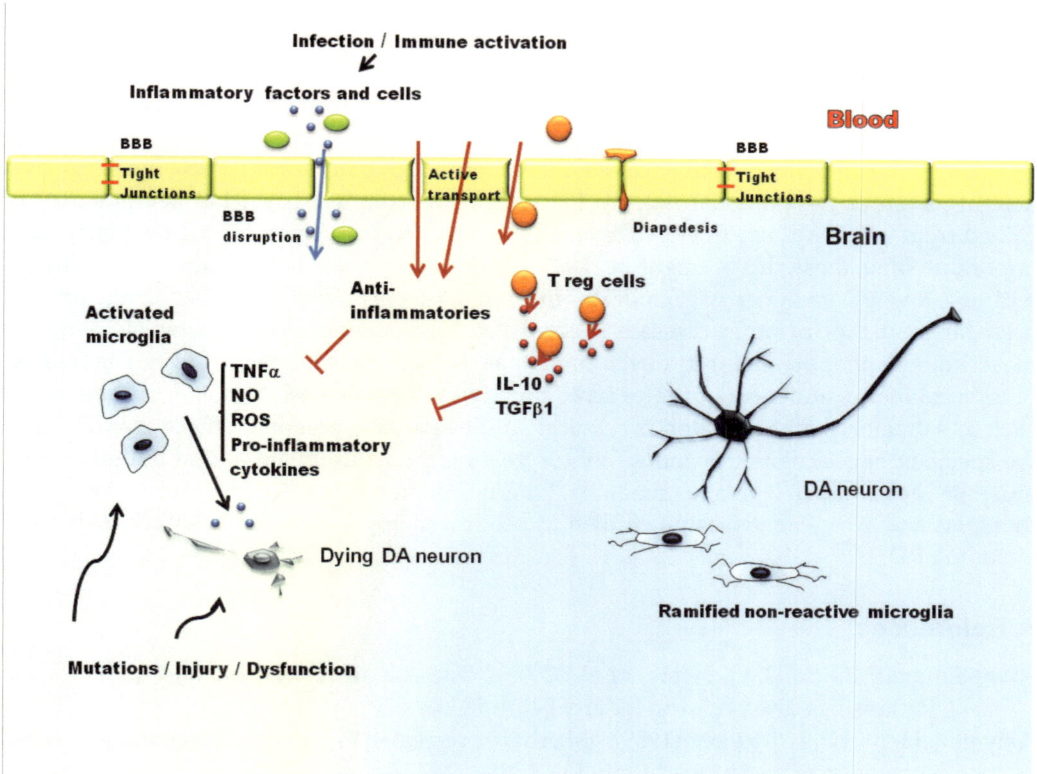

Fig. 1. Model relating chronic inflammation to dopaminergic (DA)-neuron death in Parkinson's Disease.

7. Future directions for PD therapy

Five relatively new approaches in anti-inflammatory therapy described above all show some promise for short-term or long-term therapeutics in PD. The use of exogenous anti-inflammatory cytokines such as IL10 or TGFβ1, has been shown to have potent effects in reducing neurotoxicity in both *in vitro* and in animal models of PD. However, although both cytokines are considered to be predominantly anti-inflammatory, they each can have pro-inflammatory effects in certain contexts. More thorough functional studies are needed for these anti-inflammatory cytokines, especially in the context of PD models before these might be readily used in human therapy. Particularly important factors include what form and what mode of delivery will optimize the anti-inflammatory effects of the cytokines as therapy and ameliorate any unintended negative effects. Cell-based therapies such as regulatory T cells (Tregs) offer great promise for long-term therapy in many degenerative disorders including PD. Both the use of T cells and stem cell transplantation focus on regeneration as well as intervening in neuronal death processes. However, some of the potential problems with these cell-transplant strategies are obvious since these are invasive therapies and as such carry the attendant problems associated with transplants in general as well as the specific consequences of introducing these cells into PD patients. Much remains to be determined before they become readily applicable for PD therapy. Anti-inflammatory therapies have already been developed in animal models of PD and are being used to a limited extent in human studies. The finding that the chronic use of certain NSAIDs seems to lower the risk of PD is promising for possibly reducing PD incidence. Additionally, NSAIDS (or SAIDS) might be used profitably in combinatorial therapy for PD, but the long-term use of these drugs already has well documented potential health problems. Careful determination of the potential risks to PD patients as compared to what benefits may be gained from long-term use of NSAIDS or SAIDS needs to be addressed. This is particularly important since these drugs might be well suited to combinatorial therapy in conjunction with existing PD treatments. Similarly, morphinan-based drugs, or other drugs already used for treatment of other diseases such as beta2-adrenergic receptor agonists, hold the most immediate potential for development as therapeutics to treat PD. The normal pharmacokinetics and safety profiles have already been established for some of these drugs such as salmeterol, and although preclinical studies indicate potential efficacy in PD, again the specific pharmacokinetics and safety for treating the neuroinflammation underlying PD must be determined. Orally available NF-kB inhibitors are equally attractive as PD therapies and are currently being studied in preclinical applications in a variety of diseases including PD.

8. References

Abou-Sleiman, P. M., D. G. Healy, et al. (2003). "The role of pathogenic DJ-1 mutations in Parkinson's disease." Ann Neurol 54(3): 283-6.

Akiyama, H. and P. L. McGeer (1989). "Microglial response to 6-hydroxydopamine-induced substantia nigra lesions." Brain Res 489(2): 247-53.

Albin, R. L., A. B. Young, et al. (1989). "The functional anatomy of basal ganglia disorders." Trends Neurosci 12(10): 366-75.

Angelov, D. N., S. Waibel, et al. (2003). "Therapeutic vaccine for acute and chronic motor neuron diseases: implications for amyotrophic lateral sclerosis." Proc Natl Acad Sci U S A 100(8): 4790-5.

Appel, S. H., D. R. Beers, et al. (2009). "T cell-microglial dialogue in Parkinson's disease and amyotrophic lateral sclerosis: are we listening?" Trends Immunol 31(1): 7-17.

Argaw, A. T., B. T. Gurfein, et al. (2009). "VEGF-mediated disruption of endothelial CLN-5 promotes blood-brain barrier breakdown." Proc Natl Acad Sci U S A 106(6): 1977-82.

Argaw, A. T., Y. Zhang, et al. (2006). "IL-1beta regulates blood-brain barrier permeability via reactivation of the hypoxia-angiogenesis program." J Immunol 177(8): 5574-84.

Atreya, I., R. Atreya, et al. (2008). "NF-kappaB in inflammatory bowel disease." J Intern Med 263(6): 591-6.

Barcia, C., V. Bautista, et al. (2005). "Changes in vascularization in substantia nigra pars compacta of monkeys rendered parkinsonian." J Neural Transm 112(9): 1237-48.

Barcia, C., V. de Pablos, et al. (2005). "Increased plasma levels of TNF-alpha but not of IL1-beta in MPTP-treated monkeys one year after the MPTP administration." Parkinsonism Relat Disord 11(7): 435-9.

Barcia, C., A. Sanchez Bahillo, et al. (2004). "Evidence of active microglia in substantia nigra pars compacta of parkinsonian monkeys 1 year after MPTP exposure." Glia 46(4): 402-9.

Bartels, A. L. and K. L. Leenders (2007). "Neuroinflammation in the pathophysiology of Parkinson's disease: evidence from animal models to human in vivo studies with [11C]-PK11195 PET." Mov Disord 22(13): 1852-6.

Bas, J., M. Calopa, et al. (2001). "Lymphocyte populations in Parkinson's disease and in rat models of parkinsonism." J Neuroimmunol 113(1): 146-52.

Benner, E. J., R. L. Mosley, et al. (2004). "Therapeutic immunization protects dopaminergic neurons in a mouse model of Parkinson's disease." Proc Natl Acad Sci U S A 101(25): 9435-40.

Bernardo, A., M. A. Ajmone-Cat, et al. (2005). "Nuclear receptor peroxisome proliferator-activated receptor-gamma is activated in rat microglial cells by the anti-inflammatory drug HCT1026, a derivative of flurbiprofen." J Neurochem 92(4): 895-903.

Block, M. L. and J. S. Hong (2007). "Chronic microglial activation and progressive dopaminergic neurotoxicity." Biochem Soc Trans 35(Pt 5): 1127-32.

Boka, G., P. Anglade, et al. (1994). "Immunocytochemical analysis of tumor necrosis factor and its receptors in Parkinson's disease." Neurosci Lett 172(1-2): 151-4.

Bonifati, V., Y. H. Wu-Chou, et al. (2008). "LRRK2 mutation analysis in Parkinson disease families with evidence of linkage to PARK8." Neurology 70(24): 2348; author reply 2348-9.

Bonuccelli, U., P. Del Dotto, et al. (1992). "Dextromethorphan and parkinsonism." Lancet 340(8810): 53.

Carrithers, M. D., I. Visintin, et al. (2000). "Differential adhesion molecule requirements for immune surveillance and inflammatory recruitment." Brain 123 (Pt 6): 1092-101.

Castano, A., A. J. Herrera, et al. (2002). "The degenerative effect of a single intranigral injection of LPS on the dopaminergic system is prevented by dexamethasone, and not mimicked by rh-TNF-alpha, IL-1beta and IFN-gamma." J Neurochem 81(1): 150-7.

Chao, C. C., S. Hu, et al. (1992). "Activated microglia mediate neuronal cell injury via a nitric oxide mechanism." J Immunol 149(8): 2736-41.

Chao, Y. X., B. P. He, et al. (2009). "Mesenchymal stem cell transplantation attenuates blood brain barrier damage and neuroinflammation and protects dopaminergic neurons against MPTP toxicity in the substantia nigra in a model of Parkinson's disease." J Neuroimmunol 216(1-2): 39-50.

Chen, C. C. and A. M. Manning (1995). "Transcriptional regulation of endothelial cell adhesion molecules: a dominant role for NF-kappa B." Agents Actions Suppl 47: 135-41.

Chen, H. Q., Z. Y. Jin, et al. (2008). "Luteolin protects dopaminergic neurons from inflammation-induced injury through inhibition of microglial activation." Neurosci Lett 448(2): 175-9.

Chen, W. and S. M. Wahl (2003). "TGF-beta: the missing link in CD4+CD25+ regulatory T cell-mediated immunosuppression." Cytokine Growth Factor Rev 14(2): 85-9.

Choi, D. W. (1987). "Dextrorphan and dextromethorphan attenuate glutamate neurotoxicity." Brain Res 403(2): 333-6.

Choi, D. W., M. Maulucci-Gedde, et al. (1987). "Glutamate neurotoxicity in cortical cell culture." J Neurosci 7(2): 357-68.

Choi, D. W., S. Peters, et al. (1987). "Dextrorphan and levorphanol selectively block N-methyl-D-aspartate receptor-mediated neurotoxicity on cortical neurons." J Pharmacol Exp Ther 242(2): 713-20.

Church, J., D. Lodge, et al. (1985). "Differential effects of dextrorphan and levorphanol on the excitation of rat spinal neurons by amino acids." Eur J Pharmacol 111(2): 185-90.

Cicchetti, F., J. Drouin-Ouellet, et al. (2009). "Environmental toxins and Parkinson's disease: what have we learned from pesticide-induced animal models?" Trends Pharmacol Sci 30(9): 475-83.

Cicchetti, F., N. Lapointe, et al. (2005). "Systemic exposure to paraquat and maneb models early Parkinson's disease in young adult rats." Neurobiol Dis 20(2): 360-71.

Colton, C. A. and D. L. Gilbert (1987). "Production of superoxide anions by a CNS macrophage, the microglia." FEBS Lett 223(2): 284-8.

Colton, C. A. and D. L. Gilbert (1993). "Microglia, an in vivo source of reactive oxygen species in the brain." Adv Neurol 59: 321-6.

Coxon, A., P. Rieu, et al. (1996). "A novel role for the beta 2 integrin CD11b/CD18 in neutrophil apoptosis: a homeostatic mechanism in inflammation." Immunity 5(6): 653-66.

Criswell, L. A. (2010). "Gene discovery in rheumatoid arthritis highlights the CD40/NF-kappaB signaling pathway in disease pathogenesis." Immunol Rev 233(1): 55-61.

Dauer, W. and S. Przedborski (2003). "Parkinson's disease: mechanisms and models." Neuron 39(6): 889-909.

Delgado, M., A. Chorny, et al. (2005). "Vasoactive intestinal peptide generates CD4+CD25+ regulatory T cells in vivo." J Leukoc Biol 78(6): 1327-38.

Dendorfer, U. (1996). "Molecular biology of cytokines." Artif Organs 20(5): 437-44.

Dickson, D. W. (2007). "Linking selective vulnerability to cell death mechanisms in Parkinson's disease." Am J Pathol 170(1): 16-9.

Dobbs, R. J., A. Charlett, et al. (1999). "Association of circulating TNF-alpha and IL-6 with ageing and parkinsonism." Acta Neurol Scand 100(1): 34-41.

Du, Y., Z. Ma, et al. (2001). "Minocycline prevents nigrostriatal dopaminergic neurodegeneration in the MPTP model of Parkinson's disease." Proc Natl Acad Sci U S A 98(25): 14669-74.

Engelhardt, B. and R. M. Ransohoff (2005). "The ins and outs of T-lymphocyte trafficking to the CNS: anatomical sites and molecular mechanisms." Trends Immunol 26(9): 485-95.

Fahn, S. (2003). "Description of Parkinson's disease as a clinical syndrome." Ann N Y Acad Sci 991: 1-14.

Farmer, P. and J. Pugin (2000). "beta-adrenergic agonists exert their "anti-inflammatory" effects in monocytic cells through the IkappaB/NF-kappaB pathway." Am J Physiol Lung Cell Mol Physiol 279(4): L675-82.

Farrer, M. J., K. Haugarvoll, et al. (2006). "Genomewide association, Parkinson disease, and PARK10." Am J Hum Genet 78(6): 1084-8; author reply 1092-4.

Faucheux, B. A., A. M. Bonnet, et al. (1999). "Blood vessels change in the mesencephalon of patients with Parkinson's disease." Lancet 353(9157): 981-2.

Fernandez-Checa, J. C., N. Kaplowitz, et al. (1997). "GSH transport in mitochondria: defense against TNF-induced oxidative stress and alcohol-induced defect." Am J Physiol 273(1 Pt 1): G7-17.

Fernandez-Martin, A., E. Gonzalez-Rey, et al. (2006). "Vasoactive intestinal peptide induces regulatory T cells during experimental autoimmune encephalomyelitis." Eur J Immunol 36(2): 318-26.

Flood, P. M., L. Qian, et al. (2011). "Transcriptional Factor NF-kB as a Target for Therapy in Parkinson's Disease." Inflammation and Parkinson's Disease, SAGE-Hindawi, pub. in press.

Floyd, R. A. (1999). "Antioxidants, oxidative stress, and degenerative neurological disorders." Proc Soc Exp Biol Med 222(3): 236-45.

Floyd, R. A. (1999). "Neuroinflammatory processes are important in neurodegenerative diseases: an hypothesis to explain the increased formation of reactive oxygen and nitrogen species as major factors involved in neurodegenerative disease development." Free Radic Biol Med 26(9-10): 1346-55.

Gao, H. M. and J. S. Hong (2008). "Why neurodegenerative diseases are progressive: uncontrolled inflammation drives disease progression." Trends Immunol 29(8): 357-65.

Gao, H. M., J. Jiang, et al. (2002). "Microglial activation-mediated delayed and progressive degeneration of rat nigral dopaminergic neurons: relevance to Parkinson's disease." J Neurochem 81(6): 1285-97.

Gao, H. M., B. Liu, et al. (2003). "Critical role for microglial NADPH oxidase in rotenone-induced degeneration of dopaminergic neurons." J Neurosci 23(15): 6181-7.

Gao, J., H. Miao, et al. (2011). "Influence of aging on the dopaminergic neurons in the substantia nigra pars compacta of rats." Curr Aging Sci 4(1): 19-24.

Gao, X., H. Chen, et al. (2011). "Use of ibuprofen and risk of Parkinson disease." Neurology 76(10): 863-9.

Gauss, K. A., L. K. Nelson-Overton, et al. (2007). "Role of NF-kappaB in transcriptional regulation of the phagocyte NADPH oxidase by tumor necrosis factor-alpha." J Leukoc Biol 82(3): 729-41.

Ghosh, A., A. Roy, et al. (2007). "Selective inhibition of NF-kappaB activation prevents dopaminergic neuronal loss in a mouse model of Parkinson's disease." Proc Natl Acad Sci U S A 104(47): 18754-9.

Godbout, J. P. and R. W. Johnson (2009). "Age and Neuroinflammation: A Lifetime of Psychoneuroimmune Consequences." Immunology and Allergy Clinics of North America 29(2): 321-337.

Goldberg, M. P., J. H. Weiss, et al. (1987). "N-methyl-D-aspartate receptors mediate hypoxic neuronal injury in cortical culture." J Pharmacol Exp Ther 243(2): 784-91.

Greenamyre, J. T. and C. F. O'Brien (1991). "N-methyl-D-aspartate antagonists in the treatment of Parkinson's disease." Arch Neurol 48(9): 977-81.

Groemping, Y. and K. Rittinger (2005). "Activation and assembly of the NADPH oxidase: a structural perspective." Biochem J 386(Pt 3): 401-16.

Gutierrez, E. G., W. A. Banks, et al. (1993). "Murine tumor necrosis factor alpha is transported from blood to brain in the mouse." J Neuroimmunol 47(2): 169-76.

Halliwell, B. (2006). "Oxidative stress and neurodegeneration: where are we now?" J Neurochem 97(6): 1634-58.

Henrich-Noack, P., J. H. Prehn, et al. (1996). "TGF-beta 1 protects hippocampal neurons against degeneration caused by transient global ischemia. Dose-response relationship and potential neuroprotective mechanisms." Stroke 27(9): 1609-14; discussion 1615.

Herrera, A. J., M. Tomas-Camardiel, et al. (2005). "Inflammatory process as a determinant factor for the degeneration of substantia nigra dopaminergic neurons." J Neural Transm 112(1): 111-9.

Hirsch, E. C. (2000). "Nigrostriatal system plasticity in Parkinson's disease: effect of dopaminergic denervation and treatment." Ann Neurol 47(4 Suppl 1): S115-20; discussion S120-1.

Hirsch, E. C. and S. Hunot (2009). "Neuroinflammation in Parkinson's disease: a target for neuroprotection?" Lancet Neurol 8(4): 382-97.

Hisanaga, K., M. Asagi, et al. (2001). "Increase in peripheral CD4 bright+ CD8 dull+ T cells in Parkinson disease." Arch Neurol 58(10): 1580-3.

Hu, X., D. Zhang, et al. (2008). "Macrophage antigen complex-1 mediates reactive microgliosis and progressive dopaminergic neurodegeneration in the MPTP model of Parkinson's disease." J Immunol 181(10): 7194-204.

Huusko, J., M. Merentie, et al. (2009). "The effects of VEGF-R1 and VEGF-R2 ligands on angiogenic responses and left ventricular function in mice." Cardiovasc Res.

Huxford, T. and G. Ghosh (2009). "A structural guide to proteins of the NF-kappaB signaling module." Cold Spring Harb Perspect Biol 1(3): a000075.

Imamura, K., N. Hishikawa, et al. (2003). "Distribution of major histocompatability complex 1-positive microglia and cytokine profile of Parkinson's disease brains." Acta Neuropathol 106: 518-526.

Jackson-Lewis, V. and S. Przedborski (2007). "Protocol for the MPTP mouse model of Parkinson's disease." Nat Protoc 2(1): 141-51.

Jackson-Lewis, V. and R. J. Smeyne (2005). "MPTP and SNpc DA neuronal vulnerability: role of dopamine, superoxide and nitric oxide in neurotoxicity. Minireview." Neurotox Res 7(3): 193-202.

Jellinger, K. A. (2001). "The pathology of Parkinson's disease." Adv Neurol 86: 55-72.

Jenner, P. and C. W. Olanow (1996). "Oxidative stress and the pathogenesis of Parkinson's disease." Neurology 47(6 Suppl 3): S161-70.

Jenner, P. and C. W. Olanow (1998). "Understanding cell death in Parkinson's disease." Ann Neurol 44(3 Suppl 1): S72-84.

Jenner, P. and C. W. Olanow (2006). "The pathogenesis of cell death in Parkinson's disease." Neurology 66(10 Suppl 4): S24-36.

Ji, S., G. Kronenberg, et al. (2009). "Acute neuroprotection by pioglitazone after mild brain ischemia without effect on long-term outcome." Exp Neurol 216(2): 321-8.

Jiang, H., Y. C. Wu, et al. (2007). "Parkinson's disease genetic mutations increase cell susceptibility to stress: mutant alpha-synuclein enhances H2O2- and Sin-1-induced cell death." Neurobiol Aging 28(11): 1709-17.

Johnston, L. C., X. Su, et al. (2008). "Human interleukin-10 gene transfer is protective in a rat model of Parkinson's disease." Mol Ther 16(8): 1392-9.

Kang, S. S., J. Y. Lee, et al. (2004). "Neuroprotective effects of flavones on hydrogen peroxide-induced apoptosis in SH-SY5Y neuroblostoma cells." Bioorg Med Chem Lett 14(9): 2261-4.

Keeney, P. M., J. Xie, et al. (2006). "Parkinson's disease brain mitochondrial complex I has oxidatively damaged subunits and is functionally impaired and misassembled." J Neurosci 26(19): 5256-64.

Kim, W. G., R. P. Mohney, et al. (2000). "Regional difference in susceptibility to lipopolysaccharide-induced neurotoxicity in the rat brain: role of microglia." J Neurosci 20(16): 6309-16.

Kin, N. W. and V. M. Sanders (2006). "It takes nerve to tell T and B cells what to do." J Leukoc Biol 79(6): 1093-104.

Kipnis, J. and M. Schwartz (2002). "Dual action of glatiramer acetate (Cop-1) in the treatment of CNS autoimmune and neurodegenerative disorders." Trends Mol Med 8(7): 319-23.

Kirk, S. L. and S. J. Karlik (2003). "VEGF and vascular changes in chronic neuroinflammation." Journal of Autoimmunity 21(4): 353-363.

Klockgether, T. (2004). "Parkinson's disease: clinical aspects." Cell Tissue Res 318(1): 115-20.

Knott, C., G. Stern, et al. (2000). "Inflammatory regulators in Parkinson's disease: iNOS, lipocortin-1, and cyclooxygenases-1 and -2." Mol Cell Neurosci 16(6): 724-39.

Koff, W. C., A. V. Fann, et al. (1986). "Catecholamine-induced suppression of interleukin-1 production." Lymphokine Res 5(4): 239-47.

Koh, J. Y. and D. W. Choi (1987). "Effect of anticonvulsant drugs on glutamate neurotoxicity in cortical cell culture." Neurology 37(2): 319-22.

Kohutnicka, M., E. Lewandowska, et al. (1998). "Microglial and astrocytic involvement in a murine model of Parkinson's disease induced by 1-methyl-4-phenyl-1,2,3,6-tetrahydropyridine (MPTP)." Immunopharmacology 39(3): 167-180.

Kortekaas, R., K. L. Leenders, et al. (2005). "Blood-brain barrier dysfunction in parkinsonian midbrain in vivo." Ann Neurol 57(2): 176-9.

Koto, H., J. C. Mak, et al. (1996). "Mechanisms of impaired beta-adrenoceptor-induced airway relaxation by interleukin-1beta in vivo in the rat." J Clin Invest 98(8): 1780-7.

Krige, D., M. T. Carroll, et al. (1992). "Platelet mitochondrial function in Parkinson's disease. The Royal Kings and Queens Parkinson Disease Research Group." Ann Neurol 32(6): 782-8.

Kurkowska-Jastrzebska, I., T. Litwin, et al. (2004). "Dexamethasone protects against dopaminergic neurons damage in a mouse model of Parkinson's disease." Int Immunopharmacol 4(10-11): 1307-18.

Kurkowska-Jastrzebska, I., A. Wronska, et al. (1999). "The inflammatory reaction following 1-methyl-4-phenyl-1,2,3, 6-tetrahydropyridine intoxication in mouse." Exp Neurol 156(1): 50-61.

Langston, J. W., L. S. Forno, et al. (1999). "Evidence of active nerve cell degeneration in the substantia nigra of humans years after 1-methyl-4-phenyl-1,2,3,6-tetrahydropyridine exposure." Ann Neurol 46(4): 598-605.

Lappas, M., M. Permezel, et al. (2002). "Nuclear factor kappa B regulation of proinflammatory cytokines in human gestational tissues in vitro." Biol Reprod 67(2): 668-73.

Latanich, C. A. and L. H. Toledo-Pereyra (2009). "Searching for NF-kappaB-based treatments of ischemia reperfusion injury." J Invest Surg 22(4): 301-15.

Lawrence, T. (2009). "The nuclear factor NF-kappaB pathway in inflammation." Cold Spring Harb Perspect Biol 1(6): a001651.

Lawrence, T. and C. Fong "The resolution of inflammation: anti-inflammatory roles for NF-kappaB." Int J Biochem Cell Biol 42(4): 519-23.

Lee, M., T. Cho, et al. (2010). "Depletion of GSH in glial cells induces neurotoxicity: relevance to aging and degenerative neurological diseases." The FASEB Journal 24(7): 2533-2545.

Lehnardt, S., L. Massillon, et al. (2003). "Activation of innate immunity in the CNS triggers neurodegeneration through a Toll-like receptor 4-dependent pathway." Proc Natl Acad Sci U S A 100(14): 8514-9.

Lin, M. T. and M. F. Beal (2006). "Mitochondrial dysfunction and oxidative stress in neurodegenerative diseases." Nature 443(7113): 787-95.

Litteljohn, D., E. Mangano, et al. (2011). "Inflammatory mechanisms of neurodegeneration in toxin-based models of Parkinson's disease." Parkinsons Dis 2011: 713517.

Liu, B. and J. S. Hong (2003). "Neuroprotective effect of naloxone in inflammation-mediated dopaminergic neurodegeneration. Dissociation from the involvement of opioid receptors." Methods Mol Med 79: 43-54.

Liu, J., N. Gong, et al. (2009). "Neuromodulatory activities of CD4+CD25+ regulatory T cells in a murine model of HIV-1-associated neurodegeneration." J Immunol 182(6): 3855-65.

Liu, L., E. Buchner, et al. (1996). "Amelioration of rat experimental arthritides by treatment with the alkaloid sinomenine." Int J Immunopharmacol 18(10): 529-43.

Liu, L., K. Resch, et al. (1994). "Inhibition of lymphocyte proliferation by the anti-arthritic drug sinomenine." Int J Immunopharmacol 16(8): 685-91.

Liu, Y., L. Qin, et al. (2003). "Dextromethorphan protects dopaminergic neurons against inflammation-mediated degeneration through inhibition of microglial activation." J Pharmacol Exp Ther 305(1): 212-8.

Loeffler, D. A., D. M. Camp, et al. (2006). "Complement activation in the Parkinson's disease substantia nigra: an immunocytochemical study." J Neuroinflammation 3: 29.

Lotan, M. and M. Schwartz (1994). "Cross-talk between the immune system and the nervous system in response to injury: immplications for regeneration." FASEB J 8(13): 1026-1033.

Lucking, C. B., A. Durr, et al. (2000). "Association between early-onset Parkinson's disease and mutations in the parkin gene." N Engl J Med 342(21): 1560-7.

Marshall, K. A., M. Reist, et al. (1999). "The neuronal toxicity of sulfite plus peroxynitrite is enhanced by glutathione depletion: implications for Parkinson's disease." Free Radic Biol Med 27(5-6): 515-20.

Matarese, G., V. De Rosa, et al. (2008). "Regulatory CD4 T cells: sensing the environment." Trends Immunol 29(1): 12-7.

May, M. J., R. B. Marienfeld, et al. (2002). "Characterization of the Ikappa B-kinase NEMO binding domain." J Biol Chem 277(48): 45992-6000.

McGeachy, M. J., K. S. Bak-Jensen, et al. (2007). "TGF-beta and IL-6 drive the production of IL-17 and IL-10 by T cells and restrain T(H)-17 cell-mediated pathology." Nat Immunol 8(12): 1390-7.

McGeer, P. L., S. Itagaki, et al. (1988). "Reactive microglia are positive for HLA-DR in the substantia nigra of Parkinson's and Alzheimer's disease brains." Neurology 38(8): 1285-91.

McGeer, P. L. and E. G. McGeer (2004). "Inflammation and the degenerative diseases of aging." Ann N Y Acad Sci 1035: 104-16.

McGeer, P. L., C. Schwab, et al. (2003). "Presence of reactive microglia in monkey substantia nigra years after 1-methyl-4-phenyl-1,2,3,6-tetrahydropyridine administration." Ann Neurol 54(5): 599-604.

McGeer, P. L., K. Yasojima, et al. (2001). "Inflammation in Parkinson's disease." Adv Neurol 86: 83-9.

McKeage, K. and S. J. Keam (2009). "Salmeterol/fluticasone propionate: a review of its use in asthma." Drugs 69(13): 1799-828.

Mizuno, Y., N. Hattori, et al. (2001). "Familial Parkinson's disease. Alpha-synuclein and parkin." Adv Neurol 86: 13-21.

Mogi, M., M. Harada, et al. (1994). "Interleukin-1 beta, interleukin-6, epidermal growth factor and transforming growth factor-alpha are elevated in the brain from parkinsonian patients." Neurosci Lett 180(2): 147-50.

Mogi, M., M. Harada, et al. (1996). "Interleukin (IL)-1 beta, IL-2, IL-4, IL-6 and transforming growth factor-alpha levels are elevated in ventricular cerebrospinal fluid in juvenile parkinsonism and Parkinson's disease." Neurosci Lett 211(1): 13-6.

Mogi, M., M. Harada, et al. (1994). "Tumor necrosis factor-alpha (TNF-alpha) increases both in the brain and in the cerebrospinal fluid from parkinsonian patients." Neurosci Lett 165(1-2): 208-10.

Monahan, A. J., M. Warren, et al. (2008). "Neuroinflammation and peripheral immune infiltration in Parkinson's disease: an autoimmune hypothesis." Cell Transplant 17(4): 363-72.

Montastruc, J. L., N. Fabre, et al. (1994). "N-methyl-D-aspartate (NMDA) antagonist and Parkinson's disease: a pilot study with dextromethorphan." Mov Disord 9(2): 242-3.

Moore, P. E., T. Lahiri, et al. (2001). "Selected contribution: synergism between TNF-alpha and IL-1 beta in airway smooth muscle cells: implications for beta-adrenergic responsiveness." J Appl Physiol 91(3): 1467-74.

Mosley, R. L., E. J. Benner, et al. (2006). "Neuroinflammation, Oxidative Stress and the Pathogenesis of Parkinson's Disease." Clin Neurosci Res 6(5): 261-281.

Moss, N. C., W. E. Stansfield, et al. (2007). "IKKbeta inhibition attenuates myocardial injury and dysfunction following acute ischemia-reperfusion injury." Am J Physiol Heart Circ Physiol 293(4): H2248-2253.

Nagatsu, T., M. Mogi, et al. (2000). "Changes in cytokines and neurotrophins in Parkinson's disease." J Neural Transm Suppl(60): 277-90.

Nagatsu, T., M. Mogi, et al. (2000). "Cytokines in Parkinson's disease." J Neural Transm Suppl(58): 143-51.

Nagatsu, T. and M. Sawada (2006). "Cellular and molecular mechanisms of Parkinson's disease: neurotoxins, causative genes, and inflammatory cytokines." Cell Mol Neurobiol 26(4-6): 781-802.

Naik, E. and V. M. Dixit (2011). "Mitochondrial reactive oxygen species drive proinflammatory cytokine production." The Journal of Experimental Medicine 208(3): 417-420.

Natarajan, C. and J. J. Bright (2002). "Curcumin inhibits experimental allergic encephalomyelitis by blocking IL-12 signaling through Janus kinase-STAT pathway in T lymphocytes." J Immunol 168(12): 6506-13.

Negi, G., A. Kumar, et al. (2011). "Melatonin modulates neuroinflammation and oxidative stress in experimental diabetic neuropathy: effects on NF-κB and Nrf2 cascades." Journal of Pineal Research 50(2): 124-131.

Neuwelt, E. A. and W. K. Clark (1978). "The immune system and the nervous system." Neurosurgery 3(3): 419-430.

Nguyen, M. D., T. D'Aigle, et al. (2004). "Exacerbation of motor neuron disease by chronic stimulation of innate immunity in a mouse model of amyotrophic lateral sclerosis." J Neurosci 24(6): 1340-9.

Nguyen, M. D., J. P. Julien, et al. (2002). "Innate immunity: the missing link in neuroprotection and neurodegeneration?" Nat Rev Neurosci 3(3): 216-27.

Nguyen, Q. D., S. Tatlipinar, et al. (2006). "Vascular endothelial growth factor is a critical stimulus for diabetic macular edema." Am J Ophthalmol 142(6): 961-9.

Niehaus, I. and J. H. Lange (2003). "Endotoxin: is it an environmental factor in the cause of Parkinson's disease?" Occup Environ Med 60(5): 378.

Oeckinghaus, A. and S. Ghosh (2009). "The NF-kappaB family of transcription factors and its regulation." Cold Spring Harb Perspect Biol 1(4): a000034.

Orr, C. F., D. B. Rowe, et al. (2002). "An inflammatory review of Parkinson's disease." Prog Neurobiol 68(5): 325-40.

Orr, C. F., D. B. Rowe, et al. (2005). "A possible role for humoral immunity in the pathogenesis of Parkinson's disease." Brain 128(Pt 11): 2665-74.

Owen, A. D., A. H. Schapira, et al. (1996). "Oxidative stress and Parkinson's disease." Ann N Y Acad Sci 786: 217-23.

Pachter, J. S., H. E. de Vries, et al. (2003). "The blood-brain barrier and its role in immune privilege in the central nervous system." J Neuropathol Exp Neurol 62(6): 593-604.

Pan, W. and A. J. Kastin (2002). "TNF[alpha] Transport across the Blood-Brain Barrier Is Abolished in Receptor Knockout Mice." Experimental Neurology 174(2): 193-200.

Panina-Bordignon, P., D. Mazzeo, et al. (1997). "Beta2-agonists prevent Th1 development by selective inhibition of interleukin 12." J Clin Invest 100(6): 1513-9.

Park, K. M. and W. J. Bowers (2010). "Tumor necrosis factor-alpha mediated signaling in neuronal homeostasis and dysfunction." Cell Signal 22(7): 977-83.

Pearce, R. K., A. Owen, et al. (1997). "Alterations in the distribution of glutathione in the substantia nigra in Parkinson's disease." J Neural Transm 104(6-7): 661-77.

Pei, Z., H. Pang, et al. (2007). "MAC1 mediates LPS-induced production of superoxide by microglia: the role of pattern recognition receptors in dopaminergic neurotoxicity." Glia 55(13): 1362-73.

Pereira, S. G. and F. Oakley (2008). "Nuclear factor-kappaB1: regulation and function." Int J Biochem Cell Biol 40(8): 1425-30.

Pisani, V., V. Moschella, et al. (2010). "Dynamic changes of anandamide in the cerebrospinal fluid of Parkinson's disease patients." Movement Disorders 25(7): 920-924.

Polymeropoulos, M. H., C. Lavedan, et al. (1997). "Mutation in the alpha-synuclein gene identified in families with Parkinson's disease." Science 276(5321): 2045-7.

Pope, L. E., M. H. Khalil, et al. (2004). "Pharmacokinetics of dextromethorphan after single or multiple dosing in combination with quinidine in extensive and poor metabolizers." J Clin Pharmacol 44(10): 1132-42.

Prehn, J. H. and J. Krieglstein (1994). "Opposing effects of transforming growth factor-beta 1 on glutamate neurotoxicity." Neuroscience 60(1): 7-10.

Qian, L., M. L. Block, et al. (2006). "Interleukin-10 protects lipopolysaccharide-induced neurotoxicity in primary midbrain cultures by inhibiting the function of NADPH oxidase." J Pharmacol Exp Ther 319(1): 44-52.

Qian, L. and P. M. Flood (2008). "Microglial cells and Parkinson's disease." Immunol Res 41(3): 155-64.

Qian, L., P. M. Flood, et al. (2010). "Neuroinflammation is a key player in Parkinson's disease and a prime target for therapy." J Neural Transm 117(8): 971-9.

Qian, L., X. Gao, et al. (2007). "NADPH oxidase inhibitor DPI is neuroprotective at femtomolar concentrations through inhibition of microglia over-activation." Parkinsonism Relat Disord 13 Suppl 3: S316-20.

Qian, L., K. S. Tan, et al. (2007). "Microglia-mediated neurotoxicity is inhibited by morphine through an opioid receptor-independent reduction of NADPH oxidase activity." J Immunol 179(2): 1198-209.

Qian, L., S. J. Wei, et al. (2008). "Potent anti-inflammatory and neuroprotective effects of TGF-beta1 are mediated through the inhibition of ERK and p47phox-Ser345 phosphorylation and translocation in microglia." J Immunol 181(1): 660-8.

Qian, L., H. M. Wu, et al. (2011). "{beta}2-Adrenergic Receptor Activation Prevents Rodent Dopaminergic Neurotoxicity by Inhibiting Microglia via a Novel Signaling Pathway." J Immunol. 186: 4443-4454.

Qian, L., Z. Xu, et al. (2007). "Sinomenine, a natural dextrorotatory morphinan analog, is anti-inflammatory and neuroprotective through inhibition of microglial NADPH oxidase." J Neuroinflammation 4: 23.

Qin, L., Y. Liu, et al. (2004). "NADPH oxidase mediates lipopolysaccharide-induced neurotoxicity and proinflammatory gene expression in activated microglia." J Biol Chem 279(2): 1415-21.

Qin, L., X. Wu, et al. (2007). "Systemic LPS causes chronic neuroinflammation and progressive neurodegeneration." Glia 55(5): 453-62.

Qureshi, G. A., S. Baig, et al. (1995). "Increased cerebrospinal fluid concentration of nitrite in Parkinson's disease." Neuroreport 6(12): 1642-4.

Ransohoff, R. M. and V. H. Perry (2009). "Microglial physiology: unique stimuli, specialized responses." Annu Rev Immunol 27: 119-45.

Reale, M., N. H. Greig, et al. (2009). "Peripheral chemo-cytokine profiles in Alzheimer's and Parkinson's diseases." Mini Rev Med Chem 9(10): 1229-41.

Reuther-Madrid, J. Y., D. Kashatus, et al. (2002). "The p65/RelA subunit of NF-kappaB suppresses the sustained, antiapoptotic activity of Jun kinase induced by tumor necrosis factor." Mol Cell Biol 22(23): 8175-83.

Reynolds, A. D., R. Banerjee, et al. (2007). "Neuroprotective activities of CD4+CD25+ regulatory T cells in an animal model of Parkinson's disease." J Leukoc Biol 82(5): 1083-94.

Reynolds, A. D., D. K. Stone, et al. (2010). "Regulatory T cells attenuate Th17 cell-mediated nigrostriatal dopaminergic neurodegeneration in a model of Parkinson's disease." J Immunol 184(5): 2261-71.

Reynolds, A. D., D. K. Stone, et al. (2009). "Nitrated {alpha}-synuclein-induced alterations in microglial immunity are regulated by CD4+ T cell subsets." J Immunol 182(7): 4137-49.

Rite, I., A. Machado, et al. (2007). "Blood-brain barrier disruption induces in vivo degeneration of nigral dopaminergic neurons." J Neurochem 101(6): 1567-82.

Roebuck, K. A. (1999). "Regulation of interleukin-8 gene expression." J Interferon Cytokine Res 19(5): 429-38.

Roebuck, K. A., L. R. Carpenter, et al. (1999). "Stimulus-specific regulation of chemokine expression involves differential activation of the redox-responsive transcription factors AP-1 and NF-kappaB." J Leukoc Biol 65(3): 291-8.

Rudolph, D., W. C. Yeh, et al. (2000). "Severe liver degeneration and lack of NF-kappaB activation in NEMO/IKKgamma-deficient mice." Genes Dev 14(7): 854-62.

Ruocco, A., O. Nicole, et al. (1999). "A transforming growth factor-beta antagonist unmasks the neuroprotective role of this endogenous cytokine in excitotoxic and ischemic brain injury." J Cereb Blood Flow Metab 19(12): 1345-53.

Ryu, J. K. and J. G. McLarnon (2008). "VEGF receptor antagonist Cyclo-VEGI reduces inflammatory reactivity and vascular leakiness and is neuroprotective against acute excitotoxic striatal insult." J Neuroinflammation 5: 18.

Sairam, K., K. S. Saravanan, et al. (2003). "Non-steroidal anti-inflammatory drug sodium salicylate, but not diclofenac or celecoxib, protects against 1-methyl-4-phenyl pyridinium-induced dopaminergic neurotoxicity in rats." Brain Res 966(2): 245-52.

Sawada, M., K. Imamura, et al. (2006). "Role of cytokines in inflammatory process in Parkinson's disease." J Neural Transm Suppl(70): 373-81.

Schapira, A. H. (1994). "Mitochondrial function and neurotoxicity." Curr Opin Neurol 7(6): 531-4.

Schapira, A. H. (2006). "Etiology of Parkinson's disease." Neurology 66(10 Suppl 4): S10-23.

Schapira, A. H., J. M. Cooper, et al. (1989). "Mitochondrial complex I deficiency in Parkinson's disease." Lancet 1(8649): 1269.

Schwartz, M. (2004). "Protective autoimmunity and prospects for therapeutic vaccination against self-perpetuating neurodegeneration." Ernst Schering Res Found Workshop(47): 133-54.

Sekut, L., B. R. Champion, et al. (1995). "Anti-inflammatory activity of salmeterol: down-regulation of cytokine production." Clin Exp Immunol 99(3): 461-6.

Sen, R. and D. Baltimore (1986). "Inducibility of kappa immunoglobulin enhancer-binding protein Nf-kappa B by a posttranslational mechanism." Cell 47(6): 921-8.

Sen, R. and D. Baltimore (1986). "Multiple nuclear factors interact with the immunoglobulin enhancer sequences." Cell 46(5): 705-16.

Severn, A., N. T. Rapson, et al. (1992). "Regulation of tumor necrosis factor production by adrenaline and beta-adrenergic agonists." J Immunol 148(11): 3441-5.

Sherer, T. B., R. Betarbet, et al. (2002). "Environment, mitochondria, and Parkinson's disease." Neuroscientist 8(3): 192-7.

Singh, S., K. Singh, et al. (2008). "Nicotine and caffeine-mediated modulation in the expression of toxicant responsive genes and vesicular monoamine transporter-2 in 1-methyl 4-phenyl-1,2,3,6-tetrahydropyridine-induced Parkinson's disease phenotype in mouse." Brain Res 1207: 193-206.

Sizemore, N., A. Agarwal, et al. (2004). "Inhibitor of kappaB kinase is required to activate a subset of interferon gamma-stimulated genes." Proc Natl Acad Sci U S A 101(21): 7994-8.

Sizemore, N., N. Lerner, et al. (2002). "Distinct roles of the Ikappa B kinase alpha and beta subunits in liberating nuclear factor kappa B (NF-kappa B) from Ikappa B and in phosphorylating the p65 subunit of NF-kappa B." J Biol Chem 277(6): 3863-9.

Smeyne, M., Y. Jiao, et al. (2005). "Glia cell number modulates sensitivity to MPTP in mice." Glia 52(2): 144-52.

Smith, A. D. and M. J. Zigmond (2003). "Can the brain be protected through exercise? Lessons from an animal model of parkinsonism." Exp Neurol 184(1): 31-9.

Smith, T. W., U. DeGirolami, et al. (1992). "Neuropathology of immunosuppression." Brain Pathol 2(3): 183-194.

Sofic, E., K. W. Lange, et al. (1992). "Reduced and oxidized glutathione in the substantia nigra of patients with Parkinson's disease." Neurosci Lett 142(2): 128-30.

Spencer, J. P., P. Jenner, et al. (1998). "Conjugates of catecholamines with cysteine and GSH in Parkinson's disease: possible mechanisms of formation involving reactive oxygen species." J Neurochem 71(5): 2112-22.

Stamatovic, S. M., R. F. Keep, et al. (2008). "Brain endothelial cell-cell junctions: how to "open" the blood brain barrier." Curr Neuropharmacol 6(3): 179-92.

Strle, K., J. H. Zhou, et al. (2001). "Interleukin-10 in the brain." Crit Rev Immunol 21(5): 427-49.

Suidan, G. L., J. W. Dickerson, et al. (2010). "CD8 T cell-initiated vascular endothelial growth factor expression promotes central nervous system vascular permeability under neuroinflammatory conditions." J Immunol 184(2): 1031-40.

Sun, M., J. C. Latourelle, et al. (2006). "Influence of heterozygosity for parkin mutation on onset age in familial Parkinson disease: the GenePD study." Arch Neurol 63(6): 826-32.

Szczepanik, M., M. Tutaj, et al. (2005). "Epicutaneously induced TGF-beta-dependent tolerance inhibits experimental autoimmune encephalomyelitis." J Neuroimmunol 164(1-2): 105-14.

Tak, P. P. and G. S. Firestein (2001). "NF-kappaB: a key role in inflammatory diseases." J Clin Invest 107(1): 7-11.

Tanaka, K. F., H. Kashima, et al. (2002). "Existence of functional beta1- and beta2-adrenergic receptors on microglia." J Neurosci Res 70(2): 232-7.

Tanner, C. M. (2003). "Is the cause of Parkinson's disease environmental or hereditary? Evidence from twin studies." Adv Neurol 91: 133-42.

Tansey, M. G., M. K. McCoy, et al. (2007). "Neuroinflammatory mechanisms in Parkinson's disease: potential environmental triggers, pathways, and targets for early therapeutic intervention." Exp Neurol 208(1): 1-25.

Tashkin, D. P. and C. B. Cooper (2004). "The role of long-acting bronchodilators in the management of stable COPD." Chest 125(1): 249-59.

Taylor, D. L., F. Jones, et al. (2005). "Stimulation of microglial metabotropic glutamate receptor mGlu2 triggers tumor necrosis factor alpha-induced neurotoxicity in concert with microglial-derived Fas ligand." J Neurosci 25(11): 2952-64.

Teismann, P. and J. B. Schulz (2004). "Cellular pathology of Parkinson's disease: astrocytes, microglia and inflammation." Cell Tissue Res 318(1): 149-61.

Tetrud, J. W., J. W. Langston, et al. (1989). "Mild parkinsonism in persons exposed to 1-methyl-4-phenyl-1,2,3,6-tetrahydropyridine (MPTP)." Neurology 39(11): 1483-7.

Thomas, M. P., K. Chartrand, et al. (2007). "Ion channel blockade attenuates aggregated alpha synuclein induction of microglial reactive oxygen species: relevance for the pathogenesis of Parkinson's disease." J Neurochem 100(2): 503-19.

Tortella, F. C., J. W. Ferkany, et al. (1988). "Anticonvulsant effects of dextrorphan in rats: possible involvement in dextromethorphan-induced seizure protection." Life Sci 42(24): 2509-14.

Tsoulfas, G. and D. A. Geller (2001). "NF-kappaB in transplantation: friend or foe?" Transpl Infect Dis 3(4): 212-9.

Unsicker, K. and K. Krieglstein (2002). "TGF-betas and their roles in the regulation of neuron survival." Adv Exp Med Biol 513: 353-74.

Van der Heiden, K., S. Cuhlmann, et al. "Role of nuclear factor kappaB in cardiovascular health and disease." Clin Sci (Lond) 118(10): 593-605.

van der Poll, T., J. Jansen, et al. (1994). "Noradrenaline inhibits lipopolysaccharide-induced tumor necrosis factor and interleukin 6 production in human whole blood." Infect Immun 62(5): 2046-50.

Van Snick, J. (1990). "Interleukin-6: an overview." Annu Rev Immunol 8: 253-78.

Vandenbroeck, K., I. Alloza, et al. (2004). "Inhibiting cytokines of the interleukin-12 family: recent advances and novel challenges." J Pharm Pharmacol 56(2): 145-60.

Verhagen Metman, L., P. J. Blanchet, et al. (1998). "A trial of dextromethorphan in parkinsonian patients with motor response complications." Mov Disord 13(3): 414-7.

Verhagen Metman, L., P. Del Dotto, et al. (1998). "Dextromethorphan improves levodopa-induced dyskinesias in Parkinson's disease." Neurology 51(1): 203-6.

Vilar, R., H. Coelho, et al. (2007). "Association of A313 G polymorphism (GSTP1*B) in the glutathione-S-transferase P1 gene with sporadic Parkinson's disease." Eur J Neurol 14(2): 156-61.

Wada, K., H. Arai, et al. (2006). "Expression levels of vascular endothelial growth factor and its receptors in Parkinson's disease." Neuroreport 17(7): 705-9.

Wang, M. S., S. Boddapati, et al. "Curcumin reduces alpha-synuclein induced cytotoxicity in Parkinson's disease cell model." BMC Neurosci 11: 57.

Webster, S. D., M. D. Galvan, et al. (2001). "Antibody-mediated phagocytosis of the amyloid beta-peptide in microglia is differentially modulated by C1q." J Immunol 166(12): 7496-503.

Weng, Y. H., Y. H. Chou, et al. (2007). "PINK1 mutation in Taiwanese early-onset parkinsonism : clinical, genetic, and dopamine transporter studies." J Neurol 254(10): 1347-55.

Werling, L. L., E. C. Lauterbach, et al. (2007). "Dextromethorphan as a potential neuroprotective agent with unique mechanisms of action." Neurologist 13(5): 272-93.

Whitton, P. S. (2007). "Inflammation as a causative factor in the aetiology of Parkinson's disease." Br J Pharmacol 150(8): 963-76.

Wu, D. C., V. Jackson-Lewis, et al. (2002). "Blockade of microglial activation is neuroprotective in the 1-methyl-4-phenyl-1,2,3,6-tetrahydropyridine mouse model of Parkinson disease." J Neurosci 22(5): 1763-71.

Wyss-Coray, T. and L. Mucke (2002). "Inflammation in neurodegenerative disease--a double-edged sword." Neuron 35(3): 419-32.

Xia, Y., M. E. Pauza, et al. (1997). "RelB regulation of chemokine expression modulates local inflammation." Am J Pathol 151(2): 375-87.

Yamada, T., J. K. Chong, et al. (1993). "Concentration of neural thread protein in cerebrospinal fluid from progressive supranuclear palsy and Parkinson's disease." Jpn J Psychiatry Neurol 47(3): 631-5.

Yamada, T., P. L. McGeer, et al. (1992). "Lewy bodies in Parkinson's disease are recognized by antibodies to complement proteins." Acta Neuropathol 84(1): 100-4.

Yang, S., D. Zhang, et al. (2008). "Curcumin protects dopaminergic neuron against LPS induced neurotoxicity in primary rat neuron/glia culture." Neurochem Res 33(10): 2044-53.

Yazdani, U., D. C. German, et al. (2006). "Rat model of Parkinson's disease: chronic central delivery of 1-methyl-4-phenylpyridinium (MPP+)." Exp Neurol 200(1): 172-83.

Zhang, F., L. Qian, et al. (2010). "Inhibition of IkappaB kinase-beta protects dopamine neurons against lipopolysaccharide-induced neurotoxicity." J Pharmacol Exp Ther 333(3): 822-33.

Zhang, S. X., J. J. Wang, et al. (2006). "Pigment epithelium-derived factor (PEDF) is an endogenous antiinflammatory factor." FASEB J 20(2): 323-5.

Zhang, W., S. Dallas, et al. (2007). "Microglial PHOX and Mac-1 are essential to the enhanced dopaminergic neurodegeneration elicited by A30P and A53T mutant alpha-synuclein." Glia 55(11): 1178-88.

Zhang, W., L. Qin, et al. (2005). "3-hydroxymorphinan is neurotrophic to dopaminergic neurons and is also neuroprotective against LPS-induced neurotoxicity." FASEB J 19(3): 395-7.

Zhang, W., E. J. Shin, et al. (2006). "3-Hydroxymorphinan, a metabolite of dextromethorphan, protects nigrostriatal pathway against MPTP-elicited damage both in vivo and in vitro." FASEB J 20(14): 2496-511.

Zhang, W., T. Wang, et al. (2004). "Neuroprotective effect of dextromethorphan in the MPTP Parkinson's disease model: role of NADPH oxidase." FASEB J 18(3): 589-91.

Zhang, Z. G., L. Zhang, et al. (2000). "VEGF enhances angiogenesis and promotes blood-brain barrier leakage in the ischemic brain." J Clin Invest 106(7): 829-38.

Zhou, Y., Y. Wang, et al. (2005). "Microglial activation induced by neurodegeneration: a proteomic analysis." Mol Cell Proteomics 4(10): 1471-9.

Zhu, Y., G. Y. Yang, et al. (2002). "Transforming growth factor-beta 1 increases bad phosphorylation and protects neurons against damage." J Neurosci 22(10): 3898-909.

Zlokovic, B. V. (2008). "The blood-brain barrier in health and chronic neurodegenerative disorders." Neuron 57(2): 178-201.

18

Mathematical Models: Interactions Between Serotonin and Dopamine in Parkinson's Disease

Janet Best[1], Grant Oakley[1], Michael Reed[2] and H. Frederik Nijhout[2]

[1]*Ohio State University*

[2]*Duke University*

USA

1. Introduction

Parkinson's disease (PD) has traditionally been thought of as a dysfunction in the dopamine (DA) signaling system caused primarily by cell death in the substantia nigra pars compacta (SNc). However, strong evidence has been accumulating that the serotonin (5-HT) signaling system is also involved. First, 5-HT influences normal motor function through a dense innervation of the striatum. Second, substantial cell death of serotonergic neurons occurs in PD and in some cases may occur earlier than DA cell death. And, finally, there are indications that interactions between the 5-HT system and the DA system may be responsible for some of the symptoms of PD and some of the side effects of treatment by levodopa. Some of the evidence for these assertions is reviewed below.

The 5-HT system is itself very complex. The serotonergic neurons in the raphe nuclei (RN) send ascending projections to a large number of different brain regions including medial prefrontal cortex (mPFC), motor cortex, hypothalamus, hippocampus, amygdala, and the basal ganglia. And, some of these brain regions, substantia nigra, amygdala, mPFC, and hypothalamus send projections back to the RN (Monti, 2010). Thus it is not surprising that 5-HT is linked to so many behaviors including feeding and body-weight regulation, social hierarchies, aggression and suicidality, obsessive compulsive disorder, alcoholism, anxiety, and affective disorders (Feldman et al., 1997). Since the pharmacology and the electrophysiology of both the serotonergic and the dopaminergic systems are only partially understood, it is a daunting task to understand how these two systems affect one another. This is particularly true in the presence of a degenerative disease that involves massive cell death in both systems.

In this complicated situation, mathematical models can potentially provide insight into mechanisms and interactions. The purpose of the models is not to summarize what is already known. The purpose is to provide a platform for *in silico* biological experimentation. Using models one can try out ideas, validate or refute hypotheses, settle disputes in the literature, and sometimes discover new phenomena. Of course, to be useful the models have to be well-grounded in real physiology and the creation of such models is not easy. However, if one has a model that represents (part of) the underlying physiology well, then *in silico* experiments are quick and inexpensive. The model provides a quantitative way of thinking about the phenomena being investigated and may suggest new hypotheses that can be checked by animal experiments. Thus, modeling, when combined with animal experiments and clinical trials, can shed some light on the complicated pharmacological, electrophysiological, and behavioral issues in PD.

In Section 2, we discuss the evidence for the role of 5-HT in PD and the side effects of levodopa therapy and in Section 3 we discuss possible mechanisms. In Section 4, we describe a mathematical model that we recently created to study homeostatic mechanisms in serotonergic signaling. In Section 5 we use the model, and a previous model of a DA terminal, to discuss the effects of gene polymorphisms, the stability of extracellular DA in the striatum in the face of cell death in the substantia nigra, and the mechanism of action of selective serotonin reuptake inhibitors. Finally, in Section 6 we outline how we plan to use existing models and new models to investigate the interactions between the 5-HT system and the DA system in PD.

2. PD and the serotonergic system

Tremor, rigidity, and bradykinesia, the classical motor symptoms of ideopathic PD, primarily result from loss of dopaminergic neurons in the SNc. However, neural degeneration also occurs in other sites of the brain, ranging from the brain stem to cortex, as the synaptic protein α-synuclein accumulates pathologically to form Lewy bodies (LB) or Lewy neurites. The clinical diagnosis of PD is based upon presence of the motor symptoms indicating dopamine deficiency (Chaudhuri et al., 2006; Jankovic, 2008). Postmortem analysis finds LB not only in remaining substantia nigra cells but in other specific brain regions where cells are lost (Gibb & Lees, 1988). Braak and colleagues (Braak et al., 2003) have proposed a scheme of six stages describing the development of ideopathic PD, characterized by the spatial extent of LB inclusions. Braak stage 1 involves LB inclusions in the region of the brain stem; neurodegeneration of the substantia nigra does not begin until stage 3. Braak's hypothesis concerning the progression of PD predicts that symptoms such as diminished olfactory sensitivity (Lim et al., 2009) or REM behavior disorder (Ahlskog, 2004) should precede the cardinal motor symptoms of the disease, a pattern observed in some but not all cases of PD (Linazasoro, 2007). Indeed, the retrospective nature of Braak's study obscures the actual course of progression (Halliday & McCann, 2010). In a longitudinal study, Halliday & McCann (2010) found that approximately half of ideopathic PD cases follow Braak's scheme. In all cases studied by Halliday and McCann, LB occurred not only in the substantia nigra but also in other brain areas including brain stem. Thus, extra-nigral aspects are always present in PD, and their significance can rival that of the cardinal motor symptoms (Chaudhuri et al., 2006).

Ahlskog (2004) reports that LB have been found in pontomedullary neurons of brains without substantia nigra pathology but that the reverse has not been observed. Among the nondopaminergic systems profoundly affected in PD is the serotonergic system. The extent of damage to the serotonergic system in PD is variable and is less severe than the loss of dopamine: Kish found that, while striatal dopamine concentrations decreased by more than 80%, serotonin markers decreased by less than 70% (Kish et al., 2008). It has not been clearly established to what extent this reduction in serotonin markers is due to raphe cell loss

(Jellinger, 1991), serotonergic terminal loss in the striatum, or molecular regulatory changes (Kish et al., 2008).

In post-mortem analyses of brains from PD patients, Kish et al. (2008) found that serotonin and dopamine have substantially different patterns of loss within the striatum. Serotonin markers show greater loss in the caudate than in putamen, while the dopamine loss is greater in the putamen. Thus the striatal subdivision with the more severe dopamine loss (putamen) was less affected by loss of serotonin markers, possibly reflecting compensatory sprouting of 5-HT terminals (Maeda et al., 2003). Serotonergic responses to dopamine depletion may also be evident in changes in the electrical activity of serotonergic neurons. Zhang et al. (2007) reports that, in an animal model of PD, raphe neurons have altered firing rates and fire bursts more frequently. Under levodopa administration, DA may also be released in bursts from these serotonergic neurons.

One of the clearest and best-studied involvements of 5-HT in PD symptoms is in the motor symptoms, including tremor and especially levodopa induced dyskinesias (LID). Experiments have found that the serotonergic system plays an essential role in both symptoms. Brooks (2007) reports that in order to generate tremors with the characteristic PD frequency of 3-5 Hz in animal models it is necessary to lesion not just nigro-striatal dopaminergic projections but also the midbrain tegmentum, which contains serotonergic cell bodies in the median raphe, rubrospinal, and dentatothalamic tracts. He also notes that loss of midbrain serotonin 5-HT_{1A} binding correlates with tremor severity in PD, unlike loss of striatal dopaminergic function. He speculates that this may explain why some parkinsonian tremors are relatively resistant to dopaminergic medications. 5-HT may not be equally involved in all motor symptoms of PD: it has been observed clinically that rigidity and bradykinesia are more responsive to dopaminergic drugs than is tremor (Fox et al., 2009).

Upon diagnosis of PD, patients can often use levodopa to effectively relieve symptoms for several years. However, more than 50% of patients develop motor complications in response to levodopa administration within 5 years (Olanow et al., 2000); after 10 years, the percentage is approximately 90% (Ahlskog & Muenter, 2001). These complications include a narrowing of the temporal window of efficacy (*i.e.*, the duration of benefit after a given dose of levodopa becomes progressively shorter until it approximates the plasma half-life of levodopa) (Olanow et al., 2006), sudden failures of efficacy known as "on-off fluctuations" (Nicholson & Brotchie, 2002) and, most troublesome, the appearance of involuntary movements (LID) (Carta et al., 2008; Nicholson & Brotchie, 2002).

3. Possible mechanisms of serotonergic involvement in PD motor symptoms

In order to understand the emergence of LID, it is useful to first review how levodopa may achieve therapeutic effect. The idea of administering levodopa is to provide dopamine replacement therapy. Dopamine itself is unable to pass the blood brain barrier, but its immediate precursor, levodopa, is able to reach the brain following peripheral administration when given in combination with a decarboxylase inhibitor to prevent metabolism while in the blood stream (Carta et al., 2008). The motor symptoms of PD typically emerge when a sufficient proportion of dopaminergic cells in SNc have been lost that dopaminergic terminals in the striatum are no longer able to maintain a high enough concentration of extracellular DA. Supplemental levodopa can be taken into the remaining dopaminergic terminals, converted to DA and stored in vesicles for synaptic release.

As the number of remaining dopaminergic cells continues to decrease, the levodopa may increasingly be taken up by other cell types including serotonergic neurons and glial cells. Serotonergic cells may play a special role here, as they also express the enzymes used in dopaminergic cells to convert levodopa to DA (amino acid aromatic decarboxylase, AADC) and to package DA into vesicles (vesicular monoamine transporter 2, MAT). Indeed, experiments have verified that serotonergic cells can store and release DA in vivo and in vitro (Nicholson & Brotchie, 2002). Evidence that serotonergic cells may be playing a role in LID comes from animal models of PD. (Tanaka et al., 1999) showed that, in levodopa treatment of a hemiparkinsonian rat, extracellular DA (eDA) decreased substantially when the serotonergic system was lesioned. Glial cells also contain AADC and so could contribute to the conversion of levodopa to DA; however, experiments by Kannari et al. (2000) in which he used reserpine to block vesicular packaging showed a great reduction of eDA, suggesting that most of the levodopa-derived DA is released by exocytosis of vesicles rather than by glia, at least at physiological levels of levodopa administration. Carta et al. (2007) have provided further evidence implicating serotonergic cells in LID in a rat model by showing that either toxic lesion of the serotonergic system or pharmacological impairment of the system with selective serotonin autoreceptor (5-HT_{1A} and 5-HT_{1B}) agonists resulted in a nearly complete elimination of LID.

The observation that LID becomes increasingly problematic as the disease progresses suggests that LID may result from the fact that DA released from serotonergic cells is not subject to the DA homeostatic mechanisms present in dopaminergic cells. Many approaches to eliminating LID therefore tend to focus instead on manipulating factors that regulate serotonergic cell activity, such as serotonergic autoreceptors that participate in serotonergic homeostatic mechanisms. Simply decreasing serotonergic cell activity by administering serotonin autoreceptor agonists has the drawback of also reducing the amount of dopamine released into the extracellular space, tending to worsen PD symptoms (Iravani et al., 2006). Carta et al. (2008) argue that it is reasonable to use 5-HT autoreceptor agonists especially because the DA intermixed with the 5-HT released by the serotonergic cell effectively lowers the binding of 5-HT to 5-HT autoreceptors and induces the cells to be over-active. A more detailed look at the serotonergic system, using mathematical models, may help suggest more nuanced approaches.

There are many types of serotonin receptors. 5-HT_{1A} receptors are present on the cell body and dendrites of serotonergic neurons in the dorsal and median raphe; they function as autoreceptors and they decrease firing as extracellular 5-HT (e5-HT) goes up. 5-HT_{1B} receptors are present on axon terminals in serotonin projection regions where they function as autoreceptors and decrease the release of serotonin as e5-HT goes up in the terminal region. Applying agonists only to 5-HT_{1A} or only to 5-HT_{1B} autoreceptors in a rat model of PD treated with levodopa can partially reduce LID (Bibbiani et al., 2001; Jackson et al., 2004). Carta et al. (2007) found that providing subthreshold doses of both 5-HT_{1A} and 5-HT_{1B} agonists (that is, doses that would have little or no effect alone) could completely eliminate LID. This is very strong evidence that the absence of the normal control mechanisms by the DA autoreceptors is connected to LID.

Post-synaptic mechanisms may play a role in LID. Given that serotonergic cells may be responsible for releasing much of the levodopa-derived DA in advanced PD and that these cells lack DA homeostatic mechanisms, the intermittent administration of levodopa may

result in large swings in the extracellular concentration of DA. The resulting pulsatile stimulation of striatal DA receptors may be the proximate cause of abnormal movements (de la Fuente-Fernandez et al., 2001) and may induce post-synaptic changes. In animal models of PD, alterations have been identified in the D_1 signaling pathway as well as in NMDA and AMPA receptor function and distribution (Bibbiani et al., 2005; Hallett et al., 2005; Robelet et al., 2004), and these changes have been linked to the induction and maintenance of abnormal movements (Gardoni et al., 2006; Hallett et al., 2005; Picconi et al., 2008; Santini et al., 2007). In fact, studies utilizing pumps to provide a fairly continuous dosing with levodopa or DA agonists have found fewer side effects (Nutt et al., 2000).
Changes in gene expression also have been found following treatment with levodopa (Santini et al., 2007), and these may relate to the phenomenon of priming. Some PD patients can be treated with DA receptor agonists without developing dyskinesias. But eventually, as the disease progresses, they generally need to add levodopa in order to achieve relief from symptoms. The phenomenon of priming is that patients started on levodopa and then moved to DA agonists will exhibit dyskinesias even if placed on DA agonists without levodopa (Nicholson & Brotchie, 2002).

4. Mathematical modeling of dopaminergic and serotonergic systems

As a first step in using mathematics to help understand the serotonergic and dopaminergic systems, we have created mathematical models of a serotonin terminal (Best et al., 2010b) and a dopamine terminal (Best et al., 2009). Here we briefly describe the model for a serotonin terminal and in the next section give applications. The substrates in the model are indicated in Figure 1 by the pink boxes and the blue ellipses contain the acronyms of enzymes or transporters. Blood tryptophan is considered a (possibly time-varying) input to the model and there are differential equations for the other nine substrates. Each differential equation is just a quantitative expression of mass balance; i.e. the rate of change of the concentration of a substrate is simply the sum of the rates of the reactions by which it is made minus the sum of the rates of the reactions in which it is used. For example, the concentration of 5-hydroxytryptophan, [5htp], satisfies:

$$\frac{d[5htp]}{dt} = V_{\text{TPH}}(trp, bh4, e5ht) - V_{\text{AADC}}(5htp) \quad (1)$$

where V_{TPH} is the velocity of the TPH reaction and V_{AADC} is the velocity of the AADC reaction. One must specify exactly how these velocities depend on the current values of various substrates. V_{TPH} is given by:

$$V_{\text{TPH}} = \frac{V_{max}(trp)(bh4)}{(K_{trp} + (trp) + \frac{(trp)^2}{K_i})(K_{bh4} + (bh4))} \cdot \left(1.5 - \frac{(e5ht)^2}{((.000768)^2 + (e5ht)^2)}\right). \quad (2)$$

The first term on the right is of Michaelis-Menten form and gives the dependence of the velocity on the concentrations of trp and $bh4$. The enzyme TPH shows substrate inhibition (Best et al., 2010a; Friedman et al., 1974; McKinney et al., 2005), which is the reason for the $(trp)^2$ term in the denominator. The second term on the right expresses how the concentration of extracellular 5-HT influences the rate of synthesis via the autoreceptors. At normal e5-HT concentration (.768 nM) this factor equals one. As e5-HT goes up the factor can go as low as 0.5

and as e5-HT goes down, the factor can go as high as 1.5. We chose K_m and K_i values from the literature and chose the V_{max} so that the normal velocity of the the TPH reaction is in the range given by experiments. The form of the second factor is more speculative. Though it is certain that increasing extracellular concentrations of 5-HT inhibit synthesis via the autoreceptors (Adell et al., 2002), there is relatively little information in the literature about the range of e5-HT concentrations over which the effect takes place and about the strength of the effect in the low nanomolar range. Here, as in other choices of parameters and functional forms, we base our choices as much as possible on the experimental literature. Full details of the model can be found in Best et al. (2010b).

The model can be used to show how the steady state values of concentrations and rates change if parameters, like serotonin transporter (SERT) density, or inputs, like serum tryptophan, change. One can also compute the time courses of the concentrations and rates on long time scales (hours) or very short time scales (msec) as the system responds to the release of 5-HT due to individual action potentials. However, the model has limitations. Various physiological processes known to be important are not included, for example the movement of vesicles or SERTs from the interior of the terminal to and from the synaptic membrane. The detailed biophysics of the autoreceptors is not included; instead the model has terms that represent the effect of e5-HT on TPH and on release from the vesicles. And finally, this is a model for a terminal and thus has limited value in studying network questions about the full serotonergic system.

It is important to keep in mind that there is no such thing as *the* serotonergic terminal. Important parameters vary considerably from one projection region to another. For example, SERT density (which corresponds roughly to the V_{max} of V_{SERT}) varies by about a factor of 5 (Bunin et al., 1998; Daws et al., 2005; Lin et al., 2004). And, functional polymorphisms for the TPH, SERT, and MAO genes are known to exist. Indeed, one of the strengths of the model is that it can be used to study the likely effects of such variations on the functional behavior of serotonergic terminals.

5. Applying the models

In this section we describe several applications of our 5-HT and DA terminal models to show how they can be used. The DA terminal model is similar in structure to the 5-HT model, though the details of the kinetics are different (Best et al., 2009).

5.1 Homeostatic effects of the autoreceptors

It is clear that the 5-HT autoreceptors create homeostasis by providing a kind of end-product inhibition. If firing rate goes up, then e5-HT will go up, which reduces synthesis and release via the autoreceptors. If firing rate goes down, then e5-HT will go down, which increases synthesis and release via the autoreceptors. Thus, the autoreceptors ensure that the average extracellular 5-HT in projections regions due to tonic firing of dorsal raphe neurons does not change very much.

It has been much less remarked in the literature that the autoreceptors provide another kind of homeostasis. The genes for many of the key proteins in the 5-HT system, for example TPH2, SERT, and MAO, have common functional polymorphisms. However, because of the autoreceptors, the polymorphisms have a much smaller effect on e5-HT than one might think. For, example the P449R polymorphism and the R441H polymorphism of TPH2 reduce its

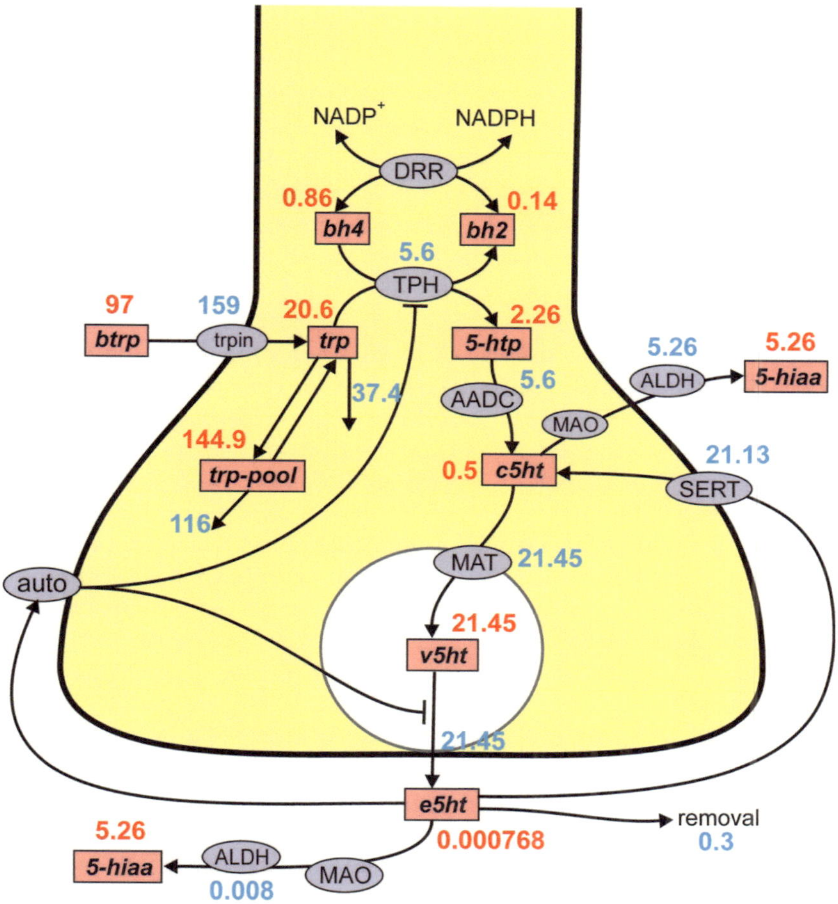

Fig. 1. Steady state concentrations and fluxes in the 5-HT terminal model. The figure shows the reactions in the model. The pink rectangular boxes indicate substrates and blue ellipses contain the acronyms of enzymes or transporters; steady state values in the model are indicated. Concentrations (red) have units of μM and rates (blue) have units of μM/hr. Full names of the substrates are: bh2, dihydrobiopterin; bh4, tetrahydrobiopterin; trp, tryptophan; btrp, serum tryptophan; 5htp, 5-hydroxytryptophan; c5ht, cytosolic 5-HT; v5ht, vesicular 5-HT; e5ht; extracellular 5-HT; 5-hiaa, 5-hydroxyindoleacetic acid; *trp—pool*, the tryptophan pool. Names of enzymes and transporters are: Trpin, neutral amino acid transporter; DRR, dihydrobiopterin reductase; TPH, tryptophan hydroxylase; AADC, aromatic amino acid decarboxylase; MAT, vesicular monoamine transporter; SERT, 5-HT reuptake transporter; auto, 5-HT autoreceptors; MAO, monoamine oxidase; ALDH, aldehyde dehydrogenase. Removal means uptake by capillaries or glial cells or diffusion out of the system.

activity to 65% and 19% of wild type, respectively. But the model predicts that e5-HT will decrease to 90% and 45% of wild type in these two cases; see Figure 4 of (Best et al., 2010b). Similarly, we show in (Best et al., 2009) that the D2 autoreceptors make extracellular DA much less sensitive to the expression level or activity of tyrosine hydroxylase (TH).

5.2 Passive stabilization of DA in the striatum

An interesting and important feature of PD is that symptoms do not appear until a very large percentage (typically 60-90%) of the cells in the SNc have died (Agid, 1991; Zygmond et al., 1990). Animal models have shown that tissue levels of DA in the striatum decline proportionally to cell loss, but eDA remains essentially normal until 85% of the SNc cells have died (Bergstrom & Garris, 2003; Bezard et al., 2001; Dentresangle et al., 2001), and this is widely believed to be the reason that symptoms do not appear until very late in the degeneration of the SNc.

A number of researchers have proposed that this homeostasis of eDA results from active adaptive mechanisms such as increased DA synthesis and the formation of new terminals (Hornykiewicz, 1966; Stanic et al., 2003; Zygmond et al., 1990; 1984). However, Garris and co-workers proposed that the homeostasis is due to passive mechanisms such as release and reuptake and provided some experimental confirmation (Bergstrom & Garris, 2003; Garris et al., 1997; Garris & Wightman, 1994). Their idea is as follows. DA is released in the striatum and is then taken back up into the terminals by the DA transporters (DATs). As the cells in the SNc die the amount of DA released in the striatum decreases proportionally, but the number of DATs available for reuptake has also decreased proportionally. Thus a released DA molecule will spend about the same amount of time in the extracellular space no matter how many SNc cells have died. Garris and co-workers called this "passive stabilization." They did not explain why this homeostasis breaks down when the fraction, f, of SNc cells that are alive becomes small.

We investigated these proposals with our mathematical model of a DA terminal (Reed et al., 2009). We found that the passive stabilization mechanism proposed by Garris works as proposed and we determined why the mechanism breaks down when f is small. Not all released DA molecules are put back into DA terminals by the DATs. Some are taken up by glial cells or blood vessels and some diffuse out of the striatum. As SNc cells die and the DA terminals in the striatum become more sparse, a greater percentage of released DA is lost through these mechanisms. This is why the Garris passive stabilization mechanism breaks down when f is small. We provided quantitative calculations about these effects and showed that passive stabilization itself keeps eDA almost constant when f is between $\frac{1}{2}$ and 1. When more than half of the SNc cells have died, the terminal autoreceptors contribute substantially to the homeostasis of eDA. And, only when f is as low as .15 or .1 are the combined homeostatic effects of passive stabilization and the autoreceptors overwhelmed by the removal of DA from the striatum by the mechanisms discussed above. For details, see (Reed et al., 2009).

5.3 Burst firing in the raphe nuclei and SSRIs

The etiology of depressive illness remains unknown despite a large body of research. A hypothesis that has been central to much work in pharmacology and electrophysiology is that depression is caused by dysfunction in the serotonergic signaling system (Feldman et al.,

1997; Schildkraut, 1965). This hypothesis led to the development of monoamine oxidase inhibitors (MAOIs), tricyclic anti-depressants and the selective serotonin reuptake inhibitors (SSRIs). The idea of the MAOIs is that by preventing the degradation of 5-HT, more will be available for packaging into synaptic vesicles. The idea of the tri-cyclics and the SSRIs is that they block SERTs and inhibit reuptake of 5-HT from the extracellular space, therefore increasing "serotonergic signaling." These drugs have shown some efficacy in the treatment of depression, but the causal chain of events and the reasons why they benefit some patients and not others are unknown.

The simple hypothesis that SSRIs would raise the level of 5-HT in serotonergic synapses by blocking reuptake was thrown into doubt by the discovery that the cell bodies of most 5-HT neurons also release 5-HT and have SERTs. Furthermore, increased e5-HT in the RN decreases the tonic firing rate of those cells via the 5-HT_{1A} autoreceptors (Adell et al., 2002; Gartside et al., 1995). Thus, there are two conflicting effects. Blocking the SERTs in the terminal region would tend to raise e5-HT there, and blocking the SERTs in the raphe nuclei (RN) would tend to decrease e5-HT in the terminal region. The balance between the two effects will depend on the densities of 5-HT_{1A} autoreceptors on different 5-HT populations in the RN and on the densities of SERTs in different projection regions, both quite variable. Thus one would expect that experimental results would depend on dose and on the projection regions being studied, and this was found to be true (Bel & Artigas, 1992; Hervas & Artigas, 1998; Malagie et al., 1995). In some cases, acute doses of SSRIs even decreased e5-HT in projection regions.

The next hypothesis focused on the 5-HT_{1A} autoreceptors on the RN cell bodies. It was shown that giving 5-HT_{1A} antagonists or knocking out the autoreceptors entirely potentiates the SSRI-induced increase of e5-HT in projection regions. Similarly, 5-HT_{1A} knockouts show increased release in projection regions (Chaput et al., 1986; Knobelman et al., 2001). Furthermore, a number of studies showed that chronic treatment with SSRIs desensitizes the 5-HT_{1A} autoreceptors in the RN (Blier et al., 1987; Chaput et al., 1986; Hervas et al., 2001; Invernizzi et al., 1992). And thus, one could explain the improvements of patients on the time scale of 3-6 weeks by the slow desensitization of autoreceptors. However, when e5-HT was measured in projection regions during the entire course of chronic SSRI treatment, it was found that e5-HT concentrations went up initially and then plateaued or declined somewhat over the course of treatment (Anderson et al., 2005; Smith et al., 2000). Thus the autoreceptor desensitization hypothesis seems unlikely to explain the delay of beneficial effects of SSRI treatments.

In (Best et al., 2011) we propose a new hypothesis for the efficacy of SSRIs and provide calculations with the 5-HT terminal model to support our ideas. The 5-HT cells in the RN fire tonically at about 1 Hz and occasionally individual spikes are replaced by short bursts (Feldman et al., 1997; Hajos et al., 1995; Heyn et al., 1982). Our physiological point of view is that tonic firing by the 5-HT neurons in the RN maintains 5-HT tone in target tissues by volume transmission and burst firing conveys specific information to one-on-one synapses that are known to exist (Maley et al., 1990; Parnavelas & Papadopoulos, 1989). Our hypothesis is that chronic treatment of depressed patients with SSRIs returns the response to bursts arriving in terminal regions to normal and we show that this is true in our model. The model behavior depends on the down regulation of SERTs on terminal membranes known to be caused by chronic exposure to SSRIs (Benmansour et al., 2002; Gould et al., 2003; Lau et al., 2008; Mizra et al., 2007). For details, see (Best et al., 2011).

6. Future work

We indicate briefly here some of the ideas that we plan to pursue. We plan to use our current model of a 5-HT terminal described above to investigate the consequences of levodopa uptake by 5-HT terminals. Both 5-HTP and levodopa will compete for AADC that will turn them into 5-HT and DA respectively, and the monoamine transporter will package them together into vesicles. Since there is leakage out of the vesicles driven by concentration gradients, the competition will limit the amounts of 5-HT and DA available for release. Our physiological point of view is that normal 5-HT or DA neurons maintain 5-HT or DA tone in target tissues by volume transmission and convey specific information via burst firing. The autoreceptors on DA neurons inhibit release when the extracellular concentration of DA goes up due to a burst, bringing the concentration back to the normal tonic level rapidly. However, levodopa therapy partially turns 5-HT neurons into DA neurons that do not have DA autoreceptors and one expects that stimulation of the 5-HT system will therefore cause larger than normal swings in extracellular DA in the striatum after levodopa therapy. This effect will be compounded by the fact that cell death in the SNc implies that there will be many fewer DATs in the striatum to take up the released DA. We plan to investigate this situation with our model. Finally, we are currently extending our models to include the competition between tyrosine, tryptophan, leucine, isoleucine, and valine at the blood-brain barrier. When this is completed we can study the tryptophan depletion and tryptophan loading experiments described in (Scholtissen et al., 2006).

We are particularly interested in how levodopa therapy could produce dyskinesis and have some ideas that can be tried out through mathematical modeling. (Carta et al., 2007) provided strong evidence that release of DA from 5-HT neurons causes LID by showing that 5-HT_{1A} agonists that reduce RN firing and/or 5-HT_{1B} agonists that reduce release in the striatum both reduce the incidence of LID in an animal model. We plan to extend our 5-HT terminal model to include the cell body in the RN so that we can study release of DA in the striatum in the presence of either 5-HT_{1A} or 5-HT_{1B} agonists (or both) after cell death in the SNc reduces the number of DATs. This will provide a platform for trying out *in silico* the experiments in (Carta et al., 2007).

There is another intriguing possibility that we plan to investigate by modeling. Recall that the 5-HT neurons in the raphe nuclei release 5-HT from their cell bodies when they fire. The released 5-HT binds to the 5-HT_{1A} autoreceptors on the cell bodies and inhibits RN firing (Adell et al., 2002). This is a kind of lateral inhibition in the RN that limits total firing. However, in the presence of levodopa, the cell bodies will release a combination of 5-HT and DA, and the lower extracellular concentration of 5-HT will provide much less lateral inhibition. Thus is it likely that the 5-HT neurons in the RN fire more frequently after levodopa therapy and there is evidence for altered firing patterns (Zhang et al., 2007). This would have the effect of releasing more DA in the striatum. Notice, however, that raphe neurons project to many brain regions that send inhibitory projections back to the RN (for example the mPFC; see (Celada et al., 2001)). Such negative feedback systems often exhibit oscillations if they are forced hard enough, and such oscillations would mean periodic oscillations in the amount of firing of 5-HT neurons in the RN and thus periodic oscillations in the amount of DA released in the striatum. It is tempting to speculate that such oscillations may contribute to LID and that they could be initiated by intermittent levodopa therapy (Nutt et al., 2000; Olanow et al., 2006; 2000). We plan to investigate this hypothesis by developing mathematical models of the

lateral inhibition by diffusion of extracellular 5-HT in the RN and a model of the projections to the mPFC with negative feedback from the mPFC to the RN.
Finally, it is well-known that the brain is capable of rewiring itself after injury to use available neurons for new purposes. Note that, in a certain sense, that is what levodopa therapy is stimulating, the use of 5-HT neurons as DA neurons. And, it is known that lesioning the SNc causes hyperinnervation by 5-HT neurons in the striatum (Maeda et al., 2003). Such retraining and rewiring takes time, of course, and it is possible that it can't happen fast enough to compensate for the degeneration in PD, but the possibility is intriguing. Not enough is known presently for mathematical modeling to be helpful here. However, if and when anatomical and electrophysiological information becomes available about such compensatory processes, mathematical models, developed along the lines that we have indicated, could perhaps suggest treatment strategies that would facilitate the compensatory processes.

7. Acknowledgements

This work was supported by NSF grants DMS-061670 (MR,HFN) and EF-1038593 (HFN,MR), NSF CAREER grant DMS-0956057 (JB), and NSF agreement 0112050 through the Mathematical Biosciences Institute (JB, MR). JB is an Alfred P. Sloan Research Foundation Fellow. The authors thank Shira Rubin for a close reading of the manuscript.

8. References

Adell, A., Celada, P., Abella, M. T. & Artigasa, F. (2002). Origin and functional role of the extracellular serotonin in the midbrain raphe nuclei, *Brain Res Rev* 39: 154–180.

Agid, Y. (1991). Parkinson's disease: pathophysiology, *Lancet* 337: 1321–1324.

Ahlskog, J. E. (2004). Challenging conventional wisdom: The etiologic role of dopamine oxidative stress in Parkinson's disease, *Movement Disorders* 20(3): 271–282.

Ahlskog, J. E. & Muenter, M. D. (2001). Frequency of levodopa-related dyskinesias and motor fluctuations as estimated from the cumulative literature, *Movement Disorders* 16(3): 448–458.

Anderson, G. M., Barr, C. S., Lindell, S., Durham, A. C., Shifrovich, I. & Higley, J. D. (2005). Time course of the effects of the serotonin-selective reuptake inhibitor sertraline on central and peripheral serotonin neurochemistry in the rhesus monkey, *Phycopharma* 178: 339–346.

Bel, N. & Artigas, F. (1992). Fluoxetine preferentially increases extracellular 5-hydroxytryptamine in the raphe nuclei: an in vivo microdialysis study, *Eur. J. Pharmacol.* 229: 101–103.

Benmansour, S., Owens, W. A., Cecchi, M., Morilak, D. & Frazer, A. (2002). Serotonin clearance in vivo is altered to a greater extent by antidepressant-induced downregulation of the serotonin transporter than by acute blockade of the transporter, *J. Neurosci.* 22(15): 6766–6772.

Bergstrom, B. & Garris, P. (2003). 'Passive stabilization' of striatal extracellular dopamine across the lesion spectrum encompassing the presymptomatic phase of Parkinson's disease: a voltametric study in the 6-OHDA-lesioned rat, *J. Neurochem* 87: 1224–36.

Best, J. A., Nijhout, H. F. & Reed, M. C. (2009). Homeostatic mechanisms in dopamine synthesis and release: a mathematical model, *Theor Biol Med Model* 6: 21.

Best, J. A., Nijhout, H. F. & Reed, M. C. (2010a). Models of dopaminergic and serotonergic signaling, *Pharmacopsychiatry* 43(Supp. 1): 561–566.

Best, J. A., Nijhout, H. F. & Reed, M. C. (2010b). Serotonin synthesis, release and reuptake in terminals: a mathematical model, *Theor Biol Med Model* 7: 34–.

Best, J., Reed, M. & Nijhout, H. F. (2011). Bursts and the efficacy of selective serotonin reuptake inhibitors, *Pharmacopsychiatry* 44(Suppl.1):S76-S83.

Bezard, E., Dovero, S., C, C. P., Ravenscroft, P., Chalon, S., Guilloteau, D., Crossman, A. R., Bioulac, B., Brotchie, J. M. & Gross, C. E. (2001). Relationship between the appearance of symptoms and the level nigrostriatal degeneration in a progressive 1-methyl-4-phenyl-1,2,3,6-tetrahydropyridine-lesioned macaque model of Parkinson's disease, *J Neurosci* 21: 6853–6861.

Bibbiani, F., Oh, J. D. & Chase, T. N. (2001). Serotonin 5-HT1a agonist improves motor complications in rodent and primate Parkinsonian models, *Neurology* 57: 1829–1834.

Bibbiani, F., Oh, J. D., Kielaite, A., Collins, M. A., Smith, C. & Chase, T. N. (2005). Combined blockade of AMPA and NMDA glutamate receptors reduces levodopa-induced motor complications in animal models of PD, *Experimental Neurology* 196: 422–429.

Blier, P., de Montigny, C. & Chaput, Y. (1987). Modifications of the serotonin system by antidepressant treatment: implications for the therapeutic response in major depression, *J. Clin. Psychoharmaco1.* 7: 24S–35S.

Braak, H., Rüb, U., Gai, W. & Tredici, K. D. (2003). Idiopathic Parkinson's disease: possible routes by which vulnerable neuronal types may be subject to neuroinvasion by an unknown pathogen, *J Neural Transmission* 110: 517–536.

Brooks, D. J. (2007). Imaging non-dopaminergic function in Parkinson's disease, *Molecular Imaging and Biology* 9: 217–222.

Bunin, M., Prioleau, C., Mailman, R. & Wightman, R. (1998). Release and uptake rates of 5-hydroxytryptamine in the dorsal raphe and substantia nigra of the rat brain, *J Neurochem* 70: 1077–1087.

Carta, M., Carlsson, T., Kirik, D. & Björklund, A. (2007). Dopamine released from 5-HT terminals is the cause of l-dopa-induced dyskinesia in Parkinsonian rats, *Brain* 130: 1819–1833.

Carta, M., Carlsson, T., Muñoz, A., Kirik, D. & Björklund, A. (2008). Serotonin–dopamine interaction in the induction and maintenance of l-dopa-induced dyskinesias, *Prog. Brain Res.* 172: 465–478.

Celada, P., Puig, M. V., Casanovas, J. M., Guillazo, G. & Artigas, F. (2001). Control of dorsal raphe serotonergic neurons by the medial prefrontal cortex: Involvement of serotonin-1a, GABAa, and glutamate receptors, *J. Neurosci* 15: 9917–9929.

Chaput, Y., Blier, P. & de Montigny, C. (1986). In vivo electrophysiological evidence for the regulatory role of autoreceptors on serotonergic terminals, *J. Neurosci* 6(10): 2796–2801.

Chaudhuri, K. R., Healy, D. G. & Schapira, A. H. V. (2006). Non-motor symptoms of Parkinson's disease: diagnosis and management, *Lancet/Neurology* 5: 235–245.

Daws, L., Montenez, S., Owens, W., Gould, G., Frazer, A., Toney, G. & Gerhardt, G. (2005). Transport mechanisms governing serotonin clearance in vivo revealed by high speed chronoamperometry, *J Neurosci Meth* 143: 49–62.

de la Fuente-Fernandez, R., Lu, J.-Q., Sossi, V., Jivan, S., Schulzer, M., Holden, J. E., Lee, C. S., Ruth, T. J., Donald, Calne, B. & Stoessl, A. J. (2001). Biochemical variations in the synaptic level of dopamine precede motor fluctuations in Parkinson's disease: PET evidence of increased dopamine turnover, *Annals of Neurology* 49(3): 298–303.

Dentresangle, C., Cavorsin, M. L., Savasta, M. & Leviel, V. (2001). Increased extracellular DA and normal evoked DA release in the rat striatum after a partial lesion of the substantia nigra, *Brain Res* 893(178-185).

Feldman, R., Meyer, J. & Quenzer, L. (1997). *Principles of Neuropharmacology*, Sinauer Associates, Inc, Sunderland, MA.

Fox, S. H., Chuang, R. & Brotchie, J. M. (2009). Serotonin and Parkinson's disease: On movement, mood, and madness, *Movement Disorders* 24: 1255–1266.

Friedman, P. A., Kappelman, A. H. & Kaufman, S. (1974). Partial purification and characterization of tryptophan hydroxylase from rabbit hindbrain, *J Biol Chem* 247: 1465–1473.

Gardoni, F., Picconi, B., Ghiglieri, V., Polli, F., Bagetta, V., Bernardi, G., Cattabeni, F., Luca, M. D. & Calabresi, P. (2006). A critical interaction between NR2B and MAGUK in l-dopa induced dyskinesia, *The Journal of Neuroscience* 26(11): 2914–2922.

Garris, P., Walker, Q. & Wightman, R. (1997). Dopamine release and uptake both decrease in the partially denervated striatum in proportion to the loss of dopamine terminals, *Brain Res* 753: 225–234.

Garris, P. & Wightman, R. (1994). Different kinetics govern dopaminergic neurotransmission in the amygdala, prefrontal cortex, and striatum: an in vivo voltametric study, *J. Neurosci* 14: 442–450.

Gartside, S. E., Umbers, V., Hajos, M. & Sharp, T. (1995). Interaction between a selective 5-HT1a receptor antagonist and an SSRI in vivo: effects on 5-HT cell firing and extracellular 5-HT, *Br. J. Pharmacol.* 115: 1064–1070.

Gibb, W. R. G. & Lees, A. J. (1988). The relevance of the Lewy body to the pathogenesis of idiopathic Parkinson's disease, *J of Neurology, Neurosurgery, and Psychiatry* 51: 745–752.

Gould, G. G., Pardon, M. C., Morilak, D. A. & Frazer, A. (2003). Regulatory effects of reboxetine treatment alone, or following paroxetine treatment, on brain noradrenergic and serotonergic systems., *Neuropsychopharmacology* 28: 1633–1644.

Hajos, M., Gartside, S. E., Villa, A. E. P. & Sharp, T. (1995). Evidence for a repetitive (burst) firing pattern in a sub-population of 5-hydroxytryptamine neurons in the dorsal and median raphe nuclei of the rat, *Neuroscience* 69: 189–197.

Hallett, P. J., Dunah, A. W., Ravenscroft, P., Zhou, S., Bezard, E., Crossman, A. R., Brotchie, J. M. & Standaert, D. G. (2005). Alterations of striatal NMDA receptor subunits associated with the development of dyskinesia in the MPTP-lesioned primate model of Parkinson's disease, *Neuropharmacology* 48: 503–516.

Halliday, G. M. & McCann, H. (2010). The progression of pathology in Parkinson's disease, *Ann. N.Y. Acad. Sci.* 1184: 188–195.

Hervas, I. & Artigas, F. (1998). Effect of fluoxetine on extracellular 5-hydroxytryptamine in rat brain. Role of 5HT autoreceptors., *Eur. J. Pharmacol.* 358: 9–18.

Hervas, I., Velaro, M. T., Romero, L., Mengod, G. & Artigas, F. (2001). Desensitization of 5-HT1a autoreceptors by a low chronic fluoxetine dose. Effect of the concurrent administration of WAY-100635, *Neuropsychopharmacology* 24: 11–20.

Heyn, J., Steinfels, G. F. & Jacobs, B. J. (1982). Activity of serotonin-containing neurons in the nucleus raphe pallidus of freely moving cats, *Brain Res.* 251: 259–276.

Hornykiewicz, O. (1966). Dopamine (3-hydroxytyramine) and brain function, *Pharmacol. Rev.* 18: 925–964.

Invernizzi, R., Bramante, M. & Samanin, R. (1992). Citalopram's ability to increase the extracellular concentrations of serotonin in the dorsal raphe prevents the drug's effect in the frontal cortex, *Brain Res.* 260: 322–324.

Iravani, M. M., Tayarani-Binazir, K., Chu, W. B., Jackson, M. J. & Jenner, P. (2006). In MPTP treated primates, the selective 5-HT1a agonist (R)- (+)-8-hydroxy-DPAT inhibits levodopa-induced dyskinesia but only with increased motor disability, *J Pharmacology and Experimental Therapeutics* 319: 1225–1234.

Jackson, M. J., Al-Barghouthy, G., Pearce, R. K. B., Smith, L., Hagan, J. J. & Jenner, P. (2004). Effect of 5-HT1b/d receptor agonist and antagonist administration on motor function in haloperidol and MPTP-treated common marmosets, *Pharmacology, Biochemistry and Behavior* 79: 391–400.

Jankovic, J. (2008). Parkinson's disease: clinical features and diagnosis, *J Neurol Neurosurg Psychiatry* 79: 368–376.

Jellinger, K. A. (1991). Pathology of Parkinson's disease: Changes other than the nigrostriatal pathway, *Molecular and Chemical Neuropathology* 14: 153–197.

Kannari, K., Tanaka, H., Maeda, T., Tomiyama, M., Suda, T. & Matsunaga, M. (2000). Reserpine pretreatment prevents increases in extracellular striatal dopamine following l-dopa administration in rats with nigrostriatal denervation, *J Neurochem* 74: 263–269.

Kish, S. J., Tong, J., Hornykiewicz, O., Rajput, A., Chang, L.-J., Guttman, M. & Furukawa, Y. (2008). Preferential loss of serotonin markers in caudate versus putamen in Parkinson's disease, *Brain* 131: 120–131.

Knobelman, D. A., Hen, R. & Lucki, I. (2001). Genetic regulation of extracellular serotonin by 5-hydroxtryptamine-1a and 5-hydroxytryptamine-1b autoreceptors in different brain regions of the mouse, *J. Pharmacol. Exper. Therap.* 298: 1083–1091.

Lau, T., Horschitz, S., Berger, S., Bartsch, D. & Schloss, P. (2008). Antidepressant-induced internalization of the serotonin transporter in serotonergic neurons, *FASEB J* 22: 1702–1714.

Lim, S.-Y., Fox, S. H. & Lang, A. E. (2009). Overview of the extranigral aspects of Parkinson disease, *Arch. Neurol.* 66(2): 167–172.

Lin, K.-J., Yen, T.-C., Wey, S.-P., Hwang, J.-J., Ye, X.-X., Tzen, K.-Y., Fu, Y.-K. & Chen, J.-C. (2004). Characterization of the binding sites 123I-ADAM and the relationship to the serotonin transporter in rat and mouse brains using quantitative autoradiography, *J. Nuc. Med.* 45: 673–681.

Linazasoro, G. (2007). Classical Parkinson disease versus Parkinson complex – reflections against staging and in favour of heterogeneity, *European Journal of Neurology* 14: 721–728.

Maeda, T., Kannari, K., H, H. S., Arai, A., Tomiyama, M., Matsunaga, M. & Suda, T. (2003). Rapid induction of serotonergic hyperinnervation in the adult rat striatum with extensive dopaminergic denervation., *Neurosci. Lett.* 343: 17–20.

Malagie, I., Trillat, A. C., Jacquot, C. & Gardier, A. M. (1995). Effects of acute fluoxetine on extracellular serotonin levels in the raphe: an in vivo microdialysis study, *Eur. J. Pharmacol.* 286: 213–217.

Maley, B. E., Engle, M. G., Humphreys, S., Vascik, D. A., Howes, K. A., Newton, B. W. & Elde, R. P. (1990). Monoamine synaptic structure and localization in the central nervous system, *J. Electron Micros. Tech.* 15: 20–33.

McKinney, J., Knappskog, P. M. & Haavik, J. (2005). Different properties of the central and peripheral forms of human tryptophan hydroxylase, *J Neurochem* 92: 311–320.

Mizra, N. R., Nielson, E. O. & Troelsen, K. B. (2007). Serotonin transporter density and anxiolytic-like effects of antidepressants in mice, *Prog. Neuropsycho. Biol. Psych.* 31: 858–866.

Monti, J. M. (2010). The structure of the dorsal raphe nucleus and its relevance to the regulation of sleep and wakefulness, *Sleep Med. Rev.* 14: 307–317.

Nicholson, S. L. & Brotchie, J. M. (2002). 5-hydroxytryptamine (5HTt, serotonin) and Parkinson's disease - opportunities for novel therapeutics to reduce problems of levodopa therapy, *European Journal of Neurology* 9(Suppl. 3): 1–6.

Nutt, J., Obesio, J. A. & Stocchi, F. (2000). Continuous dopamine-receptor stimulation in advanced Parkinson's disease, *TINS* 23: S109–S115.

Olanow, C. W., Obeso, J. A. & Stocchi, F. (2006). Continuous dopamine-receptor treatment of Parkinson's disease: scientific rationale and clinical implications, *Lancet/Neurology* 5: 677–687.

Olanow, C. W., Schapira, A. H. V. & Rascol, O. (2000). Continuous dopamine-receptor stimulation in early Parkinson's disease, *TINS* 23: S117–S126.

Parnavelas, J. G. & Papadopoulos, G. C. (1989). The monoaminergic innervation of the cerebral cortex is not diffuse and non-specific, *TINS* 12: 315–319.

Picconi, B., Paillé, V., Ghiglieri, V., Bagetta, V., Barone, I., Lindgren, H. S., Bernardi, G., Cenci, M. A. & Calabresi, P. (2008). L-dopa dosage is critically involved in dyskinesia via loss of synaptic depotentiation, *Neurobiology of Disease* 29: 327–335.

Reed, M., Best, J. & Nijhout, H. (2009). Passive and active stabilization of dopamine in the striatum, *BioScience Hypotheses* 2: 240–244.

Robelet, S., Melon, C., Guillet, B., Salin, P. & Goff, L. K.-L. (2004). Chronic l-dopa treatment increases extracellular glutamate levels and GLT1 expression in the basal ganglia in a rat model of Parkinson's disease, *European Journal of Neuroscience* 20: 1255–1266.

Santini, E., Valjent, E., Usiello, A., Carta, M., Borgkvist, A., Girault, J.-A., Hervé, D., Greengard, P. & Fisone, G. (2007). Critical involvement of CAMP/DARPP-32 and extracellular signal-regulated protein kinase signaling in l-dopa-induced dyskinesia, *The Journal of Neuroscience* 27(26): 6995–7005.

Schildkraut, J. J. (1965). The catecholamine hypothesis of affective disorders: a review of supporting evidence, *Amer. J. Psych.* 122: 509–522.

Scholtissen, B., Verhey, F. R. J., Steinbusch, H. W. M. & Leentjens, A. F. G. (2006). Serotonergic mechanisms in Parkinson's disease: opposing results from preclinical and clinical data, *J. Neural Trans.* 113: 59–73.

Smith, T., Kuczenski, R., George-Friedman, K., Malley, J. D. & Foote, S. L. (2000). In vivo microdialysis assessment of extracellular serotonin and dopamine levels in awake monkeys during sustained fluoxetine administration, *Synapse* 38: 460–470.

Stanic, D., Parish, C. L., Zhu, W. L., Krstew, E. V., Lawrence, A. J., Drago, J. & Finkelstein, D. I. (2003). Changes in function and ultrastructure of striatal dopaminergic terminals that regenerate following partial lesions of the SNpc, *J Neurochem* 86(329-343).

Tanaka, H., Kannari, K., Maeda, T., Tomiyama, M., Suda, T. & Matsunaga, M. (1999). Role of serotonergic neurons in l-dopa- derived extracellular dopamine in the striatum of 6-OHDA-lesioned rats, *NeuroReport* 10: 631–634.

Zhang, Q.-J., Gao, R., Liu, J., Liu, Y.-P. & Wang, S. (2007). Changes in the firing activity of serotonergic neurons in the dorsal raphe nucleus in a rat model of Parkinson's disease, *Acta Physiologica Sinica* 59(2): 183–189.

Zygmond, M., Abercrombie, E. D., Berger, T. W., Grace, A. A. & Stricker, E. M. (1990). Compensation after lesions of central dopaminergic neurons: some clinical and basic implications, *TINS* 13: 290–296.

Zygmond, M. J., Acheson, A. L., Stachowiak, M. K. & Stricker, E. M. (1984). Neurochemical compensation after nigrostriatal bundle injury in an animal model of preclinical Parkinsonism, *Arch. Neurol.* 41: 856–861.

19

Dopaminergic Control of the Neurotransmitter Release in the Subthalamic Nucleus: Implications for Parkinson's Disease Treatment Strategies

Ben Ampe, Anissa El Arfani, Yvette Michotte and Sophie Sarre
Vrije Universiteit Brussel,
Belgium

1. Introduction

A critical role of the subthalamic nucleus (STN) in the control of movement has been proposed based on the observations that its lesion or high-frequency stimulation, aimed at altering its activity, is effective in alleviating clinical features of Parkinson's disease (Bergman et al,. 1990; Bennazouz et al., 1993; Pollak et al., 1993, Benazzouz et al., 2000). Indeed, overactivity of the subthalamic neurons due to the loss of midbrain dopaminergic neurons is believed to be a key feature in Parkinson's disease. Several studies indicate that the activity of STN neurons can be influenced directly by dopamine and its receptor agonists/antagonists. Indeed, the STN receives a direct dopaminergic input arising in the substantia nigra pars compacta (SNc) and both dopamine D1- and D2-like receptors are present in the STN (Canteras et al., 1990; Hassani et al., 1997; Flores et al., 1999). Understanding the position of the STN within the basal ganglia and the possible direct effects of dopamine and its ligands at the level of this nucleus in normal and parkinsonian states may be important in the development of new therapies for Parkinson's disease. The purpose of this chapter is to give an overview of the current position of the STN in the basal ganglia motorloop and to clarify the role of dopamine at the level of the STN in both normal conditions and in parkinsonian experimental animal models.

2. The subthalamic nucleus and its connections

Despite the small size of this biconvex-shaped structure, the STN has an important role in the modulation of the basal ganglia output and thus movement control (DeLong & Wichmann, 2007; Obeso et al., 2008; Gubbelini et al., 2009). Indeed, together with the striatum, the STN forms the major input to the basal ganglia and is considered an important relay nucleus of the indirect pathway. In this section, the role of the STN within the basal ganglia and its connections are described.

2.1 The subthalamic nucleus as a part of the basal ganglia

The basal ganglia consist of five interconnected nuclei including the caudate nucleus, the putamen [which forms together with the caudate nucleus the striatum], the globus pallidus (pars interna (GPi) and externa (GPe)) the SN (SNc and substantia nigra pars reticulata (SNr)) and the STN (DeLong, 1990; Blandini et al., 2000). Albin and DeLong proposed a schematic view of the basal ganglia organisation which has been used for many years as a reference for understanding their functioning in physiological and pathological conditions (Albin et al., 1989; DeLong, 1990; Gubellini et al., 2009). Currently, this view has been replaced by a more recent representation of the organisation of the basal ganglia based on novel anatomical, neurochemical and physiological data (Levy et al., 1997; Gubellini et al., 2009). In this representation, the striatum and STN are considered as the two major input structures of the basal ganglia. Both nuclei receive input from the cerebral cortex, whereas the GPi and SNr provide output of the basal ganglia to the thalamus and brainstem (DeLong & Wichmann, 2007; Obeso et al., 2008). The striatum is connected with these output structures via a monosynaptic direct pathway and a polysynaptic indirect pathway which includes the GPe and the STN. The striatal direct pathway neurons also receive input from the intralaminar nuclei of the thalamus. The STN is directly connected with the output nuclei.

Besides motor functions, the basal ganglia are involved in cognition and emotion (Alexander et al., 1990; Smith et al., 1998). Indeed, the basal ganglia can be functionally divided into different cortico-subcortical circuits: the motor loop, the associative loop and the limbic loop. Each circuit originates from individual cortical areas, innervates the respective regions of the striatum, GP and SN and, via the thalamus, terminates in their respective cortical areas of origin (Hamani et al., 2004; DeLong & Wichmann, 2007). Like the other structures of the basal ganglia, the STN is subdivided into different major parts: a motor, an associative and a limbic part (Hamani et al., 2004; Benarroch, 2008). The motor part is represented by the large dorsolateral portion of the STN whereas the associative and the limbic part are represented by respectively the ventromedial portion and the medial tip of the STN. Currently, the best characterized cortico-subcortical circuit is the motor circuit.

The motor loop (figure 1) originates from the motor cortex and sends glutamatergic projections to both input nuclei, the striatum and the STN (DeLong & Wichmann, 2007; Obeso et al., 2008). Striatal efferent neurons are γ-aminobutyric acid (GABA)-ergic and are connected, as mentioned before, with the output nuclei, GPi and SNr, by the direct or the indirect pathway. Neurons from the direct pathway, which bear dopamine D1 receptors (excitatory receptors), project directly to the output nuclei. Neurons from the indirect pathway express dopamine D2 receptors (inhibitory receptors) and send GABA-ergic projections to the GPe. The GPe in turn influences the STN by GABA-ergic projections. The STN, which is a glutamatergic structure, provides excitatory input to the output nuclei of the basal ganglia. The balance within the basal ganglia is regulated by the dopaminergic neurons from the SNc. Release of dopamine in the striatum leads to an increase in activity of the direct pathway via the D1 receptors, whereas the activity of the indirect pathway is decreased via the D2 receptors. This dopamine release results in a reduction in the activity of the output nuclei and thus facilitates movement. In Parkinson's disease, nigrostriatal degeneration leads to hyperactivity of the STN and thus to an increase of the output nuclei activity which in turn results in inhibition of ongoing movement.

2.2 Subthalamic nucleus afferents and efferents

As described above, the STN has a pivotal position in the motor circuitry. Indeed, it is part of a complex organisation within the basal ganglia and is connected with a wide range of structures. It is the only glutamatergic nucleus of the basal ganglia (Smith & Parent, 1988; Blandini et al., 2000; Hamani et al., 2004). The STN provides a strong excitatory input to the two output structures, GPi and SNr, but also to the GPe. Via its excitatory input to the SNc, it influences the regulation of the dopamine release (Smith et al., 1990; Parent & Hazrati, 1995; Hamani et al., 2004). Besides the main efferent projections described above, the STN is connected with the peduncolopontine nucleus and the ventral tegmental area through which it influences the processing of emotional information (Smith et al., 1990; Parent & Hazrati, 1995; Haegelen et al., 2009). Furthermore, the STN sends poor glutamatergic projections to the striatum and the motor cortex (Smith et al., 1990; Blandini et al., 2000).

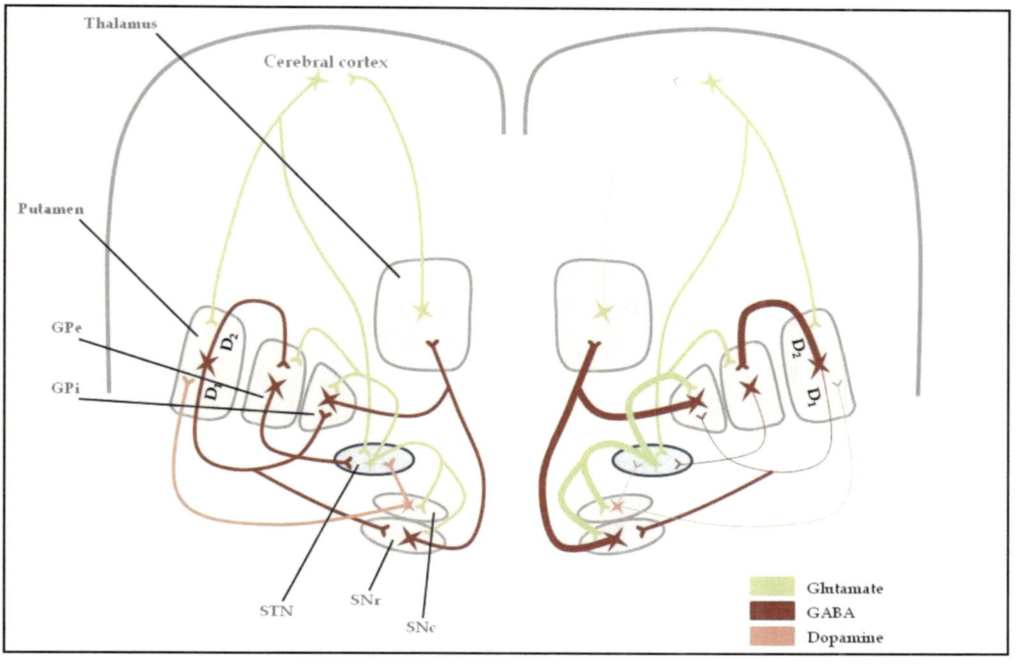

Fig. 1. Left brain hemisphere: motor loop in a normal condition. Right brain hemisphere: motor loop in Parkinson's disease. The motor loop originates from the motor cortex and sends glutamatergic projections to both input nuclei, the striatum and the STN. Striatal neurons from the direct pathway (contain D1 receptors) project directly to the output nuclei whereas neurons from the indirect pathway (contain D2 receptors) send GABA-ergic projections to the GPe. The GPe in turn influences the STN by GABA-ergic projections. The STN provides excitatory input to the output nuclei. Release of dopamine in the striatum leads to an increase in activity of the direct pathway via the D1 receptors whereas the activity of the indirect pathway is decreased via the D2 receptors. Dopamine release results in a reduction in the activity of the output nuclei and, via the thalamus, leads to glutamatergic projections to the cortex which facilitates movement. In Parkinson's disease, dopaminergic degeneration of the SNc leads to hyperactivity of the STN and thus an increase of the output nuclei activity which in turn results in inhibition of ongoing movement. The thickness of the depicted projections reflects their activity.

Neurons of the STN receive two major projections: a direct excitatory glutamatergic input from the cerebral cortex and an important inhibitory GABA-ergic innervation from the GPe (Blandini et al., 2000; Hamani et al., 2004; DeLong & Wichmann, 2007). It also receives inhibitory projections from the GPi, SNr and striatum. Another source of excitatory input to the STN is the centromedian-parafascicular nucleus of the thalamus. Furthermore, glutamatergic and cholinergic projections arise from the pedunculopontine nucleus to the STN. Besides the main glutamatergic and GABA-ergic afferents to the STN, dopaminergic neurons from the SNc also innervate the STN (Campbell et al., 1985; Canteras et al., 1990;

Hassani et al., 1996). These neurons modulate the activity of glutamatergic and GABA-ergic afferents arising from respectively the cortex and the pallidum to the STN. In addition, the STN receives serotonergic projections from the dorsal raphe nucleus which may also be involved in the modulation of the STN activity (Blandini et al., 2000; Hamani et al., 2004; DeLong & Wichmann, 2007). In this chapter, the importance of the dopaminergic input from the SNc to the STN will be described.

3. Dopamine receptors in the subthalamic nucleus

Because of their relevance in Parkinson's disease, large research efforts have been made to investigate the presence and localisation of dopamine receptors in the central nervous system, especially since the mid to late eighties (Wamsley et al., 1989). These receptors consist of a large family of D1-like dopamine receptors, divided into D1 and D5 receptors, and D2-like dopamine receptors, divided into D2, D3 and D4 receptors (Niznik, 1987; Niznik et al., 1992; Sibley et al., 1992; Gingrich et al., 1993). In general, D1 receptors are known to be positively coupled to adenylatecyclase via a Gs protein, whereas D2 receptors are either uncoupled or negatively coupled to adenylatecyclase (Onali et al., 1985; Memo et al., 1986). Both the D1-like and the D2-like dopamine receptors are known to be abundantly expressed and widely distributed throughout different basal ganglia nuclei. A series of experimental studies indicate that functional dopamine receptors are expressed and localised in the STN but there is still debate concerning the receptor subtypes.

The occurance of D1 receptors in the STN has been reported in a number of histological studies (Brown et al., 1979; Dubois et al., 1986; Fremeau et al., 1991; Mansour et al., 1992). However, Johnson et al. reported that D1 receptors are not located within the borders of the STN but are situated in the cerebral peduncles (Johnson et al., 1994). By means of autoradiography in rats, Kreiss et al. confirmed the presence of D1 dopamine receptors along the ventral edge of the STN which borders the cerebral peduncle. This was confirmed in a morphological study showing that the dendrites of STN neurons extend across the ventral STN borders into the peduncles (Kita et al., 1983). D1 receptors were not observed in the dorsal regions of the STN (Kreiss et al., 1996). Another autoradiographic study confirmed the presence of D1 receptors in the STN and found that there was a clear dorsoventral gradient in D1 binding sites at the level of the STN (Flores et al., 1999). Dopamine D2 receptors have also been shown to be present at the level of the rat STN by several groups (Boyson et al., 1986; Bouthenet et al., 1987; Johnson et al., 1994). Flores et al. were able to show the presence of all three subtypes of the D2-like receptors, although the amounts of D3 dopamine receptors were very low (Flores et al., 1999). However, no dopamine D1, D2, D3 nor D4 mRNA was detected by several investigators in both rat and human STN (Fremeau et al., 1991; Mansour et al., 1992; Augood et al., 2000). Nevertheless, Bouthenet et al. showed the presence of both D2 and D3 mRNA at the level of the STN with in situ histochemistry (Bouthenet et al., 1991). Moreover, using reverse transcriptase polymerase chain reaction the presence of D1 receptor mRNA was confirmed (Flores et al., 1999), together with the expression of the mRNA encoding for D2 and D3 receptors. By means of in situ hybridisation, high levels of D5 dopamine receptor mRNA were found at the level of the STN (Svenningson & Le Moine, 2002). However, they were unable to detect mRNA levels for all other dopamine receptor subtypes. Baufreton et al. also showed the presence of D5 dopamine receptors on burst competent STN neurons with single-cell reverse transcription-PCR profiling. They also used an antibody raised against a peptide sequence of cloned D5 receptor and detected immunoreactivity in the STN cell bodies (Baufreton et al., 2003).

Thus, using an array of techniques, all dopamine receptor subtypes have been detected in STN. However, the data remain inconsistent and more research is warranted.

4. Role of dopamine at the level of the subthalamic nucleus

Numerous studies in the past have suggested a direct role of dopamine and its receptor ligands at the level of the STN. As described above, the presence of both D1- and D2-like dopamine receptors in the STN has been demonstrated. Several anatomical studies provided evidence for a direct and substantial nigrosubthalamic dopaminergic projection in rats (Campbell et al., 1985; Canteras et al., 1990; Hassani et al., 1996). Moreover, we and others have shown that dopamine is released within the STN in vivo (Cragg et al., 2004; Ampe et al., 2007). However, despite numerous investigations, many discrepancies still exist with regard to the effect of dopamine and its receptor agonists on the activity of STN neurons. In the classical model of the basal ganglia motorloop, dopamine is widely assumed to exert an inhibitory influence on STN neuronal activity (Albin et al., 1995) and dopamine should reduce excitability of STN neurons in parkinsonian brain (DeLong, 1990; Bergman et al., 1994). A variety of in vitro an in vivo experimental studies have addressed this issue.

Several in vitro electrophysiological studies have shown inhibitory effects of dopamine on STN neuronal activity (Campbell et al., 1985; Hassani et al., 1999). However, others have found dopaminergic agonists to excite the activity of STN neurons. Indeed, Zhu et al. (2002a) showed that a dopamine bath application significantly increased the firing rates of STN neurons in a concentration-dependent fashion in both intact and 6-hydroxydopamine (6-OHDA) lesioned rats. They also showed that this excitatory effect of dopamine was largely mimicked by application of the dopamine D2 receptor agonist quinpirole. The dopamine D1 receptor agonist SKF-38393 showed a trend towards an increase in STN firing rate, but this effect was only significant in the 6-OHDA lesioned group. They concluded that dopamine exerts an excitatory influence on STN neuronal activity and that this effect is likely to be established by stimulation of D2 receptors. They also observed that dopamine, in 6-OHDA lesioned rats, in addition to the firing rates, also changes the irregular firing pattern into a more regular pacemaker pattern at the level of the STN (Zhu et al., 2002a). The same group also demonstrated that dopamine increases the firing rates of action potentials and produces inward currents in STN neurons. Together with the fact that these inward currents persisted when excitatory synaptic transmission was blocked, illustrated that dopamine exerted a direct excitatory effect at the level of the STN (Zhu et al., 2002b). In another in vitro electrophysiological study, Tofighy et al. (2003) showed that dopamine caused modest, but reliable, increases in the firing rates of STN neurons and considered this effect likely to be a direct excitatory action on STN neurons. The dopamine D2 receptor agonists quinpirole and bromocriptine caused concentration-dependent increases in the firing rates of STN neurons, whereas the mixed dopamine D1/D2 receptor agonist apomorphine caused only weak and less reproducible responses in STN firing rates. The dopamine D1 receptor agonist, SKF 38393 was without effect on STN firing rates. These results initially suggested an excitatory effect of dopamine on the STN neurons through a direct D2 receptor mediated mechanism. However, due to the fact that the effective concentration of all agonists was high, the authors stated that the effects could well be non-specific. This, together with the inconsistent effects of apomorphine and the inability of dopamine D2 (nor D1) receptor antagonists to reduce the observed excitatory effects led the authors to conclude that these effects probably cannot be assigned to dopamine receptors but to non-catecholaminergic receptors (Tofighy et al., 2003). Baufreton et al., by means of in vitro electrophysiological recordings, showed that activating D1 and D2 dopamine receptors with D1 and D2 agonists promotes pace making at the level of the STN by increasing the firing frequency of neurons that exhibit tonic firing capacity and by changing firing in burst-competent and spontaneously burst-firing neurons. Moreover, they also showed that D5 dopamine receptors may potentiate burst-firing in STN neurons by modulating L-type calcium channels in the absence of dopamine (Baufreton et al., 2003; Baufreton et al., 2005). Finally, Loucif et al. showed that dopamine clearly produces subthalamic membrane depolarisation leading towards an increase in firing rate. This effect seemed to be due to action on D1-like dopamine receptor mediated activation of a cyclic-nucleotide gated non-specific cation conductance. This conductance also contributed to the membrane depolarisation changing STN neuronal bursting towards a regular activity (Loucif et al., 2008). Thus, in vitro studies suggest that dopamine at the level of the STN exerts excitatory effects, possibly via D2 receptors. More recent studies, however, suggest D1-like mediated effects.

Several in vivo studies showed an inhibitory effect of dopamine on the activity of STN neurons. Campbell et al., using horseradish peroxidase and microiontophoresis, suggested that dopamine suppresses STN activity (Campbell et al., 1985). Injection of the mixed D1/D2 agonist apomorphine into the STN of intact rats decreased the mean firing rates of STN neurons significantly. However, an increase of firing rates was observed in 6-OHDA lesioned rats (Hassani et al., 1999). The selective D1 dopamine receptor agonist SKF 82958, when injected into the STN, decreased the activity of STN neurons in both intact and 6-OHDA lesioned rats. Injection of the selective D2 dopamine receptor agonist quinpirole decreased the firing rate of STN neurons, whereas in 6-OHDA lesioned animals it significantly increased firing rates. Hassani and colleagues concluded that dopamine receptor agonists probably have an inhibitory effect on STN neurons of intact rats via a D1 dopamine receptor mediated mechanism, whereas in 6-OHDA lesioned animals dopamine receptor agonists stimulate the STN via D2 dopamine receptors and inhibit activity via D1 dopamine receptors (Hassani et al., 1999). On the other hand, several other in vivo studies suggested a facilitatory effect of dopamine at the level of the STN. Glucose utilization was decreased in the STN following systemic administration of the dopamine D1 receptor antagonist SCH23390 (Trugman et al., 1993) whereas it was increased following systemic administration of the mixed D1/D2 dopamine receptor agonist apomorphine or following amphetamine (Brown et al., 1978; Wechsler et al., 1979; Trugman et al., 1993). Kreiss et al. described predominantly D1 mediated excitatory effects since neuronal firing rates in the STN of intact rats was increased following a systemic administration of apomorphine. Systemic administration of the dopamine D2 receptor agonist quinpirole did not alter STN firing rates, whereas the dopamine D1 receptor agonists SKF 38393 and SKF 82958 clearly increased STN firing rates. Local administration of the dopamine D1 receptor agonist SKF 82958 also increased firing rates (Kreiss et al, 1996). Using microiontophoresis, a clear excitatory effect of dopamine on the majority of STN neurons in both intact and 6-OHDA lesioned rats was observed (Ni et al., 2001). The excitatory effect of dopamine in the 6-OHDA lesioned rats was similar to that in intact rats. Their results were in good agreement with previous studies using the same technique also showing that dopamine induced an increase in firing rate of almost all STN neurons of intact rats (Mintz et al, 1986). Selective dopamine depletion by injection of 6-OHDA in the STN resulted in a clear decrease of the firing rate together with a change in firing pattern, reinforcing the evidence of an excitatory effect of dopamine at the level of the STN (Ni et al. 2001). Finally, we were the first to study the in vivo release of dopamine and glutamate in the STN using in vivo microdialysis (Ampe et al., 2007). We were able to establish that perfusion of the STN with NMDA enhanced dopamine and glutamate release in a concentration dependent manner. We showed that this release was dependent on both D1 and D2 receptors since the NMDA-mediated effects were blocked by local perfusion of both the dopamine D1 receptor antagonist SCH 23390 and the dopamine D2 receptor antagonist raclopride, confirming the presence of this type of receptors in the STN. The importance of the dopaminergic innervation to the STN in these effects was demonstrated by the fact that depletion of dopamine by 6-OHDA lesioning of the SNc resulted in an absence of the effects of NMDA in the STN (Ampe et al., 2007). More recently, we showed that perfusion of the STN with dopamine or its D1 receptor agonist SKF38393 results in excitation of the STN since extracellular glutamate is increased. Again, 6-OHDA lesioning abolished these effects (Ampe et al., submitted elsewhere). Taken together, the majority of the available in vivo data clearly suggest an excitatory effect of dopamine on STN neurons that is mediated via dopamine D1 receptors.

	Intact		6-OHDA	
	STN inhibition	**STN activation**	**STN inhibition**	**STN activation**
In Vitro	**DA** *Campbell et al., 1985* *Hassani et al., 1999*	**DA** *Zhu et al., 2002a* *Zhu et al., 2002b* **D2 - quinpirole** *Zhu et al., 2002a* *Tofighy et al., 2003* **D1/D5-SKF82958;SKF 81297** *Baufreton et al., 2003*		**DA** *Zhu et al., 2002b* **D2 - quinpirole** *Zhu et al., 2002a* *Baufreton et al., 2005* **D1/D5-SKF38393 ; SKF82958; SKF 81297** *Baufreton et al., 2005* *Loucif et al, 2008*
In Vivo	**DA** *Campbell et al., 1985* **amphetamine** *Welchsler et al.,1979* **D1/D2 - apomorphine** *Brown et al., 1978* *Hassani et al., 1999* **D1/D5 - SKF82958** *Hassani et al., 1999* **D2 - quinpirole** *Hassani et al., 1999*	**DA** *Mintz et al., 1986* *Ni et al., 2001* **D1/D2 - apomorphine** *Trugmann et al.,1993* *Kreiss et al., 1996* **D1/D5-SKF38393 ; SKF82958** *Ni et al., 2001* *Kreiss et al., 1996*	**D1/D5 - SKF82958** *Hassani et al., 1999*	**DA** *Ni et al., 2001* **D2 - quinpirole** *Hassani et al., 1999* *Ni et al., 2001* **D1/D5-SKF38393** *Ni et al., 2001*

Table 1. Overview of different publications regarding the effects of dopamine and its agonists on subthalamic activity in both intact and 6-OHDA lesioned rats.

5. Implications for Parkinson's disease treatment strategies

The existence of a direct nigrosubthalamic dopaminergic pathway is nowadays a well established fact. Moreover, dopamine receptors of both D1 and D2 like families have been shown to be present at the level of the STN. Otheiatal level, it is now clear that dopamine exerts direct effects at the level of other basal ganglia nuclei of which the STN plays a pivotal role in Parkinson's disease. Since altered neuronal output from the STN plays a central role in the pathophysiology of Parkinson's disease and overactivity of subthalamic neurons due to the loss of dopaminergic neurons contributes to increased excitation of the main output nuclei, effects of dopaminergic drugs (still the main drug treatment for Parkinson's disease) on subthalamic neuronal activity is highly important. It has been shown in different studies that dopamine and its agonists can alter subthalamic activity in both intact and parkinsonian animals. However, discrepancies still exist regarding the effects of dopaminergic stimulation. In the pathological state, most in vitro and in vivo studies agree on an excitatory effect of dopamine at the subthalamic level. Surprisingly, this opposes the current hypothesis that dopamine receptor stimulation alleviates symptoms of Parkinson's disease by reducing STN output (DeLong, 1990). The receptor subtypes by which dopamine exerts these excitatory effects differ between studies and different effects are seen depending on the receptor subtype. Moreover, not only effects on firing rates but also effects on subthalamic firing patterns were seen after dopamine application, further strengthening the hypothesis that dopamine clearly alters neuronal output at the subthalamic level. Dopamine replacement therapy remains the standard therapy for Parkinson's disease. Most of the dopamine agonists used to treat the symptoms of Parkinson's disease are non-specific for one or the other receptor subtype. We also know that after the so-called "honeymoon period" the effective response to dopamine wears off, and that undesirable side effects, like dyskinesia, occur. Further investigation towards an even better understanding of the effects of dopamine at the subthalamic level, and the receptor subtypes involved in these effects, can lead towards the development of better targeted drugs for the treatment of Parkinson's disease. Therefore, future studies investigating the effects of selective ligands of different dopamine receptor subtypes in experimental Parkinson's disease models, combining investigation towards electrophysiological effects and effects on neurotransmitter release of these ligands at the level of the STN, are necessary for developing more specific and selective drugs to treat different stages of Parkinson's disease.

6. References

Albin, R.L.; Young, A.B. & Penney, J.B. (1989). The functional anatomy of basal ganglia disorders. *Trends in neurosciences,* Vol.12, No.10, (October 1989), pp. 366-75, ISSN 0166-2236

Albin, R.L.; Young, A.B. & Penney, J. B. (1995). The functional anatomy of disorders of the basal ganglia. *Trends in neurosciences*, Vol.18, No.2, (February 1995), pp. 63-4, ISSN 0166-2236

Alexander, G.E.; Crutcher, M.D. & DeLong, M.R. (1990). Basal ganglia-thalamocortical circuits: parallel substrates for motor, oculomotor, "prefrontal" and "limbic" functions. *Progress in brain research,* Vol.85, (1990), pp. 119-46, ISSN 0079-6123

Ampe, B.; Massie, A.; D'Haens, J.; Ebinger, G.; Michotte, Y. & Sarre, S. (2007). NMDA-mediated release of glutamate and GABA in the subthalamic nucleus is mediated by dopamine: an in vivo microdialysis study in rats. *Journal of neurochemistry,* Vol.103, No.3, (November 2007), pp. 1063-74, ISSN 0022-3042

Augood, S.J.; Hollingsworth, Z.R.; Standaert, D.G.; Emson, P.C. & Penney, J.B. Jr. (2000). Localization of dopaminergic markers in the human subthalamic nucleus. *The Journal of comparative neurology,* Vol.421, No.2, (May 2000), pp. 247-55., ISSN 0021-9967

Baufreton, J.; Garret, M.; Rivera, A.; de la Calle, A.; Gonon, F.; Dufy, B.; Bioulac, B. & Taupignon, A.L. (2003). A D5 (not D1) dopamine receptors potentiate burst-firing in neurones of the subthalamic nucleus by modulating an L-type calcium conductance. *Journal of Neuroscience,* Vol.23, No.3, (February 2003), pp. 816–825, ISSN 0270-6474

Baufreton, J.; Zhu, Z.T.; Garret, M.; Bioulac, B.; Johnson, S.W. & Taupignon, A.L. (2005). Dopamine receptors set the pattern of activity generated in subthalamic neurons. *The FASEB Journal,* Vol.19, No.13, (November 2005), pp. 1771-7, ISSN 0892-6638

Benarroch, E.E. (2008). Subthalamic nucleus and its connections: Anatomic substrate for the network effects of deep brain stimulation. *Neurology,* Vol.70, No.21, (May 2008), pp. 1991-5, ISSN 0028-3878

Benazzouz, A.; Gross, C.; Féger, J.; Boraud, T. & Bioulac, B. (1993). Reversal of rigidity and improvement in motor performance by subthalamic high-frequency stimulation in MPTP-treated monkeys. *The European journal of neuroscience,* Vol.5, No.4, (April 1993), pp. 382-9, ISSN 0953-816X

Benazzouz, A.; Piallat, B.; Ni, Z.G.; Koudsie, A.; Pollak, P. & Benabid, A.L. (2000) Implication of the subthalamic nucleus in the pathophysiology and pathogenesis of Parkinson's disease. *Cell Transplant* 9, 215-221, 0963-6897.

Bergman, H.; Wichmann, T. & DeLong, M.R. (1990). Reversal of experimental parkinsonism by lesions of the subthalamic nucleus. *Science,* Vol.249, No.4975, (September 1990), pp. 1436-8, ISSN 0036-8075

Bergman, H.; Wichmann, T.; Karmon, B. & DeLong, M.R. (1994). The primate subthalamic nucleus. II. Neuronal activity in the MPTP model of parkinsonism. *Journal of neurophysiology,* Vol.72, No.2, (August 1994), pp. 507–20, ISSN 0022-3077

Bouthenet, M.L.; Matres, M.P.; Sales, N. & Schwartz, J.C. (1987). A detailed mapping of dopamine D2 receptors in rat central nervous system by autoradiography with (125I)iodosulpiride. *Neuroscience,* Vol.20, No. 1, (January 1987), pp. 117-55, ISSN 0306-4522

Bouthenet, M.L.; Souil, E.; Matres, M.P.; Sokoloff, P.; Giros, B. & Schwartz, J.C. (1991). Localisation of dopamine D3 receptor mRNA in the rat brain using in situ histochemistry: comparison with dopamine D2 receptor mRNA. *Brain research,* Vol. 564, No.2, (November 1991), pp. 203-19, ISSN:0006-8993

Boyson, S.J.; McGonigle, P. & Molinoff, P.B. (1986). Quantitative autoradiographic localization of the D1 and D2 subtypes of dopamine receptors in rat brain. *The Journal of neuroscience,* Vol. 6, No.11, (November 1986), pp. 3177-88, ISSN 0270-6474

Blandini, F.; Nappi, G.; Tassorelli, C. & Martignoni, E. (2000). Functional changes of the basal ganglia circuitry in Parkinson's disease. *Progress in neurobiology,* Vol.62, No.1, (September 2000), pp. 63-88, ISSN 0555-4047

Brown, L.L. & Wolfson, L.I. (1978). Apomorphine increases glucose utilization in the substantia nigra, subthalamic nucleus, and corpus striatum of rat. *Brain research,* Vol.140, No.1, (January 1978), pp. 188-93, ISSN 0006-8993

Brown, L.L.; Maakman, M.H.; Wolfson, L.I.; Dvorkin, B.; Warner C. & Katzman, R. (1979). A direct role of dopamine in the rat subthalamic nucleus and an adjacent intrapeduncular area. *Science,* Vol.206, No.4425, (December 1979), pp. 1416-8, ISSN 0036-8075

Campbell, G.A.; Eckardt, M.J. & Weight, F.F. (1985). Dopaminergic mechanisms in the subthalamic nucleus of rat: analysis using horseradish peroxidase and microiontophoresis. *Brain Research,* Vol.333, No.2, (May 1985), pp. 261-70, ISSN 0006-8993

Canteras, N.S.; Shammah-Lagnado, S.J.; Silva, B.A. & Ricardo, J.A. (1990). Afferent connections of the subthalamic nucleus: a combined retrograde and anterograde horseradish peroxidase study in the rat. *Brain Research,* Vol.513, No.1, (April 1990), pp. 43-59, ISSN 0006-8993

Cragg, S.J.; Baufreton, J.; Xue, Y.;Bolam, J.P. & Bevan, M.D. (2004). Synaptic release of dopamine in the subthalamic nucleus. *European Journal of Neuroscience,* Vol.20, No.7, (October 2004), pp. 1788-802, ISSN 0953-816X

DeLong, M.R. (1990). Primate models of movement disorders of basal ganglia origin. *Trends in Neuroscience,* Vol.13, No.7, (July 1990), pp. 281-5, ISSN 0166-2236

DeLong, M.R. & Wichmann, T. (2007). Circuits and circuit disorders of the basal ganglia. *Archives of neurology,* Vol.64, No.1, (January 2007), pp. 20-4, ISSN 0003-9942

Dubois, A.; Savasta, M.; Curet, O. & Scatton, B. (1986). Autoradiographic distribution of the D1 agonist (3H)SKF38393 in the rat brain and spinal cord. Comparison with the distribution of D2 receptors. *Neuroscience,* Vol.19, No.1, (September 1986), pp. 125-37, ISSN 0306-4522

Flores, G.; Liang, J.J.; Sierra, A.; Martinez-Fong, D.; Quiron, R.; Aceves, J. & Srivastava, L.K. (1999). Expression of dopamine receptors in the subthalamic nucleus of the rat: characterisation using reverse transcriptase-polymerase chain reaction and autoradiography. *Neuroscience,* Vol.91, No.2, (1999), pp. 549-56, ISSN 0306-4522

Fremeau, R.T.; Duncan, G.E.; Fornaretto, M.G; Dearry, A.; Gingrich, J.A.; Breese, G.R. & Caron, M.G. (1991). Localization of D1 dopamine receptor mRNA in brain supports a role in cognitive, affective and neuroendocrine aspects of dopaminergic neurotransmission. *Proceedings of the National Academy of Sciences of the United States of America,* Vol.88, No.9, (May 1991), pp. 3772-6, ISSN 0027-8424

Gingrich, J.A. and Caron, M.G. (1993). Recent advances in the molecular biology of dopamine receptors. *Annual review of neuroscience,* Vol.16, (1993), pp. 299-321, ISSN 0147-006X

Gubellini, P.; Salin, P.; Kerkerian-Le Goff, L. & Baunez, C. (2009). Deep brain stimulation in neurological diseases and experimental models: from molecule to complex behavior. *Progress in neurobiology,* Vol.89, No.1, (September 2009), pp. 79-123, ISSN 0555-4047

Haegelen, C.; Rouaud, T.; Darnault, P. & Morandi, X. (2009). The subthalamic nucleus is a key-structure of limbic basal ganglia functions. *Medical hypotheses,* Vol.72, No.4, (April 2009), pp. 421-6, ISSN 0306-9877

Hamani, C.; Saint-Cyr, JA.; Fraser, J.; Kaplitt, M. & Lozano, AM. (2004). The subthalamic nucleus in the context of movement disorders. *Brain,* Vol.127, No. 1, (January 2004), pp. 4-20, ISSN 0006-8950

Hassani, O.K.; Mouroux, M. & Féger, J. (1996). Increased subthalamic neuronal activity after nigral dopaminergic lesion independent of disinhibition via the globus pallidus. *Neuroscience,* Vol.72, No.1, (May 1996), pp. 105-15, ISSN 0306-4522

Hassani, O.K.; Francois, C.; Yelnik, J.; Féger J. (1997) Evidence for a dopaminergic innervation of the subthalamic nucleus in the rat. *Brain Res*. 749, 88-94, ISSN 0006-8993.

Hassani, O.K. & Féger, J. (1999). Effects of intra-subthalamic injection of dopamine receptor agonists on subthalamic neurones in normal and 6-hydroxydopamine lesioned rats:

an electrophysiological and C-Fos study. *Neuroscience,* Vol.92, No.2, (1999), pp. 533-43, ISSN 0306-4522

Johnson, A.E; Coirini, H.; Kallstrom, L. & Wiesel, F.A. (1994). Characterization of dopamine receptor binding sites in the subthalamic nucleus. *Neuroreport,* Vol.5, No.14, (September 1994), pp. 1836-8, ISSN 0959-4965

Kita, H.; Chang, H.T. & Kitai, S.T. (1983). The morphology of intracellulary labeled rat subthalamic neurons; a light microscopic analysis. *The Journal of comparative neurology,* Vol.215, No.3, (April 1983), pp. 245-57, ISSN 0021-9967

Kreiss, D.S.; Anderson, L.A. & Walters, J.R. (1996). Apomorphine and dopamine D(1) receptor agonists increase the firing rates of subthalamic nucleus neurons. *Neuroscience,* Vol.72, No.3, (June 1996), pp. 863-76, ISSN 0306-4522

Levy, R.; Hazrati, L.N.; Herrero, M.T.; Vila, M.; Hassani, O.K.; Mouroux, M.; Ruberg, M.; Asensi, H.; Agid, Y.; Féger, J.; Obeso, J.A.; Parent, A. & Hirsch, E.C. (1997). Re-evaluation of the functional anatomy of the basal ganglia in normal and Parkinsonian states. *Neuroscience,* Vol.76, No.2, (January 1997), pp. 335-43, ISSN 0306-4522

Loucif, A.J.; Woodhall, G.L.; Sehirli, U.S.; Stanford, I.M. (2008). Depolarisation and suppression of burst activity in the mouse subthalamic nucleus by dopamine D1/D5 receptor activation of a cyclic-nucleotide gated non-specific cation conductance. *Neuropharmacology,* Vol. 55, No.1 (July 2008), pp. 94-105, ISSN 0028-3908

Mansour, A.; Meador-Woodruff, J.H.; Zhou, Q.; Civello, O.; Akil, H. & Watson, S.J. (1992). A comparison of D1 receptor binding and mRNA in rat brain using receptor autoradiography and in situ hybridization techniques. *Neuroscience,* Vol.46, No.4, (1992), pp. 959-71, ISSN 0306-4522

Memo, M.; Missale, C.; Carruba, M.O. & Spano, P.F. (1986). D2 dopamine receptors associated with inhibition of dopamine release from rat neostriatum are independent of cyclic AMP. *Neuroscience letters,* Vol.71, No.2, (November 1986), pp. 192-6, ISSN 0304-3940

Mintz, I.; Hammond, C. & Féger, J. (1986). Excitatory effect of iontophoretically applied dopamine on identified neurones of the rat subthalamic nucleus. *Brain Research,* Vol.375, No.1, (June 1986), pp. 172-5, ISSN 0006-8993

Ni, Z.G.; Gao, D.M.; Bouali-Benazzouz, R.; Benabid, A.L. & Benazzouz, A. (2001). Effect of microionotophoretic application of dopamine on subthalamic nucleus neuronal activity in normal rats and in rats with unilateral lesion of the nigrostriatal pathway. *European Journal of Neuroscience,* Vol.14, No.2, (July 2001), pp. 373-81, ISSN 0953-816X

Niznik, H.B. (1987). Dopamine receptors: molecular structure and function. *Molecular and cellular endocrinology,* Vol.54, No.1, (November 1987), pp. 1-22, ISSN 0303-7207

Niznik, H.B. & Van Tol, H.H. (1992). Dopamine receptor genes: new tools for molecular psychiatry. *Journal of psychiatry & neuroscience : JPN,* Vol.17, No.4, (October 1992), pp. 158-80, ISSN 1180-4882

Obeso, J.A.; Rodríguez-Oroz, M.C.; Benitez-Temino, B.; Blesa, F.J.; Guridi, J.; Marin, C. & Rodriguez, M. (2008). Functional organization of the basal ganglia: therapeutic implications for Parkinson's disease. *Movement disorders : official journal of the Movement Disorder Society,* Vol.23, No.3, (2008), pp. 548-59, ISSN 0885-3185

Onali, P.; Olianas, M.C. and Gessa, G.L. (1985). Characterization of dopamine receptors mediating inhibition of adenylatecyclase in rat striatum. *Molecular pharmacology*, Vol.28, No.2, (August 1985), pp. 138-45, ISSN 0026-895X

Parent, A. & Hazrati, L.N. (1995). Functional anatomy of the basal ganglia. II. The place of subthalamic nucleus and external pallidum in basal ganglia circuitry. *Brain research reviews*, Vol.20, No.1, (January 1995), pp. 128-54, ISSN 0165-0173

Pollak, P.; Benabid, A.L.; Gervason, C.L.; Hoffmann, D.; Seigneuret, E. & Perret, J. (1993). Long-term effects of chronic stimulation of the ventral intermediate thalamic nucleus in different types of tremor. *Advances in neurology*, Vol.60, (1993), pp. 408-13, ISSN 0091-3952

Sibley, D.R. & Monsma, F.J. Jr. (1992). Molecular biology of dopamine receptors. *Trends in pharmacological sciences*, Vol.13, No.2, (February 1992), pp. 61-9, ISSN 0165-6147

Smith, Y. & Parent, A. (1988). Neurons of the subthalamic nucleus in primates display glutamate but not GABA immunoreactivity. *Brain research*, Vol.453, No.1-2, (June 1988), pp. 353-6, ISSN 0006-8993

Smith, Y.; Hazrati, L.N. & Parent, A. (1990). Efferent projections of the subthalamic nucleus in the squirrel monkey as studied by the PHA-L anterograde tracing method. *The Journal of comparative neurology*, Vol.294, No.2, (April 1990), pp. 306-23, ISSN 0021-9967

Smith, Y.; Bevan, M.D.; Shink, E. & Bolam, J.P. (1998). Microcircuitry of the direct and indirect pathways of the basal ganglia. *Neuroscience*, Vol.86, No.2, (September 1998), pp. 353-87, ISSN 0306-4522

Svenningsson, P. & Le Moine, C. (2002). Dopamine D1/5 receptor stimulation induces c-fos expression in the subthalamic nucleus: possible involvement of local D5 receptors. *The European journal of neuroscience*, Vol.15, No.1, (January 2002), pp. 133-42, ISSN 0953-816X

Tofighy, A.; Abbott, A.; Centonze, D.; Cooper, A.J.; Noor, E.; Pearce, S.M.; Puntis, M.; Stanford, I.M.; Wigmore, M.A. & Lacey, M.G. (2003). Excitation by dopamine of rat subthalamic nucleus neurones in vitro - a direct action with unconventional pharmacology. *Neuroscience*, Vol.116, No.1, (2003), pp. 157-66, ISSN 0306-4522

Trugman, J.M. and James, C.L. (1993). D1 dopamine agonist and antagonist effects on regional cerebral glucose utilization in rats with intact dopaminergic innervation. *Brain research*, Vol.607, No.1-2, (April 1993), pp. 270-4, ISSN 0006-8993

Wamsley, J.K.; Gehrelt, D.R.; Filloux, F.M. & Dawson, T.M. (1989). Comparison of the distribution of D1 and D2 dopamine receptors in the rat brain. *Journal of chemical neuroanatomy*, Vol.2, No.3, (May-June 1989), pp. 119-37, ISSN 0891-0618

Wechsler, L.R.; Savaki, H.E. & Sokoloff, L. (1979). Effects of D-and L-amphetamine on local cerebral glucose utilization in the conscious rat. *Journal of neurochemistry*, Vol.32, No.1, (January 1979), pp. 15-22, ISSN 0022-3042

Zhu, Z.; Bartol, M.; Shen, K. & Johnson, S.W. (2002a). Excitatory effects of dopamine on subthalamic nucleus neurones: in vitro study of rats pretreated with 6-hydroxydopamine and levodopa. *Brain Research*, Vol.945, No.1, (July 2002), pp. 31-40, ISSN 0006-8993

Zhu, Z.T.; Shen, K.Z. & Johnson, S.W. (2002b). Pharmacological identification of inward current evoked by dopamine in rat subthalamic neurones in vitro. *Neuropharmacology*, Vol.42, No.6, (May 2002), pp. 772-81, ISSN 0028-3908

20

Possible Contribution of the Basal Ganglia Brainstem System to the Pathogenesis of Parkinson's Disease

Kaoru Takakusaki[1], Kazuhiro Obara[1] and Toshikatsu Okumura[2]

[1]Research Center for Brain Function and Medical Engineering,
[2]Department of General Medicine,
Asahikawa Medical University, School of Medicine,
Japan

1. Introduction

Insight into the organization of the motor and non-motor symptoms in Parkinson's disease (PD) is critical for understanding the role of basal ganglia in the control of behavioral expression. Motor symptoms are generally characterized by hypokinesia-bradykinesia, resting tremor, muscular rigidity and posture-gait disabilities (Morris et al., 1994; Murrey et al., 1978). Sleep disturbances are major non-motor symptoms, which include insomnia, narcolepsy-like sleep attack and rapid eye movement (REM) sleep behavioral disorder (RBD) (Ferini-Strambi & Zucconi, 2000; Iranzo et al., 2006; Postuma et al., 2010; Schenck, 1996), in addition to disturbances of emotional expression and impairments of cognitive and executive functions (Aarsland et al., 2010).

It has been well established that the cortico-basal ganglia loops (C-BG loop) contribute to the volitional and intentional control of movements (Delong & Wichmann, 2007). Basal ganglia outflow directly toward to the midbrain of the brainstem (basal ganglia-brainstem system; BG-BS system) has been recently recognized with respect to the regulation of muscle tone and posture-gait synergy (Takakusaki et al., 2003a, 2004c). It has been suggested that the BG-BS may also contribute to the modulation of vigilance states (Takakusaki et al., 2004c, 2005). Fundamental structures involved in the control of posture and locomotion and those in the muscle tone regulation during awake-sleep states exist in the brainstem and spinal cord (Chase & Morales 1990; Takakusaki et al., 1993, 1994, 2004a, 2006). The importance of the midbrain area including the pedunculopontine tegmental nucleus (PPN) has been particularly recognized in relation to these functions (Palphill & Lozano 2000; Datta, 2002; Rye 1997). The PPN and a vicinity of this nucleus (PPN area) receive excitatory projections from the cortical motor areas (Matsumura et al., 2000) and the limbic system via the hypothalamus. The PPN is also a major target of GABAergic projections from the basal ganglia output nuclei (Moriizumi et al., 1988; Rye et al., 1987; Span & Grofova, 1991; Lavoie & Parent 1994).

The purpose of this review is to facilitate understanding the pathophysiological mechanism of motor and non-motor functions in PD. For this, we first refer general framework in the central nervous system for movement control in relation to volitional, emotional and automatic aspects. In the second section we demonstrated recent findings obtained in animal experimentation how BG-BS system controlled postural muscle tone and locomotion. Then we propose hypothetical models that can provide rational explanations of motor disturbances in PD. In the third, final, section, we consider the role of the BG-BS systems in non-motor functions with special reference to the regulation of arousal state and awake-sleep states.

2. General framework of movement control

2.1 Fundamental mechanisms of gait control

Activation of different areas in the forebrain evokes different types of goal directed behaviors. On the basis of findings of our studies (Takakusaki et al., 2004b, 2006) as well as those of previous works (Grillner 1981, Mori 1987, Rossignol 1996), current perception of the neuronal pathways involved in locomotor control is illustrated in Fig.1A.

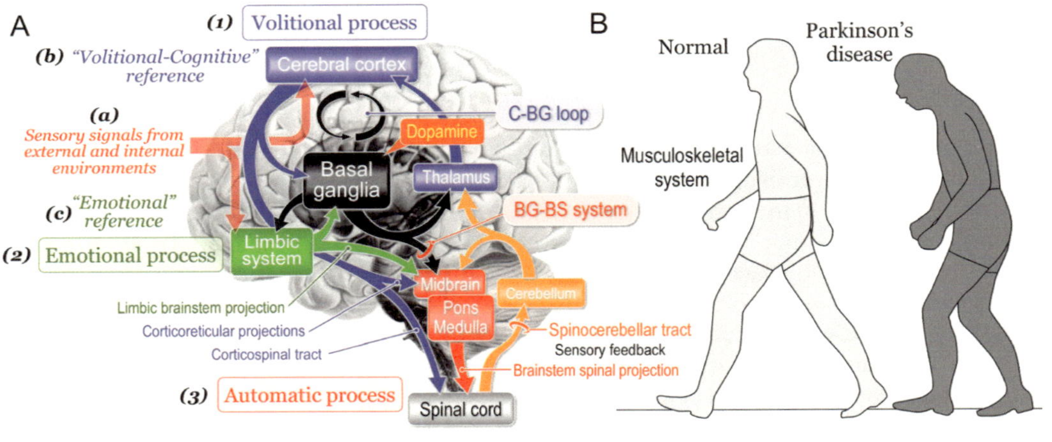

Fig. 1. Fundamental signal flows involved in gait control
A. Schematic illustrations of basic signal flows involved in gait control. (a) - (c) Sensory signals (a) act on the cerebral cortex and the limbic system generate "volitional and cognitive reference" (b) and "emotional reference" (c), respectively. (1) Volitional process requires cortical information processing. (2) Projection from the limbic system to the brainstem is responsible for emotional processes. (3) The brainstem (midbrain, pons and medulla) and spinal cord are involved in automatic processes. The basal ganglia and the cerebellum control volitional and automatic processes via cortico-basal ganglia (C-BG) loop and basal ganglia-brainstem (BG-BS) system, respectively. B. Posture of normal (left) and parkinsonian (right) states.

Motor behaviors require the recruitment of the activities of the entire nervous system (Fig.1A) and musculoskeletal systems (Fig.1B). Sensory signals, derived from both external stimuli and internal visceral information (Fig.1Aa), have the following dual functions (Takakusaki, 2008). One is to generate cognitive information processing that is utilized for working memory to guide future behavior (Fig.1Ab). Another may affect the emotional and arousal states (Fig.1Ac). Accordingly, animals initiate movements depending on either a *"volitional or cognitive reference"* or an *"emotional reference"* (Takakusaki 2008). Goal-directed behaviors therefore may require following the three processes; *"volitional process"* (Fig.1A(1)), *"emotional process"* (Fig.1A(2)) and *"automatic processes"* (Fig.1A(3)). The volitional process is derived from intentionally-elicited motor commands arising from the cerebral cortex based on volitional and cognitive references. This process requires cortical information processing and is executed by the corticoreticular and corticospinal projections. The emotional process is elicited by emotional reference via projections from the limbic-hypothalamus to the brainstem. This contributes to the emotional motor behaviors including fight or flight reactions. Regardless of whether the locomotion is volitional or emotional, it is accompanied by the automatic processes that are evoked by sequential activation of basic motor programs in the brainstem and spinal cord. The cerebellum regulates volitional and automatic processes by acting on the cerebral cortex and the brainstem, respectively. Sensory feedback via spinocerebellar tract plays an important role in this operation. The basal ganglia control these processes via loops with the cerebral cortex, brainstem and the limbic system. Because output of the basal ganglia is altered in basal ganglia disorders, all these movement processes can be disturbed.

2.2 Mechanisms of integrating posture and locomotion by subcortical structures

In animal experiments, decerebrate cat preparation has been used to examine subcortical mechanisms of controlling posture and locomotion. When the decerebration was made at the precollicular-postmammillary level (x in Fig.2A), a cat maintained reflex standing posture due to decerebrate rigidity (mesencephalic cat). Repetitive microelectrical stimulation (50 Hz, 30 μA) applied to the cuneiform nucleus (CNF; a blue point in Fig.2B) bilaterally increased the level of extensor (soleus) muscle tone, and then elicited stepping movements which were developed to locomotion by moving a treadmill (an arrowhead in Fig.2Ba). However the same type of stimuli applied to the ventral part of the PPN (red point in Fig.2B) induced muscular atonia, which lasted even after termination of the stimulation (Fig. 2Bc). Stimulation between these two sites (a green point in Fig.2C) evoked stepping movements followed by muscular atonia (Fig.2Bb). Stimulation of the locus coeruleus (LC, an orange point in Fig.2B) bilaterally increased extensor muscle tone (Fig.2Bd). Generally the locomotion evoking sites (blue circles in Fig.2D), i.e. the midbrain locomotor region (MLR), were located in the CNF, while the inhibitory region was located in the PPN (red circles in in Fig.2C). Neurons between these regions may be involved in both locomotion and muscular atonia. As show in Fig.2D, cholinergic neurons were abundantly distributed in the area corresponding to the inhibitory region, indicating that an activation of cholinergic neurons requires muscle tone suppression (Takakusaki et al., 2003a).
Our current perception of neuronal mechanisms of controlling postural muscle tone and locomotion is shown in Fig.3A on the basis of previous studies (Grillner 1981; Mori 1987; Rossignol 1996; Takakusaki et al., 2004b, 2006). Three locomotor regions are identified. They are the MLR, the subthalamic locomotor region (SLR) and the cerebellar locomotor region (CLR). Signals from the MLR may activate "muscle tone excitatory system" and "locomotor system or rhythm generating system". The former is composed of monoaminergic descending pathways such as the coerulospinal and raphespinal tracts, and excitatory reticulospinal tract arising from the ventromedial medullary reticular formation (v-MRF) which approximately corresponds to the nucleus reticularis magnocellularis. The latter is composed of the excitatory reticulospinal tract and central pattern generators (CPG) in the spinal cord. Cortical projections to the MLR have not yet been identified. It is possibly

mediated by connections via the SLR (Rossignol, 1996). If decerebration was made at precollicular-premammillary level (y in Fig.2A), the cat spontaneously walked without stimulation. Thus the SLR exists between two decerebrate levels, and mostly corresponds to the lateral hypothalamus, and it may contribute to emotional behaviors (Griller et al. 1997). Signals from the SLR activate the locomotor system either directly or indirectly via the MLR (Grillner et al., 1997). The CLR corresponds to the mid-part of cerebellar white matter which contains massive fibers connecting bilateral fastigial nuclei. (Mori et al., 1999).

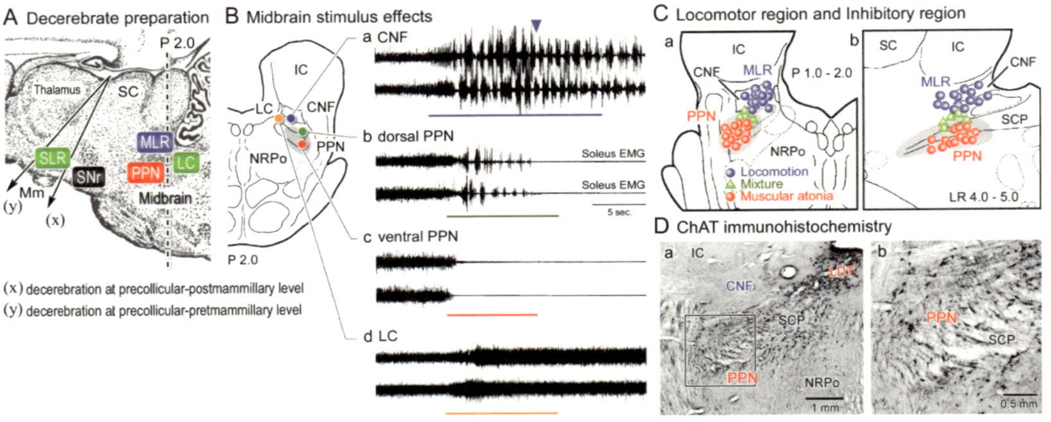

Fig. 2. Midbrain control of locomotion and muscle tone in decerebrate cat preparation

A. Two decerebrate levels (x and y) in parasagittal plane of the cat brainstem. B. Stimulus sites on coronal plane of the mesopontine tegmentum, which is indicated by dashed line in (A; at P 2.0). (a) - (d) Locomotion (a, b) and muscle tone alteration (b, c, d) induced by repetitive stimuli (30 μA, 50 Hz) applied to each site. Stimulus period is indicated under each record. C. Effective sites where stimulation evoked locomotion (blue circles), muscular atonia (red circles) and a mixture of both (green triangles) on coronal (a) and parasagittal (b) planes of the brainstem. D. Microphotographic presentation of cholinergic neurons identified by choline-acetyltransferase (ChAT) immunohistochemistry with lower (a) and higher (b) magnification of the mesopontine tegmentum. Abbreviations, EMG; electromyograms, IC; inferior colliculus, LDT; laterodorsal tegmental nucleus, LR; left and right, MLR; midbrain locomotor region, Mm; mammillary body, NRPo; nucleus reticularis pontis oralis, PPN; pedunculopontine tegmental nucleus, SC; superior colliculus, SCP; superior cerebellar peduncle, SLR; subthalamic locomotor region, SNr; substantia nigra pars reticulata.

Muscle tone control regions also exist in the brainstem. One is muscle tone inhibitory region in the PPN (Figs.2 and 3A). Cholinergic neurons in the PPN may activate "muscle tone inhibitory system", which is composed of cholinoceptive pontine reticular formation (PRF) neurons (Takakusaki et al., 2003a), reticulospinal neurons arising from the dorsomedial MRF corresponding to the nucleus reticularis gigantocellularis, and spinal inhibitory interneurons in the lamina VII of Rexed (Takakusaki et al., 1994, 2003b). This system then inhibits α- and γ-motoneurons innervating extensor and flexor muscles in parallel to interneurons mediating reflex pathways (Takakusaki et al., 2001). Because CPG is composed of spinal interneuronal circuits, an activation of the inhibitory system can simultaneously

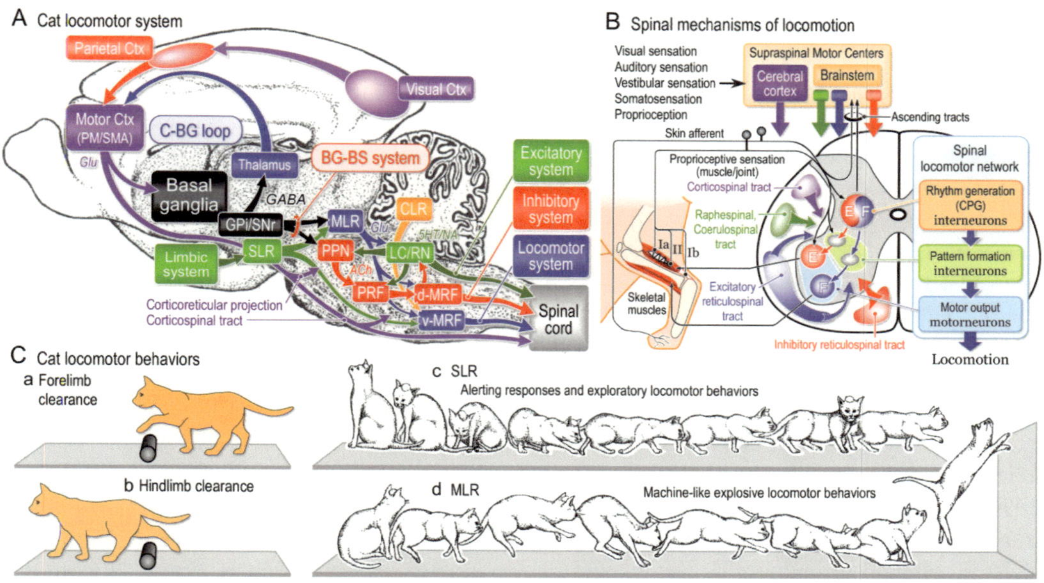

Fig. 3. Neuronal mechanism of locomotion in cats
A. Cat locomotor system. Signals from the MLR activate muscle tone excitatory system and locomotor system. Locomotor system is composed of excitatory reticulospinal tract from the ventromedial medullary reticular formation (v-MRF) and central pattern generator (CPG) in spinal cord. The excitatory reticulospinal tract also operates as the muscle tone excitatory system as well as the coerulospinal tract from the LC and raphespinal tract from the raphe nuclei (RN). Signals from the SLR and the cerebellar locomotor region (CLR) act on these systems to evoke locomotion. Cholinergic neurons in the PPN activate muscle tone inhibitory system, which arises from the pontine reticular formation (PRF) neurons and inhibitory reticulospinal tract neurons in the dorsomedial MRF (d-MRF). GABAergic output from the SNr to the MLR/PPN controls locomotion and muscle tone. Output from the basal ganglia to the thalamocortical neurons controls intentional and volitional gait behaviors. Visuospatial information from the visual cortex (Ctx) to motor Ctx via the parietal Ctx requires for programing accurate postural-gait synergy. B. Central and peripheral inputs to spinal locomotor network. Locomotor rhythm and pattern are generated by spinal interneurons. Activity of spinal neurons is modified by corticospinal tract, locomotor system (excitatory reticulospinal system) and muscle tone control systems (raphespinal, coerulospinal and inhibitory reticulospinal tracts). C. Obstacle clearance by forelimb (a) and hindlimb (b) during locomotion. Locomotor behaviors elicited by stimulating the SLR (c) and MLR (d) in cats with chronically implanted stimulating electrodes. Each picture was depicted at 0.5 sec and 0.1 sec intervals in (c) and (d), respectively. A and B are modified Takakusaki et al., 2008. (c) and (d) in C are modified Mori et al. 1989.

suppress postural muscle tone and locomotor rhythm (Takakusaki et al., 2003b). This inhibitory system is also thought to induce muscular atonia during the rapid eye movement (REM) sleep (Chase & Morales 1990; Takakusaki et al., 1993). There are serotonergic projections to the PPN (Honda & Semba, 1994) and to the cholinoceptive area of the PRF (Semba, 1993). Serotonergic projections to the PPN likely inhibit cholinergic neurons

(Leonald & Llinás, 1994), and those to the PRF may reduce activity of the inhibitory system (Takakusaki et al., 1994). In contrast, the inhibitory system suppresses the activity of the coerulospinal tract (Mileykovskiy et al., 2000). Accordingly muscle tone can be regulated by a counterbalance between the inhibitory and the excitatory systems (Takakusaki et al., 2006). It was reported that a patient with a lesion in the dorsolateral mesopontine tegmentum did not lose muscle tone during REM sleep ("REM without atonia") (Boeve et al., 2007; Culebras & Moore 1989). Also, a patient with a lesion in the dorsal part of mesopontine tegmentum could not stand and walk (Masdeu et al., 1994). These clinical case reports suggest that both a muscle tone inhibitory region and a MLR are realities in the mesopontine tegmentum of the human.

Spinal mechanisms of locomotor control are schematically illustrated in Fig.3B. Signals from the cerebral cortex and the brainstem, and those from peripheral sensory afferents are integrated at spinal cord to achieve appropriate locomotor control. Various combinations of spinal reflexes operate during locomotion. Those mediating flexion reflex and crossed extension reflex undertake major roles in the generation of locomotor rhythm (Rossignol 1996; Rossignol et al., 2006; Takakusaki et al., 2001, 2003b; McCrea & Rybak, 2008). Spinal interneurons that constitute CPG generate detailed locomotor rhythm. The locomotor rhythm is then translated to next order interneuronal groups which shape "locomotor pattern". Finally signals are sent to last-order interneurons, including reciprocal Ia interneurons, Ib interneurons and Renshaw cells. They are located in lamina IV-VII of Rexed and project to target motoneurons. Lamina VIII interneurons project to the contralateral side of spinal cord and may control alternating limb movements (Matsuyama & Takakusaki, 2008). Signals generated by spinal locomotor network are then transmitted back to the cerebral cortex, the brainstem and the cerebellum so that they monitor events in the spinal cord (Fig.3B).

2.3 Initiation of movements by the forebrain structures

2.3.1 Cortical control of locomotor behaviors

Drew et al. (1996) demonstrated, in cats with chronically implanted electrodes in the cerebral cortex, that a majority of motor cortical neurons exhibited simple rhythmic firing in relation to step cycles during steady-state locomotion. However their discharge rates considerably increased when the cats initiated to walk and had to accurately step over obstacles. Thus, commitment of cortical processing seems unnecessary during the automatic locomotor movements. On the other hand, stepping movements that accompany accurate foot placement resemble to the forelimb reaching of higher primates (Drew et al., 2004; Georgopoulos & Grillner, 1989). Such an accurate movement requires visuomotor cognitive processes (Fig.3A), which are controlled by neural circuits involving the cerebral cortex, basal ganglia, and cerebellum (Middleton & Strick, 2000). Subjects are aware of the locations of obstacles around them, and they are able to alter their stepping patterns even without available visual information of the location of the obstacles relative to the body (Fig.3C). McVea & Pearson (2007) reported that perturbing walking cats in a consistent manner evoked lasting changes to the walking pattern that were expressed only in the context in which walking was disturbed. Moreover, cats that had stepped over an obstacle by forelimb (Fig.3Ca) remembered the location of the obstacle and could use working memory to guide stepping for the hindlimb (Fig.3Cb). Therefore, sensory inputs that signal context –the surrounding visual and auditory environment- play an important role in shaping the basic pattern of locomotion. Lajoie & Drew (2007) observed, after unilateral lesion of area 5 of the posterior parietal cortex, that cats frequently hit the obstacle as they stepped over it. They also frequently hit the obstacle with their hindlimbs even when the forelimbs negotiated the obstacle successfully. These findings suggest an important role for the posterior parietal cortex in the coordination of the forelimbs and hindlimbs and in the planning and programming of visually-guided gait modification (Fig.3C). Neuroanatomical studies indicate that the posterior parietal cortex sends selected projections to the motor cortical areas from layer III, while those to the lateral cerebellum via the pontine nuclei arise from layer V (Andujar & Drew, 2007). Neurons in the primary motor cortex and those in the premotor/supplementary motor areas (PM/SMA) mainly project to the spinal cord and the reticular formation via corticospinal and corticoreticular projections, respectively (Matsuyama & Drew 1997).

2.3.2 Emotional locomotor behaviors

The MLR was initially established as a functional region involved in the initiation of locomotion on the basis of its connections with limbic structures and the basal ganglia (Armstrong, 1986; Megensen et al., 1991). Regardless of the nature of emotional stimuli, they usually elicit alert responses that produce stereotyped movements such as increased postural muscle tone and/or locomotion that accompanies autonomic sympathetic responses. The limbic-hypothalamic systems play crucial roles in these processes. Sinnamon (1993) proposed the following three types of locomotor systems that function in different behavioral or motivational contexts; an appetitive system, a primary defensive system, and an exploratory system. In cats with chronically implanted electrodes, stimulation of the SLR elicited alerting responses followed by exploratory (searching) or defensive behaviors (Fig.3Cc; Mori et al., 1989). Signals from the SLR are mediated by dense fibers in the medial forebrain bundle projecting to the midbrain (Rossignol, 1996). On the other hand, stimulation of the MLR abruptly elicited machine-like explosive locomotion (Fig.3Cd). Neural circuits connecting the nucleus accumbens (the oldest part of the striatum), the hippocampus, and the amygdala, are involved in emotional memory, and projections from the nucleus accumbens to the MLR may contribute to the expression of exploratory behaviors (Mogenson, 1991). In addition, projections from the lateral and the medial hypothalamic areas to the MLR are thought to operate as defensive and appetitive systems, respectively (Grillner et al., 1997; Jordan, 1998). The orexin-containing neurons located in the prefornical lateral hypothalamic area are considered to control appetite, energy balance, and vigilance states via projections to various areas in the nervous system (Peyron et al., 1998; Sakurai, 2002; Siegel, 2004). The orexinergic projections to the MLR facilitated the activity of the locomotor system (Takakusaki et al., 2005), indicating that the hypothalamic orexinergic system contributes to appetitive behaviors.

3. Basal ganglia control of movements and motor disturbances by the basal ganglia dysfunction

It is established that the C-BG loop is required for volitional movement (Delong & Wichmann, 2007; Middleton & Strick, 2000). Neural circuits between the prefrontal cortex and the caudate nucleus (cognitive loop) are involved in the regulation of complex, visually-guided limb movements and the planning and programming those movements. Neural circuits between motor cortical areas, including the primary motor cortex, PM and SMA, and the putamen (motor loop) contribute to the regulation of voluntary, discrete, ipsilateral limb movements. In addition the BG-BS system may control automatic and steady-state locomotor movements. This section first refers how the BG-BS system controls posture and locomotion and then considers how BG-BS contributes to pathophysiological mechanisms of motor disturbances in PD.

3.1 BG-BS system controls postural muscle tone and locomotion

How do the basal ganglia control locomotion and muscle tone via the BG-BS system? To answer this question, we employed decerebrate cat preparation where only the substantia nigra was preserved, whereas most basal ganglia structures were removed (Fig.4A). Then we examined how GABAergic output from the basal ganglia to the brainstem modulated the PPN/MLR-activated movements by manipulating the activity of neurons in the substantia nigra pars reticulata (SNr). Repetitive stimuli applied to the ventrolateral part of the PPN (red circles in Fig.4Ac) abolished muscle tone (Fig.4Ba). While stimulation of the lateral part of the SNr (filled squares in Fig.4Ab) alone did not alter muscle tone, it completely blocked the PPN-effects (Fig.4Bb). Stimulation of the MLR (blue circles in Fig.4Ac) increased muscle tone and evoked stepping movements on stationary surface (Fig.4Ca). But stimulation of the medial part of the SNr, indicated by filled squares in Fig.4Ab, arrested the MLR-activated locomotion (Fig.4Cb). It was re-established after termination of the SNr stimulation. In immobilized decerebrate preparation, MLR stimulation first depolarized the membrane potential and then generated rhythmic membrane oscillations associating with bursting firing, which corresponded to step cycles, in hindlimb motoneurons (fictive locomotion). During SNr stimulation, the rhythmic oscillation was arrested, and membrane potential was maintained at the depolarizing state in both extensor and flexor motoneurons, indicating that SNr stimulation co-contracts agonistic and antagonistic muscles, leading to disturbing rhythmic limb movements. Because these effects by SNr stimulation were blocked by injections of bicuculline (a $GABA_A$-receptor antagonist) into the PPN/MLR, the SNr stimulus effects can be mediated by GABAergic projections to these areas. These findings suggest that the BG-BS system controls steady state (e.g., rhythmic limb movements) and dynamic state (e.g., initiation and termination) of locomotion. It should be noted that the effects of SNr stimulation was depend on stimulus parameters. Step cycles and onset of MLR-activated locomotion was prolonged by increasing SNr stimulus intensity (Fig.4Da). However frequency more than 140 Hz was less effective while frequencies between 50 and 100 Hz were prominently inhibited locomotor activity (Takakusaki et al., 2003a). Similar findings were observed in the nigral control of muscle tone (Takakusaki et al., 2004c). Frequency between 50-100 Hz is almost the same as the spontaneous firing rates SNr neurons in alert monkey (Hikosaka & Wurtz, 1985). A frequency within this range can be a critical determinant in the control of muscle tone, locomotion and saccadic eye movements (Hikosaka et al., 2000).
Next we injected muscimol, a $GABA_A$ receptor agonist, into the SNr in order to inhibit neuronal activity. It was observed that muscimol injections into the lateral part of the SNr suppressed postural muscle tone (Fig.4Bc) and those into the medial part of the SNr evoked locomotion (Fig.4Cc). Judging from the relationship between effective stimulus sites in the SNr (Fig.4Ab) and those in the mesopontine tegmentum (Fig.4Ac), there exist functional topography in the nigrotegmental projections; lateral SNr controls muscle tone and the medial SNr controls locomotion. It follows that the BG-BS system can control locomotion and postural muscle tone independently.

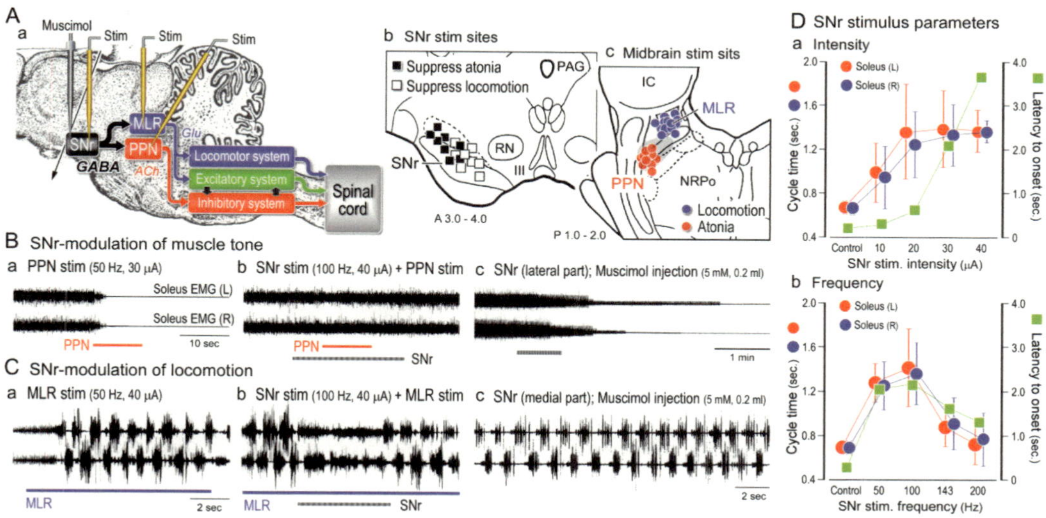

Fig. 4. Nigral stimulus effects on PPN/MLR-induced muscle tone suppression and locomotion in decerebrate cats
A. (a) Experimental design in decerebrate cat preparation. (b) Effective stimulus sites in the SNr for inhibition of the PPN (filled squares) and the MLR (open squares) effects. (c) Effective stimulus sites for evoking muscular atonia (PPN; red circles) and locomotion (MLR; blue circles) in the mesopontine tegmentum. B. (a) PPN-induced muscular atonia. (b) Inhibition of the PPN-induced atonia by SNr stimulation. (c) Muscular atonia induced by an injection of muscimol into the lateral part of the SNr. C. (a) MLR-activated stepping movements. (b) Inhibition of MLR-activated stepping by SNr stimulation. (c) Locomotion induced by an injection of muscimol into the medial part of the SNr. D. Changes in step cycles and gait onset of the MLR-activated locomotion following changes in stimulus intensity (a) and frequency (b) applied to the SNr. Abbreviations, III; oculomotor nerve, PAG; periaqueductal grey, RN; red nucleus.

3.2 Role of the C-BG loop and BG-BS system in relation to the gait control

As illustrated in Fig.5A, output from the SNr and the internal segment of globus pallidus (GPi) is regulated by hyper-direct, direct and indirect pathways in the basal ganglia circuits (Delong & Wichmann, 2007; Hikosaka et al., 2000; Numbu, 2004). Neurons in the GPi/SNr inhibit target neurons in the thalamus and brainstem with their tonic, high background activity, thus preventing unnecessary movements. To initiate movements, motor commands from the motor cortices first increase the basal ganglia output by an activation of the hyper-direct pathway to the subthalamic nucleus (STN) so that the excitability of target systems would be further reduced (Fig.5Ba). Signals via the direct pathway from the striatum to the GPi/SNr remove this sustained inhibition, resulting in a disinhibition of the target systems (Fig.5Bb). The phasic activity of GABAergic output neurons in the striatum, which are mostly silent, interrupts the tonic GPi/SNr inhibition, and movements are allowed to occur. Finally, signals through the indirect pathway, involving the external segment of the globus pallidus (GPe) and the STN, can further re-enhance the inhibition of the target systems (Fig.5Bc). This sequential information processing, an enhancement of tonic inhibition and disinhibition, would enhance the temporal contrast of the excitability of the target systems so that only the selected motor program could be initiated, executed and terminated at the appropriate timing, whereas other competing programs can be cancelled (Hikosaka et al., 2000; Numbu, 2004). This is the "first key mechanism" of movement control by the basal ganglia.

The above mechanisms may act on brainstem networks, including the locomotor system and muscle tone control systems (Fig.5A, lower right). Therefore the brainstem networks could be combined with basal ganglia motor circuits. In this "hybrid model", output of the basal ganglia controls the MLR for locomotion and the PPN for muscle tone via GABAergic projection. When locomotor movement is being prepared, tonic activity of SNr neurons would continuously inhibit both systems. When a trigger signal occurred, the hyper-direct pathway would enhance the inhibition. Then the direct pathway would release the activity of these systems, resulting in an initiation of locomotion that would be followed by a smooth reduction of the level of muscle tone. To terminate the locomotion, the direct pathway would inhibit each system, resulting in a cessation of rhythmic locomotor movements and an accompanying increase in the level of muscle tone (muscle co-contraction). A parallel organization from the SNr to the MLR/PPN would be therefore assist regulation of the level of muscle tone which was appropriate for the initiation and termination of locomotion.

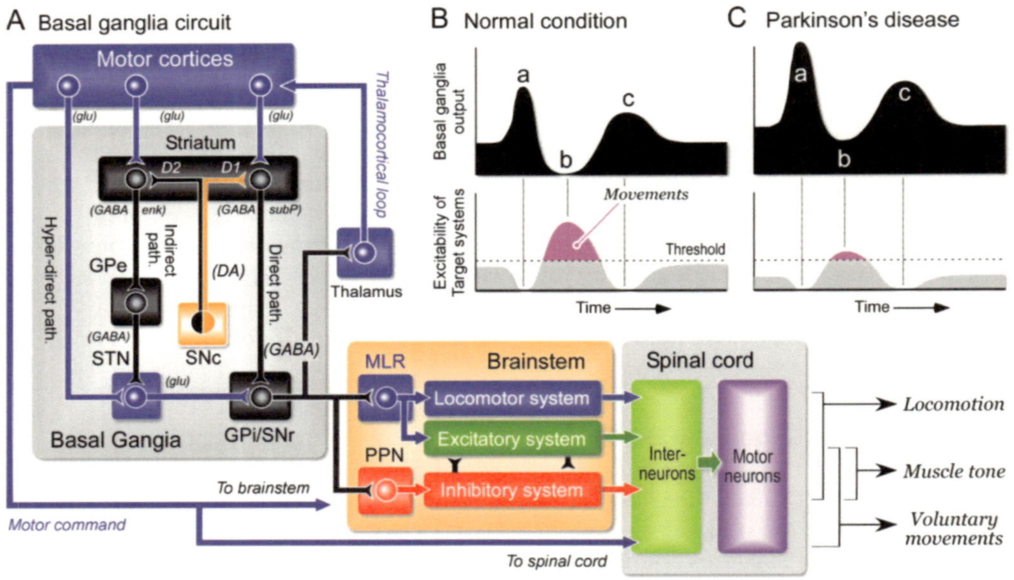

Fig. 5. Hybrid model of C-BG loop and BG-BS system
A. Left; basal ganglia motor circuits. Lower right; BG-BS system for controlling locomotion and muscle tone. B and C. Changes in the basal ganglia output and in the excitability of target systems following sequential information processing of hyper-direct (a), direct (b) and indirect (c) pathways. When excitability of target systems goes beyond the threshold, movements occur. Excitability of direct and indirect pathways is modified by dopaminergic projections from the SNc to the striatum. B. Normal condition. C. Parkinson's disease. Abbreviations, D1 and D2; D1 and D2-dopamine receptors, DA; dopamine, enk; enkephaline, Glu; glutamate, GPe; external segment of globus pallidus subP; substance P, STN; subthalamic nucleus

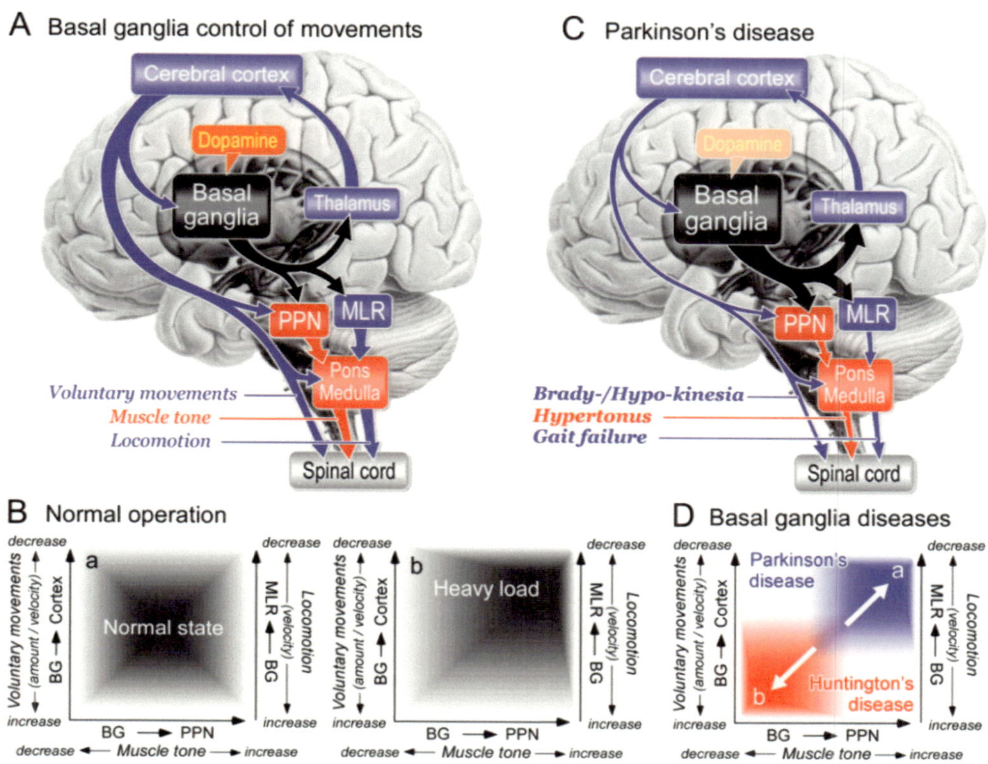

Fig. 6. Hypothetical models for movement control by the basal ganglia
A. GABAergic basal ganglia projections to the thalamocortical neurons are involved in the volitional control of movements, while those to the MLR and the PPN may be responsible for the automatic control of locomotion and muscle tone. B. Normal operation of the basal ganglia control of voluntary movements, locomotion and muscle tone. C. Pathophysiological changes in the activities of the cortico-BG loop and BG-BS system in PD. Loss of dopamine results in an increase in the basal ganglia output to the cerebral cortex, the limbic system and the brainstem. Consequently, voluntary and cognitive activities of the cerebral cortex and emotional expression can be reduced. Reduced cortical output results in bradykinesia and hypokinesia. Reduced activity in the MLR-locomotor system may induce gait failure. Inhibition of the PPN-muscle tone inhibitory system may induce hypertonus. D. Motor disturbances in basal ganglia disorders. (a) Parkinson disease. (b) Huntington's disease. Regardless of whether an increase or a decrease in the basal ganglia output, degree of freedom of movements may be restricted.

Given the above consideration, we propose a hypothetical model in Fig.6A for the basal ganglia control of movements. The motor cortical neurons that receive basal ganglia output may control the velocity and the amount of voluntary movement (Turner & Anderson, 1997), which is indicated in the ordinate on the left of the graph in Fig.6Ba. The GABAergic basal ganglia output to the MLR reduced the drive from the MLR, resulting in disruption of the activity of CPGs in the spinal cord. Basal ganglia efferents to the MLR may therefore control the locomotor pattern (ordinate on the right in Fig.6Ba). In addition, basal ganglia efferents to the PPN may determine the level of muscle tone via the muscle tone control systems (abscissa). Because the basal ganglia output is variable in a normal condition (Fig.6Ba), the degree of freedom for the amount and the velocity of movement, the locomotor velocity, and the muscle tone, can be large. Each parameter can take any of the coordinates within the frame in Fig.6Ba. For example, when a subject needs to adapt to a heavy load during walking, the subject may unconsciously select an appropriate gait pattern which is associated with a higher level of muscle tone and slower walking speed. Such a gait pattern could be realized by an increase in sustained SNr output to the PPN and the MLR. This would result in a decrease in the excitabilities of the inhibitory system and locomotor system (Fig.6Bb). Consequently, a sustained basal ganglia output may control the degree of freedom of the excitability of the target systems during movements. This can be the "second key mechanism" of motor control by the basal ganglia.

3.3 Pathophysiological mechanisms of motor disturbances in basal ganglia disorders

Gait disturbances and postural instability are observed in PD patients (Morris et al., 1994; Murray et al., 1978). These are delays in gait onset including freezing of gait (FOG), an increase in the stance phase in locomotor cycles, tiny steps and a decrease in gait velocity. Neurodegeneration of dopamine neurons in PD patients leads to higher activity in the hyper-direct and indirect pathways (Fig.5Ca and Cc) and lower activity of the direct pathway (Fig.5Cb). Therefore the GABAergic basal ganglia output is thought to be overactive in PD (Fig.6C). Excessive inhibitory actions on the target systems can consequently produce motor disturbances. For example, the excessive inhibition upon thalamocortical neurons may suppress cortical information processing (dysfunction of C-BG loop). A decrease in the output from the primary motor cortex reduces the amount (hypokinesia) and the velocity of movement (bradykinesia), leading to tiny step with a decrease in gait velocity. Moreover, reduced activities in the prefrontal cortex and PM/SMA may disturb planning and motor programming, respectively (Hanakawa et al. 1999). This may further disturb intentional gait control (gait initiation, precise hoot placement and obstacle avoidance), resulting in FOG. In the brainstem, the excessive inhibition of the MLR together with a decrease in cortical excitation of the reticular formation may decrease the activity of locomotor system and then disturb automatic aspect of steady-state gait control (rhythmic limb movements). Similarly, an increase in basal ganglia inhibition together with a decrease in cortical excitation of the PPN may reduce the activity of inhibitory system, which, in turn, facilitates excitatory systems. As a result, muscle tone would be increased (hypertonus). Therefore muscular rigidity, one of the most prominent symptoms of PD, can be the result of inhibition of the muscle tone inhibitory system that reduces the inhibition to α- and γ-motoneurons. As shown in Fig.4C, MLR-activated locomotion was arrested but the muscle tone was maintained at higher level during the period of SNr stimulation, indicating that muscle rigidity is a cause of gait disturbances. We postulate that dysfunction of the BG-BS system can be the primary basis for gait impairments of PD.

In contrast, an output from the basal ganglia is decreased in Huntington's disease (HD) because of increased activity of the direct pathway. This may extremely facilitate cortical information processing, thus unnecessary motor programs cannot be cancelled, resulting in hyperkinesia and involuntary movements (Chorea). The decrease in the basal ganglia output to the PPN may reduce muscle tone (hypotonus). It should be noted, regardless of PD or HD, the degree of freedom of movements would be reduced and restricted. The frame moves to the upper right for PD (Fig.6Da) and to lower left for HD (Fig.6Db). From these considerations, the reduction of the degree of freedom of movements could exist in the background of PD and HD. Consequently, dysfunction of the BG-BS system together with that of the C-BG loop may underlie the pathogenesis of the motor disturbances in these basal ganglia diseases.

Dystonia is a syndrome characterized by abnormal postures, muscle spasms and tremor, due to involuntary muscle co-contractions. Some dystonia are task specific, and patients only develop muscular co-contraction when performing skilled movements such as writing (Van der Kamp et al. 1989). By using positron emission tomography an inappropriate over-activity of the basal ganglia projections to the premotor and dorsal prefrontal cortex has been observed (Brooks 1995). However the activity of the primary sensorimotor and caudal premotor cortices is rather attenuated (Hutchins et al. 1988). Although alterations of noradrenaline and DA levels in brainstem structures have been reported in two cases (Hornykiewicz et al., 1986), most studies, by contrast, have not found abnormalities in the brainstem. This evidence suggests that the activity of the BG-BS system and that of the C-BG loop are controlled separately in dystonia.

Recently PPN/MLR area became one of targets of deep brain stimulation (DBS) for neurosurgical therapy for PD (PPN-DBS) (Stefani et al., 2007; Pierantozzi et al., 2008; Alessandro et al., 2010). Low frequency stimulation (~25Hz) applied to the above area ameliorated postural disturbance and gait failure. On the other hand, DBS applied to the SNr (SNr-DBS) with high frequency (135-190 Hz), which possibly intervened to the output from the SNr, also ameliorated axial symptoms such as gait akinesia and postural disturbances (Chasetan et al. 2009). Although evidence of the PPN-DBS and the SNr-DBS is still limited, these clinical findings agree well with our results suggesting that the BG-BS system contributes to the postural and locomotor synergies in human.

4. Disturbances of non-motor functions in Parkinson's disease

Disturbances in cognitive and psychotic processes have been observed in patients with degenerative disorders that involve primarily the basal ganglia such as PD (Mellers et al., 1995; Taylor et al., 1986) and HD (McHugh & Folsten, 1975). Awake-sleep states were also impaired in PD (Bliwise et al., 2000; Eisensehr et al., 2001). It is also reported that PD is preceded and accompanied by daytime sleep attacks, nocturnal insomnia, REM sleep behavior disorder, hallucinations and depression, symptoms which are frequently as troublesome as the motor symptoms of this disease. All these symptoms are present in narcolepsy (Thannical et al., 2007). These clinical evidences corroborate that the basal ganglia and their connections with the brainstem are also involved in the expression of non-motor function. In this section, we focus on the roles played by the BG-BS system in the regulation of vigilance states, arousal state, attention and cognition in relation to non-motor symptoms in PD.

4.1 Does output of the basal ganglia modulate sleep?

Cholinergic neurons in the PPN and laterodorsal tegmental nucleus are thought to be involved in not only the maintenance of arousal state but also generation of REM sleep (Datta and Siwek, 2002; Koyama & Sakai, 2000; Maloney et al., 1999). Therefore, we elucidated how GABAergic SNr-PPN projection altered the activities of the REM generator and the muscle tone inhibitory system (Takakusaki et al., 2004c). Summary of the results are shown in Fig.7. Stimulation of inhibitory region of the PPN induced REM which was associated with muscular atonia in decerebrate cats (REM and atonia; Fig.7Ba). Conditioning stimuli applied to the lateral part of the SNr (blue circles in Fig.7C) completely abolished the PPN-induced REM with atonia (Fig.7Bb). On the other hand, stimulation of the SNr, denoted by black squares in Fig.7C, only inhibited REM (Fig.7Bd). It was also observed that stimuli applied to the sites which were indicated by red circles in Fig.7C did not block REM but attenuated the muscular atonia (Fig.7Bc), i.e., REM without atonia (Sanford, 1994), which is considered to be relevant to RBD in human (Culebras & Moore, 1989), was evoked. These findings indicate that neurons in the PPN that are responsible for generation of REM sleep are affected by GABAergic projections from the SNr.

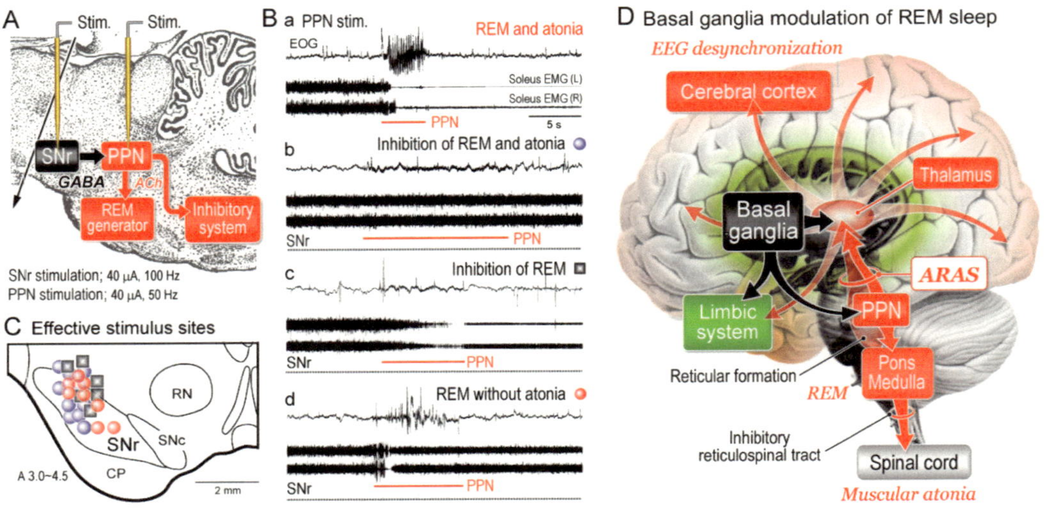

Fig. 7. Possible mechanisms of basal ganglia modulation of REM sleep
A. Experimental design in decerebrate cats. B. (a) Stimulation of the PPN induced REM and atonia. (b) ~ (d) Effects of stimuli applied to various sites of the SNr on the PPN-induced REM and atonia. (b) Stimulation of the sites indicated by blue circles in C inhibited both REM and atonia. (c) Stimulation of the sites indicated by black squares in C. only inhibited REM. (d) Stimulation of the sites indicated by red circles in C inhibited atonia but not REM (REM without atonia). C. Effective sites for modulating the eye movements and muscular atonia were located in the lateral part of the SNr. D. Possible mechanisms of basal ganglia modulation of REM sleep. Abbreviations, ARAS; ascending reticular activating system, REM; rapid eye movement.

4.2 Possible mechanisms of sleep disturbances in Parkinson's disease

4.2.1 Disturbance of REM sleep (REM sleep behavior disorder; RBD)

Sleep disturbance is one of early signs of PD (Askenasy, 2001; Ferini-Strambi & Zucconi, 2000; Larsen & Tandberg, 2001). There are several reports suggesting that nearly half number of PD patients who were diagnosed as idiopathic RBD but free of neurodegenerative diseases had developed PD (Boeve, 2007; Iranzo, 2006; Schenck, 1996). Postuma et al. (2010) conclude that severity of REM atonia loss in idiopathic RBD predicts PD. Neuronal loss in the PPN was reported in PD (Hirsch et al., 1987; Jellinger, 1988; Zweig et al., 1989), and loss of cholinergic neurons in the PPN is possibly related to disability of PD patients (Rinne et al., 2008).

Several mechanisms are postulated in relation to the basal ganglia regulation of sleep. On one hand, recent brain imaging studies revealed that damage of brainstem, particularly the reticular formation, is critically involved in the pathogenesis of RBD (Unger et al., 2010). The brainstem damage could also explain some non-motor symptoms in this disease, which often precede diagnosis, such as autonomic dysfunction and sleep disorders. On the other hand, roles of dopaminergic influence on the basal ganglia in the control of sleep-wake behavior are suggested (Mena-Segovia J et al., 2008). It is also possible that basal ganglia efferents to the non-specific thalamic nuclei may affect awake-sleep states by modulating the activity of ascending reticular activating system (ARAS). Since the classical study of Moruzzi and Magoun (1949), the pontomesencephalic reticular formation has been known to comprise the ARAS. The PPN has been considered as a part of the ARAS (Garcia-Rill, 1991; Inglis & Winn, 1995; Jones, 1991).

The SNr has a direct projection to the thalamic nuclei (Parent et al., 1983; Pare´ et al., 1990) in addition to the PPN (Fig.7D). Because PPN has dense projections to the midbrain dopaminergic neurons, activity of the PPN neurons may affect awake-sleep states by modulating dopaminergic systems projecting to the basal ganglia and extra-basal ganglia areas. Consequently, our idea is that basal ganglia output from the SNr may affect awake–sleep cycles by modulating the activity of the ARAS through dual mechanisms (Fig.7D). One is through direct nigro-thalamic projection, and the other, which is considered in this study, is though indirect connections via the PPN (Takakusaki et al. 2004c, 2006).

4.2.2 Narcolepsy-like symptoms

The presence in PD patients of narcolepsy-like features, such as daytime REM sleep intrusions associated with visual hallucinations, has led some authors to suggest that a mechanism similar to that of narcolepsy might underlie excessive daytime sleepiness (EDS) in PD (Arnulf et al., 2000). Thannickal et al. (2007) demonstrated that a massive loss of orexin neurons was found in PD patients and suggested that it was a cause of the narcolepsy-like symptoms. However, Compta et al. (2009) showed that orexin-A level was normal in the cerebrospinal fluid and it was unrelated to severity of sleepiness or the cognitive status of PD patients. Therefore alternative mechanisms other than dysfunction of orexin neurons might be responsible for EDS and the disturbance of sleep architecture in PD. In animal experiments, midbrain strucutes, including the SNr, the PPN and the MLR, receive orexinergic efferents from the perifornical lateral hypothalams (Nambu et al., 1999; Peyron et al., 1998). Therefore it is interesting to elucidate how orexinergic projections to the midbrain are involved in alteration of sleep-awake states. Then we examined effects of injections of orexin-A into the MLR, PPN and the SNr upon motor behaviors in decerebrate cats (Takakusaki et al., 2005). Microinjections of orexin into the MLR facilitated locomotion, while those into either the PPN or the SNr suppressed PPN-induced muscular atonia. The latter effects were reversed by subsequent injection of bicuculline into the PPN. Thus the excitability seems to be higher in the locomotor system than in the atonia system in the presence of orexin. On the contrary the excitability of the muscle tone inhibitory system may be higher than that of the locomotor system in the absence of orexin. Accordingly GABAergic projection from the SNr to the PPN/MLR area (BG-BS system) may underlie orexin-mediated vigilance state regulation and its dysfunction may be one of pathophysiological mechanisms of narcolepsy-like features of PD (Takakusaki 2008).

4.3 Disturbances of arousal state, attention and cognition

Behavioral arousal requires an activation of dopaminergic projections arising from the SNc to the striatum and the ventral tegmental area (VTA) to the prefrontal cortex and the limbic system. The nigrostriatal projection is responsible for basal ganglia related motor functions. The mesocortical projection contributes to volitional expression and attention, and the mesolimbic projection is involved in emotional expression. On the other hand, ARAS plays a major role in the electroencephalographic arousal. An activation of the two arousal systems is required to maintain arousal state that enables alert, attention and cognition (Jones 1991). Because PPN has dense cholinergic and non-cholinergic excitatory connections with dopamine (DA) neurons in the SNc and other basal ganglia nuclei (Futami et al., 1994; Kitai, 1998; Takakusaki et al., 1996), these projections appear to play a role in more specific subcortical integration of motor and non-motor functions such as behavioral arousal, attention and reward (Kitai, 1998). For example, an injection of muscimol into the PPN reduced the speed and amount of arm movements and delayed the onset of movements but the accuracy was rather maintained (Matsumura and Kojima, 2001). Moreover, Kojima et al. (1997) demonstrated that kainic acid-induced lesion in the unilateral PPN induced hemiparkisonism which was observed in the contralateral side of the injection. From these findings they suggest that the PPN may thus facilitate the voluntary limb movements through its excitatory connections with the DA neurons.

Midbrain DA neurons are also involved in the predictive reward which is specifically linked with reinforcement behaviors. DA neurons are activated by rewarding events that are better than predicted, remain uninfluenced by events that are worse than predicted (Hikosaka et al., 2000; Schultz, 1998). Kobayashi et al. (2002) demonstrated that PPN neurons showed multi-modal activities during saccade tasks in alert monkey; their activities were related to the arousal levels, execution and preparation of movements, the level of task performance, and reward. Therefore the PPN may serve as an integrative interface between the various signals required for performing purposive behaviors (Kobayashi et al., 2004). We postulate that the PPN facilitates, possibly via dopaminergic systems, the central processes for motor command generation and extrinsic sensory processing by modulating arousal and attentive states.

In non-human primate, limited lesions of the striatum induce deficits in rule acquisition (Divac 1972), cognition (Taylor et al., 1990), working memory performance (Goldman-Rakic, 1987) and selected attention (Battig et al., 1962). Laplane et al. (1984) reported a patient with restricted bilateral pallidal lesions who was appeared apathetic and unconcerned or attention deficits, and his affect was flattened and emotional responses were blunted in the absence of any motor disorder or pure psychic akinesia. These symptoms were also described in progressive supranuclear palsy (PSP) in which major lesions were observed in the subcortical areas including the PPN. Because loss of cholinergic PPN neurons were observed not only in PSP (75-80%) but also PD (43-57%) (Hirsch et al., 1987; Jellinger, 1988; Zweig et al., 1987, 1989), the loss of cholinergic PPN neurons in both diseases could attribute to attentive and cognitive impairments and sleep deficiencies in these diseases (Scarnati & Florio, 1997).

Both neuroanatomical (von Krosigk et al., 1992; Smith & Bolam, 1990) and electrophysiological (Häusser & Yung, 1994; Saitoh et al., 2004; Paladini et al., 1999) studies demonstrated that dopaminergic neurons, as well as cholinergic neurons, receive GABAergic inhibitory effects from the basal ganglia, particularly from the SNr. Consequently a BG-BS system appears to involve the interdigitation of motor information with information relating to reward and reinforcement by modulating the excitability of both dopaminergic and cholinergic systems.

5. Concluding thoughts

The basal ganglia controls various function by acting on thalamocortical loop (C-BG loop) and the brainstem (BG-BS system). There are two key mechanisms for the operation by the basal ganglia circuit. One is sequential information processing, which would enhance the temporal contrast of the excitability of the target systems so that only the selected motor program could be appropriately executed, whereas other competing programs can be cancelled. The other is sustained output from the basal ganglia, which may control the degree of freedom of the excitability of the target systems during movements. We suggest that following roles can be played by the BG-BS system. First this system is involved in the automatic or unconscious control of movements that accompany voluntary movements. Second, the BG-BS systems may be involved in the maintenance of arousal and attentive states and in the regulation of REM sleep. Because output from the basal ganglia is thought to be overactive in PD, dysfunction of the BG-BS system in addition to that of C-BG loop can be seriously involved in motor and non-motor functions in this disease.

6. Acknowledgment

This work is supported by Grants-in-Aid for Challenging Exploratory Research (Project # 23650202) and Priority Areas "Emergence of Adaptive Motor Function through Interaction between Body, Brain and Environment (Area #454)" from the Japanese Ministry of Education, Culture, Sports, Science and Technology to K.T. We express sincere appreciation to Ms. Mihoko Ebisawa for preparation of this manuscript.

7. References

Aarsland, D., Bronnick, K., Williams-Gray, C., Weintraub, D., Marder, K., Kulisevsky, J., Burn, D., Barone, P., Pagonabarraga, J., Allcock, L., Santangelo, G., Foltynie, T., Janvin, C., Larsen, JP., Barker, RA. & Emre, M. (2010) Mild cognitive impairment in Parkinson disease: a multicenter pooled analysis. *Neurology*, Vol. 75, No.12,(September 21), pp. 1062-1069, ISSN 0028-3878.

Arnulf, I., Bonnet, AM., Damier, P., Bejjani, BP., Seilhean, D., Derenne, JP. & Agid, Y. (2000) Hallucinations, REM sleep, and Parkinson's disease: a medical hypothesis. *Neurology*, Vol. 55, No.2, (July 25), pp. 281-288, ISSN 0028-3878 .

Alessandro, S., Ceravolo, R., Brusa, L., Pierantozzi, M., Costa, A., Galati, S., Placidi, F., Romigi, A., Iani, C., Marzetti, F. & Peppe, A. (2010) Non-motor functions in parkinsonian patients implanted in the pedunculopontine nucleus: focus on sleep and cognitive domains. *J. Neurol. Sci.*, Vol. 289, No. 1-2, (Feb. 15) pp. 44-48, ISSN 0022-510X.

Andujar, J-E. & Drew, T. (2007) Organization of the projections from the posterior parietal cortex to the rostral and caudal regions of the motor cortex of the cat. *J. Comp. Neurol.* Vol. 504, No.1, (Sep. 1), pp. 17–41, ISSN 0092-7317.

Armstrong, DM. (1986) Supraspinal contribution to the initiation and control of locomotion in the cat. *Prog. Neurobiol.*, 26, (n.d.), pp. 273-361, ISSN 0301-0082.

Askenasy, JJ. (2001) Approaching disturbed sleep in late Parkinson's disease: first step toward a proposal for a revised UPDRS. *Parkinsonism Relat. Disord.*, Vol.8, No.2, (October) pp. 123–131, ISSN 1353-8020.

Battig, K., Rosvold, HE. & Mishkin, M. (1962) Comparison of the effects of frontal and caudate lesions on discrimination learning in monkeys. *J. Comp. Physiol. Psychol.*, Vol. 55, (August), pp. 458-463, ISSN 0021-9940.

Bliwise, DL., Willians, ML., Irbe, D., Ansari, FP. & Rye, DB. (2000) Inter-rater reliability for identification of REM sleep in Parkinson's disease. *Sleep*, Vol. 23, No 1, (August 1) pp. 671–676, ISSN 0161-8105.

Boeve, BF., Silber, MH., Saper, CB., Ferman, TJ., Dickson, DW., Parisi, JE., Benarroch, EE., Ahlskog, JE., Smith, GE., Caselli, RC., Tippman-Peikert, M., Olson, EJ., Lin S-C., Young, T., Wszolek, Z., Schenck, CH., Mahowald, MW., Castillo, PR., Del Tredici, K. & Braak, H. (2007) Pathophysiology of REM sleep behaviour disorder and relevance to neurodegenerative disease. *Brain*, Vol.130, Pt.11, (November), pp. 2770-2788, ISSN 0006-8950.

Brooks, DJ. (1995) The role of the basal ganglia in motor control: contributions from PET. *J. Neurol. Sci.*, Vol. 128, No. 1, (January), pp. 1-13, ISSN 0022-510X.

Chase, MH. & Morales, FR. (1990) The atonia and myoclonia of active (REM) sleep. *Annu. Rev. Psychol.*, Vol. 41, (n.d.), pp. 557–584, ISSN 0066-4308.

Chastan, N., Westby, GW., Yelnik, J., Bardinet, E., Do, MC., Agid, Y. & Welter, ML. (2009) Effects of nigral stimulation on locomotion and postural stability in patients with Parkinson's disease. *Brain*, 132, Pt.1, (January), pp. 172-184, ISSN 0006-8950.

Compta, Y., Santamaria, J., Ratti, L., Tolosa, E., Iranzo, A., Muñoz, E., Valldeoriola, F., Casamitjana, R., Ríos, J. & Marti, MJ. (2009) Cerebrospinal hypocretin, daytime sleepiness and sleep architecture in Parkinson's disease dementia. *Brain*, Vol. 132, Pt. 12, (December), pp. 3308-3317, ISSN 0006-8950.

Culebras, A, Moore, JT. (1989) Magnetic resonance findings in REM sleep behavior disorder. *Neurology*, Vol. 39, No. 11, (November), pp. 1519–1523, ISSN 0028-3878.

Datta, S. (2002). Evidence that REM sleep is controlled by the activation of brain stem pedunculopontine tegmental kainate receptor. *J. Neurophysiol.*, Vol. 87, No. 4, (April), pp. 1790–1978, ISSN 0022-3077.

Datta, S. & Siwek, DF. (2002) Single cell activity patterns of pedunculopontine tegmentum neurons across the sleep-wake cycle in the freely moving rats. *J. Neurosci. Res.*, Vol.70, No. 4, (November 15), pp. 611-621, ISSN 0168-0102.

DeLong, MR. & Wichmann, T. (2007) Circuits and circuit disorders of the basal ganglia. *Arch. Neurol.*, Vol. 64, No. 1, (January), pp. 20-24, ISSN 0003-9942.

Divac, I. (1972) Neostriatum and functions of the prefrontal cortex. *Acta Neurobiol. Exp.*, Vol. 32, No. 2, (n.d.), pp. 461-477,ISSN 0065-1400.

Drew, T., Jiang, W., Kably, B. & Lavoie, S. (1996) Role of the motor cortex in the control of visually triggered gait modifications. *Can J. Physiol. Pharmacol.*, Vol. 74, No. 4, (April), pp. 426-442, ISSN 0008-4212.

Drew, T., Prentice, S. & Schepens, B. (2004) Cortical and brainstem control of locomotion. Prog. Brain Res., Vol. 143, (n.d.), pp. 251-261, ISSN 0079-6123.

Eisensehr, I., Lindeiner, H., Jager, M. & Noachtar, S. (2001) REM sleep behavior disorder in sleep-disordered patients with versus without Parkinson's disease: is there a need for polysomnography? *J. Neurol. Sci.*, Vol. 186, No. 1-2, (May 1), pp. 7–11, ISSN 0022-510X.

Ferini-Strambi, L. & Zucconi, M. (2000) REM sleep behavior disorder. *Clin. Neurophysiol.*, Vol. 111, Suppl. 2, (September), S136-140, ISSN 1388-2457.

Futami, T., Takakusaki, K., Kitai, ST. (1995) Glutamatergic and cholinergic inputs from the pedunculopontine tegmental nucleus to dopamine neurons in the substantia nigra pars compacta. *Neurosci. Res.*, Vol. 21, No. 4, (February), pp. 331-342, ISSN 0168-0102.

Garcia-Rill, E. (1991) The pedunculopontine tegmental nucleus. *Prog. Neurobiol.*, Vol. 36, No. 5, (n.d.), pp. 363-389, ISSN 0301-0082.

Georgopoulos, AP. & Grillner, S. (1989) Visuomotor coordination in reaching and locomotion. *Science*, 245, pp.1209-1210, ISSN 0036-8075.

Goldman-Rakic, PS. (1987) Circuitry of primate prefrontal cortex and regulation of behavior by representational memory. In: *Handbook of Physiology*, the Nervous System V, F. Plum (Ed.), 273-416, ISBN 019-520662-2, American Physiological Society Press, Bethesda.

Grillner, S. (1981) Control of locomotion in bipeds, tetrapods, and fish. In: *Handbook of Physiology*, the Nervous System II, V.B. Brooks, (Ed.), 1179-1236, ISBN 10: 0195206592, ISBN 13: 9780195206593, (Published November 30, 1980), American Physiological Society Press, Bethesda.

Grillner, S., Georgopoulos, A.P. & Jordan L.M. (1997) Selection and initiation of motor behavior. In: *Neurons, Networks, and Motor Behavior*, P.S.G. Stein, S. Grillner, A.I. Selverson, D.G. Stuart, (Eds.), 3-19, ISBN-10: 0-262-19390-6, MIT Press.

Hanakawa, T., Katsumi, Y., Fukuyama, H., Honda, M., Hayashi, T., Kimura, J. & Shibasaki, H. (1999) Mechanisms underlying gait disturbance in Parkinson's disease: a single photon emission computed tomography study. *Brain*, Vol. 122, Pt.7, (July), pp. 1271-1282, ISSN 0006-8950.

Häusser, MA. & Yung, WH. (1994) Inhibitory synaptic potentials in guinea-pig substantia nigra dopamine neurones in vitro. *J. Physiol.*, Vol. 479, Pt.3, (September 15), pp. 401-422, ISSN 0022-3751.

Hikosaka, O., Takikawa, Y. & Kawgoe, R. (2000) Role of the basal ganglia in the control of purposive saccadic eye movements. *Physiol. Rev.*, Vol. 80, No. 3, (July), pp. 954–978, ISSN 00319333.

Hikosaka, O. & Wurtz, RH. (1985) Modification of saccadic eye movements by GABA-related substances: II. Effects of muscimol in monkey substantia nigra pars reticulata. *J. Neurophysiol.*, Vol. 53, No. 1, (January), pp. 292-308, ISSN 0022-3077.

Hirsch, EC., Graybiel, AM. ,Duyckaerts, C. & Javoy-Agid, F. (1987) Neuronal loss in the pedunculopontine tegmental nucleus in Parkinson disease and in progressive supranuclear palsy. *PNAS, USA*, Vol. 84, No. 16, (August), pp. 5976-5980, ISSN 0027-8424.

Honda, T. & Semba, K. (1994) Serotonergic synaptic input to cholinergic neurons in the rat mesopontine tegmentum. *Brain Res.*, Vol. 647, N0. 2, (Jun 6), pp. 299-306, ISSN 0006-8993.

Hornykiewicz, O., Kish, S.J., Becker, L.E., Farley, I. & Shannak, K. (1986) Brain neurotransmitters in dystonia musculorum deformans. *New Engl. J. Med.,* Vol. 315, No. 6. (August), pp. 347-353, ISSN 0028-4793.

Hutchins, KD., Martino, AM. & Strick, PL. (1988) Corticospinal projections from the medial wall of the hemisphere. *Exp. Brain Res.,* Vol. 71, No3, (n.d.), pp. 667-672, ISSN 0735-7044.

Inglis, WL. & Winn, P. (1995). The pedunculopontine tegmental nucleus: where the striatum meets the reticular formation. *Prog. Neurobiol.,* Vol. 47, No.1, (September), pp. 1–29, ISSN 0301-0082.

Iranzo, A., Molinuevo, JL., Santamaría, J., Serradell, M., Martí, MJ., Valldeoriola, F. & Tolosa, E. (2006) Rapid-eye movement sleep behaviour disorder as an early marker for a neurodegenerative disorder: a descriptive study. *Lancet Neurol.,* Vol. 5, No. 7, (July), pp. 572–577, ISSN 1474-4422.

Jellinger, K. (1988) The pedunculopontine nucleus in Parkinson's disease, progressive supranuclear palsy and Alzheimer's disease. *J. Neurol. Neurosurg. Psychiatry,* Vo. 51, No. 4, (April), pp. 540-543, ISSN 0022-3050.

Jones, BE. (1991) Paradoxical sleep and its chemical/structural substrates in the brain. *Neuroscience,* Vo. 40, No. 3, (n.d.) pp. 637–656, ISSN 0306-4522.

Jordan, LM. (1998). Initiation of locomotion in mammals. *Ann. NY. Acad. Sci.,* Vol. 860, (November 16), pp. 83-93, ISSN 0077-8923.

Kitai, ST. (1998) Afferent control of substantia nigra compacta dopamine neurons: anatomical perspective and role of glutamatergic and cholinergic inputs. *Advances in Pharmacology,* Vol. 42, (n.d.), pp. 700-702.

Kobayashi, Y., Inoue, Y. & Isa, T. (2004) Pedunculopontine control of visually guided saccades. *Prog. Brain Res.,* Vol. 143, (n.d.), pp. 439-145, ISSN 0079-6123.

Kobayashi, Y., Inoue, Y., Yamamoto, M., Isa, T. & Aizawa, H. (2002) Contribution of pedunculopontine tegmental nucleus neurons to performance of visually guided saccade tasks in monkeys. *J. Neurophysiol.,* Vol. 88, No. 2, (August), pp. 715-731, ISSN 0022-3077.

Kojima. J., Yamaji. Y., Matsumura. M., Nambu. A., Inase. M., Tokuno. H., Takada. M. & Imai. H. (1997) Excitotoxic lesions of the pedunculopontine tegmental nucleus produce contralateral hemiparkinsonism in the monkey. *Neurosci. Lett.,* Vol. 226, No.2, (April 25) pp. 111- 114, ISSN 0304-3940.

Koyama, Y. & Sakai, K. (2000) Modulation of presumed cholinergic mesopontine tegmental neurons by acetylcholine and monoamines applied iontophoretically in unanesthetized cats. *Neuroscience,* Vol. 96, No. 4, (n.d.) pp. 723-733, ISSN 0306-4522.

Lajoie, K. & Drew T. (2007) Lesions of area 5 of the posterior parietal cortex in the cat produce errors in the accuracy of paw placement during visually guided locomotion. *J. Neurophysiol.,* Vol. 97, No. 3, (March), pp. 2339-2354, ISSN 0022-3077.

Laplane, D., Baulac, M., Widlocher, D. & Dubois, B. (1984). Pure psychic akinesia with bilateral lesions of basal ganglia. *J. Neurol. Neurosurg. Psychiatry,* Vol. 47, No. 4, (April), pp. 377-385, ISSN 0022-3050.

Larsen, JP. & Tandberg, E. (2001) Sleep disorders in patients with Parkinson's disease: epidemiology and management. *CNS Drugs,* Vol. 15, No. 4, (n.d.), pp. 267-75, ISSN 1172-7047.

Lavoie, B. & Parent, A. (1994) Pedunculopontine nucleus in the squirrel monkey: projections to the basal ganglia as revealed by anterograde tract-tracing methods. *J. Comp. Neurol.*, Vol. 344, No. 2, (Jun 8), pp. 210-231, ISSN 0021-9967.

Leonald, CS. & Llinás, R. (1994) Serotonergic and cholinergic inhibition of mesopontine cholinergic neurons controlling REM sleep; an in vitro electrophysiological study. *Neuroscience* Vol. 59, No. 2, (March), pp. 309-330, ISSN 0306-4522.

Maloney, KJ., Mainville, L. & Jones, BE. (1999) Differential c-Fos expression cholinergic, monoaminergic and GABAergic cell groups of the pontomesencephalic tegmentum after paradoxical sleep deprivation and recovery. *J. Neurosci.*, Vol. 19, No. 8, (April 15), pp. 3057-3072, ISSN0306-4522.

Masdeu, JC., Alampur, U., Cavaliere, R. & Tavoulareas, G. (1994) Astasia and gait failure with damage of the pontomesencephalic locomotor region. *Ann. Neurol.*, Vo. 35, No.5, (May), pp. 619-621, ISSN 0364-5134.

Matsumura, M. & Kojima, J. (2001) The role of the pedunculopontine tegmental nucleus in experimental parkinsonism in primates. *Stereotactic and Functional Neurosurgery*, Vol. 77, No. 1-4, (n.d.), pp.108- 115, ISSN 1011-6125.

Matsumura, M., Nambu, A., Yamaji, Y., Watanabe, K., Imai, H., Inase, M., Tokuno, H. & Takada, M. (2000). Organization of somatic motor inputs from the frontal lobe to the pedunculopontine tegmental nucleus in the macaque monkey. *Neuroscience*, Vol. 98, No.1, (n.d.) pp. 97- 110, ISSN 0306-4522.

Matsuyama, K. & Drew, T. (1997) Organization of the projections from the pericruciate cortex to the pontomedullary brainstem of the cat: a study using the anterograde tracer Phaseolus vulgaris- leucoagglutinin. *J.Comp. Neurol.*, Vol. 389, No. 4, (December 29), pp. 617-641, ISSN 0021-9967.

Matsuyama, K. & Takakusaki, K. (2009) Organizing principles of axonal projections of the long descending reticulospinal pathway and its target spinal lamina VIII commissural neurons: with special reference to the locomotor function. In: *Handbook on White Matter: Structure, Function and Changes, Chapter XVIII*, T.B. Westland, R.N. Calton (eds). 335-356, (n.d.), Nova Science Publishing Co. New York, USA, ISBN: 978-1-61668-975-9.

McCrea, DA. & Rybak, IA. (2008) Organization of mammalian locomotor rhythm and pattern generation. *Brain Res. Rev.*, Vol. 57, No. 1, (January), pp. 134-146, ISSN 0165-0173.

McHugh, PR. & Folsten, MF. (1975) Psychiatric syndromes of Huntington's chorea: a clinical and phenomenologic study. In: *Psychiatric aspects of neurological disease. vol. 13*, F. Beston, D. Blumer (Eds.), 267-286, (n.d.), Grune & Stratton, New York. ISBN13: 978-0-19-530943-0, ISBN10: 0-19-530943-X

McVea, DA. & Pearson, KG. (2007) Long-lasting, context-dependent modification of stepping in the cat after repeated stumbling-corrective responses. *J. Neurophysiol.*, Vo. 97, No.1, (January), pp. 659-669, ISSN 0022-3077.

Mellers, JD., Quinn, NP. & Ron, MA. (1995) Psychotic and depressive symptoms in Parkinson's disease. A study of the growth hormone response to apomorphine. *Br. J. Psychiatry*, Vol. 167, No. 4, (October), pp. 522-526, ISSN 0007-1250.

Mena-Segovia, J., Winn, P. & Bolam, JP. (2008) Cholinergic modulation of midbrain dopaminergic systems. *Brain Res. Rev.*, Vol. 58, No. 2, (August), pp. 265–271, ISSN 0165-0173.

Middleton, FA. & Strick, PL (2000) Basal ganglia and cerebellar loops: motor and cognitive circuits. *Brain Res. Rev.*, Vol. 31, No. 2-3, (March), pp. 236–250, ISSN 0165-0173.

Mileykovskiy, BY., Kiyashchenko, LI., Kodama, T., Lai, YY. & Siegel, JM. (2000) Activation of pontine and medullary motor inhibitory regions reduces discharge in neurons located in the locus coeruleus and the anatomical equivalent of the midbrain locomotor region. *J. Neurosci.*, Vol. 20, No. 22, (November 15), pp. 8551-8558, ISSN 0270-6474.

Mogenson, GI. (1991) The role of mesolimbic dopamine projections to the ventral striatum in response initiation. In: *Neurobiological Basis of Human Locomotion*, M. Shimamura, S. Grillner, V.R. Edgarton (Eds.), 33-44, (October) Japan Scientific Press, Tokyo. ISBN 4762246468.

Mori, S. (1987) Integration of posture and locomotion in acute decerebrate cats and in awake, free moving cats. *Prog. Neurobiol.*, Vol. 28, No. 2, (n.d.), pp. 161-196, ISSN 0301-0082.

Mori, S., Matsui, T., Kuze, B., Asanome, M., Nakajima, K. & Matsuyama, K. (1999) Stimulation of a restricted region in the midline cerebellar white matter evokes coordinated quadrupedal locomotion in the decerebrate cat. *J. Neurophysiol.*, Vol. 82, No. 1, (July), pp. 290-300, ISSN 0022-3077.

Mori, S., Sakamoto, T., Ohta, Y., Takakusaki, K. and Matsuyama, K (1989) Site-specific postural and locomotor changes evoked in awake, freely moving intact cats by stimulating the brainstem. *Brain Res.*, Vol. 505, No. 1, (December 25), pp. 66-74, ISSN 0006-8993.

Morris, ME, Iansek R, Matyas, TA & Summers, JJ. (1994) The pathogenesis of gait hypokinesia in Parkinson's disease. *Brain,* Vol. 117, Pt. 5, (October), pp. 1169-1181, ISSN 0006-8950.

Moriizumi, T., Nakamura, Y., Tokuno, H., Kitao, Y. & Kudo, M. (1988) Topographic projections from the basal ganglia to the nucleus tegmenti pedunculopontinus pars compacta of the cat with special reference to pallidal projections. *Exp. Brain Res.*, Vol. 71, No. 2, (n.d.), pp. 298–306, ISSN 0932-4011.

Moruzzi, G. & Magoun, HW (1949) Brain stem reticular formation and activation of the EEG. *Clin. Neurophysiol.*, Vol. 1, No. 4, (November), 455-473, ISSN 1388-2457.

Murray, MP, Sepic, SB, Gardner, GM & Downs, WJ. (1978) Walking patterns of men with parkinsonism. *Am. J. Phys. Med.*, Vol. 57, No. 6, (December), pp. 278-294, ISSN 0002-9491.

Nambu A. (2004) A new dynamic model of the cortico-basal ganglia loop. *Prog. Brain Res.*, 143, (n.d.), pp. 461-466, ISSN 0079-6123.

Nambu, T., Sakurai, T., Mizukami, K., Hosoya, Y., Yanagisawa, M. & Goto, K. (1999) Distribution of orexin neurons in the adult rat brain. *Brain Res.*,Vol. 827, No. 1-2, (May 8), pp. 243-260, ISSN 0006-8993.

Pahapill, PA. & Lozano, AM. (2000) The pedunculopontine nucleus and Parkinson's disease. *Brain*, Vol. 123, Pt. 9, (September), pp. 1767-1783, ISSN 0006-8950.

Paladini, CA., Iribe, Y. & Tepper, JM. (1999). $GABA_A$ receptor stimulation blocks NMDA-induced bursting of dopaminergic neurons in vitro by decreasing input resistance. *Brain Res.*, Vol. 832, No. 1-2, (Jun 19), pp. 145-151, ISSN 0006-8993.

Paré, D., Curro-Dossi, R., Datta, S. & Steriade, M (1990) Brainstem genesis of reserpine - induced ponto-geniculo-occipital waves: an electrophysiological and morphological investigation. *Exp. Brain Res.*, Vol. 81, No. 3, (n.d.), pp. 533-544, ISSN 0932-4011.

Parent, A., Mackey, A., Smith, Y. & Boucher, R. (1983) The output organization of the substantia nigra in primate as revealed by a retrograde double labeling method. *Brain Res. Bull.*, Vol. 10, No. 4, (April), pp. 529-537, ISSN 0361-9230.

Peyron, C., Tighe, DK., van den Pol, AN., de Lecea, L., Heller, HC., Sutcliffe, JG. & Kilduff, TS. (1998) Neurons containing hypocretin (orexin) project to multiple neuronal systems. *J. Neurosci.*, Vol. 18, No. 23, (December 1), pp. 9996-10015, ISSN 0270-6474.

Pierantozzi, M., Palmieri, MG., Galati, S., Stanzione, P., Peppe, A., Tropepi, D., Brusa, L., Pisani, A., Moschella, V., Marciani. MG., Mazzone, P. & Stefani A. (2008) Pedunculopontine nucleus deep brain stimulation changes spinal cord excitability in Parkinson's disease patients. *J. Neural Transm.*, Vol. 115, No. 5, (May), pp. 731-735, ISSN 0300-9564.

Postuma, RB., Gagnon, JF., Rompré, S. & Montplaisir, JY. (2010) Severity of REM atonia loss in idiopathic REM sleep behavior disorder predicts Parkinson disease. *Neurology*, Vol. 74, No. 3, (January 19) pp. 239-244, ISSN 0028-3878.

Rinne, JO., Ma, SY., Lee, MS., Collan, Y. & Röyttä, M. (2008) Loss of cholinergic neurons in the pedunculopontine nucleus in Parkinson's disease is related to disability of the patients. *Parkinsonism Relat. Disord*, Vol. 14, No. 7, (November), pp. 553-557, ISSN 1353-8020.

Rossignol, S. (1996) Neural control of stereotypic limb movements. In: *Handbook of Physiology, sec. 12,* L.B. Rowell, J.T. Shepherd (Eds.), 173-216, (n.d.), New York: Oxford University Press, ISBN 019-509174-4

Rossignol, S , Dubuc, R. & Gossard, JP. (2006) Dynamic sensorimotor interactions in locomotion. *Physiological Reviews,* Vol. 86, No. 1, (January), pp. 89-154, ISSN 0031-9333.

Rye, DB (1997) Contributions of the pedunculopontine region to normal and altered REM sleep. *Sleep*, Vol. 20, No. 9, (September), pp. 757–788, ISSN 0161-8105.

Rye DB., Saper CB., Lee HJ. & Wainer, BH. (1987) Pedunculopontine tegmental nucleus of the rat: cytoarchitecture, cytochemistry, and some extrapyramidal connections of the mesopontine tegmentum. *J.Comp. Neurol.*, Vol. 259, No. 4, (May 22), pp. 483–528, ISSN 0028-3878.

Saitoh, K., Isa, T. & Takakusaki, K. (2004) Nigral GABAergic inhibition upon mesencephalic dopaminergic cell groups in rats. *Eur. J. Neurosci.*, Vol. 19, No. 9, (May), pp. 2399-2409, ISSN 0953-816X.

Sakurai, T. (2002) Roles of orexins in regulation of feeding and wakefulness. *Neuroreport,* Vol. 13, No. 8, (Jun 12), pp. 987–995, ISSN 0959-4965.

Sanford, RD., Morrison, AD., Mann, GL., Harris, JS., Yoo, L. & Ross, RJ. (1994) Sleep pattern and behaviour in cats with pontine lesions creating REM without atonia. *J. Sleep Res.*, Vol. 3, No. 4, (December), pp. 233–240, ISSN 0962-1105.

Scarnati, E. & Florio, T. (1997) The pedunculopontine nucleus and related structures. Functional organization. *Adv. Neurol.*, 74, (n.d.), pp. 97-110, ISSN 0091-3952.

Schenck, CH., Bundlie, SR. & Mahowald, MW. (1996) Delayed emergence of a parkinsonian disorder in 38% of 29 older men initially diagnosed with idiopathic rapid eye movement sleep behaviour disorder. *Neurology*, Vol. 46, No. 2, (February), pp.388 - 393, ISSN 0028-3878.

Schultz, W. (1998) Predictive reward signals of dopamine neurons. *J. Neurophysiol.*, Vol. 80, No. 1, (July), pp. 1-27, ISSN 0022-3077.

Semba, K. (1993) Aminergic and cholinergic afferents to REM sleep induction regions of the pontine reticular formation in the rat. *J. Comp. Neurol.*, Vol. 330, No. 4, (April 22), pp. 543–556, ISSN 0021-9967.

Siegel, JM. (2004) Hypocretin (orexn): Role in normal behavior and neuropathology. *Annu. Rev. Psychol.*, 55, (n.d.), pp. 125-148, ISSN 0066-4308.

Sinnamon, HM. (1993) Preoptic and hypothalamic neurons and initiation of locomotion in the anesthetized rat. *Prog. Neurobiol.*, Vol. 41, No. 3, (September), pp. 323-344, ISSN 0301-0082.

Smith, Y. & Bolam, JP. (1990) The output neurones and the dopaminergic neurones of the substantia nigra receive a GABA-containing input from the globus pallidus in the rat. *J. Comp. Neurol.*, Vol. 296, No. 1, (Jun 1), pp. 47-64, ISSN 0021-9967.

Spann, BM. & Grofova, I. (1991) Nigro-pedunculopontine projection in the rat: an anterograde tracing study with Phaseolus Vulgaris-Leucoagglutinin (PHA-L). *J. Comp. Neurol.*, Vol. 311, No.3, (September 15), pp. 375–388, ISSN 0021-9967.

Stefani, A., Lozano, AM., Peppe, A., Stanzione, P., Galati, S., Tropepi, D., Pierantozzi, M., Brusa, L., Scarnati, E. & Mazzone, P. (2007) Bilateral deep brain stimulation of the pedunculopontine and subthalamic nuclei in severe Parkinson's disease. *Brain*, Vol. 130, Pt. 6, (Jun), pp. 1596-1607, ISSN 0006-8950.

Takakusaki, K. (2008) Forebrain control of locomotor behaviors. *Brain Res. Rev.*, Vol. 57, No. 1, (January), pp. 192-198, ISSN 0165-0173.

Takakusaki, K., Habaguchi, T., Ohtinata-Sugimoto, J., Saitoh, K. & Sakamoto, T. (2003a) Basal ganglia efferents to the brainstem centers controlling postural muscle tone and locomotion; A new concept for understanding motor disorders in basal ganglia dysfunction. *Neuroscience*, Vol. 119, No. 1, (n.d.),pp. 293-308, ISSN 0306-4522.

Takakusaki, K., Habaguchi, T., Saitoh, K. & Kohyama, J. (2004a) Changes in the excitability of hindlimb motoneurons during muscular atonia induced by stimulating the pedunculopontine tegmental nucleus in cats. *Neuroscience*, Vol. 124, No. 2, (n.d.), pp. 467-480, ISSN 0306-4522.

Takakusaki, K., Kohyama, J. & Matsuyama, K. (2003b) Medullary reticulospinal tract mediating a generalized motor inhibition in cats: III. Functional organization of spinal interneurons in the lower lumbar segments. *Neuroscience*, Vol. 121, No. 3, (n.d.), pp. 731-746, ISSN 0306-4522.

Takakusaki, K., Kohyama, J., Matsuyama, K. & Mori, S. (1993) Synaptic mechanisms acting on lumbar motoneurons during postural augmentation induced by serotonin injection into the rostral pontine reticular formation in decerebrate cats. *Exp. Brain Res.*, Vol. 93, No. 3, (n.d.), pp. 471-82, ISSN 0932-4011.

Takakusaki, K., Kohyama, J., Matsuyama, K., Mori, S. (2001) Medullary reticulospinal tract mediating the generalized motor inhibition in cats: parallel inhibitory mechanisms acting on motoneurons and on interneuronal transmission in reflex pathways. *Neuroscience,* Vol. 103, No. 2, (n.d.), pp. 511–527, ISSN 0306-4522.

Takakusaki, K., Saitoh, K., Harada H. & Kashiwayanagi, M (2004b) Role of basal ganglia – brainstem pathways in the control of motor behaviors *Neurosci. Res.,* Vol. 50, No. 2, (October), pp. 137-151, ISSN 0168-0102.

Takakusaki, K., Saitoh, K., Harada, H., Okumura, T. & Sakamoto T. (2004c) Evidence for a role of basal ganglia in the regulation of rapid eye movement sleep by electrical and chemical stimulation for the pedunculopontine tegmental nucleus and the substantia nigra pars reticulata in decerebrate cats. *Neuroscience,* Vol. 124, No. 1, (n.d.), pp. 207-220, ISSN 0306-4522.

Takakusaki, K., Saitoh, K., Nonaka, S., Okumura, T., Miyokawa, N. & Koyama, Y. (2006) Neurobiological basis of state-dependent control of motor behavior. *Sleep and Biological Rhythms,* 4, (n.d.), pp. 87-104, ISSN 1446-9235.

Takakusaki, K., Shimoda, N., Matsuyama, K. & Mori, S. (1994) Discharge properties of medullary reticulospinal neurons during postural changes induced by intrapontine injections of carbachol, atropine and serotonin, and their functional linkages to hindlimb motoneurons in cats. *Exp. Brain Res.,* Vol. 99, No. 3, (n.d.), pp. 361–374, ISSN 0932-4011.

Takakusaki, K., Shiroyama, T., Yamamoto, T., Kitai, ST. (1996) Cholinergic and noncholinergic tegmental pedunculopontine projection neurons in rats revealed by intracellular labeling. *J. Comp. Neurol.,* Vol. 371, No. 3, (July 29), pp. 345-361, ISSN 0021-9967.

Takakusaki, K., Takahashi, K., Saitoh, K., Harada, H., Okumura, T., Kayama, Y. & Koyama, Y. (2005) Orexinergic projections to the cat midbrain mediate alternation of emotional behavioural states from locomotion to cataplexy. *J. Physiol.,* Vol. 568, Pt. 3, (November 1), pp. 1003–1020, ISSN 0022-3751.

Taylor, JR., Elsworth, JD., Roth, RH., Slodek, JR. & Redmond, DE. (1990) Cognitive and motor deficits in the acquisition of an object retrieval/detour task in MPTP-treated monkeys. *Brain,* Vol. 113, Pt. 3, (Jun), pp. 617-637, ISSN 0006-8950..

Taylor, JR., Saint-Cyr, JA. & Lang, AE. (1986) Frontal lobe dysfunction in Parkinson's disease. *Brain,* Vol. 109, Pt.5, (October), pp. 845-883, ISSN 0006-8950..

Thannickal, TC., Lai, YY. & Siegel, JM. (2007) Hypocretin (orexin) cell loss in Parkinson's disease. *Brain,* Vol. 130, Pt. 6, (Jun), pp. 1586-1595, ISSN 0006-8950.

Turner, RS. & Anderson, ME. (1997) Pallidal discharge related to the kinematics of reaching movements in two dimensions. *J. Neurophysiol.,* Vol. 77, No. 3, (March), pp. 1051-1074, ISSN 0022-3077.

Unger, MM., Belke, M., Menzler, K., Heverhagen, JT., Keil, B., Stiasny-Kolster, K., Rosenow, F., Diederich, NJ., Mayer, G., Möller, JC., Oertel, WH. & Knake S. (2010) Diffusion tensor imaging in idiopathic REM sleep behavior disorder reveals microstructural changes in the brainstem, substantia nigra, olfactory region, and other brain regions. *Sleep,* Vol. 33, No. 6, (Jun 1)pp. 767-773, ISSN 0161-8105.

Van der Kamp, W., Berardelli, A., Rothwell, JC., Thompson, PD., Day, BL. & Marsden, CD. (1989) Rapid elbow movements in patients with torsion dystonia. *J. Neurol., Neurosurg. Psychiatry*, Vol. 52, No. 9, (September), 1043-1049, ISSN 0022-3050.

von Krosigk, M., Smith, Y., Bolam, JP. & Smith, AD. (1992) Synaptic organization of GABAergic inputs from the striatum and the globus pallidus onto neurons in the substantia nigra and retrorubral field which project to the medullary reticular formation. *Neuroscience*, Vol. 50, No. 3, (October), pp. 531-549, ISSN 0306-4522.

Zweig, RM., Jankel, WR., Hedreen, JC., Mayeux, R. & Price, DL. (1989) The pedunculopontine nucleus in Parkinson's disease. *Ann. Neurol.*, Vol. 26, No. 1, (July)pp. 41-46, ISSN 0364-5134.

Zweig, RM., Whitehouse, PJ., Casanova, MF., Walker, LC., Jankel, WR. & Price, DL. (1987) Loss of pedunculopontine neurons in progressive supranuclear palsy. *Ann. Neurol.*, Vol. 22, No. 1SN 0364-5134.

21

Role of Lysosomal Enzymes in Parkinson's Disease: Lesson from Gaucher's Disease

Tommaso Beccari et al.*
Dipartimento di SEEA, Università di Perugia, Italy

1. Introduction

The lysosome, initially discovered by Christian de Duve in 1955, is an intracellular organelle responsible of the ordered degradation of proteins, glycoproteins, proteoglycans, lipids, and other macromolecules originated from autophagy, endocytosis and phagocytosis. It is characterize by a limiting external membrane containing intraluminal vesicles. These organelles are estimated to contain 50-60 soluble acidic hydrolases (Journet et al., 2002), 55 membrane-associated proteins and 215 integral membrane proteins (Bagshaw et al., 2005). The macromolecules are scomposed by acid hydrolases in small molecules that are transported back in the cytosol by specific transporter proteins and then catabolized or re-used by anabolic processes. Lysosomal hydrolases are synthetized as N-glycosylated precursors in the endoplasmatic reticulum and are transported to the lysosomes via a vectorial transport dependent on mannose 6-phosphate. Lysosomes are involved in many cellular processes like cholesterol homeostasis, autophagy, membrane repair, pathogen defense, cell signaling, apoptosys and bone/tissue remodelling; it is a foundamental organelle for cell life and not only the wastebasket of the cell. Microscopic identification of lysosomes is hard due to heterogeneity of organelles morphology dependent on their function as digestive organelles. The size and quantity of lysosomes varies in different cell types and can increase when the lysosomes accumulate non-digested material. Functional deficit of hydrolases, membrane-associated or integral membrane proteins causes lysosomal storage disorders (LSDs), a group of inherited metabolic pathologies characterized by intralysosomal deposition of undegraded macromolecules and by multisystemic phenotype (Saftig, 2006). The absence or reduced activity of a specific lysosomal hydrolase or other lysosomal proteins cause an abnormal function of the entire endosomal/lysosomal system (Bellettato & Scarpa, 2010).

More than 50 lysosomal storage disorders (LSD) are known with a total incidence of 1:7,000-1:9,000 (Fletcher, 2006). Two thirds of them involve the central nervous system (Meikle et al.,

*Chiara Balducci[1], Silvia Paciotti[1], Emanuele Persichetti[1], Davide Chiasserini[2], Anna Castrioto[2], Nicola Tambasco[2], Aroldo Rossi[2], Paolo Calabresi[2], Veronica Pagliardini[3], Bruno Bembi[4] and Lucilla Parnetti[2]
[1]*Dipartimento di SEEA, Università di Perugia, Italy*
[2]*Clinica Neurologica, Ospedale S. Maria della Misericordia, Università di Perugia, Italy*
[3]*Dipartimento di Pediatria, Università di Torino, Italy*
[4]*Centro Regionale per le malattie Rare, Ospedale Universitario 'Santa Maria della Misericordia', Italy*

1999). The LSD can be classified in sphingolipidoses, mucopolysaccharidoses, mucolipidoses, lipid storage disease, glycogen storage disease type II and lysosomal transport defects. Different LSD displayed different symptoms severity and different age onset and it depend on the organs affected and the residual enzyme activity. Generally, mutation leaving very low residual enzyme activity cause the most severe onset form of the pathologies; contrary higher residual enzyme activity delays disease onset (Kolter & Sandhoff, 1999). The disease course and severity are different in late-onset forms and can be variable even among affected siblings in the same family (Zhao & Grabowski, 2002). LSDs are often multisystemic disorders and many of these displayed a severe, progressive and untreatable neurological impairment. Almost all LSDs are related to devastating, progressive and untreatable effects on central nervous system (CNS). Neuronal loss occurs in the advanced stages of the diseases and is due to apoptosis or necrosis. The neurological symptoms are mental retardation, progressive neurodegeneration, dementia. Most LSDs show CNS involvment althought the undegraded material concentration is lower in the brain than in other organs. It seems that neurons are more vulnerable than other cellular type probably for a limited cell regeneration potential or for the absence of compensatory pathways (Bellettato & Scarpa, 2010). The Neuronal Ceroid Lipofuscinoses (NCLs) are lysosomal storage diseases affecting the CNS, with progressive loss of vision, decreasing cognitive and motor skills, epileptic seizures and premature death, with dementia without visual loss prominent in the rarer adult forms (Kohan et al., 2011). GM1 type 3 Gangliosidosis is an autosomal recessive lysosomal storage disorder caused by β-galactosidase deficiency, patients were recently found to be affected by generalized dystonia associated to akinetic-rigid parkinsonism (Roze et al., 2005). The San Filippo Syndrome type B is a LSDs due to mutation in the gene encoding α-N-acetylglucosaminidase with an accumulation of heparan sulfate. Affected children shown mental retardation, dementia, behavior problems. The analysis of mutant mice showed cytoplasmic inclusion of P-tau aggregates, characteristic of tauopathies, a group of age-related dementia that include Alzheimer disease (Ohmi et al., 2009).

In some adult neurodegenerative disorders like Alzheimer's disease, Parkinson's disease and Huntington' s disease the clical features are similar to those found in LSDs: accumulation of undegraded material, abnormal inflammatory response in the brain and changes in neurons morphology and functionality (Bellettato et al., 2010). In Parkinson's disease was found an involvement of cathepsin D, a lysosomal enzyme, in α-synuclein degradation and formation of carboxy-terminally truncated α-synuclein. Recent works suggest that impaired cathepsin D activity would result in incresed a-synuclein levels that cause its aggregation (Sevlever et al., 2008). In Huntington's disease N-terminal mutant huntingtin fragments form inclusions that lead to cell death. Some protease, like cathepsin D, B and L, help to degrade mutant huntingtin but increase N-terminal fragment formation and inclusions deposition inducing neuronal disruption (Kim et al., 2006).

2. Gaucher's disease: An overview

Gaucher's disease (GD) is an inherited autosomal recessive metabolic disorder, resulting from a deficiency of the lysosomal enzyme β-glucocerebrosidase (also called acid β-glucosidase, GCase) (EC 3.2.1.45).

GD was first described as a systemic disease by Philippe Gaucher in 1882, but only in 1965 this disorder was related to the deficiency of β-glucocerebrosidase (Patrick, 1965; Brady et al.

1965). This enzyme is involved in the catabolic pathway of glycosphingolipids and is responsible for the cleavage of the β-glucosidic bond on the glucosylceramide (or glucocerebroside) (Fig. 1).
The human β-glucosidase is encoded by a gene (GBA) located on chromosome 1 (1q21) (Barneveld et al., 1983) which comprises 11 exons and 10 introns, spanning 7.6 kb of sequence. A non processed pseudogene (GBAP), which shares 96% exonic sequence homology, is located 16 kb downstream of the functional β-glucocerebrosidase gene (Horowitz et al., 1989).
The lack of GCase activity leads to accumulation of glycolipid substrates, primarily glucocerebroside and its nonacylated analog, glucosylsphingosine, in all organs, particularly in spleen, liver, lungs and bone marrow (Cox & Shofield, 1997; Beutler & Grabowski, 2001). The material stored is the product of the arrested breakdown of gangliosides, glycosphingolipids and globosides, which derived from the cellular turnover of membranes.

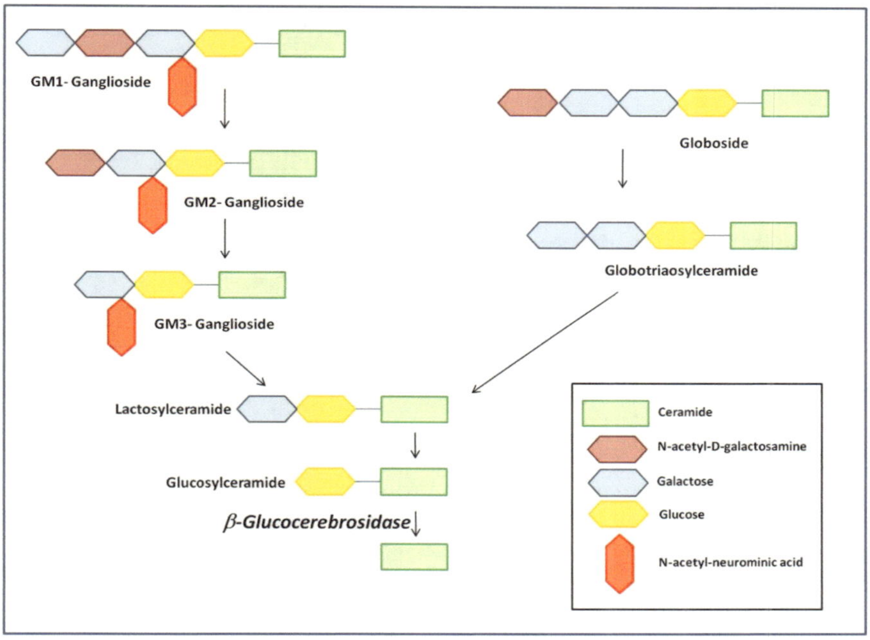

Fig. 1. Involvement β-glucocerebrosidase in the catabolic pathway of glycosphingolipids

Although in the patients the GCase is inactive in all cells, glucocerebroside accumulation occurs principally within the lysosomes of macrophages which adopt a characteristic "Gaucher's cell" morphology. Disease manifestations are related to the migration and accumulation of the Gaucher's cells, which displace healthy cells in the tissues. Furthermore the abnormal material stored in the cells of the reticuloendothelial system induces the release of inflammatory factors, including chemokines and cytokines, which leads to the cascade of pathological changes (Beutler & Grabowski, 2001; Cox, 2001; Aerts & Hollak, 1997; Moran et al., 2000; Jmoudiak & Futerman, 2005; Nilsson & Svennerhol, 1982; Pelled et al., 2005; Futerman & van Meer, 2004) (Table 1).
Gaucher's disease may occur at any age in any human population (Beutler & Grabowski, 2001; Zimran et al., 1992; Cox & Shofield, 1997; Erikson, 1986). Although the birth frequency

of Gaucher's disease is one case per 60,000 live births in the general population (Meikle et al., 1999), it is the most frequent genetic disease in the Ashkenazi Jewish people where epidemiological data, based on estimated gene frequencies, show a prevalence of one case per 850 live births (Beutler et al., 1993).

GD has a highly variable phenotype, and even though a recent trend is to consider GD as a continuum of disease states (Goker-Alpan et al., 2003), three basic clinical forms are conventionally distinguished on the basis of the neurological involvement: the non neuronopathic form (type 1), the acutely neuronopathic form (type 2) and the subacute neurophatic form (type 3).

Products	Functions
Lysozyme	Antibacterial
Angiotensin-converting enzyme	Vasopressor
Lysosomal acid hydrolases	Digestion
Interleukin-1b, TNFa	Diverse host defence: fever, weight loss
Interleukin 6	Acute phase response, B-cell stimulation, bone resorption, trophic for mieloma cells
Interleukin 8	Granulocyte chemoattractant
Interleukin 10	Inhibits pro-inflammatory cytokines

Table 1. Macrophage secretory products icreased in Gaucher's disease

Type 1 GD (OMIM 230800) is the most frequent form of Gaucher's disease and account 94% of all registered cases according to Gaucher Registry. It is a chronic multisystem storage disorder which, by definition, does not involve the central nervous system. Nevertheless recent studies have shown a possible correlation between type 1 GD and some neurological manifestations (Sindransky, 2004; Cherin, 2006; Biegstraaten et al., 2008). In a number of cases these symptoms can be the consequence of secondary complications of the primary disease (e.g. compression of bone marrow or root nerve as a result of vertebral crush fractures caused by osteonecrosis), whereas in other ones they can be the product of specific GBA gene mutations, particularly in patients presenting parkinsonian syndromes (Aharon-Peretz et al., 2004; Bembi et al., 2003; Clark et al., 2005; Gan-Or et al., 2008; Machaczka et al., 1999; McKeran et al., 1985; Tayeby et al. 2003; Ziegler et al. 2007).

The type 1 GD course is slowly progressive. Generally the symptoms develop in adulthood even though various clinical manifestation may emerge in childhood. The clinical spectrum is vast and includes the complete absence of symptoms as well as the severe organ involvement with disability and occasionally fatal outcome. The patients show hepatosplenomegaly, with thrombocytopenia, anemia and leucopenia. Although in most patients these complications are not life-threatening and may go unrecognized for many years (some subjects remain asymptomatic up to the age of 70 or 80 years) (Berrebi et al., 1984), in other ones this metabolic defect can cause bruising, bleeding and high risk of infection as consequence of pancytopenia and respiratory insufficiency due to diffuse infiltration of Gaucher's cells into the alveolar spaces, perivascular, peribronchial, and into the septal regions (Schneider et al., 1977; Lee, 1982). Asthenia and fatigability are constant and seem independent of anemia, but rather to reflect an alteration of basal metabolism and cytokine secretion (Allen et al., 1997). Moreover degenerative changes in skeleton are the leading cause of bone pain and disability in patients with type 1 disease. The infiltration of Gaucher's cells in the bone marrow causes osteonecrosis, particularly during growth and leads to impaired function of large joints, including hip, knee, and shoulder. Other bone symptoms include local swelling (Gaucheromas) and osteolysis as well as generalized demineralization and osteoporosis with consequent risk of fractures. Furthermore patients may show abnormal diffuse yellow-brawn skin pigmentation and delays of growth, menarche and dentition. In rare cases there can be also renal involvement, pulmonary hypertension (Theise & Ursell, 1990), and cardiac abnormalities.

Type 2 (OMIM 230900) is the most severe form of Gaucher's disease which accounts for fewer than 1% cases. It manifests in early childhood; neurological deterioration progresses quickly and death generally occurs within the age of two years, in a context of psychomotor decline (Brady et al., 1993). The majority of cases of type 2 GD emerges around age of 3 months. The presenting sign is usually hepatosplenomegaly. By 6 months, neurologic complications develop. The first diagnostic simptoms are frequently supranuclear horizontal oculomotor paralysis or bilateral fixed strabismus accompanied by trismus, retroflection of the head, progressive spasticity, hyperreflexia, positive Babinski signs and other phatologic reflexes. Other symptoms can be dysphagia and difficulty in handling secretions developed, often followed by aspiration pneumonia. Death occurs by either apnea or aspiration pneumonia.

Gaucher's disease type 3 (OMIM 231000) is particularly frequent in Norbottnian Swedes (Erikson, 1986). It leads to subacute neurological symptoms that are less severe than those of type 2 disease. It is characterized by the presence of a later onset and a slow progressive neurological syndrome. The clinical manifestations vary. Systemic symptoms precede neurologic abnormalities and usually are similar to those seen in type 1 GD. Neurologic deterioration includes cerebellar ataxia, spastic paraperesis, psychomotor seizures, horizontal supranuclear ophthalmoplegia, myoclonic epilepsy and dementia.

Over 300 mutations of the β-glucosidase gene have been described (Beutler & Gelbart, 1996; Geabowski & Horowitz, 1997, Hruska et al., 2008). The most common are c.1226A>G (N370S), c.1448T>C (L444P), IVS2+1G>A and 84insG. The frequency and distribution of mutations vary with the population studied; in the Ashkenazi population N370S is found in 78% of patients whereas in non-Jewish populations the most frequent mutation is L444P (36%), followed by N370S (29%) (Beutler, 2006).

Although molecular analysis of the glucocerebrosidase gene in patients with Gaucher's disease has permitted broad correlations between genotype and phenotype, this does not consent a confident prediction of clinical phenotype (Cox & Sholfield, 1997; Germain, 2004). Many studies have shown the enormous clinical variation between patients who have the same genotype including monozygotic twins (Sidransky, 2004; Lachmann et al., 2004). Nevertheless the presence of N370S on one or both alleles is associated with type 1 GD and it seems to protect against neurological symptoms, except for Parkinson-like syndromes (Charrow et al., 2000; Cherin et al., 2006). On the contrary the presence of the L444P/L444P mutation is associated with the development of neurological manifestations, above all in Gaucher's disease type 3 (75% of cases) (Charrow et al., 2000). Other mutations, including 84insG, IVS2+1G>A, c.754T>A (F213I) and c.1297G>T (V394L), are generally responsible for the emergence of a neurological form, when associated with mutation L444P either alone or integrated in a complex allele.

3. Gaucher's and Parkinson's disease: Theories of a link

Parkinson's disease (PD) is the one of the common movement disorders and the second most common human neurodegenerative disease. The major diagnostic neuropathological features of the pathologiy are loss of dopaminergic neurons and the appearance of Lewy bodies (LB), which are intraneuronal inclusions composed by α-synuclein and abnormal ubiquitinated proteins aggregates.

The first associations of the glucocerebrosidase enzyme with parkinsonism were discovered through careful clinical observation of people affecting by GD, who in several cases developed Parkinson's disease. Although in recent years GBA mutations were found to be a major risk factor for the development of Parkinson's disease (Sidransky et al., 2009), it is not clear how these are related. However many findings suggest that GBA protein and α-synuclein are implicated in a common cellular pathway and different hypothesis have been created to explain the linkage between them.

Recent studies have shown as some mutations in the GBA gene can lead to the misfolded protein formation (Sawkar et al., 2005), contributing to parkinsonism by leading to lysosomal insufficiency, as a result of impairing autophagic pathways necessary to prevent the synucleopathies, or by crushing the ubiquitin-proteasome system.

During the life span of a protein, cellular systems continuously check on the quality of the protein and take care of its repair or removal from the cell if there is any abnormality. The advancement during the past decades in understanding the quality control system of cellular proteins has allowed the identification of unequivocal links between malfunctioning of these systems and some severe human pathologies, including major neurodegenerative disease as Parkinson's (PD) and Alzheimer's (AD).

Many newly synthesized proteins are incorrectly translated or wrongly folded as a result of errors in their sequence due to either genetic mutations or alterations during the synthesis process (Wheatley & Inglis, 1980; Vabulas & Hartl, 2005; Shubert et al., 2000; Yewdell, 2005). The role of protein catabolism in protecting cells from defective, misfolded proteins is essential to avoid the risk of long term accumulation of proteins which frequently develop abnormal intermolecular interaction, forming insoluble aggregates toxic for the cells (Squier, 2001; Kourie & Henry, 2001). So it is evident the involvement of the quality control system in maintaining cell homeostasis as well as the association between the alteration of the protein turnover and many disease states (Kundu & Thompson, 2008). The autophagy-lysosome and the ubiquitin-proteasome pathways are the two main routes of the quality control system in eukaryotic.

Autophagy-lysosomal degradation pathway is a complex system tightly regulated by series of signaling events that promote the efficient delivery of macronutrients and organelles to lysosomes for degradation by acidic hydrolases (Levine & Klionsky, 2004). It is implicated in the catabolism and recycling of long-lived proteins and organelles and it is thought to be involved in many physiological processes, including the response to starvation, cell growth control, antiaging mechanisms and innate immunity. Some years ago the authophagy-lysosome pathway was considered as a non selective form of catabolism, while now the view is changed and it is thought as a specialized system that distinguishes the substrates and chooses the route by which they reach the lysosomes. Three types of autophagy have been described: macroautophagy, microautophagy and chaperon mediated autophagy (CMA) (Cuervo, 2004). They share a common endpoint, the lysosome, but differ in substrates targeted, their regulation and the conditions in which each of them is preferentially activated.

Macroautophagy process is activated to generate essential macromolecules and energy in condition of nutritional scarcity (Mizushima, 2005) or as a mechanism to remove the altered intracellular components (Levine & Klionsky, 2004). It can be induced also by hypoxia, neurotrophic factor deprivation, excitotoxins and accumulation of protein aggregates through PI3K and ERK-mediated pathways (Zhu t al., 2007; Boland & Nixon, 2006). Macroautophagy is described as the sequestration of complete regions of the cytosol, including not only soluble proteins, but also complete organelles, into a double membrane vescicle known as autophagosome, which is considered an immature form of autophagic vacuole (AV) (Seglen et al., 1996; Mortimore et al., 1996). The limiting double membrane is thought to arise from the endoplasmatic reticulum, although the Golgi complex has also been indicated as a source (Levine & Klionsky, 2004; Mijaljica et al., 2006). Because these vesicles lack any enzyme, the trapped contents are not degradated until the autophagosome founds with a lysosome, forming a single membrane autophagolysosome.

Macroautophagy is regulated by the action of a family of molecules, known as autophagy-related proteins (Atg), which participates in each of the different steps of this process (Klionsky et al., 2003). A series of conjugation events (protein-to-lipid and protein-to-protein) and several members of intracellular kinase families are involved (Klionsky, 2005; Ohsumi, 2001).

One hypotheses has been proposed to explain the role of dysregulated autophagy in PD pathogenesis, in patients affected to Gaucher's disease. This theory ("offensive metabolite theory") is based on the ceramide activity in the process of autophagic pathway modulation (Scarlatti et al., 2004). Ceramide is a sphingolipid mediator with an essential role in different situations correlated with authophagic system, such as cell growth, cell death, proliferation and stress response (Klionsky & Emr, 2000). Studies have shown as ceramide interferes with the inhibitory class I PI3K signaling pathway and induces the expression of a autophagy-related gene beclin 1, stimuling the autophagyc process.

It's possible that the lack of β-glucocerebrosidase activity and the accumulation of glucocerebroside may interfere with the ceramide modulation system, destroing cellular pathways necessary for autophagic-lysosomal degradation and leading to the LB formation.

The other types of described autophagy are microautophagy and CMA. The first one consists of direct engulfment of small volumes of cytosol (constituted by soluble proteins but also by complete organelles) by lysosomes (Ahlberg et al., 1982) through invaginations or tabulations that "pinch off" from the membrane into the lysosomal lumen where they are rapidly degraded (Marzella et al., 1981). Microautophagy participates in the continuous turnover of long-lived proteins inside many types of cells (Mortimore et al., 1988); in addition a number of studies have shown as a particular form of microautophagy can lead to preferential degradation of peroxisomes (micropexophagy) (Farre and Subramani, 2004; Mukaiyama et al., 2002; Veenhuis et al., 2000).

Chaperon-mediated autophagy is characterized by selectivity; about 30% of cytosolic proteins are degraded by this pathway. Through CMA particular cytosolic proteins are recognized by a chaperone in the cytosol, which delivers the proteins directly to the surface of the lysosome (Dice, 1990; Majeski & Dice, 2004, Massey et al., 2006). A distinctive feature of this pathway is that all substrate proteins contain in their amino acid sequence a motif, biochemically related to the pentapeptide KFERQ, required for targeting to the lysosomal compartment (Dice, 1990). A heat shock protein, hsc73 (Chiang et al., 1989) , recognizes the substrates containing the motif, and brings them to the lysosome membrane, where it binds to the receptor protein, lamp2 (lysosome-associated membrane protein type 2a) (Cuervo & Dice, 1996). The substrate interacts direcly with lamp2, and once unfolded, it is transported in the lysosome lumen (Salvador et al., 2000) where it is degraded.

Substrates for CMA consist of a very heterogeneous pool of cytosolic proteins, different for structure and function, but having all the same KFERQ motif. CMA acts in the degradation of many different substrates (i.e. several glycolitic enzymes, glutathione transferase, ribonuclease A) and damaged proteins: its selective role allows removal of the altered proteins without affecting neighbouring healty ones (Kiffin et al., 2004; Cuervo et al., 1999). Many studies have shown as this autophagic pathway is activated when stress condition occurs in the cells, such as prolonged nutrient deprivation or exposure to toxic compounds (Cuervo & Dice, 1998).

Independently of the autophagic pathway, all substrates are brought to the lysosome lumen where several different lysosomal hydrolases rapidly degrade them. These enzymes are synthesized in the endoplasmatic reticulum, sorted to the trans-Golgi network by mannose-6-phosphate receptors, transported through the endosome to arrive to their lysosomal destination, where they are activated upon the exposure to the acid environment (Jadot et al., 1997). The proteolytic capacity of lysosomes comprises a mixture of endo- and exo-peptidases, called cathepsins, which act in concert to degrade proteins to a mixture of amino acids and dipeptides. Expression, activation and inhibition of these cathepsins are differentially regulated, and individual cathepsins often have non-redundant functions in normal and disease states (Kroemer & Jaattela, 2005). In addition to peptidases activity, intralysosomal conditions and other lysosomal components (i.e. glycosidase, lipases, phospholipases, solphatases, nucleases and phosphatases) are designed to favor the complete degradation of the internalized products.

One route of degradation of the α-synuclein is via CMA pathway (Cuervo et al., 2004). Studies have revealed as impaired lysosomal function seems to be involved in familial forms of PD, as consequence of reduced α-synuclein degradation. So one theory is that disturbances in the lysosome (i.e. the alteration in the GCase function) contribute to reduce α-synuclein degradation and consequently promote its aggregation. This may be possible since ceramide can activate cathepsin D (aspartate protease), which in turn is responsible for the proteolytic activation of other lysosomal proteins (Heinrich et al., 1999). So the reduced activity of one protease can spark off the decremented action of other acid hydrolases causing an α-synuclein accumulation and contributing in LB formation.

The other α-synuclein degradation pathway is the ubiquitin-proteasome system (UPS). It serves as the primary route for the degradation of thousands of short-lived proteins and provides the specificity and temporal control needed for tuning the stady-state levels of many regulatory proteins (Ciechanover et al., 2000). UPS-mediated catabolism is also essential to preserve amino acid pools in acute starvation and contributes significantly to the degradation of defective proteins (Ciechanover & Brudin, 2003; Whealtley & Inglis, 1980; Vabulas & Hartl, 2005). UPS contributes also to diverse cellular processes, such as protein quality control, cell-cycle progression, signal transduction, and development (Kerscher et al., 2006).

Substrates of the ubiquitin/proteasome system (UPS) get post-translationally modified by covalent attachment of multiple ubiquitin molecules at internal lysine residues. This polyubiquitylation of substrate proteins involves three enzymes: ubiquitin-activating enzymes (E1), ubiquitin-conjugating enzymes (E2), and ubiquitin protein ligases (E3). E1 hydrolyses ATP and forms a thioester-linked conjugate between itself and ubiquitin; E2 receives ubiquitin from E1 and forms a similar thioester intermediate with ubiquitin; and E3 binds both E2 and the substrate, and transfers the ubiquitin to the substrate. A chain made of four to six ubiquitin moieties targets the conjugated substrate for degradation by the 26S proteasome (Richly et al., 2005; Zhang et al., 2009).

The UPS can only degrade proteins when they are in a soluble state or as a part of reversible protein complexes that can be disassembled into single protein units (Finkbeiner et al., 2006; Kopito, 2000). So any type of irreversible oligomeric structures, preaggregates, and protein aggregates cannot be handled by UPS, instead they can be degraded by the autophagic-lysosomal pathway.

A different theory ("misfolded protein theory") to explain the linkage between Gaucher's and Parkinson's disease, is that mutant misfolded glucocerebrosidase might overwhelm the UPS, causing a delay in the degradation of accumulated proteins, including α-synuclein (Dawson, 2006). Ron et al. have shown that misfolded GCase endures endoplasmatic reticulum associated degradation (ERAD) (Ron and Horowitz, 2005). In this process, mutant proteins are identified as misfolded by the ER quality control system and retrotraslocated from ER to cytosol, ubiquitinated and eliminated by the ubiquitin-proteasome system. The same authors proposed that mutated GBA protein (but not WT GBA) undergoes parkin (E3-ligase)-mediated ubiquitination, creating an imbalance in protein degradation resulting in secondary toxicity. It is likely that, since GCase is not a natural substrate of parkin, the enduringly ER retention and proteasomal degradation of mutant β-glucosidase, mediated by parkin, affect its activity toward its natural substrates. Accumulation during the years of these proteins can lead to the death of cells in substantia nigra and eventually, to the development of PD.

The theories described above, cannot explain completely the correlation between the diseases. In the "offensive metabolite theory" the reducing of the released ceramide inhibits the autophagic-lysosomal functions. This can explain the development of LB and parkinsonism in Gaucher patients, but not in GBA mutations carriers.

Moreover in Gaucher patients where mutations in GBA result in no protein product (i.e. c.84dupG and IVS2+1G>A) the risk to develop PD is high. So the "misfolded protein theory" also cannot clear fully the question, even if it is probably that very truncated forms of the mutant protein still might induce endoplasmic reticulum stress and guide to crashing of UPS.

4. Genetic studies and neuropathological data

The first indication of a relationship between parkinsonism and GD was due to sporadic case reports in the literarture (Neudorfer et al., 1996; Machaczka et al., 1999; Tayebi et al., 2001). In these papers it was highlighted how in some GD patients the enzyme deficiency itself could predisposed to the susceptibility to parkinsonisms.

These observations of occurrence of Parkinson's disease in some patients with non-neuropathic type 1 Gaucher disease and in their first degree relatives has led to the identification of GBA1 heterozigous mutations as a genetic risk factor for idiopathic Parkinson's disease.

In these subjects the mean age at onset of parkinsonian symptoms is lower than in patients without GD1, becoming evident at an average age of 48 years compared with 71 years in the general population (Elbaz et al., 2003).

These early observations led to several studies which revealed that patients with idiopathic PD had a higher probability of harboring GBA1 mutations compared to the general population.

The first large study was conducted by Lwin et al. (2004), using sequence analyses on brain samples from 57 subjects of different nationality, GBA alterations were detected in 12 sample (21%).

Subsequently Aharon-Peretz et al. (2004), explored the association between six GBA mutations (N370S, L444P, c.84dupG, IVS+1A>G, R496H, V394L) and PD in Ashkenazi Jews population. From the screening of 99 patients and 1,543 healty people they identified these mutations in 31.3% of patients with PD versus 6.2% of healty controls.
Many studies have been conducted in the years, some of these have been screened PD patients for common GBA mutations (Clarck et al., 2005; Sato et al., 2005; Tan et al., 2007; Wu et al., 2007; De Marco et al., 2008; Spitz et al., 2008; Mata et al., 2008; Gan-Or et al., 2008), others have been sequenced the entire GBA gene (Eblan et al., 2006; Ziegler et al., 2007; Clark et al., 2007; Bras & Singleton, 2009; Kalinderi et al., 2009; Neumann et al., 2009).
All of these studies evidenced a higher frequency of GBA mutations among PD patients than in matched controls, but the frequency of GBA mutations varies in relation with the study's design (popolation, number and type of mutations screened or whole GBA scanning).
Toft et al. (2006) searched the association between two mutations (N370S and L444P) and PD in Norwegian population. From the analyses of 311 patients and 474 controls they found these mutations in 2.3% of subjects with PD versus 1.7% of controls.
The frequency of GBA mutations ranges between 10.7% and 31.3% in PD patients from Ashkenazi Jewish and between 2.3% and 9.4% in patients from other populations.
Most of these studies were conducted on sporadic PD patients, recently Nichols et al. (2009) and Mitsui et al. (2009) specifically investigated familial PD. They demonstrated an association between GBA variants and familial PD cases as well as sporadic disease.
Most of these studies have independently reached similar results demonstrating that GBA mutations are found in patients with PD at a higher frequency than expected.
A large meta-analysis was conducted by Sidransky et al. (2009) pooling genotypic data from 16 different centers across the world. A total of 5,691 genotyped patients with Parkinson disease and 4,898 controls were evaluated; full sequencing was performed on 1859 patient and 1674 control samples. Overall, the odds ratio for carryng a GBA mutation in subjects with PD was 5.43 (95% CI 3.89-7.57), selecting mutations in GBA gene as a common risk factor for PD.
Investigators extended their studies to analyses whether GBA mutations are related with other Lewy bodies disorders. Goker-Alpan et al. (2006), analyzing the coding region of GBA gene in 75 brain's sample of autopsy cases with pathologically confirmed Lewy body disorders, found GBA mutations in 23% of LBD patients, 4% of PD patients and none within Multiple System Atrophy patients (MSA).
Afterward Mata et al. (2008), Farrer et al. (2009) and Clark et al. (2009) showed a correlation between GBA mutations and LBD, while was found no significant difference in GBA mutations incidence between MSA patients and controls (Segarane et al., 2009).
Considering the spectrum of PD clinical manifestations in GD1 patients, a wide range of symptoms have been described, varying from the more aggressive, early-onset disease, with poor response to L-dopa therapy, to the more typical PD disease (presenting with asymmetric onset of resting tremor, bradykinesia, rigidity, gait and balance disturbance, weakness, pain, cognitive decline, and depression), responsive to L-dopa (Neudorfer et al., 1996; Tayebi et al, 2003; Bembi et al., 2003; Tayebi et al, 2001; Halperin et al. 2006; Gan-Or et al., 2008; Bultron et al., 2010; Chérin et al., 2010;). The emerging evidence of the association between GBA mutations and a variety of synucleinopathyes may account for the wide phenotype variability (Hruska at al., 2006; Velayati et al, 2010). Even if different studies described early-onset (< 50 years) as an element that characterizes this association, this observation might be influenced by the small number of patients involved in each study.

Trying to find an answer to this issue, Gan-Or et al. (2008) performed a study analysing a large cohort of 420 unrelated Jewish Ashkenazi PD patients, which evidenced a strong correlation between GD1 and early-onset of PD symptoms (average age at onset of 51.2 years, versus 60.7 years of the noncarriers PD population), while GBA carriers showed an average age of 57.2 years at PD onset.

They also analysed the different effects of mutation severity, observing a higher risk for PD in patients carrying severe GBA mutations as well as a decreased age of symptoms onset. Finally, when they analysed clinical PD manifestations among GBA carriers and non-carriers, they observed a reduced presence of rigidity (16.90% vs 28.57%) and an increase of weakness (16.90% vs 7.14%) in GBA carriers.

Another recent large observational study of 444 consecutive GD1 patients (Bultron et al., 2010), aiming to analyse the risk of PD occurrence, showed 11 patients (2.47%) who developed the disease at a mean age of 55.0 ± 8.8 years (range 40-65 years). Analysing GD overall severe score index (SSI) and bone disease score (Hermann score) in the overall population, they found both of them significantly higher in PD patients (SSI: 10.8±0.8 vs 6.9±3.7, p=0.02; Herman score: 4.6±0.5 vs 2.5±1.5, p=0.002).

Moreover, these authors estimated age and gender-adjusted risk to develop PD in three different groups of GD1 patients, finding that the range of risk was increased 11.0 to 31.3 fold in male patients and 5.7 to 13.8 fold in female patients, with an overall relative risk to develop PD in GD1 patients of 21.4 (95% CI, 10.7-38.3).

As regard the clinical response to ERT in GD1 patients with PD, all published experiences demonstrated its effectiveness on hematological and systemic involvement, while they were ineffective in correcting PD symptoms (Neudorfer et al., 1996; Tayebi et al, 2003; Bembi et al., 2003; Tayebi et al, 2001; Itokawa et al., 2006; Bultron et al., 2010). The new era of substrate reducing and chaperone therapies with small molecules that are able to cross the blood-brain barrier may open new perspectives in the treatment of central nervous system involvement in GD, including PD symptoms. A recent report of Hughes et al. (2007) that showed an improvement in the clinical conditions of a PD patient during SRT with Miglustat, introduces a new possible therapeutic approach.

5. Expression of GBA and other lysosomal enzyme in animal models of Parkinson's disease

The majority of sporadic PD cases result from interaction between genes and environment but the age remains the greatest risk factor. The first evidence of a genetic involvement in PD manifestations was the identification of three missense mutations on the α-synuclein gene, SNCA. These mutations (A30P, E46K, A53T) segregate with the disease in unrelated families and caused PD with high penetrance (Polymeropoulos et al., 1997; Kruger et al., 1998; Zarranz et al., 2004). Afterward duplication and triplication of the SNCA gene has been shown to cause PD, suggesting that high level expression of α-synuclein may also be pathogenic (Singleton et al., 2003; Ibanez et al., 2004). The degree of overexpression was found to correlate with the degree of severity of the pathology. The effects of point mutation and duplication-triplication of SNCA gene have been investigated using transgenic technology and viral infection and different mouse models were created. All PD animal models are based on the concept that parkinsonian signs are linked to dopaminergic nigral cell loss and even if they show many of the symptoms of the disease they don't display all the complexity of the neurological pathology. A lot of mouse line expressing wild-type or

mutant α-synuclein (Masliah et al., 2000; Lee et al., 2002; Richfield et al., 2002) was found to lead to the develp of granular deposits, but none of these results in the involvment of dopaminergic nerve cellsof the substantia nigra. Previous data demonstrated that truncated α-synuclein (1-120) was aboundantly presents in Lewy bodies extracts (Tofaris et al., 2003).
There are two different animal models of Parkinson's disease: the first one is a mouse model that express a truncated human α-synuclein (1-120) under the rat tyrosine hydroxylase promoter on a mouse α-synuclein null background (Tofaris et al., 2006). In this mouse model (TG Syn 120) were found pathological inclusions in substantia nigra and olfactory bulb, a reduction in dopamine levels in the striatum and in spontaneous locomotion and a better response to amphetamine. C-terminally truncated α-synuclein aggregates more quickly than full-lenght protein and has been found in Lewy bodies in human patients. The second one is a rat model (6OH-DA) with the lesion of the ascending nigrostriatal dopamine pathway due to 6-hydroxydopamine injection in the unilateral substantia nigra (Rozas et al., 1997; Picconi et al., 2003). These rats displayed some feautures of parkinsonian pathology. This rat model has been initially used to understand the behavioral functions of the basal ganglia, and to evaluate the brain's ability to compensate for specific neurochemical depletions. Now this model is use has strument to understand the mechanisms of PD pathology and as an experimental basis to develop new antiparkinsonian drugs and treatment strategies, or surgical approaches (Rozas et al., 1997). To deepen the involvement of lysosomal enzyme in Parkinson's disease, a comparative analysis of the activity of β-glucocerebrosidase (EC 3.2.1.45), α-mannosidase (EC 3.2.1.24), β-mannosidase (EC 3.2.1.25), β-hexosaminidase (EC 3.2.1.52) and β-galactosidase (EC 3.2.1.23) have been performed in different brain sections of the two animal's model.
In particular lysosomal enzymatic activities were determined in cerebellum, cortex and brain-stem. The obtained results show a different expression in these sections of central nervous system of TG Syn 120 mouse model compared to control mice, with a decreased activity of all the enzymes in brain-stem, and an increased activity in the cerebellum. In the cortex all the enzymatic activities remain invariated.

		Beta-hexosaminidase	Alpha-mannosidase	Beta-mannosidase	Beta-galactosidase	Beta-glucosidase
brain-stem	Wistar	20.37±4.33	0.45±0.17	0.32±0.08	3.70±1.22	0.15±0.1
	6OH-DA	17.61±5.75	0.31±0.1	0.23±0.1	2.82±0.91	0.15±0.08
cerebellum	Wistar	16.43±3.42	0.51±0.23	0.36±0.13	3.88±0.83	0.1±0.04
	6OH-DA	11.27*±2.5	0.25*±0.05	0.22*±0.05	2.64*±0.81	0.08±0.02
cortico-striatal	Wistar	18.81±3.64	0.3±0.05	0.39±0.29	1.30±0.83	0.1±0.04
	6OH-DA	12.85*±0.92	0.167*±0.03	0.11*±0.03	0.48±0.38	0.05*±0.022

Table 2. Lysosomal enzyme specific activities (μmol min^{-1}/mg total protein x 1000) in, cerebellum, cortico-striatal and brain-stem of control and 6OH-DA rats. Mean ± SD are given. *$p<0.05$ versus control.

A more pronunced differences in lysosomal enzyme expressions were observed in 6OH-DA rats (table 2). A clear reduction of enzyme activities were found in brain-stem, cerebellum and cortico-striatal. The chemical model show a profound involvement of the brain's areas and this is, probably, a consequence of the 6-hydroxydopamine treatment, infact the neurotoxins destroied selectively and rapidly catecholaminergic neurons whereas the PD pathogenensis in human and in the mouse model follows a progressive course over decades. The results obtained in this rat model might explain the reduction on alpha-mannosidase, beta-glucosidase, and beta-mannosidse activities observed in the CSF od PD patients (Balducci et al., 2007).

6. CSF lysosomal enzyme activities as possible marker of synucleinopathies

Recently it became evident that accumulation of unwanted and misfolded protein play a central role in the PD pathogenesis. An involvement of the lysosomal system has been postulated. Lysosomal activity decreased over the lifespan and a lysosomal malfunction has been linked with cronic neurodegenerative disorders (Terman, 2006; Pan et al., 2008). This assumption has been confirmed by the selective inhibition of lysosomal enzyme in different cellular models that leads to protein aggregation, synaptic loss and neuronal death (Felbor et al., 2002; Bendiske & Bahr, 2003). Furthermore, in experimental system, has been noted that α-synuclein aggregation leads to inhibition of lysosomal functions, triggering a vicious cycle (Bennett et al., 2005; Cuervo et al., 2004). On the basis of these evidences was performed a comparative analysis of the activity of β–glucocerebrosidase (EC 3.2.1.45), α-mannosidase (EC 3.2.1.24), β-mannosidase (EC 3.2.1.25), β-hexosaminidase (EC 3.2.1.52) and β-galactosidase (EC 3.2.1.23) in cerebrospinal fluid (CSF) of Parkinson's disease (PD) subjects and age matched controls first (Balducci et al., 2007), and then in Dementia with Lewy bodies (DLB), Alzheimer's disease (AD) and Frontotemporal Dementia (FTD) patients as well as in age matched controls (Parnetti et al., 2009). The framekork is different in the different neurodegenerative diseases, in PD patients a reduced activity of β-glucocerebrosidase, β-mannosidase and α-mannosidase was found, whereas β-galactosidase and β-hexosaminidase remain unchanged. In DLB patients, all the enzymes tested showed a decrease activity with β–glucocerebrosidase with the lower value. In FTD patients, only α-mannosidase activity was lower than controls, while the other enzymes showed unchanged acticities. α-mannosidase and β-hexosaminidase are the only two enzyme that showed reduced activity in AD patients.

The data suggest a significant involvement of the ensosomal-lysosomal system in the neurodegenerative diseases examined. Moreover, the different pattern of lysosomal activity can reflect the diverse implication of the lysosomal apparatous in the distinct neurodegenerative pathologies. It has also been hypotized that ameliorate the activity of the lysosomal system can be a possible therapeutic strategy for these disorders characterized by misfolding and aggregation of wild-type or mutant protein in the cytoplas of neuronal cells (Lee et al., 2004).

7. Conclusion

Clinical and genetic studies suggest that mutations in the glucocerebrosidase gene are an important risk factor for the development of parkinsonism and related didorders. While Gaucher disease is an autosomal inherited disorder, patients with parkinson's disease can be Gaucher heterozygotes or homozygotes. The involvment of the lysosomal system in parkinson's disease has also been further demonstated by the different expression of lysosomal enzymes, such as β-glucosidase, α-mannosidase, β-mannosidase, and β-galactosidase in CSF and in the brain of animal models. The elucidation of the molecular basis of this association may contribute to understand the development of parkinsonism. Anyway it is still unclear which is the common cellular pathway that links Gaucher and Parkinson diseases.

8. References

Aerts, J.M. & Hollak, C.E. (1997). Plasma and metabolic abnormalities in Gaucher's disease. *Bailliere's Clinical Haematology,* Vol.10, No.4, (Dec), pp. 691-709, ISSN 0950-3536

Aharon-Peretz, J., Rosenbaum, H. & Gershoni-Baruch, R. (2004). Mutations in the glucocerebrosidase gene and Parkinson's disease in Ashkenazi Jews. *The New England Journal of Medcine,* Vol.351, No.19 (Nov), pp. 1972-7, ISSN 0028-4793

Ahlberg, J., Marzella, L. & Glaumann, H. (1982). Uptake and degradation of proteins by isolated rat liver lysosomes. Suggestion of a microautophagic pathway of proteolysis. *Laboratory Investigation,* Vol.47, No.6, (Dec), pp. 523-32, ISSN 0023-6837

Allen, M.J., Myer, B.J., Khokher, A.M., Rushton, N. & Cox, T.M. (1997). Pro-inflammatory cytokines and the pathogenesis of Gaucher's disease: increased release of interleukin-6 and interleukin-10. *QJM: monthly journal of the Association of Physicians,* Vol.90, No.1, (Jan), pp. 19-25, ISSN 1460-2725

Altered dynamics of the lysosomal receptor for chaperone-mediated autophagy with age. *Journal of Cell Science,* Vol.120, No.5, (Mar), pp. 782-91, ISSN 0021-9533

Bagshaw, R.D., Mahuran, D.J. & Callahan, J.W. (2005). Lysosomal membrane proteomics and biogenesis of lysosomes. *Molecular Neurobiology,* Vol. 32, No. 1, (Aug), pp. 27-41, ISSN:0893-7648

Balducci, C., Pierguidi, L., Persichetti, E., Parnetti, L., Sbaragli, M., Tassi, C., Orlacchio, A., Calabresi, P., Beccari, T. & Rossi, A. (2007). Lysosomal hydrolases in cerebrospinal fluid from subjects with Parkinson's disease. *Movement Disorder,* Vol.22, No.10, (Jul), pp. 1481-84, ISSN 0885-3185

Barneveld, R.A., Keijzer, W., Tegelaers, F.P., Ginns, E.I., Geurts van Kessel, A., Brady, R.O., Barranger, J.A., Tager, J.M., Galjaard, H., Westerveld, A. & Reuser, A.J. (1983). Assignment of the gene coding for human beta-glucocerebrosidase to the region q21-q31 of chromosome 1 using monoclonal antibodies. *Human Genetics,* Vol.64, No.3, pp. 227-31, ISSN 0340-6717

Bellettato, C.M. & Scarpa, M. (2010). Pathophysiology of neuropathic lysosomal storage disorders. *Journal of Inherited and Metabolic Disorders,* Vol.33, No.4, (Aug), pp. 347-62, ISSN 0141-8955

Bembi, B., Zambito Marsala, S., Sidransky, E., Ciana, G., Carrozzi, M., Zorzon, M., Martini, C., Gioulis, M., Pittis, M.G. & Capus, L. (2003). Gaucher's disease with Parkinson's disease: clinical and pathological aspects. *Neurology,* Vol.61, No.1, (Jul), pp. 99-101, ISSN 0028-3878

Bendiske, J. & Bahr, B.A. (2003). Lysosomal activation is a compensatory response against protein accumulation and associated synaptopathogenesis--an approach for slowing Alzheimer disease? *Journal of Neuropathology and Experimental Neurology*, Vol.62, No.5, (May), pp. 451-463, ISSN 0022-3069

Bennett, E.J., Bence, N.F., Jayakumar, R. & Kopito, R.R. (2005). Global impairment of the ubiquitin-proteasome system by nuclear or cytoplasmic protein aggregates precedes inclusion body formation. *Molecular Cell*, Vol.17, No.3, (Feb), pp. 351-365, ISSN 1097-2765

Berrebi, A., Wishnitzer, R. & Von-der-Walde, U. (1984). Gaucher's disease: unexpected diagnosis in three patients over seventy years old. *Nouvelle Revue Francaise d'Hematologie*, Vol.26, No.3, pp. 201-3, ISSN 0029-4810

Beutler, E., Nguyen, N.J., Henneberger, M.W., Smolec, J.M., McPherson, R.A., West, C. & Gelbart, T. (1993). Gaucher disease: gene frequencies in the Ashkenazi Jewish population. *The American Journal of Human Genetics*, Vol.52, No.1, (Jan), pp. 85-8, ISSN 0002-9297

Beutler, E. & Gelbart, T. (1996). Glucocerebrosidase (Gaucher disease). *Human Mutation*, Vol.8, No.3, pp. 207-13, ISSN 1059-7794.

Beutler, E. & Grabowski, G.A. (2001). Gaucher disease. *The Metabolic and Molecular Basis of Inherited Disease Vol. III, 8th* ed. Scriver CR., Beaudet AL., Sly WS., Valle D., editors, 3635–68, NY, McGraw-Hill, New York

Beutler, E. (2006). Gaucher disease: multiple lessons from a single gene disorder. *Acta Paediatrica Supplement*, Vol.95, No.451, (Apr), pp. 103-9, ISSN 0803-5326

Biegstraaten, M., van Schaik, I.N., Aerts, J.M. & Hollak, C.E. (2008). 'Non-neuronopathic' Gaucher disease reconsidered. Prevalence of neurological manifestations in a Dutch cohort of type I Gaucher disease patients and a systematic review of the literature. *Journal of Inherited Metabolic Disease*, Vol.31, No.3, (Jun), pp. 337-49, ISSN 0141-8955

Boland, B. & Nixon, R.A. (2006). Neuronal macroautophagy: from development to degeneration. *Molecular Aspects of Medicine*, Vol.27, No.5-6, (Oct-Dec), pp. 503-19, ISSN 0098-2997.

Brady, R.O., Kanfer, J.N. & Shapiro, D. (1965). Metabolism of glucocerebrosides. II. Evidence of an Enzymatic deficiency in Gaucher's disease. *Biochemical and Biophysical Research Communication*, Vol.18, pp. 221-5, ISSN 0006-291X

Brady, R.O., Barton, N.W. & Grabowski, G.A. (1993). The role of neurogenetics in Gaucher disease. *Archives of Neurology*, Vol.50, No.11, (Nov), pp. 1212-24, ISSN 003-9942

Bras, J.M. & Singleton, A. (2009). Genetic susceptibility in Parkinson's disease. *Biochimica et biophysica acta*, Vol. 1792, No. 7, (Jul), pp. 597-603, ISSN 0006-3002

Bultron, G., Kacena,K., Pearson, D., Boxer, M., Yang, R., Sathe, S., Pastores, G. & Mistry, P.K. (2010). The risk of Parkinson's disease in type 1 Gaucher disease. *Journal of Inherited Metabolic Disease*, Vol. 33, No. 2 (Apr), pp. 167-73, ISSN 0141-8955

Charrow, J., Andersson, H.C., Kaplan, P., Kolodny, E.H., Mistry, P., Pastores, G., Rosenbloom, B.E., Scott, C.R., Wappner, R.S., Weinreb, N.J. & Zimran, A. (2000). The Gaucher registry: demographics and disease characteristics of 1698 patients with Gaucher disease. *Archives of Internal Medicine*, Vol.160, No.18, (Oct), pp. 2835-43, ISSN 0003-9926

Chérin, P., Sedel, F., Mignot, C., Schupbach, M., Gourfinkel-An, I., Verny, M. & Baumann, N. (2006). Neurological manifestations of type 1 Gaucher's disease: Is a revision of disease classification needed?. *Revue Neurologique*, Vol.162, No.11, (Nov), pp. 1076-83, ISSN 0035-3787

Chérin, P., Rose, C., de Roux-Serratrice, C., Tardy, D., Dobbelaere, D., Grosbois, B., Hachulla, E., Jaussaud, R., Javier, R.M., Noël, E., Clerson, P. & Hartmann, A. (2010). The neurological manifestations of Gaucher disease type 1: the French Observatoire on Gaucher disease (FROG). *Journal of Inherited Metabolic Disease*, Vol. 33, No. 4, (Aug), pp. 331-8, , ISSN 0141-8955

Chiang, H.L., Terlecky, S.R., Plant, C.P. & Dice, J.F. (1989). A role for a 70-kilodalton heat shock protein in lysosomal degradation of intracellular proteins. *Science*. Vol.246, No.4928, (Nov), pp. 382-5, ISSN 0036-8075

Ciechanover, A., Orian, A. & Schwartz, A.L. (2000). Ubiquitin-mediated proteolysis: biological regulation via destruction. *Bioessays*, Vol.22, No.5, (May), pp. 442-51, ISSN 0265-9247

Ciechanover, A. & Brundin, P. (2003). The ubiquitin proteasome system in neurodegenerative diseases: sometimes the chicken, sometimes the egg. *Neuron*, Vol.40, No.2, (Oct), pp. 427-46, ISSN 0896-6273

Clark, L.N., Nicolai, A., Afridi, S., Harris, J., Mejia-Santana, H., Strug, L., Cote, L.J., Louis, E.D., Andrews, H., Waters, C., Ford, B., Frucht, S., Fahn, S., Mayeux, R., Ottman, R. & Marder, K. (2005). Pilot association study of the beta-glucocerebrosidase N370S allele and Parkinson's disease in subjects of Jewish ethnicity. *Movement Disorders*, Vol.20, No.1, (Jan), pp. 100-3, ISSN 0885-3185

Clark, L.N., Ross, B.M., Wang, Y., Mejia-Santana, H., Harris, J., Louis, E.D., Cote, L.J., Andrews, H., Fahn, S., Waters, C., Ford, B., Frucht S., Ottman, R. & Marder, K. (2007). Mutations in the glucocerebrosidase gene are associated with early-onset Parkinson disease. *Neurology*, Vol.18, No.12, (Sep), pp. 1270-1277, ISSN:0028-3878

Clark, L.N., Kartsaklis, L.A., Wolf Gilbert, R., Dorado, B., Ross, B.M., Kisselev, S., Verbitsky, M., Mejia-Santana, H., Cote, L.J., Andrews, H., Vonsattel, J.P., Fahn, S., Mayeux, R., Honig, L.S. & Marder, K. (2009). Association of glucocerebrosidase mutations with dementia with lewy bodies. *Archives of Neurology*, Vol.66, No.5, (May), pp.578-583, ISSN 0003-9942

Cox, T.M. & Schofield, J.P. (1997). Gaucher's disease: clinical features and natural history. *Bailliere's Clinical Haematology*, Vol.10, No.4, (Dec), pp. 657-89, ISSN 0950-3536

Cox, T.M. (2001). Gaucher disease: understanding the molecular pathogenesis of sphingolipidoses. *Journal of Inherited Metabolic Disease*, Vol.24, Suppl.2, pp. 106-21, discussion 87-8, ISSN 0141-8955

Cuervo, A.M. & Dice, J.F.(1996). A receptor for the selective uptake and degradation of proteins by lysosomes. *Science*, Vol.273, No.5274, (Jul), pp. 501-3, ISSN 0036-8075

Cuervo, A.M. & Dice, J.F. (1998). Lysosomes, a meeting point of proteins, chaperones, and proteases. *Journal of Molecular Medicine*, Vol.76, No.1, (Jan), pp. 6-12, ISSN 0377-046X

Cuervo, A.M., Hildebrand, H., Bomhard, E.M. & Dice, J.F. (1999). Direct lysosomal uptake of alpha 2-microglobulin contributes to chemically induced nephropathy. *Kidney International*, Vol.55, No.2, (Feb), pp. 529-45, ISSN 0085-2538

Cuervo, A.M. (2004). Autophagy: many paths to the same end. *Molecular and Cellular Biochemistry*, Vol.263, No.1-2, (Aug), pp. 55-72, ISSN 0300-8177

Cuervo, A.M., Stefanis, L., Fredenburg, R., Lansbury, P.T. & Sulzer, D. (2004). Impaired degradation of mutant alpha-synuclein by chaperone-mediated autophagy. *Science,* Vol.305, No.5688, (Aug), pp. 1292-5, ISSN 0036-8075.

Dawson, T.M. (2006). Parkin and defective ubiquitination in Parkinson's disease. *Journal of Neural Transmission Supplement,* No.70, pp. 209-13, ISSN 0303-6995

De Duve, C., Pressman, B.C., Gianetto, R., Wattiaux, R. & Appelmans, F. (1955). Tissue fractionation studies. 6. Intracellular distribution patterns of enzymes in rat-liver tissue. *The Biochemical Journal,* Vol.60, No.4, (Aug), pp. 604-617, ISSN 0264-6021

De Marco, E.V., Annesi, G., Tarantino, P., Rocca, F.E., Provenzano, G., Civitelli, D., Cirò Candiano, I.C., Annesi, F., Carrideo, S., Condino, F., Nicoletti, G., Messina, D., Novellino, F., Morelli, M. & Quattrone, A. (2008). Glucocerebrosidase gene mutations are associated with Parkinson's disease in southern Italy. *Movement disorders* , Vol.23, No.3, (Feb), pp. 46046-3, ISSN 0885-3185

Dice, J.F. (1990). Peptide sequences that target cytosolic proteins for lysosomal proteolysis. *Trends in Biochemical Science,* Vol.15, No.8, (Aug), pp. 305-9, ISSN 0968-0004

Eblan, M.J., Nguyen, J., Ziegler, S.G., Lwin, A., Hanson, M., Gallardo, M., Weiser, R., De Lucca, M., Singleton, A. & Sidransky, E. (2006). Glucocerebrosidase mutations are also found in subjects with early-onset parkinsonism from Venezuela. *Movement Disorder,* Vol.21, No.2, (Feb), pp. 282-3, ISSN 0885-3185

Elbaz, A., Bower, J.H., Peterson, B.J., Maraganore, D.M., McDonnell, S.K., Ahlskog, J.E., Schaid, D.J. & Rocca, W.A. (2003). Survival study of Parkinson disease in Olmsted County, Minnesota. *Archives of Neurology,* Vol.60, No.1, (Jan), pp. 91-6, ISSN 0003-9942

Erikson, A. (1986). Gaucher disease-Norrbottnian type (III). Neuropaediatric and neurobiological aspects of clinical patterns and treatment. *Acta Paediatric Scandinavica Supplement,* Vol.326, pp. 1-42, ISSN 0300-8843

Farré, J.C. & Subramani, S. (2004). Peroxisome turnover by micropexophagy: an autophagy-related process. *Trends in Cell Biology,* Vol.14, No.9, (Sep), pp. 515-23, ISSN 0962-8924

Farrer,M.J., Williams, L.N., Algom, A.A., Kachergus, J., Hulihan, M.M., Ross, O.A., Rajput, A., Papapetropoulos, S., Mash, D.C. & Dickson, D.W. (2009). Glucosidase-beta variations and Lewy body disorders. *Parkinsonism & related disorders,* Vol.15, No.6, (Jul), pp. 414-6, ISSN 1353-8020

Felbor, U., Kessler, B., Mothes, W., Goebel, H.H., Ploegh, H.L., Bronson, R.T. & Olsen, B.R. (2002). Neuronal loss and brain atrophy in mice lacking cathepsins B and L. *Proceedings of the National Academy of Sciences (USA),* Vol.99, No.12, (Jun), pp. 7883-8, ISSN 0027-8424

Finkbeiner, S., Cuervo, A.M., Morimoto, R.I. & Muchowski, P.J. (2006). Disease-modifying pathways in neurodegeneration. *J Neuroscience,* Vol.26, No.41, (Oct), pp. 10349-57, ISSN 0270-6474

Fletcher, J.M. (2006). Screening for lysosomal storage disorders--a clinical perspective.*Journal of inherited metabolic disease,* Vol.29, No.2-3 (Apr-Jun), pp. 405-8, ISSN 0141-8955

Futerman, A.H. & van Meer, G. (2004). The cell biology of lysosomal storage disorders. *Nature Reviews: Molecular and Cell Biology,* Vol.5, No.7, (Jul), pp. 554-65, ISSN 1471-0072

Gan-Or, Z., Giladi, N., Rozovski, U., Shifrin, C., Rosner, S., Gurevich, T., Bar-Shira, A. & Orr-Urtreger, A. (2008). Genotype-phenotype correlations between GBA mutations and Parkinson disease risk and onset. *Neurology*, Vol.70, No.24, (Jun), pp. 2277-83, ISSN 0028-3878

Gaucher disease and parkinsonism: a phenotypic and genotypic characterization. *Molecular Genetics and Metabolism*, Vol.73, No.4, (Aug), pp. 313-21, ISSN 1096-7192

Germain, D.P. (2004). Gaucher's disease: a paradigm for interventional genetics. *Clinical Genetics*, Vol.65, No.2, (Feb), pp. 77-86, ISSN 0009-9163

Goker-Alpan O., Schiffmann R., Park J.K., Stubblefield B.K., Tayebi N. & Sidransky E. (2003). Phenotypic continuum in neuronopathic Gaucher disease: an intermediate phenotype between type 2 and type 3. *Journal of Pediatrics*, Vol.143, No.2, (Aug), pp. 273-6, ISSN 0022-3476

Goker-Alpan, O., Giasson, B.I., Eblan, M.J., Nguyen, J., Hurtig, H.I., Lee, V.M., Trojanowski, J.Q. & Sidransky, E. (2006). Glucocerebrosidase mutations are an important risk factor for Lewy body disorders. *Neurology*, Vol.67, No.5, (Sep), pp. 908-10, ISSN 0028-3878

Goker-Alpan, O., Lopez, G., Vithayathil, J., Davis, J., Hallett, M. & Sidransky, E. (2008). The spectrum of parkinsonian manifestations associated with glucocerebrosidase mutations. *Archives of Neurology*, Vol. 65, No. 10, (Oct), pp: 1353-7, ISSN 0003-9942

Grabowski, G.A. & Horowitz, M. (1997). Gaucher's disease: molecular, genetic and enzymological aspects. *Bailliere's Clinical Haematology*, Vol.10, No.4, (Dec), pp. 635-56, 0950-3536

Halperin, A., Elstein, D. & Zimran, A. (2006). Increased incidence of Parkinson disease among relatives of patients with Gaucher disease. *Blood Cells, Molecules & Diseases*, Vol. 36, No. 3, (May-Jun), pp. 426-8, ISSN: 1079-9796

Heinrich, M., Wickel, M., Schneider-Brachert, W., Sandberg, C., Gahr, J., Schwandne,r R., Weber, T., Saftig, P., Peters, C., Brunner, J., Krönke, M. & Schütze, S.(1999). Cathepsin D targeted by acid sphingomyelinase-derived ceramide. *EMBO Journal*, Vol.18, No.19, (Oct), pp. 5252-63, ISSN 0261-4189

Horowitz, M., Wilder, S., Horowitz, Z., Reiner, O., Gelbart, T. & Beutler, E. (1989). The human glucocerebrosidase gene and pseudogene: structure and evolution. *Genomics.*, Vol.4, No.1, (Jan), pp. 87-96, ISSN 0888-7543

Hruska, K.S., Goker-Alpan, O. & Sidransky, E. (2006). Gaucher disease and the synucleinopathies. *Journal of biomedicine & biotechnology*, Vol. 3, 78549, ISSN:1110-7243

Hruska, K.S., LaMarca, M.E., Scott, C.R. & Sidransky, E. (2008). Gaucher disease: mutation and polymorphism spectrum in the glucocerebrosidase gene (GBA). *Human Mutation*, Vol.29, No.5, (May), pp. 567-83, ISSN 1059-7794

Hughes, D.A., Ginsberg, L., Bake,r R., Goodwin, S., Milligan, A., Richfield, L. & Mehta, A.B. (2007). Effective treatment of an elderly patient with Gaucher's disease and Parkinsonism: a case report of 24 months' oral substrate reduction therapy with miglustat. *Parkinsonism & related disorders*, Vol. 13, No.6, (Aug), pp. 365-8. ISSN: 1353-8020

Ibáñez, P., Bonnet, A.M., Débarges, B., Lohmann, E., Tison, F., Pollak, P., Agid, Y., Dürr, A. & Brice, A. (2004). Causal relation between alpha-synuclein gene duplication and familial Parkinson's disease. *Lancet*, Vol.364, No.9440, (Sep), pp. 1169-71, ISSN 0140-6736

Itokawa, K., Tamura, N., Kawai, N., Shimazu, K. & Ishii, K. (2006). Parkinsonism in type I Gaucher's disease. *Internal Medicine*, Vol. 45, No.20, pp. 1165-7, ISSN: 0918-2918

Jadot, M., Dubois, F., Wattiaux-De Coninck, S. & Wattiaux, R. (1997). Supramolecular assemblies from lysosomal matrix proteins and complex lipids. *European Journal of Biochemistry*, Vol.249, No.3, (Nov), pp. 862-9, ISSN 0014-2956.

Jmoudiak, M. & Futerman, A.H. (2005). Gaucher disease: pathological mechanisms and modern management. *British Journal of Haematology*, Vol.129, No.2, (Apr), pp. 178-88, ISSN 0007-1048

Journet, A., Chapel, A., Kieffer, S., Roux, F. & Garin, J. (2002). Proteomic analysis of human lysosomes: application to monocytic and breast cancer cells. *Proteomics*, Vol. 2, Np. 8, (Aug), pp. 1026-40, ISSN:1615-9853

Kalinderi, K., Bostantjopoulou, S., Paisan-Ruiz, C., Katsarou, Z., Hardy, J. & Fidani, L. (2009). Complete screening for glucocerebrosidase mutations in Parkinson disease patients from Greece. *Neurosci Letters*, Vol.452, No.2, (Mar), pp. 87-9, ISSN 0304-3940

Kerscher, O., Felberbaum, R. & Hochstrasser, M. (2006). Modification of proteins by ubiquitin and ubiquitin-like proteins. *Annual Review of Cell and Developmental Biology*, Vol.22, pp. 159-80, ISSN 1081-0706.

Kiffin, R., Christian, C., Knecht, E. & Cuervo, A.M. (2004). Activation of chaperone-mediated autophagy during oxidative stress. *Molecular Biology of the Cell*, Vol.15, No.11, (Nov), pp. 4829-40, ISSN 1059-1524

Kim, Y.J., Sapp, E., Cuiffo, B.G., Sobin, L., Yoder, J., Kegel, K.B., Qin, Z.H., Detloff, P., Aronin, N. & Di Figlia, M. (2006). Lysosomal proteases are involved in generation of N-terminal huntingtin fragments. *Neurobiology of Disease*, Vol.22, No.2, (May), pp. 346-56, ISSN 0969-9961

Klionsky, D.J. & Emr,S.D. (2000). Autophagy as a regulated pathway of cellular degradation. *Science*, Vol.290, No.5497, (Dec), pp. 1717-21, ISSN 0036-8075

Klionsky, D.J., Cregg, J.M., Dunn, W.A. Jr, Emr, S.D., Sakai,Y., Sandoval, I.V., Sibirny, A., Subramani, S., Thumm, M., Veenhuis, M. & Ohsumi, Y. (2003). A unified nomenclature for yeast autophagy-related genes. *Developmental Cell*, Vol.5, No.4, (Oct), pp. 539-45, ISSN 1534-5807

Klionsky, D.J. (2005). Autophagy. *Current Biology*, Vol.15, No.8, (Apr), pp. 282-3, ISSN 0960-9822.

Kohan, R., Cismondi, I.A., Oller-Ramirez, A.M., Guelbert, N., Anzolini, T.V., Alonso, G., Mole, S.E., de Kremer, D.R & de Halac, N.I. (2011). Therapeutic Approaches to the Challenge of Neuronal Ceroid Lipofuscinoses. *Current Pharmaceutical Biotechnology*, (Jan) [Epub ahead of print] ISSN 1389-2010

Kolter, T. & Sandhoff, K. (2006). Sphingolipid metabolism diseases. *Biochimica et Biophysica Acta*, Vol.1758, No.12, (Dec), pp. 2057-79, ISSN 0006-3002

Kopito, R.R. (2000). Aggresomes, inclusion bodies and protein aggregation. *Trends Cell Biology*, Vol.10, No.12, (Dec), pp. 524-30, ISSN 0962-8924

Kourie, J.I. & Henry, C.L. (2001). Protein aggregation and deposition: implications for ion channel formation and membrane damage. *Croat Medical Journal.*, Vol.42, No.4, (Aug), pp. 359-74, ISSN 0353-9504

Kroemer, G. & Jäättelä, M. (2005). Lysosomes and autophagy in cell death control. *Nature Reviews. Cancer*, Vol.5, No.11, (Nov), pp. 886-97, ISSN 1474-175X

Krüger, R., Kuhn, W., Müller, T., Woitalla, D., Graeber, M., Kösel, S., Przuntek, H., Epplen,J.T., Schöls, L. & Riess, O. (1998). Ala30Pro mutation in the gene encoding alpha-synuclein in Parkinson's disease. *Nature genetics*, Vol.18, No.2, (Feb), pp. 106-8, ISSN 1061-4036

Kundu, M. & Thompson, C.B. (2008). Autophagy: basic principles and relevance to disease. *Annual Review of Pathology*, Vol.3, pp. 427-55, ISSN 1553-4006

Lachmann, R.H., Grant, I.R., Halsall, D. & Cox, T.M. (2004). Twin pairs showing discordance of phenotype in adult Gaucher's disease. *QJM: monthly journal of the Association of Physicians*, Vol.97, No.4, (Apr), pp. 199-204, ISSN 1460-2725

Lee, H.J., Shin, S.Y., Choi, C., Lee, Y.H. & Lee, S.J.(2002). Formation and removal of alpha-synuclein aggregates in cells exposed to mitochondrial inhibitors. *The Journal of biological chemistry*, Vol.277, No.7, (Feb), pp. 5411-7, ISSN 0021-9258

Lee, H.J., Khoshaghideh, F., Patel, S. & Lee, S.J. (2004). Clearance of alpha-synuclein oligomeric intermediates via the lysosomal degradation pathway. *The Journal of neuroscience*, Vol.24, No.8, (Feb), pp. 1888-96, ISSN 0270-6474

Lee, R.E. (1982). The pathology of Gaucher disease. *Progress in Clinical and Biological Research*, Vol.95, pp. 177-217, ISSN 0361-7742

Levine, B. & Klionsky, D.J. (2004). Development by self-digestion: molecular mechanisms and biological functions of autophagy. *Developmental Cell*, Vol.6, No.4, (Apr), pp. 463-77, ISSN 1534-5807

Lwin, A., Orvisky, E., Goker-Alpan, O., LaMarca, M.E. & Sidransky, E. (2004). Glucocerebrosidase mutations in subjects with parkinsonism. *Molecular genetics and metabolism*, Vol.81, No.1, (Jan), pp. 70-3, ISSN 1096-7192

Machaczka, M., Rucinska, M., Skotnicki, A.B. & Jurczak, W. (1999). Parkinson's syndrome preceding clinical manifestation of Gaucher's disease. *American Journal of Hematology*, Vol.61, No.3, (Jul), pp. 216-7, ISSN 0361-8609

Majeski, A.E. & Dice, J.F. (2004). Mechanisms of chaperone-mediated autophagy. *The International Journal of Biochemistry & Cell Biology*, Vol.36, No.12, (Dec), pp. 2435-44, ISSN 1357-2725

Marzella, L., Ahlberg, J. & Glaumann, H. (1981). Autophagy, heterophagy, microautophagy and crinophagy as the means for intracellular degradation. *Virchows Arch. B, Cell Pathology Including Molecular Pathology*, Vol.36, No.2-3, pp. 219-34, ISSN 0340-6075

Masliah, E., Rockenstein, E., Veinbergs, I., Mallory, M., Hashimoto, M., Takeda, A., Sagara, Y., Sisk, A. & Mucke, L. (2000). Dopaminergic loss and inclusion body formation in alpha-synuclein mice: implications for neurodegenerative disorders. *Science*, Vol.287, No.5456, (Feb), pp. 1265-9, ISSN 0036-8075

Massey, A.C., Zhang, C. & Cuervo, A.M. (2006). Chaperone-mediated autophagy in aging and disease. *Current Topics in Developmental Biology*, Vol.73, pp. 205-35, ISSN 0070-2153

Mata, I.F., Samii, A., Schneer, S.H., Roberts, J.W., Griffith, A., Leis, B.C., Schellenberg, G.D., Sidransky, E., Bird, T.D., Leverenz, J.B., Tsuang, D. & Zabetian, C.P. (2008). Glucocerebrosidase gene mutations: a risk factor for Lewy body disorders. *Archives of neurology,* Vol.65, No.3, (Mar), pp. 379-82, ISSN 0003-9942

McKeran, R.O., Bradbury, P., Taylor, D. & Stern, G. (1985). Neurological involvement in type 1 (adult) Gaucher's disease. *Journal of Neurology, Neurosurgery, and Psychiatry,* Vol.48, No.2, (Feb), pp. 172-5, ISSN 0022-3050

Meikle, P.J., Hopwood, J.J., Clague, A.E. & Carey, W.F. (1999). Prevalence of lysosomal storage disorders. *Journal of American Medical* Association, Vol.281, No.3, (Jan), pp. 249-54, ISSN 0098-7484

Mijaljica, D., Prescott, M. & Devenish, R.J. (2006). Endoplasmic reticulum and Golgi complex: Contributions to, and turnover by, autophagy. *Traffic,* Vol.7, No.12, (Dec), pp. 1590-5, ISSN 1398-9219

Mitsui, J., Mizuta, I., Toyoda, A., Ashida, R., Takahashi, Y., Goto, J., Fukuda, Y., Date, H., Iwata, A., Yamamoto, M., Hattori, N., Murata, M., Toda, T. & Tsuji, S. (2009). Mutations for Gaucher disease confer high susceptibility to Parkinson disease. *Archives of neurology,* Vol.66, No.5, (May), pp. 571-6, ISSN 0003-9942

Mizushima, N. (2005). A(beta) generation in autophagic vacuoles. *The Journal Cell Biology,* Vol.171, No.1, (Oct), pp. 15-7, ISSN 0021-9525

Moran, M.T., Schofield, J.P., Hayman, A.R., Shi, G.P., Young, E. & Cox, T.M. (2000). Pathologic gene expression in Gaucher disease: up-regulation of cysteine proteinases including osteoclastic cathepsin K. *Blood,* Vol.96, No.5, (Sep), pp. 1969-78, ISSN 0006-4971

Mortimore, G.E., Lardeux, B.R. & Adams, C.E. (1988). Regulation of microautophagy and basal protein turnover in rat liver. Effects of short-term starvation. *The Journal of Biological Chemistry,* Vol.263, No.5, (Feb), pp. 2506-12, ISSN 0021-9258

Mortimore, G.E., Miotto, G., Venerando, R. & Kadowaki, M. (1996). Autophagy. *Sub-cellular Biochemistry,* Vol.27, pp. 93-135, ISSN 0306-0225

Mukaiyama, H., Oku, M., Baba, M., Samizo, T., Hammond, A.T., Glick, B.S., Kato, N. & Sakai, Y. (2002). Paz2 and 13 other PAZ gene products regulate vacuolar engulfment of peroxisomes during micropexophagy. *Genes to Cells: devoted to molecular & cellular mechanisms,* Vol.7, No.1, (Jan), pp. 75-90, ISSN 1356-9597

Neudorfer, O., Giladi, N., Elstein, D., Abrahamov, A., Turezkite, T., Aghai, E., Reches, A., Bembi, B. & Zimran, A. (1996). Occurrence of Parkinson's syndrome in type I Gaucher disease. *QJM : monthly journal of the Association of Physicians,* Vol.8, No. 9 (Sep), pp. 691-4, ISSN: 1460-2725

Neumann, J., Bras, J., Deas, E., O'Sullivan, S.S., Parkkinen, L., Lachmann, R.H., Li, A., Holton, J., Guerreiro, R., Paudel, R., Segarane, B., Singleton, A., Lees, A., Hardy, J., Houlden, H., Revesz, T. & Wood, N.W. (2009). Glucocerebrosidase mutations in clinical and pathologically proven Parkinson's disease. *Brain : a journal of neurology,* Vol.132, No.7, (Jul), pp. 1783-94, ISSN 0006-8950

Nichols, W.C., Pankratz, N., Marek, D.K., Pauciulo, M.W., Elsaesser, V.E., Halter, C.A., Rudolph, A., Wojcieszek, J., Pfeiffer, R.F., Foroud, T. & Parkinson Study Group-PROGENI Investigators. (2009). Mutations in GBA are associated with familial

Parkinson disease susceptibility and age at onset. *Neurology*, Vol.72, No.4, (Jan), pp.310-6, ISSN 0028-3878

Nilsson, O. & Svennerholm, L. (1982). Accumulation of glucosylceramide and glucosylsphingosine (psychosine) in cerebrum and cerebellum in infantile and juvenile Gaucher disease. *Journal of Neurochemistry*, Vol.39, No.3, (Sep), pp. 709–718, ISSN 0022-3042

Occurrence of Parkinson's syndrome in type I Gaucher disease. *QJM : monthly journal of the Association of Physicians*, Vol.89, No.9, (Sep), pp. 691-4, ISSN 1460-2725

Ohmi, K., Kudo, L.C., Ryazantsev, S., Zhao, H.Z., Karsten, S.L. & Neufeld, E.F.(2009). Sanfilippo syndrome type B, a lysosomal storage disease, is also a tauopathy. *Proceedings of the National Academy of Sciences of the United States of America*, Vol.106, No.20, (May), pp. 8332-7, ISSN 0027-8424

Ohsumi, Y. (2001). Molecular dissection of autophagy: two ubiquitin-like systems. *Nature Reviews. Molecular Cell Biology*, Vol.2, No.3, (Mar), pp. 211-6, ISSN 1471-0072

Pan, T., Kondo, S., Le, W. & Jankovic, J. (2008). The role of autophagy-lysosome pathway in neurodegeneration associated with Parkinson's disease. *Brain : a journal of neurology*, Vol.131, No.8, (Aug), pp. 1969-78, ISSN 0006-8950

Parnetti, L., Balducci, C., Pierguidi, L., De Carlo, C., Peducci, M., D'Amore, C., Padiglioni, C., Mastrocola, S., Persichetti, E., Paciotti, S., Bellomo, G., Tambasco, N., Rossi, A., Beccari, T. & Calabresi, P. (2009). Cerebrospinal fluid beta-glucocerebrosidase activity is reduced in Dementia with Lewy Bodies. *Neurobiology of Disease*, Review Vol.34, No.3, (Jun), pp. 484-6, ISSN 0969-9961

Patrick, A.D. (1965). Deficiencies of –SH-dependent enzymes in cystinosis. *Clinical Science*, Vol.28, (Jun), pp. 427-43, ISSN 0009-9287

Pelled, D., Trajkovic-Bodennec, S., Lloyd-Evans, E., Sidransky, E., Schiffmann, R. & Futerman, A.H. (2005). Enhanced calcium release in the acute neuronopathic form of Gaucher disease. *Neurobiology of Disease*, Vol.18, No.1,(Feb), pp. 83-8, ISSN 0969-9961

Picconi, B., Centonze, D., Håkansson, K., Bernardi, G., Greengard, P., Fisone, G., Cenci, M.A. & Calabresi, P. (2003) Loss of bidirectional striatal synaptic plasticity in L-DOPA-induced dyskinesia. *Nature neuroscience*, Vol.6, No.5, (May), pp. 501-6, ISSN 1097-6256

Polymeropoulos, M.H., Lavedan, C., Leroy, E., Ide, S.E., Dehejia, A., Dutra, A., Pike, B., Root, H., Rubenstein, J., Boyer, R., Stenroos, E.S., Chandrasekharappa, S., Athanassiadou, A., Papapetropoulos, T., Johnson, W.G., Lazzarini, A.M., Duvoisin, R.C., Di Iorio, G., Golbe, L.I. & Nussbaum, R.L. (1997). Mutation in the alpha-synuclein gene identified in families with Parkinson's disease. *Science*, Vol.276, No.5321, (Jun), pp. 2045-7, ISSN 0193-4511

Richfield, E.K., Thiruchelvam, M.J., Cory-Slechta, D.A., Wuertzer, C., Gainetdinov, R.R., Caron, M.G., Di Monte, D.A. & Federoff, H.J. (2002). Behavioral and neurochemical effects of wild-type and mutated human alpha-synuclein in transgenic mice. *Experimental neurology*, Vol.175, No.1, (May), pp. 35-48, ISSN 0014-4886

Richly, H., Rape, M., Braun, S., Rumpf, S., Hoege, C. & Jentsch, S. (2005). A series of ubiquitin binding factors connects CDC48/p97 to substrate multiubiquitylation and proteasomal targeting. *Cell*, Vol.120, No.1, (Jan), pp. 73-84, ISSN 0092-8674

Ron, I. & Horowitz, M. (2005). ER retention and degradation as the molecular basis underlying Gaucher disease heterogeneity. *Human Molecular Genetics,* Vol.14, No.16, (Aug), pp. 2387-98, ISSN 0964-6906

Ron, I., Rapaport, D. & Horowitz, M. (2010). Interaction between parkin and mutant glucocerebrosidase variants: a possible link between Parkinson disease and Gaucher disease. *Human Molecular Genetics,* Vol.19, No.19, (Oct), pp. 3771-81, ISSN 0964-6906

Rozas, G., Guerra, M.J. & Labandeira-García, J.L. (1997). An automated rotarod method for quantitative drug-free evaluation of overall motor deficits in rat models of parkinsonism. *Brain research. Brain research protocols,* Vol.2, No.1, (Dec), pp. 75-84, ISSN 1385-299X

Roze, E., Paschke, E., Lopez, N., Eck, T., Yoshida, K., Maurel-Ollivier, A., Doummar, D., Caillaud, C., Galanaud, D., Billette de Villemeur, T., Vidailhet, M. & Roubergue, A. (2005). Dystonia and parkinsonism in GM1 type 3 gangliosidosis. *Movement Disorders,* Vol.20, No.10, (Oct), pp. 1366-9, ISSN 0885-3185

Saftig, P. (2006). Physiology of the lysosome, In: *Fabry Disease: Perspectives from 5 Years of FOS,* Mehta A., Beck M., Sunder-Plassmann G., Oxford: Oxford PharmaGenesis; Chapter 3 ISBN-10: 1-903539-03-X, Oxford

Salvador, N., Aguado, C., Horst, M. & Knecht, E. (2000). Import of a cytosolic protein into lysosomes by chaperone-mediated autophagy depends on its folding state. *The Journal of Biological Chemistry,* Vol.275, No.35, (Sep), pp. 27447-56, ISSN 0021-9258

Sato, C., Morgan, A., Lang, A.E., Salehi-Rad, S., Kawarai, T., Meng, Y., Ray, P.N., Farrer, L.A., St George-Hyslop, P. & Rogaeva, E. (2005). Analysis of the glucocerebrosidase gene in Parkinson's disease. *Movement Disorders,* Vol.20, No.3, (Mar), pp. 367-70, ISSN 0885-3185

Sawkar, A.R., Adamski-Werner, S.L., Cheng, W.C., Wong, C.H., Beutler, E., Zimmer, K.P. & Kelly, J.W. (2005). Gaucher disease-associated glucocerebrosidases show mutation-dependent chemical chaperoning profiles. *Chemistry and Biology,* Vol.12, No.11, (Nov), pp. 1235-44, ISSN 1074-5521

Scarlatti, F., Bauvy, C., Ventruti, A., Sala, G., Cluzeaud, F., Vandewalle, A., Ghidoni, R. & Codogno, P. (2004). Ceramide-mediated macroautophagy involves inhibition of protein kinase B and up-regulation of beclin 1. *The Journal of Biological Chemistry,* Vol.279, No.18, (Apr), pp. 18384-91, ISSN 0021-9258

Schneider, E.L., Epstein, C.J., Kaback, M.J. & Brandes, D. (1977). Severe pulmonary involvement in adult Gaucher's disease. Report of three cases and review of the literature. *American Journal of Medicine,* Vol.63, No.3, (Sep), pp. 475-80, ISSN 0002-9343

Schubert, U., Antón, L.C., Gibbs, J., Norbury, C.C., Yewdell, J.W. & Bennink, J.R. (2000). Rapid degradation of a large fraction of newly synthesized proteins by proteasomes. *Nature,* Vol.404, No.6779, (Apr), pp. 770-4, ISSN 0028-0836

Segarane, B., Li, A., Paudel, R., Scholz, S., Neumann, J., Lees, A., Revesz, T., Hardy, J., Mathias, C.J., Wood, N.W., Holton, J. & Houlden, H. (2009). Glucocerebrosidase mutations in 108 neuropathologically confirmed cases of multiple system atrophy. *Neurology,* Vol.72, No.13, (Mar), pp. 1185-6, ISSN 0028-3878

Seglen, P.O., Berg, T.O., Blankson, H., Fengsrud, M., Holen, I. & Strømhaug, P.E. (1996). Structural aspects of autophagy. *Advances in Experimental Medicine and Biology*, Vol.389, pp. 103-11, ISSN 0025-2598

Sevlever, D., Jiang, P. & Yen, S.H. (2008). Cathepsin D is the main lysosomal enzyme involved in the degradation of alpha-synuclein and generation of its carboxy-terminally truncated species. *Biochemistry*, Vol.47, No.36, (Sep), pp. 9678-87, ISSN 0006-2960

Sidransky, E. (2004). Gaucher disease: complexity in a "simple" disorder. *Molecular Genetics and Metabolism*, Vol.83, No.1-2, (Sep-Oct), pp. 6-15, ISSN 1096-7192

Sidransky, E., Nalls, M.A., Aasly, J.O., Aharon-Peretz, J., Annesi G., Barbosa, E.R., Bar-Shira, A., Berg, D., Bras, J., Brice, A., Chen, C.M., Clark, L.N., Condroyer, C., De Marco, E.V., Dürr, A., Eblan, M.J., Fahn, S., Farrer, M.J., Fung, H.C., Gan-Or, Z., Gasser, T., Gershoni-Baruch, R., Giladi, N., Griffith, A., Gurevich, T., Januario, C., Kropp, P., Lang, A.E., Lee-Chen, G.J., Lesage, S., Marder, K., Mata, I.F., Mirelman, A., Mitsui, J., Mizuta, I., Nicoletti, G., Oliveira, C., Ottman, R., Orr-Urtreger, A., Pereira, L.V., Quattrone, A., Rogaeva, E., Rolfs, A., Rosenbaum, H., Rozenberg, R., Samii, A., Samaddar, T., Schulte, C., Sharma, M., Singleton, A., Spitz, M., Tan, E.K., Tayebi, N., Toda, T., Troiano, A.R., Tsuji, S., Wittstock, M., Wolfsberg, T.G., Wu, Y.R., Zabetian, C.P., Zhao, Y. & Ziegler, S.G. (2009). Multicenter analysis of glucocerebrosidase mutations in Parkinson's disease. *The New England Journal Medicine*, Vol.361, No.17, (Oct), pp. 1651-61, ISSN 0028-4793

Singleton, A.B., Farrer, M., Johnson, J., Singleton, A., Hague, S., Kachergus, J., Hulihan, M., Peuralinna, T., Dutra, A., Nussbaum, R., Lincoln, S., Crawley, A., Hanson, M., Maraganore, D., Adler, C., Cookson, M.R., Muenter, M., Baptista, M., Miller, D., Blancato, J., Hardy, J. & Gwinn-Hardy, K. (2003). alpha-Synuclein locus triplication causes Parkinson's disease. *Science*, Vol.302, No.5646, (Oct), pp. 841, ISSN 0193-4511

Spitz, M., Rozenberg, R., Pereira, L.da V. & Reis Barbosa, E. (2008). Association between Parkinson's disease and glucocerebrosidase mutations in Brazil. *Parkinsonism & related disorders*, Vol.14, No.1, (Aug), pp. 58-62, ISSN 1353-8020

Squier, T.C. (2001). Oxidative stress and protein aggregation during biological aging. *Experimental Gerontolology*, Vol.36, No.9, (Sep), pp. 1539-50, ISSN 0531-5565

Tan, E.K., Tong, J., Fook-Chong, S., Yih, Y., Wong, M.C., Pavanni, R. & Zhao, Y. (2007). Glucocerebrosidase mutations and risk of Parkinson disease in Chinese patients. *Archives of Neurology*, Vol.64, No.7, (Jul), pp. 1056-8, ISSN 0003-9942

Tayebi, N., Callahan, M., Madike, V., Stubblefield, B.K., Orvisky, E., Krasnewich, D., Fillano, J.J. & Sidransky, E. (2001) Gaucher disease and parkinsonism: a phenotypic and genotypic characterization. *Molecular Genetics and Metabolism*, Vol. 73, No 4 (Aug), pp. 313-21, ISSN 1096-7192

Tayebi, N., Walker,J., Stubblefield, B., Orvisky, E., LaMarca, M.E., Wong, K., Rosenbaum, H., Schiffmann, R., Bembi, B. & Sidransky, E. (2003). Gaucher disease with parkinsonian manifestations: does glucocerebrosidase deficiency contribute to a vulnerability to parkinsonism? *Molecular Genetics and Metabolism*, Vol.79, No.2, (Jun), pp. 104-9, ISSN 1096-7192

Terman, A. (2006). Catabolic insufficiency and aging. *Annals of the New York Academy of Sciences*, Vol.1067, (May), pp. 27-36, ISSN 0077-8923

Theise, N.D. & Ursell, P.C. (1990). Pulmonary hypertension and Gaucher's disease: logical association or mere coincidence? *The American Journal of Pediatric Hematology/Oncology*, Vol.12, No.1, (Spring), pp. 74-6, ISSN 0192-8562

Tofaris, G.K., Razzaq, A., Ghetti, B., Lilley, K.S. & Spillantini, M.G. (2003). Ubiquitination of alpha-synuclein in Lewy bodies is a pathological event not associated with impairment of proteasome function. *The Journal of Biological Chemistry*, Vol.278, No.45, (Nov), pp. 44405-11, ISSN 0021-9258

Tofaris, G.K., Garcia, Reitböck, P., Humby, T., Lambourne, S.L., O'Connell, M., Ghetti, B., Gossage, H., Emson, P.C., Wilkinson, L.S., Goedert, M. & Spillantini, M.G.(2006). Pathological changes in dopaminergic nerve cells of the substantia nigra and olfactory bulb in mice transgenic for truncated human alpha-synuclein(1-120): implications for Lewy body disorders. *The Journal of Neuroscience : the Official Journal of the Society for Neuroscience*, Vol.26, No.15, (Apr), pp. 3942-50, ISSN 0270-6474

Toft, M., Pielsticker, L., Ross, O.A., Aasly, J.O. & Farrer, M.J. (2006). Glucocerebrosidase gene mutations and Parkinson disease in the Norwegian population. *Neurology*, Vol.66, No.3, (Feb), pp. 415-7, ISSN 0028-3878

Vabulas, R.M. & Hartl, F.U. (2005). Protein synthesis upon acute nutrient restriction relies on proteasome function. *Science*, Vol. 310, No. 5756, (Dec), pp. 1960-3, ISSN 0193-4511

Veenhuis, M., Salomons, F.A. & Van Der Klei, I.J. (2000). Peroxisome biogenesis and degradation in yeast: a structure/function analysis. *Microscophy Research and Technique*, Vol.51, No.6, (Dec), pp. 584-600, ISSN 1059-910X.

Velayati, A., Yu, W.H. & Sidransky, E. (2010). The role of glucocerebrosidase mutations in Parkinson disease and Lewy body disorders. *Current Neurology and Neuroscience Reports*, Vol. 10, No. 3 (May), pp. 190-8, ISSN: 1528-4042

Wheatley, D.N., & Inglis, M.S. (1980). An intracellular perfusion system linking pools and protein synthesis. *Journal of Theoretical Biology*, Vol. 83, No. 3, (Apr), pp. 437-45, ISSN 0022-5193

Wu, Y.R., Chen, C.M., Chao, C.Y., Ro, L.S., Lyu, R.K., Chang, K.H. & Lee-Chen, G.J. (2007). Glucocerebrosidase gene mutation is a risk factor for early onset of Parkinson disease among Taiwanese. *Journal of Neurology, Neurosurgery, and Psychiatry*, Vol.78, No.9, (Sep), pp. 977-9, ISSN 0022-3050

Yewdell, J.W. (2005). Serendipity strikes twice: the discovery and rediscovery of defective ribosomal products (DRiPS). *Cellulae and Molecular Biology (Noisy-le-grand)* , Vol.51, No.7, (Dec), pp. 635-41, ISSN 0145-5680

Zarranz, J.J., Alegre, J., Gómez-Esteban, J.C., Lezcano, E., Ros, R., Ampuero, I., Vidal, L., Hoenicka, J., Rodriguez, O., Atarés, B., Llorens, V., Gomez Tortosa, E., del Ser, T., Muñoz, D.G. & de Yebenes, J.G. (2004). The new mutation, E46K, of alpha-synuclein causes Parkinson and Lewy body dementia. *Annals of Neurology*, Vol.55, No.2, (Feb), pp. 164-73, ISSN 0364-5134

Zhang, D., Chen, T., Ziv, I., Rosenzweig, R., Matiuhin, Y., Bronner, V., Glickman, M.H. & Fushman, D. (2009). Together, Rpn10 and Dsk2 can serve as a polyubiquitin chain-length sensor. *Molecular Cell*, Vol.36, No.6, (Dec), pp. 1018-33, ISSN 1097-2765

Zhao, H. & Grabowski, G.A. (2002). Gaucher disease: Perspectives on a prototype lysosomal disease. *Cellular and molecular life sciences*, Vol. 59, No. 4, (Apr), pp. 694-707, ISSN:1420-682X

Zhu, J.H., Horbinski, C., Guo, F., Watkins, S., Uchiyama, Y. & Chu, C.T. (2007). Regulation of autophagy by extracellular signal-regulated protein kinases during 1-methyl-4-phenylpyridinium-induced cell death. *The American Journal of Pathology*, Vol.170, No.1, (Jan), pp. 75-86, ISSN 0002-9440

Ziegler, S.G., Eblan, M.J., Gutti, U., Hruska, K.S., Stubblefield, B.K., Goker-Alpan, O., LaMarca, M.E. & Sidransky, E. (2007). Glucocerebrosidase mutations in Chinese subjects from Taiwan with sporadic Parkinson disease. *Molecular Genetics and Metabolism*, Vol.91, No.2, (Jun), pp. 195-200, ISSN 1096-7192

Zimran, A., Gelbart, T., Garver, P., Thurston, D., Saven, A. & Beutler, E. (1992). Gaucher disease. Clinical, laboratory, radiologic, and genetic features of 53 patients. *Medicine (Baltimore)*, Vol.71, No.6, (Nov.), pp. 337-53, ISSN 0025-7974

22

Physiological and Biomechanical Analyses of Rigidity in Parkinson's Disease

Ruiping Xia
Department of Physical Therapy, Creighton University, Omaha, Nebraska
USA

1. Introduction

Parkinson's disease is one of the most common movement disorders characterized by bradykinesia, rigidity, resting tremor and postural instability (Fahn, 2003). It affects nearly five million elderly people worldwide (de Lau & Breteler, 2006). As the population ages, the incidence and prevalence of Parkinson's disease are expected to increase dramatically (Dorsey et al., 2007; Tanner & Goldman, 1996; Tanner & Ben-Shlomo, 1999). Rigidity is one of the clinical hallmark symptoms that characterize and define Parkinson's disease. Rigidity is one form of the increased muscle tone, which is defined as a resistance to a passive movement. Rigidity is clinically characterized by an increase in muscle tone, and is felt as a constant and uniform resistance to the passive movement of a limb persisting throughout its range (Bantam, 2000; Fung & Thompson, 2002; Hallett, 2003). There are two types of rigidity: plastic or lead-pipe rigidity, in which resistance remains uniform, constant and smooth, such as experienced when bending a piece of lead; and cogwheel rigidity, in which tremor is superimposed on increased tone, giving rise to the perception of intermittent fluctuation in muscle tone. The latter is principally attributable to the combination of plastic rigidity and tremor.

In addition to being a key element of parkinsonian rigidity, increased muscle tone also characterizes spasticity which is a common motor symptom in a few other neurological disorders, such as multiple sclerosis, stroke and cerebral palsy. Spasticity is clinically described as an increased resistance to passive movement due to hyperexcitability of stretch reflex (Lance, 1980; Rymer & Katz, 1994). Rigidity and spasticity share the characteristic feature of the increased muscle tone to a passive movement. However, the unique lead-pipe resistance can distinguish the increased muscle tone in rigidity from that associated with spasticity. In particular, the differentiation between rigidity and spasticity is not straightforward in a clinical scenario (Fung & Thompson, 2002).

Rigidity generally responds well to dopaminergic medication and surgical intervention. Thus, it is used as a diagnostic criterion and to evaluate the efficacy of therapeutic interventions (Prochazka et al., 1997). Clinical examination and assessment of rigidity is determined by an examiner's perception of resistance while rotating the limb at major joints, based upon the Unified Parkinson Disease Rating Scale (Fahn & Elton, 1987; Goetz et al., 2008). A better understanding of the physiological and biomechanical characteristics of rigidity merits scientific significance and clinical implication. In this chapter, studies on elucidation of the physiological mechanisms and biomechanical quantification of parkinsonian rigidity will be reviewed and the latest research on this topic will be presented.

2. Physiological studies of parkinsonian rigidity

2.1 Reflex responses to passive stretch

The history of studying the pathophysiology of rigidity can be traced back to nearly a century ago. Forester's observation (1921) that parkinsonian rigidity is reduced by the dorsal root section suggested that rigidity could be of reflex origin, although other equally plausible explanations are possible. The most widespread view was that rigidity arose from the increased response of muscle receptors to externally imposed stretch. This view was supported by earlier experiments (Pollock & Davis, 1930; Rushworth, 1960), demonstrating that rigidity was substantially reduced by dorsal root section or local anesthetic block.

However, illustration by microneurographic recordings from muscle nerves has provided evidence that increased muscle afferent discharge (due to increased fusimotor drive) was not sufficient to explain the presence of rigidity (Burke et al., 1977). Recent studies using electrophysiological techniques demonstrated that monosynaptic segmental stretch reflexes showed no significant differences between individuals with Parkinson's disease and healthy controls (Bergui et al., 1992; Delwaide, 1985; Delwaide et al., 1986; Meara and Cody, 1993; Rothwell et al., 1983). Numerous studies on stretch reflexes have also shown that most reflexes (H-reflex, tendon jerks and tonic vibration reflex), considered to be principally mediated by Ia afferents and to be spinal in origin, appear normal in Parkinson's disease (Burke et al., 1972a; Dietrichson, 1971; Lance et al., 1973). In brief, there is no evidence that Ia muscle afferent pathway might explain the pathophysiological basis of parkinsonian rigidity.

If the response of the spinal machinery to muscle primary spindle afferent input is intact in Parkinson's disease, supraspinally mediated reflexes might well play a role in the pathophysiology of rigidity. Lee and Tatton (1975) were the first to demonstrate that long-latency stretch reflexes in forearm muscles were exaggerated in patients with Parkinson's disease. This observation was subsequently confirmed by several other investigators who studied rigidity in the same or different muscle groups (Berardelli et al., 1983; Cody et al., 1986; Mortimer & Webster, 1979; Rothwell et al., 1983). Some studies found a quantitative association between the degree of increase in long-latency stretch reflex and the clinically assessed degree of rigidity (Mortimer & Webster, 1979; Berardelli et al., 1983), whereas others found that no correlation existed between the two based on a larger number of patients (Cody et al., 1986; Rothwell et al., 1983). The lack of a consistent correlation might be because rigidity is often assessed using a sustained static stretch whereas long-latency stretch reflexes is elicited by transient and brisk muscle stretches (Marsden, 1990). However, it is certain that patients with parkinsonian rigidity show a marked increase in long-latency stretch reflexes, compared with healthy controls (Marsden, 1990; Fung & Thompson, 2002), though there is no universal agreement as to the origin of the long-latency stretch reflexes (Matthews, 1991). In addition, the tonic muscle response to slow and sustained stretch is reported to be exaggerated in Parkinson's disease (Dietrichson, 1971; Andrews et al., 1972).

Findings obtained from the aforementioned studies provide partial explanations for increased resistance, *i.e.*, one of the two elements defining parkinsonian rigidity. However, they cannot account for the constancy and uniformity of resistance which is uniquely associated with rigidity. Recent studies have shed light on the underlying mechanism of the uniform nature of parkinsonian rigidity (Xia & Rymer, 2004; Xia et al., 2011). Evidence indicates that shortening reaction and stretch-induced inhibition play pivotal roles in the genesis of lead-pipe characteristics of rigidity.

2.2 Responses to passive shortening – Shortening reaction

Besides abnormal muscle responses to stretch, anomalous reactions in the shortened muscles during a passive joint motion have also been described in Parkinson's disease. More than a century ago, Westphal (1877, 1880) observed muscular contraction in the passively shortened skeletal muscles. Before he observed this phenomenon, he had already studied the muscular contraction in lengthening or stretched muscles. Thus, he named it 'paradoxer Muskel-contraction'. At that time, he also described enhanced activation of tibialis anterior corresponding to the shortening phase in patients who had great difficulty in passively aiding imposed movement. The phenomenon he observed is often referred to as "Westphal's phenomenon". Later, Sherrington (1909) described analogous findings in both the spinal dog and the decerebrate cat under the name "shortening reaction'. This term has been used since then.

Application of electromyographic (EMG) recording method has demonstrated that inappropriate activation of shortened muscles occurs widely in basal ganglia disorders (Rondot & Metral, 1973), and most prominently in Parkinson's disease (Andrews et al., 1972; Angel, 1983; Berardelli & Hallett, 1984; Rondot & Metral, 1973; Xia & Rymer, 2004). An example of shortening reaction is illustrated in Fig. 1B (Xia et al., 2011). During the passive wrist flexion movement, flexor muscles were progressively shortened. There occurred strong muscle activations in the wrist flexor muscles. Shortening reaction has been reported to be manifested in both upper and lower limb muscles. Some investigators suggested that shortening reaction plays an important role in the pathophysiology of rigidity (Angel, 1983; Rondot & Metral, 1973), given that it represents a reflex action that agonistically assists with a passive movement in contrast to antagonistic opposition of a motion caused by stretch reflex. Correlational analysis showed that there was no direct relationship between shortening reaction and changes in muscle tone (Berardelli & Hallett, 1984).

Nevertheless, the neural mechanism of the shortening reaction was virtually unknown. Since shortening reaction was first reported a century ago, very little attention has been paid to exploring its underlying physiology. Shortening reaction is the opposite of stretch reflex, a topic that has been extensively studied for a long period of time. In contrast, only a limited number of studies were conducted to understand and characterize shortening reaction, and these previous studies simply monitored muscle electromyographic activity (Andrews et al. 1972; Angel, 1983; Berardelli et al. 1983; Berardelli and Hallett, 1984; Rondot and Metral, 1973). The importance of shortening reaction in the pathophysiology of parkinsonian rigidity is undoubtedly underestimated. Utilization of both EMG recording and joint torque measure has provided us with useful information to reveal the role of shortening reaction in mediating rigidity in Parkinson's disease (Xia & Rymer, 2004; Xia et al., 2011). A parallel mechanism responsible for mediating parkinsonian rigidity is stretch-induced inhibition which will be discussed in the next section.

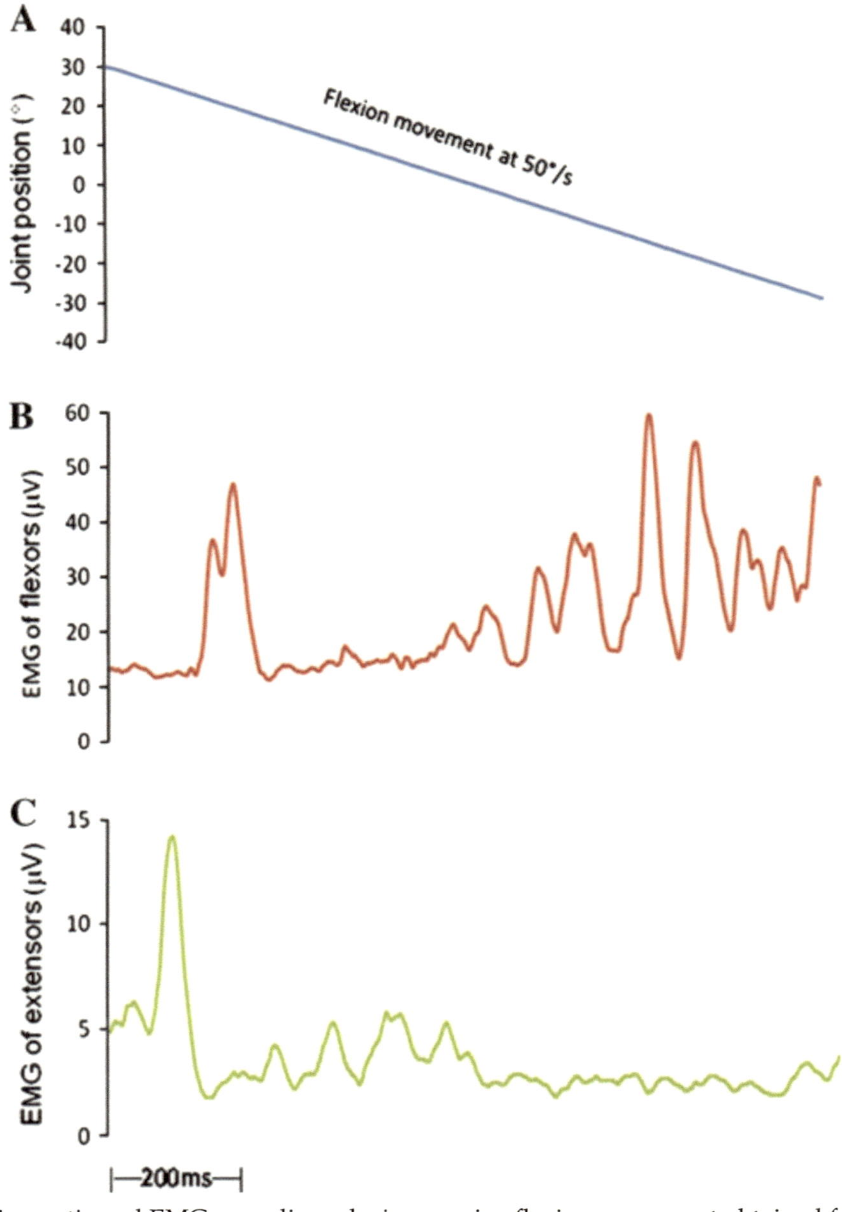

Fig. 1. Kinematic and EMG recordings during passive flexion movement obtained from a patient after an overnight withdrawal of medication (Off-medication). **A.** Wrist joint position during the passive flexion movement; the subject's wrist joint was externally rotated from 30 degree to -30 degree at 50°/s. **B.** Shortening reaction was recorded in shortened flexors in the Off-medication state in a parkinsonian subject. There was an increased EMG activation in passively shortened muscles. **C.** Stretch-induced inhibition was observed in the stretched extensor muscles during the same movement. There was an EMG reduction, when the stretch exceeded the neutral position and the muscle length was elongated [from Xia et al. (2011) with permission].

2.3 Lengthening reaction or stretch-induced inhibition

In addition to shortening reaction, Sherrington (1909) also observed in the above-noted animal preparations that *"... when an examiner bent the knee against the knee-extensor's contraction, the examiner felt the opposition offered by the extensor gave away almost abruptly at a certain pressure; the knee could then be flexed without opposition ..."*. He named this phenomenon "lengthening reaction". Lengthening reaction was demonstrated in both spinal dog and in decerebrate rigidity of the cat, yet the reaction was recognized to have differential features in the two preparations. In his monograph, he also pointed out that muscles, exhibiting shortening reaction and lengthening reaction, were all extensor muscles. The distinction of the flexor and extensor muscle groups has been documented in parkinsonian rigidity (Mera et al., 2009; Xia et al., 2006).

The well-know clasp-knife phenomenon associated with human spasticity, appears to be the equivalent of the lengthening reaction (Burke et al., 1970, 1971). The clasp-knife reflex is characterized by an abrupt decline in muscle force that occurs when a spastic limb is moved beyond a certain joint angle. There is a common ground between lengthening reaction in animal preparations (Burke et al., 1972b; Rymer et al., 1979) and clasp-knife reflex in human spasticity in that the essential feature of both phenomena is the sudden release of the resistance due to continuous stretch of the elongated muscle, hence also referred to as "stretch-induced inhibition" (Rymer et al., 1979). The physiological framework previously established or explored in the context of the lengthening reaction or stretch-induced inhibition has recently been investigated in parkinsonian rigidity (Xia & Rymer, 2004; Xia et al., 2011).

Fig. 1C illustrates a stretch-induced inhibition recorded from a parkinsonian patient in the Off-medication state. During the passive flexion movement (Fig. 1A), there was a large initial stretch reflex in the wrist extensor muscles. The initial stretch reflex was followed by a period of sustained activity and curtailed by an evident decline when the progressive movement approached at almost the neutral position and the muscle length of the extensors was elongated, demonstrating the stretch-induced inhibition (Fig. 1C). It is noted that both shortening reaction and stretch-induced inhibition occur during the same movement phase (Fig. 1). The importance and functional role stretch-induced inhibition and the above described shortening reaction may have played in parkinsonian rigidity will be explained and discussed in Section 3.

3. Pathophysiological mechanisms of lead-pipe rigidity

This session will begin with an overview of the basic principles of muscle mechanics. When an active muscle is stretched, the muscle force output increases proportionally with the increasing muscle length. The dependence of muscle force on muscle length gives rise to a "spring-like" behavior (Gordon et al., 1966; Matthews, 1959; Rack & Westbury, 1969). This spring-like property of skeletal muscle has been shown to play a key role in the maintenance of posture and control of movement. A limb's posture is maintained when the forces exerted by agonist and antagonist muscle groups are equal and opposite.

Rotational movements about human joints are promoted by a resultant torque which is a summation of the individual contributions of agonist muscles minus contributions of antagonist muscles, where a single torque is mathematically defined as the product of force times the moment arm for each muscle. The corresponding measure of rotational position is the joint angle, which determines the length of each muscle acting on the joint. Ultimately, it is the torque-angle relationship that serves to characterize the musculature of the joint as a whole (Feldman, 1966). Given the phenomenon that individual muscles are characterized by the length-tension relationship or spring-like property, thus the net torque-angle relation, arising from the summation of the stretched muscles and shortening muscles in normal subjects, manifests a steep curve. Fig. 2A shows that the net torque-angle characteristics of the joint arising from the summation of the spring-like properties of the stretched flexor muscle and shortening extensor muscle display spring-like behavior in healthy subjects, which is characterized by a steep torque-angle curve.

However, the natural spring-like property can be altered, generating a relatively flat torque-angle relationship that is equivalent to a plastic sensation perceived in parkinsonian rigidity. Such a flattened torque-angle relationship can be resulted from either the impact of a shortening reaction or a stretch-induced inhibition or a combination of the two. In the case of parkinsonian rigidity (Figs. 2B-2D), the torque produced by the stretched muscles (i.e., wrist flexors in this example) is increased due to the exaggerated long-latency stretch reflexes (Lee & Tatton, 1975) and enhanced tonic muscle responses (Dietrichson, 1971). There are two ways in which a joint could generate relatively constant torque with the changing joint position. Firstly, if there is an inappropriate shortening reaction in parkinsonian rigidity, the increasing force generated by the stretched flexor is offset by increasing activation of the shortening extensor. This muscle interaction could lead to a flat net torque-angle relationship, and promote the perception of the constant rigidity. Fig. 2B shows the potential interactions between stretched and activated shortening muscle in the presence of a shortening reaction. Another possibility, shown in Fig. 2C, is that a reduction in activation of stretched muscle at an elongated muscle length counteracts the otherwise gradual increase in muscle force (i.e., spring-like or elastic-like muscle force) as the muscle length of the stretched flexors is elongated throughout the stretch. Due to this counteracting effect, the net torque is relatively constant throughout the rotation of the limb. During the passive flexion or extension movement, one group of muscles is shortened whereas the other group is stretched. Both shortening reaction and stretch-induced inhibition have counteracting effects within a specified movement, generating the promotion of constant rigidity (uniformity) as defined in rigidity. Fig. 2D schematically illustrates the net torque resulting from a combined effect of the two mechanisms.

During passive movements, one group of muscles is shortened whereas the other group of muscles is stretched. Thus, the two mechanisms are potentially generating counteracting effects on the net torque resistance simultaneously. However, a dissociation of the two mechanisms is not readily available and technically challenging. Application of a biomechanical model (Holzbaur et al., 2005) implemented through the Software for Interactive Musculoskeletal Modeling (Delp & Loan, 1995) made it possible to quantify the torque generated by shortening muscles and by stretched muscles, separately, and to identify which mechanism predominates. Our findings obtained through the biomechanical modeling approach indicate that both shortening reaction and stretch-induced inhibition contribute significantly to the lead-pipe nature of parkinsonian rigidity (Xia et al., 2011). During the passive flexion movement, shortening reaction plays a predominant role in the genesis of lead-pipe rigidity, whereas stretch-induced inhibition is a primary contributor to the manifestation of lead-pipe rigidity during the passive extension movement. The knowledge gained from these studies provides new insights into the biomechanical and physiological underpinnings of this common symptom in patients with Parkinson's disease. The use of this approach may offer a means of assessing the efficacy of rehabilitation programs and therapeutic interventions. Efficacy of anti-Parkinson medication on the biomechanical and physiological characteristics associated with parkinsonian rigidity will be discussed in later section of this Chapter.

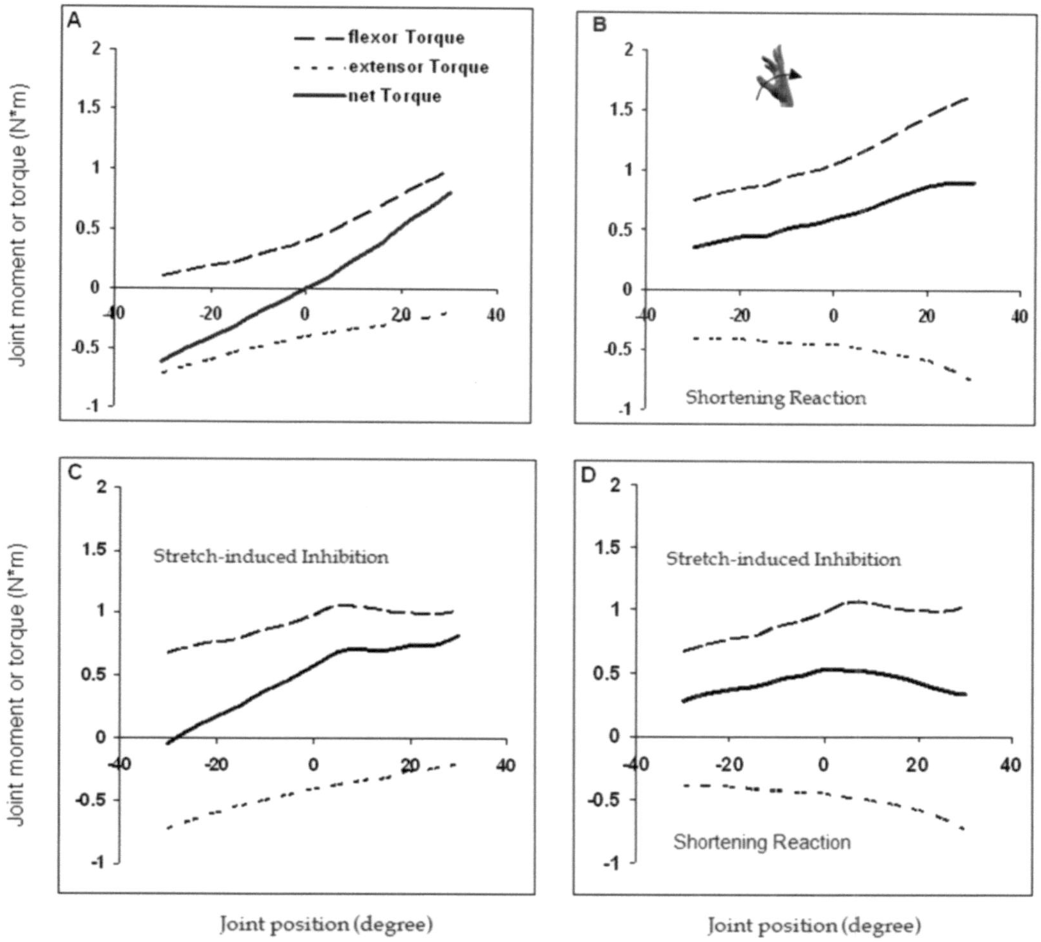

Fig. 2. Schematics of the net (solid line) torque-angle relationship showing four possible types of interactions between stretched and shortening muscles during extension of a right wrist. **A**: torque-angle relationship characterizing spring-like property of the stretched flexor and shortening extensor muscles in healthy subjects; **B**: the potential impact of a shortening reaction in the extensor muscles (contributing to extensor torque), inducing a flattened net torque-angle relation and promoting the perception of the constant rigidity; **C**: the effect of a stretch-induced inhibition in flexor muscles, causing spring-like force generated by a muscle stretch to decline as the muscle length increases. **D:** The combined effect of shortening reaction and stretch-induced inhibition on the net torque. The units and torque curves are arbitrary.

4. Non-neural factor responsible for parkinsonian rigidity

Evidence has indicated that in addition to neural-mediated abnormal muscle reflex responses, the non-neural component also contributes to parkinsonian rigidity (Dietz, 1987; Dietz et al., 1981; Watts et al., 1986). The non-neural component includes visco-elastic (i.e., mechanical) properties of muscle fiber and passive connective tissues. Dietz et al. (1981) examined ten patients with parkinsonian rigidity aiming to identify the physiological mechanism with respect to altered muscle activity to account for impaired gait pattern in Parkinson's disease. Compared to healthy control subjects, parkinsonian patients exhibited significantly stronger EMG activity in tibialis anterior during the swing phase of gait, while the strength and timing of EMG activity recorded from triceps surae were similar in two groups of participants. The authors stated that the increased muscle tone in parkinsonian rigidity cannot be explained by the electrical activity of the antagonist muscle groups of the limb, since there was no co-contraction of tibialis anterior and triceps surae muscles. It was concluded that the altered mechanical properties of muscle fibers were mainly responsible for the increased muscle tone in rigidity. This conclusion was also drawn by Watts et al. (1986) who examined elbow joint of patients with Parkinson's disease and normal controls by using a torque motor. Even in patients with relatively mild symptoms, the upper limb was stiffer than controls in the totally relaxed state with no EMG activity present. The study findings suggested that changes in the passive mechanical properties of the upper limb likely accounted for greater passive stiffness. Using the torque motor, natural progression of the disease can be quantified and followed.

Evidence indicates that neural and non-neural mechanisms operate in parallel, both contributing to parkinsonian rigidity. However, there is no simple and easy solution in differentiation and quantification of the neural and non-neural components because clinical measures of rigidity consist of the two parallel components. Using advanced technology and computational algorithm, a few sophisticated approaches have been developed to segregate the two responsible factors and quantify the individual component contributing to the overall joint stiffness (Kearney et al., 1997; Meinders et al., 1996; Sinkjaer et al., 1993; Sinkjaer & Magnussen, 1994; Zhang & Rymer, 1997). One approach, termed as parallel-cascaded system identification technique, was initially applied to separate the overall stiffness into neural reflex stiffness and non-neural mechanical stiffness at ankle joint in normal healthy adults (Kearney et al., 1997; Mirbagheri et al., 2000). Subsequently, the system identification approach has been applied to characterize the dynamic joint stiffness and to quantify the neural and non-neural contribution to the abnormal muscle tone in spasticity associated with upper motor neuron syndromes, such as stroke and spinal cord injury (Alibiglou et al., 2008; Galiana et al., 2005; Mirbagheri et al., 2001, 2009, 2010). The validity of this method has been demonstrated as well as its efficiency, accuracy and advantages by Mirbagheri et al. (2000) and Alibiglou et al. (2008).

More recently, we have applied the parallel-cascaded system identification technique to make a distinction between the neural and non-neural contributions to rigidity in patients with Parkinson's disease (Xia et al., 2010). Patients participated in the protocol under two medication states: initially under a temporary overnight withdrawal of dopaminergic medication and then after the resumption of medication. The results have shown that both neural and non-neural components contributed to parkinsonian rigidity, with the neural component being predominating over the non-neural to the overall rigidity. Medication therapy caused a reduction of torque resistance in the neural reflex torque, but did not decrease the non-neural mechanical torque. This observation appears to be attributed to the mechanism of anti-Parkinson medication therapy.

5. Biomechanical quantification of parkinsonian rigidity

In clinic, parkinsonian rigidity is examined and assessed using a numerical rating scale which is known as the Unified Parkinson Disease Rating Scale (Fahn & Elton, 1987; Goetz et al., 2008). However, the nature of this assessment tool is highly qualitative and subjective because it is largely dependent on examiners' individual interpretation and experience (Patrick et al., 2001; Prochazka et al., 1997). When the actual change in rigidity resulting from treatment is small, it may be challenging for the examiners to detect. This can limit ability for evaluation of treatment effectiveness especially in large multi-center clinical drug trials in which a large number of investigators are involved, because differences can exist between different examiners (i.e., inter-rater) and between assessments performed on different visits by a given examiner (i.e., intra-rater) with respect to the efficacy of treatment. Reliability studies have demonstrated varying degrees of inter-rater reliability with respect to rigidity component of clinical rating tools, ranging from low, moderate, very good to excellent (Martinez-Martin, 1993; Rabey et al., 1997; Richards et al., 1994; Van Dillen & Roach, 1988). A need for more accurate evaluations has been expressed to improve the management of symptoms in patients with Parkinson's disease (Obeso et al., 1996; Ondo et al., 1998; Ward et al., 1983).

During the past several decades, considerable efforts have been made aiming to quantify assessment of parkinsonian rigidity by means of biomechanical measures. A variety of quantitative methods have been developed to measure the dynamics of joint stiffness associated with rigidity (Lee et al., 2002; Prochazka et al., 1997; Teräväinen et al., 1989; Watts et al., 1986; Wiegner & Watts, 1986). The underlying approach is to measure the amount of imposed force resistance to externally generated passive movement about the examined joint. The passive movements applied in earlier studies were induced either by a torque motor (Fung et al., 2000; Mak et al., 2007; Shapiro et al., 2007; Watts et al., 1986; Xia et al., 2006) or generated by an examiner to closely resemble a clinical setting (Caligiuri, 1994; Endo et al., 2009; Patrick et al., 2001; Prochazka et al., 1997; Sepehri et al., 2007). Variables described in these previous studies included peak torque (Mak et al., 2007), impulse (i.e., an integral of torque with respect to time; Fung et al., 2000), work score which is calculated as a torque integral with respect to joint angular position (see Fig. 3; Fung et al., 2000; Mak et al., 2007; Shapiro et al., 2007; Teräväinen et al., 1989; Xia et al., 2006, 2009), elastic coefficient (Endo et al., 2009), and mechanical impedance calculated based on the force imposed and displacement of the movement (Patrick et al., 2001; Prochazka et al., 1997).

There are a few advantages of quantification by force or torque measures over quantification by EMG. Torque-based assessment of rigidity is more objective and reliable than EMG-derived evaluation. However, there are limitations in estimation of using surface EMGs as its measures are susceptible to the placement of electrodes, condition of soft tissues and concerns of cross-talk. Biomechanical measures using torque can avoid the limitations inherent in EMG measures. In addition, non-neural contribution to parkinsonian rigidity is also included in torque measures but is not reflected in EMG recordings. Previous studies have shown that correlation is relatively weak between clinical degree of rigidity and EMG quantification of rigidity while correlation is found to be much stronger between clinical degree of rigidity and torque quantification of rigidity (Endo et al., 2009; Levin et al., 2009;

Park et al., 2010; Teräväinen et al., 1989). Evidence indicates that torque measure has proven to be a more objective and robust way for assessing rigidity, compared to EMG evaluation of rigidity.

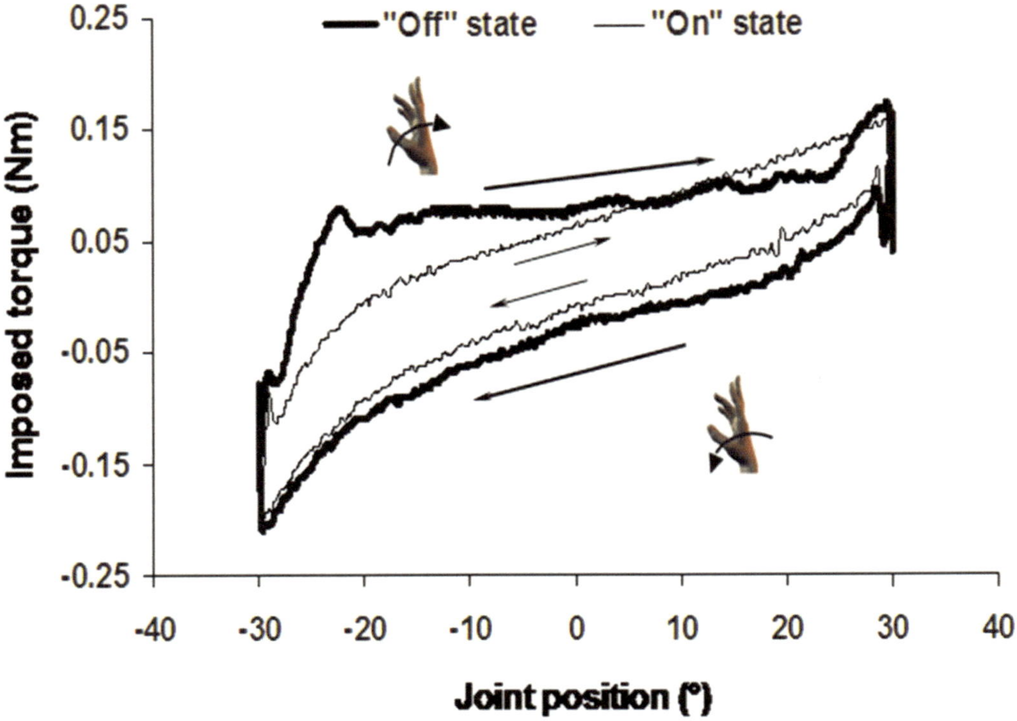

Fig. 3. Torque-angle relationship in a parkinsonian subject in the Off-medication (thicker line) and On-medication (thinner line) states. The subject's more affected side was tested. The upper traces represent imposed extension movements and the lower traces flexion movements. The wrist joint was externally rotated at 50 °/s between 30° flexion and 30° extension shown as a loop. The subject was instructed to remain relaxed. The work, used to quantify the degree of rigidity, was equivalent to the areas inside the loop of torque-angle plots in the respective medication states [from Xia et al. (2006) with permission].

Application of biomechanical measures has also enabled us to investigate more profoundly some of the characteristics associated with parkinsonian rigidity, thus further increasing our understanding of this motor symptom. Firstly, only through the measures of torque resistance and joint position, can lead-pipe nature of rigidity be examined and revealed (Mera et al., 2009; Xia & Rymer, 2004; Xia et al., 2006, 2011). The slope of torque-angle curve was used to quantify the degree of lead-pipe property. The smaller slopes represent higher degrees of constant and uniform resistance through the range of passive movement. The torque-angle slopes are smaller when patients were tested in the untreated conditions, and become greater in the treated conditions (Xia & Rymer, 2004; Xia et al., 2006).

Secondly, rigidity has been thought to be plastic with respect to direction of the movement (Berardelli et al., 1983; Delwaide, 2001). However, recent studies employing the biomechanical measures have demonstrated that rigidity associated with extension movement is more evident as compared to rigidity during flexion movement in the upper limb including the wrist and elbow (Mera et al., 2009; Park et al., 2010; Xia et al., 2006). These authors used mechanical parameters, such as work, torque-angle slope and visco-elastic parameter, to evaluate the difference and distinction between the passive flexion and extension movements.

Thirdly, parkinsonian rigidity has traditionally been considered to be independent of velocity in contrast to spasticity which is highly velocity-dependent (Lance, 1980). The notion of velocity-independency of rigidity might be anecdotal. As such, this view has been examined by a few recent studies. Lee et al. (2002) studied hypertonia at the elbow joint in patients with Parkinson's disease and patients with hemiparesis as compared to control subjects. Four different stretching velocities were applied, ranging from 40 to 160 °/s. The authors concluded that both rigidity and spasticity have approximately equal velocity-dependent property. Quantitative measure of trunk rigidity in patients with Parkinson's disease also revealed a velocity-dependent feature (Mak et al., 2007). Our results on the effect of movement velocity on rigidity concurred with those reports. Velocity-dependency of rigidity was also demonstrated at the wrist joint of patients with Parkinson's disease (Xia et al., 2009) in which both slow velocity at 50 degree/second and fast speed at 280 °/s were applied. The results showed that the work done during the fast movement was significantly larger than the work associated with the slower movement. The accumulating evidence has pointed out the velocity-dependency of parkinsonian rigidity.

Fourthly, compared to the effect of movement velocity on quantitative analysis of parkinsonian rigidity, effect of displacement amplitude on rigidity has thus far sparsely been investigated, except for one study by Teräväinen et al. (1989). To determine the optimal angular velocity and displacement amplitude for detecting abnormal muscle tone, four movement amplitudes or central ranges of motion, ranging from ±15, ±20, ±25 to ±30 degrees, were applied to examine rigidity at the wrist joint in 29 patients with Parkinson's disease. The results showed that the larger movement amplitudes were more sensitive for detecting parkinsonian rigidity and had stronger correlation with the clinical scores of rigidity. Given the situation that some clinicians rotate the limb back and forth rapidly in the mid-range whereas others focus on the extremes of range of motion or the entire range of motion with slow stretches (Prochazka et al., 1997), it is important and significant to explore the influence of displacement amplitude on objective measurements of rigidity. We recently conducted a study aiming to examine the effect of displacement amplitude. Twenty four patients participated in the experiment under treated (On-medication) and untreated (Off-medication) conditions, with the more affected side of the wrist joint tested. Passive movements of wrist flexion and extension were imposed with two displacement amplitudes, ±30 degree and ±45 degree, respectively, at either 50 °/s or 280 °/s, and the order of movement pattern was presented in a random fashion. Figure 4 depicts and compares the torque-angle plots associated with two ranges of motion: 60 degree (Fig. 4A) and 90 degree (Fig. 4B), in a parkinsonian subject under the two medication conditions. The work score was calculated to quantify rigidity, and was normalized to the range of motion to validate the comparison. Clearly, there is a difference in the area of the torque-angle loop between the two displacement amplitudes or the ranges of motion. Figure 4B shows that the extreme joint position, the larger displacement amplitude, caused increase in rigidity work score.

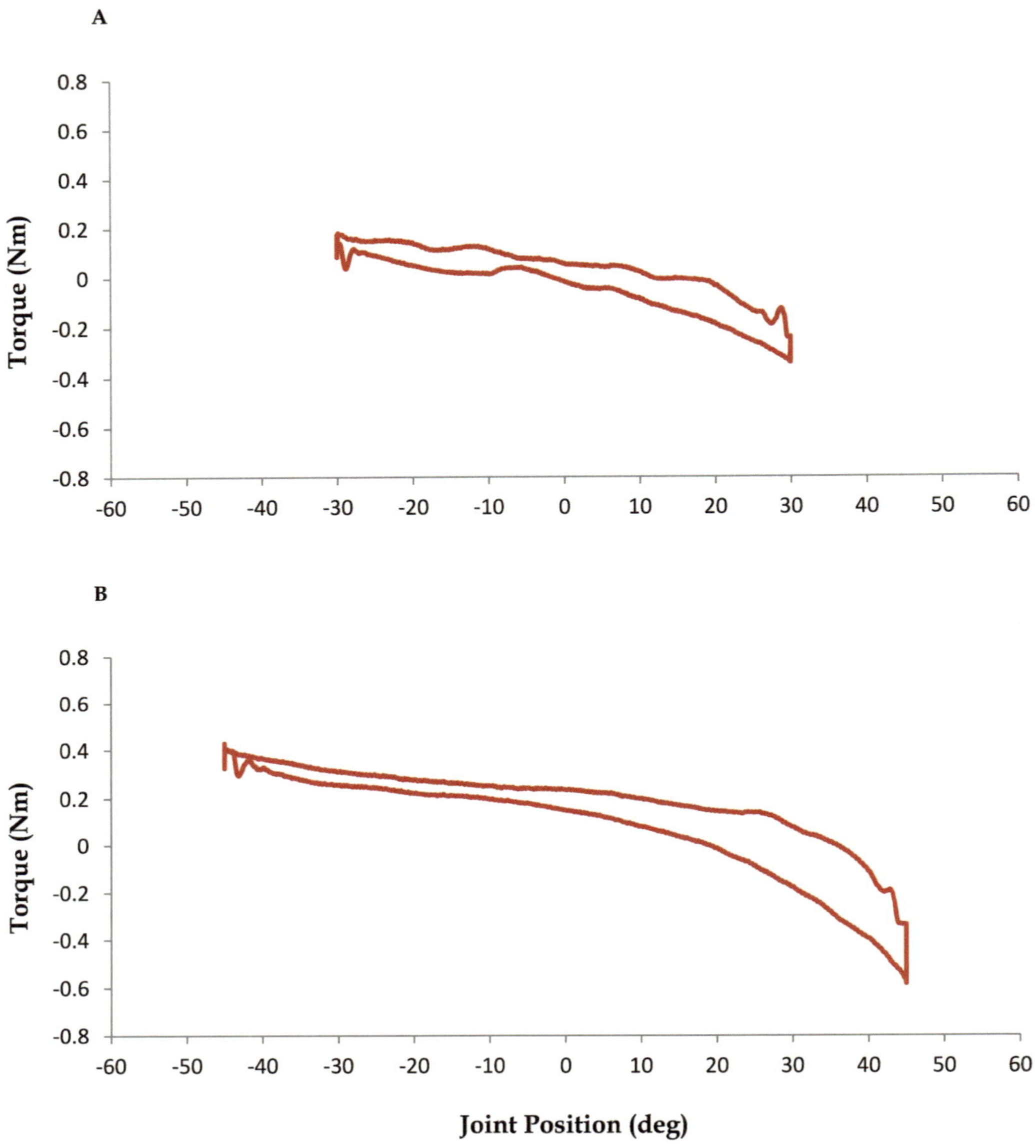

Fig. 4. Comparison of torque-position traces of passive flexion and extension movements of two ranges of motion: 60° (A) and 90° (B) at angular velocity of 50° /s from a subject with Parkinson's disease tested in the Off-medication state. The rigidity score, quantified by the integral of the torque with respect to angular position (Nm-deg), increased in response to the greater range of motion. Upper traces are associated with extension movements while lower traces are associated with flexion movements [from Powell et al. (in press) with permission].

Finally, the phenomenon that rigidity can be reinforced by a concurrent ipsi- or contralateral voluntary activation has recently been further quantified using biomechanical measures (Hong et al., 2007; Powell et al., 2011). Figure 5 illustrates torque-angle traces of the entire cycle of flexion and extension movements when a subject with PD was tested in the Off-medication condition. Torque resistance was elevated by the presence of contralateral activation (Active condition) as compared to the Passive condition. There is an obvious difference in the contained area of torque-angle plots between the Passive and Active conditions. These studies aimed to provide quantitative data and objective evaluation of clinical assessment of rigidity as a component of the Unified Parkinson Disease Rating Scale (Fahn & Elton, 1987; Goetz et al., 2008). The type of voluntary activations applied in clinical examinations include a variety of motor acts such as tapping fingers, fist opening–closing or heel tapping. The use of reinforcing maneuvers was originated and first investigated by Jules Froment, a French neurologist, in the 1920's (Broussolle et al., 2007). Froment studied muscle tone at the wrist joint while the subject was in different positions, at rest in a sitting position, and standing in stable and unstable postures. In addition to clinical examination, Fremont also conducted experiments recording activity of forearm extensors using a myograph. He described an increased resistance to passive movements of a limb about a joint during the presence of a voluntary action of a contralateral body part. Due to his contributions to the study of parkinsonian rigidity, the activation or facilitation test has been referred to as the "Froment maneuver". The impact of facilitation test is significant as it has been formalized in the motor scale of the Unified Parkinson Disease Rating Scale. The maneuver is particularly used to detect increased muscle tone at an early stage of the disease when rigidity is not otherwise manifested during the examination.

6. Effect of anti-Parkinson medication on physiological and biomechanical measures of rigidity

Rigidity generally responds well to anti-Parkinson medication. Several studies have examined the changes in muscle activation, joint torque resistance and torque-angle slope associated with rigidity reduction as a result of medication therapy (Kirollos et al., 1996; Mera et al., 2009; Powell et al., 2011; Xia & Rymer, 2004; Xia et al., 2006, 2009). Following a standard protocol, patients are tested initially in the Off-medication state, *i.e.*, 12 hours after the last dose of medication when the majority of the beneficial effects of medication therapy are eliminated (Defer et al., 1999). Twelve-hour overnight withdrawal of medication has been broadly used to examine the effect of medication on motor performance and on basal ganglia function (Brown & Marsden, 1999; Corcos et al., 1996; Jahanshahi et al., 2010; Robichaud et al., 2004; Tunik et al., 2004). After the initial tests are completed, patients are retested approximately one hour after taking their regular dose of medication in the On-medication state. These studies have demonstrated that stretch-reflex and shortening reaction are diminished following the treatment (Powell et al., 2011; Xia & Rymer, 2004). The same effects are observed in the changes associated with torque resistance (Kirollos et al., 1996; Mera et al., 2009; Xia et al., 2006, 2009). Further, torque-angle curves associated with the On-medication test become steeper, manifesting the spring-like feature and the typical length-tension relationship (Gordon et al., 1966; Matthews, 1959; Rack & Westbury, 1969; Xia et al., 2006, see Fig. 2).

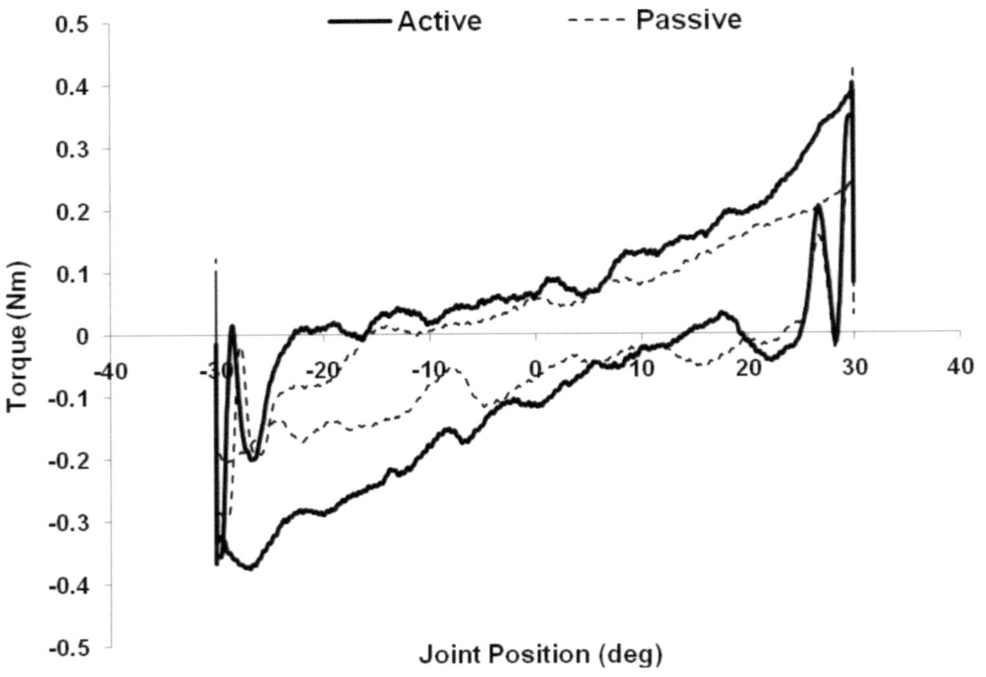

Fig. 5. Comparison of torque-angle traces between the Passive (dashed) and Active (solid) conditions recorded in a subject with Parkinson's disease under the Off-Medication condition. Under the Active condition, passive movement of the wrist joint was concurrent with a contra-lateral hand gripping activation at 20% of maximal voluntary contraction. Rigidity score, calculated as the integral of the torque with respect to position for the entire cycle of flexion and extension movements, was enhanced under the Active condition. Upper traces are associated with the passive extension movement and the lower ones with the flexion movement [from Powell et al. (2011) with permission].

Effects of deep brain stimulation of the subthalamic nucleus in conjunction with medication have also been evaluated on the work rigidity and clinical rigidity scores in patients with Parkinson's disease (Shapiro et al., 2007). Subjects' elbow joints were tested under four experimental conditions determined by various combinations of medication (Off vs. On) and deep brain stimulation (Off vs. On) status. Treatment by deep brain stimulation reduced rigidity as indicated by work score and by rigidity score on the Unified Parkinson Disease Rating Scale. The results suggested that the surgical treatment may be more effective in alleviating rigidity in the upper limb of parkinsonian patients than medications administered at pre-surgery dosage level.

7. Interaction of rigidity with other motor symptoms

Parkinson's disease is characterized by both motor and non-motor related symptoms. Motor symptoms, often referred to as cardinal symptoms, include bradykinesia (slowness and decreased amplitude of movement), muscle rigidity, tremor-at-rest, and postural instability.

According to the diagnostic criteria, clinical diagnosis is based on two cardinal features of the disease (Fahn & Sulzer, 2004; Lang & Lozano, 1998). Parkinson's disease is a heterogeneous disease both across different patients and during the natural progression of the same patient. The heterogeneity of the disease among different patients is reflected by multiple sub-types of Parkinson's disease, i.e., akinetic-rigid type, tremor-predominant type, and postural instability gait difficulty sub-type (Burn et al., 2006; Hallett, 2003; Jankovic et al., 1990). Bradykinesia is labeled as a negative symptom due to its describing the poverty and slowing of voluntary movement, whereas rigidity and tremor are referred to as positive motor symptoms.

Many clinical studies have indicated that the distinctions are significant among the hallmark motor symptoms although they share similarities and common origins (Elias et al., 2008). The distinctive nature has also been revealed by Temperli and coauthors (2003) who studied the reappearance of the clinical signs of Parkinson's disease when subthalamic nucleus deep brain stimulation was switched off in 35 patients treated with implanted deep brain stimulators. Authors reported that a sequential pattern of return of motor signs was observed, with a fast worsening of tremor within 10 to 15 minutes, followed by a smoother, slower worsening of bradykinesia and rigidity over half an hour to an hour, and finally a slow and steady worsening of axial signs over three to four hours. When switching the stimulation "on" again, all motor signs improved with a similar pattern. It was concluded that the four major parkinsonian signs may respond to brain stimulation by different mechanisms.

8. Clinical interventions of Parkinson's disease

Our knowledge and understanding of Parkinson's disease have dramatically increased over the past years, consequently shifting the descriptions of this disease. Parkinson's disease, previously considered to be characterized by only motor symptoms (bradykinesia, rigidity, resting tremor and postural instability), is now viewed as a disease affected by both motor symptoms and a range of non-motor symptoms such as depression, disturbed sleeping patterns, fatigue, hallucination, cognitive impairments, changes in ability to taste or smell and a few other domains. Only during the last couple of decades or so, non-motor related symptoms have begun receiving attention in medical and research communities. As a result, a number of clinical rating tools have been developed to target specific or general non-motor symptoms (Brown et al., 2005; Chaudhuri et al., 2007).

Rigidity is treated as part of parkinsonian motor symptoms. Among the motor symptoms of Parkinson's disease, bradykinesia and rigidity are the signs that are most responsive to medication and surgical treatments. A variety of pharmacological and surgical interventions are available for the management of Parkinson's disease. Levodopa was the first major breakthrough in the treatment of Parkinson's disease, and still remains the "gold standard" in the management of symptoms. Levodopa is converted in the brain into dopamine to replenish the brain's dwindling supply in patients with Parkinson's disease. The introduction of dopamine agonists was a milestone in the treatment of parkinsonian symptoms. In contrast to levodopa, dopamine agonists act directly on dopamine receptors in the brain, and thus can help alleviate the symptoms of Parkinson's disease. Based on preclinical observation, there is an increasingly popular theory known as continuous dopamine agonist stimulation that helps to prevent the occurrence of long-term complications.

However, with the treatment of medication on advanced stage of this progressive disease, many patients experience motor complications, which is broadly classified as "wearing off reactions", "On-Off reactions", dyskinesia, confusion, sleepiness, hallucination, and low blood pressure when standing (Stacy, 2009). In patients who are severely affected or in those who fail to respond satisfactorily to pharmacological therapy, surgical treatments have reportedly been effective in reducing symptoms and improving function. These include pallidotomy, thalamotomy and subthalamotomy, and high frequency deep brain stimulation via electrodes implanted in the globus pallidus, thalamus (a "relay station" deep in brain), or subthalamic nucleus. Rigidity can be specifically improved by subthalamic nucleus deep brain stimulation (Temperli et al., 2003).

9. Conclusion

Evidence has indicated that no single mechanism can account for parkinsonian rigidity, which is influenced by a multitude of physiological phenomena and biomechanical features. Treatment of rigidity primarily involves an administration of dopaminergic medication. However, serious side effects usually occur after a few years' drug treatment. Therefore, rehabilitative programs are highly desirable for patients with Parkinson's disease. A better understanding of the comprehensive characteristics of parkinsonian rigidity is crucial for designing effective evidence-based exercise program and physical therapy intervention. An objective assessment of rigidity is essential for evaluating the efficacy of therapeutic interventions, especially in large clinical studies in which trials are conducted across multiple centers.

10. Acknowledgments

The author would like to acknowledge support of the National Institutes of Health, Nebraska Tobacco Settlement Biomedical Research Development Fund, Health Future Foundation of Creighton University, and Faculty Development Fund of School of Pharmacy and Health Professions, Creighton University in Omaha Nebraska, USA.

11. References

Alibiglou, L.; Rymer, WZ.; Harvey, RL. & Mirbagheri MM. (2008). The relation between Ashworth scores and neuromechanical measurements of spasticity following stroke. *J Neuroeng Rehabil*, Vol.5, pp. 18-31.

Andrews, CJ.; Burke, D. & Lance, JW. (1972). The response to muscle stretch and shortening in Parkinsonian rigidity. *Brain,* Vol.95, pp. 795-812.

Angel, RW. (1983). Muscular contractions elicited by passive shortening. *Adv Neurol*, Vol.39, pp. 555-563.

Bantam Medical Dictionary (2000). 3rd edition, New York, USA: Bantam Books, Incorporated.

Berardelli, A. & Hallett, M. (1984). Shortening reaction of human tibialis anterior. *Neurology,* Vol. 34, pp. 242-246.

Berardelli, A.; Sabra, AF. & Hallett, M. (1983). Physiological mechanisms of rigidity in Parkinson's disease. *J Neurol Neurosurg Psychiatry,* Vol.46, pp. 45-53.

Broussolle, E.; Krack, P.; Thobois, S.; Xie-Brustolin, J.; Pollak, P. & Goetz, C.G. (2007). Contribution of Jules Froment to the study of parkinsonian rigidity. *Mov Disord,* Vol.22, pp. 909-14.

Brown, R.G.; Dittner, A.; Findley, L. & Wessely, S.C. (2005). The Parkinson fatigue scale. *Parkinsonism Relat Disord,* Vol. 11, pp. 49–55.

Brown, P. & Marsden, CD. (1999). Bradykinesia and impairment of EEG desynchronization in Parkinson's disease. *Mov Disord,* Vol.14, pp.423-429.

Bergui, M.; Lopiano, L.; Paglia, G.; Quattrocolo, G.; Scarzella, L. & Bergamasco, B. (1992). Stretch reflex of quadriceps femoris and its relation to rigidity in Parkinson's disease. *Acta Neurol Scand,* Vol. 86, pp. 226-229.

Burke, D.; Andrews, CJ. & Lance JW. (1972a). Tonic vibration reflex in spasticity, Parkinson's disease, and normal subjects. *J Neurol Neurosurg Psychiatry,* Vol.35, pp. 477-486.

Burke, D.; Gillies, JD. & Lance, JW. (1970). The quadriceps stretch reflex in human spasticity. *Journal of Neurology, Neurosurgery and Psychiatry,* Vol. 33, pp. 216-223.

Burke, D.; Hagbarth, KE. & Wallin, BG. (1977). Reflex mechanisms in Parkinsonian rigidity. *Scand J Rehabil Med.,* Vol.9, pp. 15-23.

Burke, D.; Knowles, L.; Andrews, C. & Ashby, P. (1972b). Spasticity, decerebrate rigidity and the clasp-knife phenomenon: an experimental study in the cat. *Brain,* Vol. 95, pp. 31-48.

Burn, DJ.; Rowan, EN.; Allan, LM.; Molloy, S.; O'Brien, JT. & McKeith, IG. (2006). Motor subtype and cognitive decline in Parkinson's disease, Parkinson's disease with dementia, and dementia with Lewy bodies. *J Neurol Neurosurg Psychiatry,* Vol. 77, pp.585-9.

Caligiuri, M.P. (1994). Portable device for quantifying parkinsonian wrist rigidity. *Mov Disord,* Vol. 9(1), pp. 57-63.

Chaudhuri KR, Martinez-Martin P, Brown RG, Sethi K, Stocchi F, Odin P, Ondo W, Abe K, Macphee G, Macmahon D, Barone P, Rabey M, Forbes A, Breen K, Tluk S, Naidu Y, Olanow W, Williams AJ, Thomas S, Rye D, Tsuboi Y, Hand A, Schapira AH 2007. The metric properties of a novel non-motor symptoms scale for Parkinson's disease: Results from an international pilot study. *Mov Disord.* Oct 15;22(13):1901-11.

Cody, FWJ.; MacDermott, N.; Matthews, PBC. & Richardson, HC. (1986). Observations on the genesis of the stretch reflex in Parkinson's disease. *Brain,* Vol.109, pp. 229-249.

Corcos, DM.; Chen, CM.; Quinn, NP.; McAuley, J. & Rothwell, JC. (1996). Strength in Parkinson's disease: relationship to rate of force generation and clinical status. *Ann Neurol,* Vol.39, pp.79-88.

De Lau, LM. & Breteler, MM. (2006). Epidemiology of Parkinson's disease. *Lancet Neurol,* Vol.5, pp. 525-535.

Defer, GL.; Widner, H.; Marié, RM.; Rémy, P. & Levivier, M. (1999). Core assessment program for surgical interventional therapies in Parkinson's disease (CAPSIT-PD). *Mov Disord,* Vol.14, pp.572-84.

Delp, SL. & Loan, JP. (1995) A graphics-based software system to develop and analyze models of musculoskeletal structures. *Comput Biol Med,* Vol. 25, pp. 21–34.

Delwaide, PJ. (1985). Are there modifications in spinal cord functions of parkinsonian patients? In: *Clinical Neurophysiology in Parkinsonism,* P.J. Delwaide, A. Agnoli, (Ed.) pp. 19- 32, Elsevier, New York, USA.

Delwaide, P.J. (2001). Parkinsonian rigidity. *Funct Neurol* Vol. 16(2), pp. 147-56.

Delwaide, PJ.; Sabbatino, M. & Delwaide, C. (1986). Some pathophysiological aspects of the parkinsonian rigidity. *J Neural Transm Suppl,* Vol.22, pp.129-39.

Dietrichson, P. (1971). Phasic ankle reflex in spasticity and Parkinsonian rigidity. The role of the fusimotor system. *Acta Neurol Scand*, Vol.47, pp. 22-51.

Dietz, V. (1987). Changes of inherent muscle stiffness in Parkinson's disease. *J Neurol Neurosurg Psychiatry*, Vol. 50, pp. 944.

Dietz, V.; Quintern, J. & Berger, W. (1981). Electrophysiological studies of gait in spasticity and rigidity. Evidence that altered mechanical properties of muscle contribute to hypertonia. *Brain*, Vol.104, pp. 431-449.

Dorsey, E.R.; Constantinescu, R.; Thompson, JP.; Biglan, KM.; Holloway, RG.; Kieburtz, K.; Marshall, FJ.; Ravina, BM.; Schifitto, G.; Siderowf, A. & Tanner, CM. (2007). Projected number of people with Parkinson disease in the most populous nations, 2005 through 2030. *Neurol*, Vol. 68(5), pp.384-6.

Elias, S.; Israel, Z. & Bergman, H. (2008). Physiology of Parkinson's disease. In: *Therapeutics of Parkinson's Disease and Other Movement Disorders*, M. Hallett, W. Poewe, (Ed). 25-36, John Wiley & Sons Ltd., ISBN 978-0-470-06648-5, West Sussex, UK.

Endo, T.; Okuno, R.; Yokoe, M.; Akazawa, K. & Sakoda, S. (2009). A novel method for systematic analysis of rigidity in Parkinson's disease. *Mov Disord*, Vol.24, pp. 2218-2224.

Fahn, S. & Elton, RL. (1987) Members of the UPDRS development committee. Unified parkinson's disease rating scale, In: *Recent developments in Parkinson's disease*, S. Fahn, D. C. Marsden, P. Jenner, P. Teychenne, (Ed). 153-164, Macmillian Healthcare, ISBN 978-088-1671-32-2, Florham, New Jersey, USA.

Fahn, S. (2003). Description of Parkinson's disease as a clinical syndrome. *Ann NY Acad Sci*, Vol.991, pp. 1-14.

Fahn, S. & Sulzer, D. (2004). Neurodegeneration and neuroprotection in Parkinson disease. *NeuroRx*, Vol. 1, pp.139-54.

Feldman, AG. (1966). Functional tuning of the nervous system on control of movement or maintenance of a steadyposture. II. Controllable parameters of the muscle. *Biophysics*, Vol.11, pp. 565-578.

Forester, O. (1921). Zur Analyse und Pathophysiologie der striaten Bewegungsstörungen. *Z Ges Neurol Psychiat*, Vol.73, pp. 1-169

Fung, VS. & Thompson, PD. (2002). Rigidity and spasticity, In: *Parkinson's disease and Movement Disorders*, J. J. Jankovic, E. Tolosa (4th. Ed.), 473-482, Lippincott Williams & Wilkins, ISBN: 0-7817-7881-6, Philadelphia, USA.

Fung, VS.; Burne, JA. & Morris, JG. (2000). Objective quantification of resting and activated parkinsonian rigidity: a comparison of angular impulse and work scores. *Mov Disord*, Vol.15, pp. 48-55

Galiana, L.; Fung, J. & Kearney, R. (2005). Identification of intrinsic and reflex ankle stiffness components in stroke patients. *Exp Brain Res*, Vol.165, pp. 422-434.

Goetz, CG.; Tilley, BC.; Shaftman, SR.; Stebbins, GT.; Fahn, S.; Martinez-Martin, P.; Poewe, W.; Sampaio, C.; Stern, MB.; Dodel, R.; Dubois, B.; Holloway, R.; Jankovic, J.; Kulisevsky, J; Lang, AE.; Lees, A.; Leurgans, S.; LeWitt, PA.; Nyenhuis, D.; Olanow, CW.; Rascol, O.; Schrag, A.; Teresi, JA.; van Hilten, JJ. & LaPelle, N. (2008). Movement Disorder Society-sponsored revision of the Unified Parkinson's Disease Rating Scale (MDS-UPDRS): scale presentation and clinimetric testing results. *Mov Disord*, Vol.23, pp. 2129-2170

Gordon, AM.; Huxley, AF. & Julian, FJ. (1966). The variation in isometric tension with sarcomere length in vertebrate muscle fibres. *J Physiol*, Vol. 184, pp. 170-192.

Hallett, M. (2003). Parkinson revisited: pathophysiology of motor signs. *Adv Neurol*, Vol.91, pp. 19-28.

Holzbaur, KR.; Murray, WM. & Delp, SL. (2005) A model of the upper extremity for simulating musculoskeletal surgery and analyzing neuromuscular control. *Ann Biomed Eng*, Vol.33. pp. 829–840.

Hong, M.; Perlmutter, J.S. & Earhart, G.M. (2007). Enhancement of rigidity in Parkinson's disease with activation. *Mov Disord*, Vol. 22, pp. 1164-8.

Jahanshahi, M.; Jones, CR.; Zijlmans, J.; Katzenschlager, R.; Lee, L.; Quinn, N.; Frith, CD. & Lees AJ. (2010). Dopaminergic modulation of striato-frontal connectivity during motor timing in Parkinson's disease. *Brain*, Vol. 133, pp.727-745.

Jankovic, J.; McDermott, M.; Carter, J.; Gauthier, S.; Goetz, C.; Golbe, L.; Huber, S.; Koller, W.; Olanow, C.; Shoulson, I. et al. (1990). Variable expression of Parkinson's disease: a base-line analysis of the DATATOP cohort. The Parkinson Study Group. *Neurol*, Vol. 40, pp.1529-34.

Kearney, RE.; Stein, RB. & Parameswaran, L. (1997). Identification of intrinsic and reflex contributions to human ankle stiffness dynamics. *IEEE Trans Biomed Eng*, Vol.44, pp. 493-504.

Kirollos, C.; Charlett, A.; O'Neill, CJ.; Kosik, R.; Mozol, K.; Purkiss, AG.; Bowes, SG.; Nicholson, PW.; Hunt, WB.; Weller, C.; Dobbs, SM. & Dobbs, RJ. (1996). Objective measurement of activation of rigidity: diagnostic, pathogenetic and therapeutic implications in parkinsonism. *Br J Clin Pharmaco*, Vol. 41, pp.557-64.

Lance, JW. (1980). Pathophysiology of spasticity and clinical experience with baclofen, In: *Spasticity: disordered motor control*, R. G. Feldman, R. R. Young, W. P. Koella, (Ed). 185-203, ISBN - 978-081-5132-40-0, Year Book Medical Publishers, Chicago, Illinois, USA.

Lance, JW.; Burke, D. & Andrews, CJ. (1973). The reflex effects of muscle vibration. In: *New Developments in Electromyography and Clinical Neurophysiology*, J. E. Desmedt (Ed), 3:44-462, ISBN 978-380-5514-09-5 Basel: Karger, Switzerland

Lang, A.E. & Lozano, A.M. (1998). Parkinson's disease. First of two parts. *N Engl J Med*, 339:1044-53.

Lee, HM.; Huang, YZ.; Chen, JJ. & Hwang, IS. (2002). Quantitative analysis of the velocity related pathophysiology of spasticity and rigidity in the elbow flexors. *J Neurol Neurosurg Psychiatry*, Vol.72, pp. 621–9.

Lee, RG. & Tatton, WG. (1975). Motor responses to sudden limb displacements in primates with specific CNS lesions and in human patients with motor system disorders. *Can J Neurol Sci*, Vol.2, pp. 285-293.

Levin, J.; Krafczyk, S.; Valkovic, P.; Eggert, T.; Claassen, J. & Bötzel, K. (2009). Objective measurement of muscle rigidity in Parkinsonian patients treated with subthalamic stimulation. *Mov Disord*, Vol.24(1), pp. 57-63.

Mak, MK.; Wong, EC. & Hui-Chan, CW. (2007). Quantitative measurement of trunk rigidity in Parkinsonian patients. *J Neurol*, Vol.254, pp. 202–209.

Martinez-Martin, P. (1993). "Rating sales in Parkinson's disease," In: *Parkinson's Disease and Movement Disorders*, 2nd ed, J. Jankovic, E. Tolosa, (Eds.), 281-292, Williams & Wilkins, Baltimore, MD, USA.

Marsden, CD. (1990). Neurophysiology. In: *Parkinson's disease*, G. Stern, (Ed.), 57-98, Johns Hopkins University Press, Baltimore, MD, USA.

Matthews, PBC. (1959). The dependence of tension upon extension in the stretch reflex of the soleus muscle of the decerebrate cat. *J Physiol*, Vol.147, pp.521-546

Matthews, PBC. (1991). The human stretch reflex and the motor cortex. *Trends Neurosci*, Vol.14, pp. 87-91

Meara, RJ. & Cody, FWJ. (1993). Stretch reflexes of individual parkinsonian patients studied during changes in clinical rigidity following medication. *Electroencephalogr Clin Neurophysiol*, Vol.89, pp. 261-268

Mera, T.O.; Johnson, M.D.; Rothe, D.; Zhang, J.; Xu, W.; Ghosh, D.; Vitek, J. & Alberts, J.L. (2009). Objective quantification of arm rigidity in MPTP-treated primates. *J Neurosci Methods*. Vol.177(1):20-29.

Meinders, M.; Price, R.; Lehmann, JF. & Questad, KA (1996). The stretch reflex response in the normal and spastic ankle: effect of ankle position. *Arch Phys Med Rehabil*, Vol. 77(5), pp. 487-92.

Mirbagheri, MM.; Barbeau, H.; Ladouceur, M. & Kearney, RE. (2001). Intrinsic and reflex stiffness in normal and spastic, spinal cord injured subjects. *Exp Brain Res*, Vol.141, pp. 446-459.

Mirbagheri, MM.; Chen, D. & Rymer W.Z. (2010). Quantification of the effects of an alpha-2 adrenergic agonist on reflex properties in spinal cord injury using a system identification technique. *J Neuroeng Rehabil*, Vol.7, pp. 29-35.

Mirbagheri, M.M.; Tsao, C. & Rymer, W.Z. (2009). Natural history of neuromuscular properties after stroke: a longitudinal study. *J Neurol Neurosurg Psychiatry*, Vol. 80, pp. 1212-1217.

Mortimer, JA. & Webster, DD. (1979). Evidence for a quantitative association between EMG stretch responses and Parkinsonian rigidity. *Brain Res.*, Vol.162, pp. 169-173.

Obeso, JA.; Linazasoro, G.; Rothwell, JC.; Jahanshahi, M. & Brown, R. (1996). Assessing the effects of pallidotomy in Parkinson's disease. *The Lancet*, Vol. 347(9013), pp. 1490

Ondo, WG.; Jankovic, J.; Lai, EC.; Sankhla, C.; Khan, M.; Ben-Arie, L.; Schwartz, K.; Grossman, RG. & Krauss, JK. (1998). Assessment of motor function after stereotactic pallidotomy. *Neurology*, Vol.50(1), pp. 266-70

Park, B.K.; Kwon, Y.; Kim, J.W.; Lee, J.H.; Eom, G.M.; Koh, S.B.; Jun, J.H. & Hong, J. (2010). Analysis of viscoelastic properties of wrist joint for quantification of Parkinsonian rigidity. *IEEE T Neur Sys Reh*, Vol.99, ISSN: 1534-4320

Patrick, S.K.; Denington, A.A.; Gauthier, M.J.; Gillard, D.M. & Prochazka, A. (2001). Quantification of the UPDRS Rigidity Scale. *IEEE Trans Neural Syst Rehabil Eng.*, Vol. 9, pp. 31-41.

Pollock. LJ. & Davis, L. (1930). Muscle tone in Parkinsonian states. *Arch Neurol Psychiatry*, Vol.23, Pp. 303- 319

Powell, D; Hanson, N.; Threlkeld, AJ.; Fang, X. & Xia, R. (2011). Enhancement of parkinsonian rigidity with contralateral hand activation. *Clin Neurophysiol* Vol.122, pp. 1595-1601.

Powell, D.; Threlkeld, AJ.; Fang, X.; Muthumani, A. & Xia, R. Amplitude- and velocity-dependency of rigidity measured at the wrist in Parkinson's disease. *Clin Neurophysiol (in press)*.

Prochazka, A.; Bennett, DJ.; Stephens. MJ.; Patrick, SK.; Sears-Duru, R.; Roberts, T, & Jhamandas, JH. (1997). Measurement of rigidity in Parkinson's disease. *Mov Disord*, Vol.12, pp. 24-32

Rabey, JM.; Bass, H.; Bonuccelli, U.; Brooks, D.; Klotz, P.; Korczyn, AD.; Kraus, P.; Martinez-Martin, P.; Morrish, P.; Van Sauten, W. & Van Hilten, B. (1997). Evaluation of the Short Parkinson's Evaluation Scale: a new friendly scale for the evaluation of Parkinson's disease in clinical drug trials. *J Neuropharmacol*, Vol.20(4), pp. 322-37.

Rack, PM. & Westbury, DR. (1969). The effects of length and stimulus rate on tension in the isometric cat soleus muscle. *J Physiol*, Vol. 204, pp. 443-460.

Richards, M.; Marder, K.; Cote, L. & Mayeux, R. (1994). Interrater reliability of the Unified Parkinson's Disease Rating Scale motor examination. *Mov Disord*, Vol.9(1), pp. 89-91.

Robichaud, JA.; Pfann, KD.; Comella, CL.; Brandabur, M. & Corcos DM. (2004). Greater impairment of extension movements as compared to flexion movements in Parkinson's disease. *Exp Brain Res*, Vol. 156, pp.240-254.

Rondot, P. & Metral, S. (1973). Analysis of the shortening reaction in man. In: *New Developments in Electromyography and Clinical Neurophysiology*, J.E. Desmedt, (Ed), 3:629-634, ISBN 978-380-5514-09-5, Basel: Karger, Switzerland

Rothwell, JC.; Obeso, JA.; Traub, MM. & Marsden, CD. (1983). The behaviour of the long-latency stretch reflex in patients with Parkinson's disease. *J Neurol Neurosurg Psychiatry*, Vol.46, pp. 35-44

Rushworth, G. (1960). Spasticity and rigidity: An experimental study and review. *J Neurol Neurosurg Psychiatry*, Vol.23, pp. 99-118

Rymer, WZ. & Katz, RT. (1994). Mechanisms of spastic hypertonia. *Phys Med Rehabil: State of the Art Reviews*, Vol.8, pp. 441-454.

Rymer, WZ.; Houk. JC. & Crago, PE. (1979). Mechanisms of the clasp-knife reflex studied in an animal model. *Exp Brain Res*, Vol.37, pp. 93-113.

Sepehri, B.; Esteki, A.; Ebrahimi-Takamjani, E.; Shahidi, GA.; Khamseh, F. & Moinodin, M. (2007). Quantification of rigidity in Parkinson's disease. *Ann Biomed Eng*, Vol.35(12), pp. 2196-203.

Shapiro, MB.; Vaillancourt, DE.; Sturman, MM.; Metman, LV.; Bakay, RA. & Corcos, DM. (2007). Effects of STN DBS on rigidity in Parkinson's disease. *IEEE Trans Neural Syst Rehabil Eng*. Vol.15, pp. 173-181.

Sherrington, CS. (1909). On plastic tonus and proprioceptive reflexes. *Q J Exp Physiol* , Vol.2, pp. 109- 156.

Sinkjaer, T. & Magnussen, I. (1994). Passive, intrinsic and reflex-mediated stiffness in the ankle extensors of hemiparetic patients. *Brain*, Vol.117, pp. 355–363.

Sinkjaer, T.; Toft, E.; Larsen, K.; Andreassen, S. & Hansen, HJ. (1993). Non-reflex and reflex mediated ankle joint stiffness in in multiple sclerosis patients with spasticity. *Muscle Nerve*, Vol.16, pp. 69–76.

Tanner, CM. & Ben-Shlomo, Y. (1999). Epidemiology of Parkinson's disease. *Adv Neurol* Vol.80, pp.153-159.

Tanner, CM. & Goldman, SM. (1996). Epidemiology of Parkinson's disease. *Neurol Clin*, Vol.14, pp.317-335.

Temperli, P.; Ghika, J.; Villemure, J.G.; Burkhard, P.R.; Bogousslavsky, J. & Vingerhoets, F.J. (2003). How do parkinsonian signs return after discontinuation of subthalamic DBS? *Neurology*, Vol.60, pp. 78-81.

Teräväinen, H.; Tsui, JKC.; Mak, E., & Calne, DB. (1989). Optimal indices for testing parkinsonian rigidity. *Can. J. Neurol Sci.*, Vol.16, pp. 180-183.

Tunik, E.; Poizner, H.; Adamovich, SV.; Levin, MF. & Feldman, AG. (2004). Deficits in adaptive upper limb control in response to trunk perturbations in Parkinson's disease. *Exp Brain Res*, Vol.159, pp.23-32.

Van Dillen, LR. & Roach, KE. (1988). Interrater reliability of a clinical scale of rigidity. *Phys Ther*, Vol.68(11), pp. 1679-81.

Ward, CD.; Sanes, JN.; Dambrosia, JM. & Calne, DB. (1983). Methods for evaluating treatment in Parkinson's disease. *Adv Neurol*, Vol. 37, pp. 1-7.

Watts, RL.; Wiegner, AW. & Young, RR. (1986). Elastic properties of muscles measured at the elbow in man: II. Patients with parkinsonian rigidity. *J Neurol Neurosurg Psychiatry*, Vol.49, pp. 1177-1181.

Westphal, C. (1877). Unterschenkelphänomen und Nervendehnung. *Archiv Fur Psychiatrie Und Nervenkrankheiten*, Vol. 7, pp. 666-670.

Westphal, C. (1880). Űber eine Art paradoxer Muskel-contraction. *Archiv Fur Psychiatrie Und Nervenkrankheiten*, Vol.10, pp. 243-248.

Wiegner, AW. & Watts, RL. (1986). Elastic properties of muscles measured at the elbow in man: I. Normal controls. *J Neurol Neurosurg Psychiatry*, Vol.49(10), pp. 1171-6.

Xia, R. & Rymer, WZ. (2004). The role of shortening reaction in mediating rigidity in Parkinson's disease. *Exp Brain Res*, Vol.156, pp. 524-528.

Xia, R.; Markopoulou, K.; Puumala, SE. & Rymer, WZ. (2006). A comparison of the effects of imposed extension and flexion movements on Parkinsonian rigidity. *Clin Neurophysiol*, Vol.117, pp. 2302-2307.

Xia, R.; Powell, D.; Rymer, WZ.; Hanson, N.; Fang, X. & Threlkeld, AJ. (2011). Differentiation of contributions between shortening reaction and stretch-induced inhibition in Parkinson's disease. *Exp Brain Res'*, Vol.209, pp.609–618 DOI 10.1007/s00221-011-2594-2.

Xia, R.; Radovic, M.; Mao, ZH. & Threlkeld, AJ. (2010). System identification and modeling approach to characterizing rigidity in Parkinson's disease: neural and non-neural contributions. *Proceedings of the 4th International Conference on Bioinformatics and Biomedical Engineering* (iCBBE 2010), Paper No. 40046 (4 pages), doi: 10.1109/ICBBE.2010.5514861

Xia, R.; Sun, J. & Threlkeld. AJ, (2009). Analysis of interactive effect of stretch reflex and shortening reaction on rigidity in Parkinson's disease. *Clin Neurophysiol*, Vol.120, pp. 1400-1407.

Zhang, LQ. & Rymer, WZ. (1997). Simultaneous and nonlinear identification of mechanical and reflex properties of human elbow joint muscles. *IEEE Trans Biomed Eng*, Vol. 44(12), pp. 1192-209.

23

Mesothalamic Dopaminergic Activity: Implications in Sleep Alterations in Parkinson's Disease

Daniele Q. M. Madureira
Laboratório Nacional de Computação Científica
Brazil

1. Introduction

Movement, sleep and cognition: three connected realms enriching to the human life. Three harmed realms limiting parkinsonian patients.

A degenerative process in dopaminergic neurons from the substantia nigra (SN) midbrain nucleus is the basic origin underlying a set of symptoms developed in patients with Parkinson's Disease (PD) (Andrade & Ferraz, 2003). The devastating motor difficulties usually do not appear isolated. Indeed, PD consists of distinct kinds of manifestations involving motor and mental rigidity as well as sleep alterations (Dubois & Pillon, 1996; Rye et al., 2000; De Cock et al., 2008; Arnulf & Leu-Semenescu, 2009).

Even though impairments in other brain nuclei also contribute to the symptoms present in PD (Braak et al., 2000), it is surprising how so distinct brain systems suffer influence of the degenerative alterations in the SN. This phenomenon may be regarded as a simple consequence of the connections between the SN and diverse brain areas. As a matter of fact, it also highlights that distinct behavioral aspects are achieved through the sharing of brain resources. Here, we examine - through a neurocomputational model - relationships between alterations in the mesothalamic dopaminergic activity (MDA) and sleep impairments in PD.

With origins in the SN, the mesothalamic pathway (MP) reaches the thalamic complex, in particular the thalamic reticular nucleus (TRN). Investigations on such dopaminergic pathway, evidenced by Freeman and colleagues (Freeman et al., 2001), have been contributing to a more global comprehension of cognitive processes in the brain. Based on experimental results (Florán et al., 2004), the mathematical model proposed in (Madureira et al., 2010) indicates a way by which the mesothalamic dopamine inhibits neurons in the TRN. And computational simulations of this model suggest that alterations in the MDA lead to inattention symptoms as observed in PD and Attention Deficit Hyperactivity Disorder (ADHD).

Thalamic neurons are able to spike under tonic and burst states (Steriade et al., 1993; Llinás & Steriade, 2006). Whenever in the tonic state, these neurons respond linearly to input stimuli. By this way, they propagate information reliably from perceptual systems to the cerebral cortex, where a more refined processing takes place. This mode of activity is crucial to the thalamocortical filtering of perceptual stimuli that allows attention focusing (Madureira et al., 2007, 2010; Carvalho, 1994).

Conversely, under the burst state thalamic neurons are no more reliable channels through which neural representations from sensorial inputs reach the cerebral cortex. As a matter of fact, this mode of activity underlies the thalamic behavior during sleep (Steriade et al., 1993; Pace-Schott & Hobson, 2002). In this case, the environmental stimuli are not perceived consciously as it occurs throughout wakefulness (Carvalho, 1994). The thalamic burst mode also permeates epileptic episodes during which environmental information is not processed reliably (Jeanmonod et al., 1996; Llinás et al., 1999). The dynamics of the ionic channels under the burst mode are different from the ones underlying the thalamic tonic state. That is why, under the burst mode, thalamic neurons spike quite autonomously, in such a way that their pattern of activity does not represent the input information.

Since the inattention symptoms addressed in (Madureira et al., 2010) concerned awakened people, the model considered the behavior of thalamic neurons under the tonic state. In the present work, we go further with the matter and scrutinize relationships between the MDA and the oscillatory state of neurons in the thalamic complex. Doing so, it becomes possible to widen the investigation to examine a possible MDA contribution to sleep alterations in PD and, to look at attention focusing aspects under a little more detailed point of view.

Clinical evidences indicating a variety of sleep alterations in PD suggest that this class of symptoms should not be considered as a secondary one: on the contrary, sleep problems certainly pertain to the core symptoms that define PD (De Cock et al., 2008; Arnulf & Leu-Semenescu, 2009). Such sleep alterations involve daytime sleepiness, inappropriate intrusion of REM sleep episodes throughout the day, and nocturne movement. In other words, parkinsonism disrupts the control of the sleep-wake cycle (Jancovic, 2002; Arnulf & Leu-Semenescu, 2009).

The question thus that naturally arises concerns the dopaminergic role in the sleep-wake cycle control. Given the clinical evidence from sleep impairments in PD, a disease whose basic neural origins is the dopaminergic neurons degeneration, we tend to conclude that dopamine does participate in the sleep regulation. Is it the case?

Up to recently, the above mentioned clinical observations have been quite disregarded. If, through PD, the dopaminergic participation in the control of the sleep cycle may be inferred (Rye, 2004), there is, on the other hand, a number of neuroscientific studies showing that the variation in the dopaminergic level throughout the sleep-wake cycle is too small to be taken into account (Jancovic, 2002).

A series of experiments undertaken by (Dzirasa et al., 2006), however, illuminated this controversy. They were capable of demonstrating that sleep-wake states are also controlled by dopamine. This seminal work shows the importance of the dopaminergic influence in the sleep regulation - even under small variations. In addition, they emphasize the relationship between dopaminergic alterations and sleep impairments in PD.

Here, we address - through a neurocomputational approach - the interference of SN neurons, particularly the degenerated ones, in the thalamocortical spiking modes. Our goal consists in investigating if the PD dopaminergic disruption alters the typical spiking patterns associated to sleep and wake states, thus compromising the normal sleep-wake cycle in PD.

We now outline the contents of this chapter. In Section 2 we introduce our hypothesis of dopaminergic influence on the control of the sleep-wake cycle, and describe the model. In Section 3, we explain how the computational simulations of the model are designed, and present the computational results. Finally, we conclude by discussing the consequences of our results in terms of sleep alterations in PD, in the context of the neuroscience of sleep.

2. The model

In (Madureira et al., 2010), we proposed a mathematical model indicating how the mesothalamic dopamine influences the thalamocortical loop, through the TRN, and thus modulates the attentional focus formation. In particular, we investigated relationships between alterations in this dopaminergic pathway and attention deficits in PD and ADHD.

Here, we extend this model to address how dopamine influences the emergence of distinct spiking modes in thalamic neurons. Since the thalamic modes of spiking are specifically related to sleep and wake neuron states, our modeling enables us to discuss if and how dopaminergic alterations in PD are related to the sleep problems observed in the disease.

Throughout the sleep-wake cycle, complex chemical and electrical networks of events occur in the thalamocortical neural circuit. They give rise to distinct patterns of neural behavior that underlies the different brain rhythms specifically associated to different sleep phases and also to the wake state (Pace-Schott & Hobson, 2002; Hobson & Pace-Schott, 2002; Diekelmann & Born, 2010).

The variety of brain rhythms extensively studied by the neuroscience of sleep (Steriade et al., 2003; De Gennaro & Ferrara, 2003; Llinás & Steriade, 2006; Steriade, 2006; Pace-Schott & Hobson, 2002; Hobson & Pace-Schott, 2002; Hobson, 2009; Diekelmann & Born, 2010) reflects the behavior of neural groups. Indeed, such brain rhythms, e.g. spindles, slow oscillation and theta activity, are measurements of field potential oscillations captured by EEGs experiments - not by single cell recordings. Therefore, they provide information from a scale above the cellular one.

Our model, on the other hand, addresses the dynamics of ionic and synaptic currents. It thus deals with information at the same level of single cell recordings, in particular, variations in the membrane electric potential.

Under this approach, it is reasonable to examine sleep issues by mathematically modeling neurons in the thalamocortical loop, and computationally simulating the action of neuromodulators throughout this brain area.

As an outcome of our neurocomputational model, we conjecture that the inhibitory action of mesothalamic dopamine in the thalamic reticular nucleus (TRN) (Florán et al., 2004) affects the spiking mode of thalamocortical neurons. This is possible whenever the dopaminergic action leads to a period of neuron hyperpolarization that activates the calcium conductance, thus changing the way by which the neuron behaves (Carvalho, 1994). Next, we present the model and develop such ideas more deeply.

2.1 The neural network

We model a thalamocortical circuit with a dopaminergic projection from SN to the TRN, according to Figure 1. We can note the excitatory and inhibitory connections in the modeled neural network. Thalamocortical and corticothalamic projections are excitatory, mediated by glutamate. Both areas send glutamatergic excitatory collateral axons to the TRN. Conversely, efferent projections from the TRN to thalamus are GABAergic inhibitory (Guillery & Harting, 2003).

With relation to the dopaminergic action, the architecture of the network incorporates results gathered together from Freeman et al. (2001) and Florán et al. (2004), which reveal the inhibitory dopaminergic projection from SN to the TRN, or the mesothalamic dopaminergic pathway. The explanation we suggest for the dopaminergic action in TRN is that dopamine acts on the calcium dependent potassium channels, possibly by increasing its conductance. By this way, the level of potassium that leaves the cell increases, which consequently inhibits neuron spiking. Thus, the GABA release becomes inhibited - for more details see (Madureira et al., 2010).

Given such a structure, external stimuli *X* and *Y* are projected through excitatory pathways to neighboring thalamic regions, T_x and T_y, respectively. Once stimulated, T_x activates TRN_x beyond collaterals of an ascending glutamatergic projection, whose final destiny is the PFC. Since our work does not model the PFC explicitly, such excitatory projection ends up in *TRN* in the model. Also, through an excitatory glutamatergic descending pathway, the cortical region enhances the activation of T_x, and also sends collateral axons to TRN_x. Thus, once activated, the TRN_x inhibits the thalamic region T_y through a GABAergic inhibitory projection. Summarizing, the thalamocortical circuit activation by an external stimulus *X* excites a central thalamic region T_x and inhibits its neighborhood, represented by the neuron T_y. As the mesothalamic dopamine inhibits neurons in *TRN*, a rise in the dopaminergic level contributes to deactivating such cells. This leads to a more active thalamic region T_y. Conversely, a reduction in the dopaminergic level activates *TRN*, and increases the inhibition of T_y. A symmetrical case involves the T_y and TRN_y neurons, as illustrated in Figure 1.

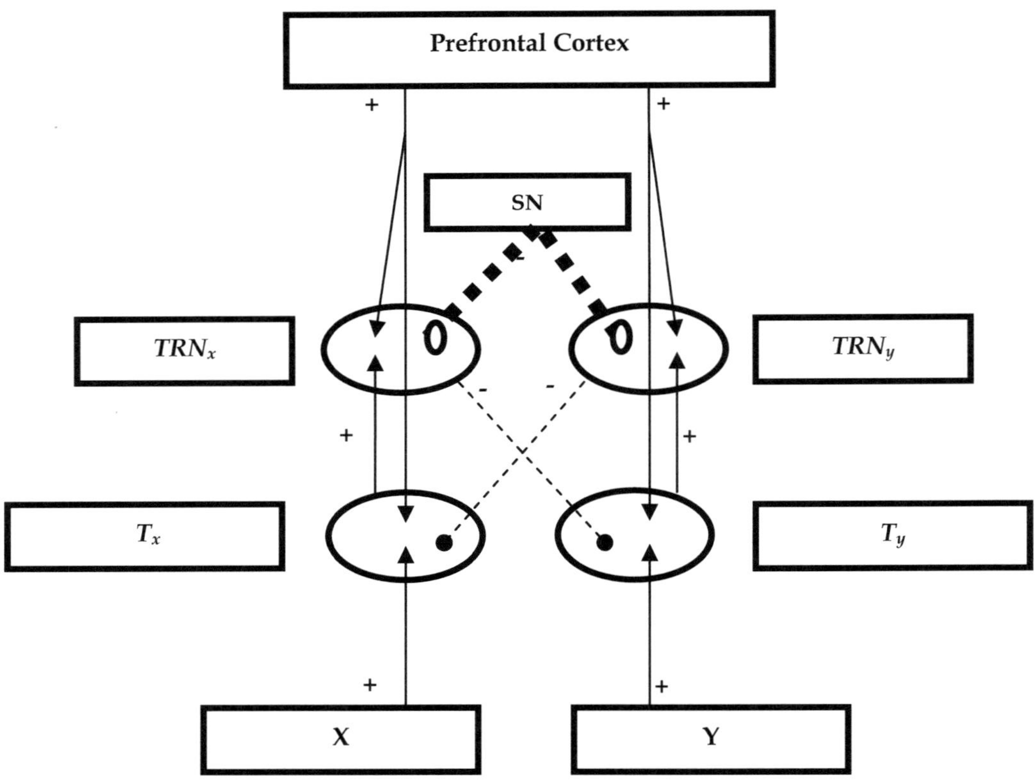

Fig. 1. The modeled thalamocortical network architecture: excitatory glutamatergic synapses (arrows), inhibitory GABAergic synapse (black sphere), inhibitory dopaminergic synapse (white sphere).

In the following, we describe the systems of equations that model the behaviors of T_x, T_y, TRN_x and TRN_y. The neural activities of the SN and the PFC, as well as the excitatory projections from X and Y are codified as temporal sequences representing their respective spiking times. As this work takes further the model presented in (Madureira et al., 2010), throughout the next section we examine specially the particular aspects of this extension.

2.2 Ionic currents

To better investigate alternate thalamic states, this model incorporates physiological features related to the tonic and the bursting modes of thalamic spikes. Thus, we address the neuron spike by considering the sodium, I_{Na}, and the calcium, I_{Ca}, currents, which depolarize the neuron, and the potassium current, I_K, which restores the cellular membrane potential (Kandel, 2000). With relation to the patterns of intervals between spikes, associated to different potassium currents (McCormick et al., 1995), our model incorporates the calcium dependent-potassium current, I_c, particularly, in the *TRN* neurons: it is a transient current, whose amplitude increases with intracellular calcium concentration, and it suffers dopaminergic influence (Florán et al., 2004; Madureira et al., 2010). Essentially associated to the bursting mode, the I_{ahp}, a current that underlies neural hyperpolarization, is modeled as described below.

The model deals with a network of ionic and synaptic events that leads to a specific mode of spiking. Particularly, under this approach we examine if dopamine is able to influence the spikes of thalamic neurons. In this model we assume that a high inhibitory dopamine action on D4 receptors in TRN neurons hyperpolarizes such cells, thus facilitating the activation of calcium currents. As a consequence, and according to thalamic properties (Carvalho, 1994), even a small membrane depolarization is capable of triggering an action potential, due to the low threshold calcium-currents. Whenever the inflow of Ca^{2+} in the cell, due to spikes, increases the Ca^{2+} concentration above a threshold, then the hyperpolarizing current I_{ahp}, becomes activated, hyperpolarizing the neuron. Therefore, the calcium currents become activate - or remain activated, depending on their previous state - and a cyclic or oscillatory behavior takes place in the TRN neuron. This is the burst thalamic mode of spiking, associated to sleep states (Steriade et al., 1993; Llinás & Steriade, 2006). It may be interrupted due to the calcium currents inactivation, which occurs whenever the neuron does not suffer hyperpolarization for around 100ms.

Based on this model, we speculate another possibility that is directly related to the PD origins: the generation of bursting in thalamic neurons, due to a strong inhibition imposed by TRN neurons. Such situation is plausible to occur in case of mesothalamic hypodopaminergy, which allows the inhibitory TRN neurons to become atypically over stimulated (Madureira et al., 2010, Florán et al., 2004).

Because of the dopaminergic modulation in the TRN, two types of neurons are modeled: the thalamic ones, T_x and T_y, and the *TRN* neurons. Both are single point spiking and are presented next.

2.2.1 Thalamic neurons

We define a simplified neuron model with a single compartment where dendrites, soma and axons are concentrated, and whose electric potential is V. The neural membrane is modeled according to the equation:

$$C_T \frac{dV}{dt} = I_k + I_{ahp} + I_{syn} + I_l ,$$

where we recall that I_k represents the potassium current, I_{ahp} the hyperpolarizing current, I_{syn} the dendritic current induced by synaptic action, and I_l the leak current, i.e., currents that are not modeled.

Considering the relation between membrane voltage and ionic currents, as

$$\begin{aligned} I_k &= g_k (E_k - V), \\ I_{ahp} &= g_{ahp} (E_k - V), \\ I_l &= g_l (E_l - V), \\ I_{syn} &= g_{syn} (E_{syn} - V) \end{aligned} \tag{1}$$

where the constants E_k, E_{ahp}, E_l and E_{syn} are reversal potentials for the currents I_k, I_{ahp}, I_l and I_{syn}, respectively, and g_k, g_{ahp}, g_l and g_{syn} represent the conductances corresponding to these currents.

The occurrence of a spike is associated to a step function $s(V)$, whose unitary value indicates the action potential depolarizing phase, depending on the I_{Na} or I_{Ca} currents:

$$s(V) = \begin{cases} 1, \text{ if } V \geq \theta_{spike} \\ 0, \text{ if } V < \theta_{spike}, \end{cases}$$

where θ_{spike} is a voltage threshold for the channel opening. It is defined as:

$$\theta_{spike} = \begin{cases} \theta_{Na}, \text{ if } I_{Ca} \text{ is inactivated} \\ \theta_{Ca}, \text{ if } I_{Ca} \text{ is activated}, \end{cases}$$

where, θ_{Na} is the voltage threshold for the sodium channels opening, and θ_{Ca} for the calcium channels. We have $\theta_{Na} > \theta_{Ca}$, and the spikes triggered by the calcium ionic channels are the low threshold spikes (LTS).

During the network activity, the membrane potential, V, is monitored. When strong inhibitory events lead to periods of hyperpolarization, around 100ms, the I_{Ca} currents become activated (Carvalho, 1994). Once in activity, I_{Ca} currents cause the LTS.

Following a spike, the conductance g_k of the restoring current I_k increases rapidly, bringing the neuron back to a resting potential. Such a process is described by

$$\frac{dg_k}{dt} = \frac{s\beta_k - g_k}{\tau_k}$$

where the constant β_k represents a variation rate of g_k, and τ_k a time constant associated to the potassium channel.

According to the frequency of spikes, the calcium concentration increases - and decreases due to calcium buffers and pumps (Carvalho & Roitman, 1995). Then, we have:

$$\frac{d[Ca]}{dt} = \frac{s\beta_{Ca} - [Ca]}{\tau_{Ca}} \tag{2}$$

where β_{Ca} represents the rate of calcium concentration variation, and τ_{Ca} a time constant.
If the intracellular calcium concentration reaches a given threshold Θ_{Ca}, the potassium channels related to the hyperpolarizing current are opened. The step function f([Ca]) describes such event as:

$$f([Ca]) = \begin{cases} 1, \text{ if } [Ca] \geq \Theta_{Ca} \\ 0, \text{ if } [Ca] < \Theta_{Ca}. \end{cases}$$

The following equation describes how its conductance, g_{ahp}, behaves with respect to the I_{ahp} current:

$$\frac{d g_{ahp}}{dt} = \frac{f\beta_{ahp} - g_{ahp}}{\tau_{ahp}}$$

where β_{ahp} represents a variation rate of g_{ahp}, and τ_{ahp} a time constant.
Once in the activated state, the I_{Ca} current facilitates the occurrence of LTS, and the consequent increase of the calcium concentration, *[Ca]*. As a result, the conductance g_{ahp} grows, and the neuron suffers a hyperpolarization.

2.2.2 *TRN* neurons

Since TRN and thalamic neurons main properties are similar, the equations for the *TRN* neuron are quite similar to the ones considered in 2.2.1, except for the inclusion of the calcium-dependent potassium current I_c.
We assume the final target of dopaminergic action is the calcium-dependent potassium channel, whose ionic current is I_c (Madureira et al., 2010; Florán et al., 2004). Thus, the membrane equation for the *TRN* neuron incorporates the ionic current I_c as:

$$C_{TRN}\frac{dV}{dt} = I_k + I_{ahp} + I_c + I_{syn} + I_l$$

Indeed, $I_c = g_c\,(E_k - V)$, where E_k represents the potassium reversal potential, and g_c the conductance of ionic current I_c.
The conductance g_c suffers dopaminergic influence, via D4 receptor, and depends on the intracellular calcium concentration. Thus, $g_c = \hat{g}_c\, D_4^*\, S(\,[Ca]\,)$, where $\hat{g}_c$ is a constant, D_4^* stands for the dopaminergic action on g_c, and $S(\,[Ca]\,)$ stands for a sigmoid function of the intracellular calcium concentration, which increases by virtue of a neural spiking. We set

$$S([Ca]) = \frac{1}{1 + \exp(-a[Ca])}$$

where the constant a controls the slope of S, and rhe calcium concentration behaves according to the equation (2). Indeed, in (2) the term s raises the calcium concentration whenever there is a neural spiking. Therefore g_c increases and inhibits the cell, if the cell is excited beyond a threshold.

The dopaminergic action on g_c is modeled by the summation of alpha functions (Carvalho, 1994) representing the rise and the decrease of the dopaminergic level, in each of the N presynaptic spikes that occurred at times t_i, before t, with $1 \leq i \leq N$:

$$D_4^* = \hat{g}_{d4} \sum_{i=1}^{N} (t - t_i)\exp[-(t - t_i) \; / \, t_{pd}]$$

Here, the constant t_{pd} stands for the peak time for the alpha function, and $\hat{g}_{d4}$ is the conductance constant of the dopaminergic projection. For further details, see ref. (Madureira et al., 2010).

2.3 Synaptic projections

Finally, we present the synaptic modeling (Carvalho, 1994). For the synaptic conductance g_{syn}, appearing in Equation (1), it follows that

$$g_{syn} = \hat{g}_{syn} \sum_{i=1}^{N} (t - t_i)\exp\left[-(t - t_i) \; / \, t_p\right]$$

where $\hat{g}_{syn}$ is the maximal conductance, which assumes different values for each particular synapse. In fact, each modeled synapse has a specific associated conductance, reflecting its influence: $\hat{g}_{c\text{-}trn}$ and $\hat{g}_{c\text{-}t}$ for synapses between the cortex and the TRN, and between the cortex and the thalamus, respectively; $\hat{g}_{t\text{-}trn}$ and $\hat{g}_{trn\text{-}t}$ for synapses between the thalamus and the TRN, and vice versa; and $\hat{g}_{e\text{-}t}$ for synapses between somatosensory projections and the thalamus.

The synaptic conductance g_{syn} is also represented by a summation of alpha functions, for each of the N presynaptic spikes that occurred at times t_i before t, for $1 \leq I \leq N$. We denote by t_p the peak time for the alpha function, and it assumes the values t_{pe} and t_{pi} for excitatory and inhibitory synapses respectively.

We used the ANSI C ® programming language to implement the model. The differential equations are integrated by the Euler's method. Ref. (Madureira et al., 2010) and Table 1 present glossaries with all necessary parameter values.

I_{ahp}	Hyperpolarizing potassium current	(μA.cm^{-2})
g_{ahp}	Conductance of I_{ahp}	(m.mhos.cm^{-2})
θ_{Ca}	Threshold for calcium channel's opening	(0 mV)
θ_{Na}	Threshold for sodium channel's opening	(1 mV)
Θ_{Ca}	Intracellular calcium concentration threshold for I_{ahp} activation	(mM)
β_{ahp}	Variation rate of g_{ahp}	(100)
τ_{ahp}	Time constant of g_{ahp}	(2 ms)

Table 1. Glossary of parameters.

3. Computational simulations

Due to a mechanism of inhibitory feedback between thalamic and TRN neurons in the thalamocortical circuit, when a projected stimulus on the central thalamic area T_x is propagated for posterior cortical processing, its neighboring thalamic area T_y suffers inhibition from *TRN*. This property was highly explored in (Madureira et al., 2010), because our major concern was the attentional focus formation.

Here, we explore such inhibitory feedback to inspect how the activity degree in the TRN influences the thalamic excitatory state. Summarizing, our simulations illustrate how dopamine modulates the activation of TRN neurons and, consequently, that of the thalamic cells.

With relation to the dopaminergic action in the TRN, we assume a relationship between the level of mesothalamic dopamine released in the TRN and the nigral spiking frequency. Consequently, we simulate variations in the level of dopamine released in the TRN by varying the SN spiking pattern. We also address the dopamine receptor D4 degree of activity, through the term $\hat{g}_{d4}$ in (3). Indeed, $\hat{g}_{d4}$ model the weight of the connection between the SN and *TRN* neurons. Then, $\hat{g}_{d4}$ tells us how much receptor D4, in the TRN, is affected by the dopamine release due to a nerve impulse from SN, or due to the action of exogenous factors as drugs that alter the dopamine level throughout synaptic clefts.

Overall, throughout these simulations our major concern is the dopaminergic effect on the thalamocortical dynamics. We do not intend to focus our exploration on the consequences of variations in external or cortical stimuli.

3.1 Asymmetrical architecture

In this section, we describe a series of simulations performed using an artificial neural network that presents the architecture illustrated in the Figure 2. Since such network is the one used in (Madureira et al., 2010), we set it as our departure point.

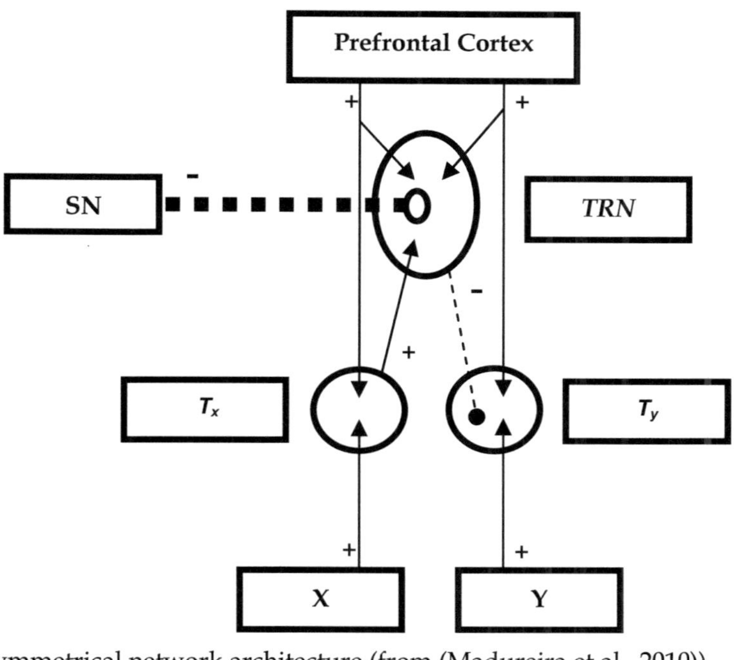

Fig. 2. The asymmetrical network architecture (from (Madureira et al., 2010)).

Here, we investigate if variations in the activity of receptor D4 in the TRN may influence the mode of spiking in neurons of the thalamic complex, along different SN spiking frequencies. We impose a drastic decrease in the nigral dopamine level, reflecting a disturbance in the mesothalamic system, and raise the dopaminergic level afterwards. Through the 500ms-simulations, variations in the dopaminergic receptor activation are modeled by altering the parameter $\hat{g}_{d4}$ after 250ms.

Table 2 describes all simulated variations in the SN spiking frequency, the imposed changes on receptor D4 activation, as well as the characteristic spike modes related to each situation. From these results, we gather that the bursting mode was elicited in two opposing situations: increase of D4 activation under mesothalamic hypoactivity (interval between spikes in SN equals 50 and above) and, decrease of D4 activation under mesothalamic hyperactivity (interval between spikes in SN equals 5).

In the first case, the mesothalamic hypoactivity turns the TRN_x neuron so highly excited, that T_y becomes strongly inhibited, thus activating the calcium current. The posterior increase of the D4 activity, plausibly representing the effect of some dopaminergic agonist, was able to elicit LTSs. Consequently, the calcium concentration reached a threshold value that activated the hyperpolarizing current, promoting the oscillatory pattern in the thalamic cell T_y.

Interval between Spikes in SN (ms)	Changes in the Activity of Dopamine Receptor D4 ($\hat{g}_{d4}$)	Neuron	Spike Mode
100, 150 and 200	1.0 to 1.2	T_y	Tonic to Bursting
50	1.0 to 1.2	T_y	Tonic to Bursting
10	1.0 to 1.2	-	Tonic
5	1.0 to 0.8	TRN	Tonic to Bursting

Table 2. Spiking modes examined through an asymmetrical network.

Conversely, in the second case, the mesothalamic hyperactivity generated the strong inhibition in the TRN neuron, which enabled the calcium currents activation. Then, the imposed decrease of D4 activity was sufficient to diminish the TRN inhibition, thus allowing LTSs and, finally, the bursting mode of spiking.

3.2 Symmetrical architecture

Following the first series of experiments, we extend the network architecture to incorporate the symmetry between neighboring thalamic areas. The symmetrical architecture is represented in the Figure 1.

3.2.1 SN spiking frequency and the attentional focus

We start exploring the extended architecture by addressing the dopaminergic action in neurons under the tonic mode of spiking. Therefore, as a first approximation, we apply the mathematical model developed in (Madureira et al., 2010). In this set of simulations, a weaker stimulus X is presented to the network before the a stronger one, Y. Again, we initiate with a low SN spike frequency, characterizing the mesothalamic dopamine hypoactivity, and raise the SN activity in successive steps. Table 3 presents our simulations results. Overall, we gather that as the mesothalamic dopaminergic activity decreases, the *TRN* neurons become more excited. Also, T_x becomes be more inhibited than T_y, enlarging thus the difference between the activations of T_x and T_y, as showed in Table 4. Therefore the mesothalamic dopamine hypoactivity forces the attention to focus on the stimulus *Y*, implying in attentional shifting difficulty and mental rigidity. On the other hand, the almost identical neural activity of T_x and T_y, enhanced by the mesothalamic dopamine hyperactivity, lead to a no-winner competition between stimuli *X* and *Y*, which may represent distraction or lack of attentional focus. These results are compatible with the ones provided by our previous model.

Interval between Spikes in SN (ms)	Spikes in 100ms			
	T_x	T_y	TRN_x	TRN_y
	(100ms - 200ms)			
	(400ms - 500ms)			
50	11	0	25	14
	2	14	14	28
30	14	0	23	9
	4	14	16	25
20	12	0	21	10
	7	13	13	21
10	18	0	17	0
	10	15	5	10
5	18	0	0	0
	18	19	0	0

Table 3. SN spiking frequency and the thalamic tonic state.

3.2.2 Receptor D4 activity and the attentional focus

In the next series of experiments, we keep up our focus on the tonic mode of spiking. And, for each imposed SN spike frequency, we examine the effects of changes in the receptor D4 activation. Since the different degrees of D4 activation can be associated to not modeled exogenous or endogenous factors, that are not modeled, this approach makes it possible to speculate plausible outcomes of the dopaminergic agonists (or antagonists) action at the synaptic cleft. The simulations results are summarized in Table 4. First, we may note that the results presented in the column relative to $\hat{g}_{d4} = 1.0$ agree with the previous set of experiments. It is more interesting, however, to observe that as the receptor D4 activity diminishes, the thalamic neurons become less active, thus reaching a completely inhibited state. Conversely, as the receptor D4 activity increases, thalamic neurons become more active and tend to spike at the same frequency. Finally, we highlight that, except for the baseline case where the interval between spikes in SN equals 10, when $\hat{g}_{d4}$ assumes values lower than 1.0, the differences between T_x and T_y spiking frequencies disappear. So, the mesothalamic hypoactivity does not impose the attention to focus on the stimulus *Y* anymore.

Interval between Spikes in SN (ms)		Spikes in 100ms					
		Activity of Dopamine Receptor D4 ($\hat{g}_{d4}$)					
		0.4	0.6	0.8	1.0	1.2	1.4
50	T_x	-	0	2	2	11	14
	T_y	-	0	2	14	16	19
	TRN_x	-	46	32	14	9	4
	TRN_y	-	46	32	28	15	6
30	T_x	-	0	4	4	12	15
	T_y	-	0	4	13	17	18
	TRN_x	-	42	30	25	12	2
	TRN_y	-	42	30	25	12	5
20	T_x	-	0	5	7	12	18
	T_y	-	0	5	13	15	18
	TRN_x	-	40	30	13	10	5
	TRN_y	-	40	30	21	12	2
10	T_x	0	0	0	10	16	18
	T_y	0	6	10	15	17	19
	TRN_x	52	30	20	5	5	0
	TRN_y	50	30	30	10	4	0
5	T_x	0	5	15	18	18	-
	T_y	0	5	15	19	19	-
	TRN_x	40	25	10	0	0	-
	TRN_y	40	20	5	0	0	-

Table 4. Receptor D4 activity and the thalamic tonic state.

3.2.3 Dopaminergic activity and the oscillatory state

Next, we simulate the mathematical model described in Section 2 through the extended symmetrical network illustrated in the Figure 1. In this set of experiments, two identical, external stimuli, *X* and *Y*, activate the network simultaneously. As in the previous experiments, we impose different SN spiking frequencies. We observe, in Table 5, that extreme and opposing situations lead to the bursting spiking mode in the thalamic complex: the drastic mesothalamic dopamine hypoactivity caused the oscillatory pattern in the T_x and T_y neurons, whereas the mesothalamic dopamine hyperactivity made the TRN neurons to spike through bursts. With relation to the T_x and T_y neurons, the appearance of the bursting mode comes from the strong inhibition they suffered through the GABAergic projection from the TRN neurons, which were over activated due to the low dopaminergic activity. Conversely, the oscillatory behavior of the TRN_x and TRN_y neurons originated from the inhibition suffered by the TRN due to the high dopaminergic level. The dynamics of the ionic currents involved in such processes are the same described in Subsection 2.2. Figure 3 illustrates the changes in the T_x behavior due to the diminishing of the receptor D4 activation, throughout the dopamine hypoactivity case, described in the first line of Table 5.

Interval between Spikes in SN (ms)	Activity of Dopamine Receptor D_4^* ($\hat{g}_{d4}$)	Neurons	Spike Mode
100	0.8	T_x and T_y	Bursting
	0.9	all	Tonic
	1.0	all	Tonic
50	0.8	all	Tonic
	0.9	all	Tonic
	1.0	all	Tonic
40, 30, 20, 10	1.0	all	Tonic
5	1.0	TRN_x and TRN_y	Bursting

Table 5. Distinct dopaminergic activities in presence of similar stimuli.

3.2.4 Variations in the dopaminergic activity and the oscillatory state

In our last series of simulations, we deepen our investigations on the changes in the spiking mode. Now, we repeat the strategy undertaken in Subsection 3.2.1, where a stimulus X is presented to the asymmetrical network before a stronger one, Y. Through the extended mathematical model we propose in Section 2, here we look for situations where changes in the dopaminergic action lead to the burst mode in neurons of the thalamic complex. In this set of simulations, we examine only extreme cases of dopaminergic alterations. Such option was because all previous experiments indicated these extreme situations as the more plausible to initiate the ionic events that underlie the burst mode occurrence. Table 6 summarizes our results.

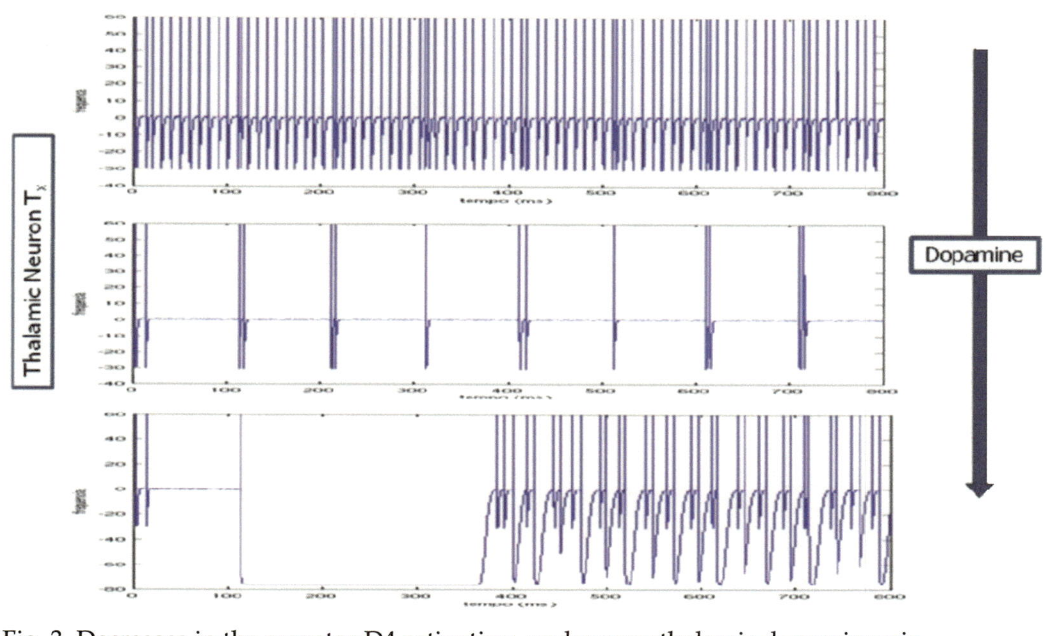

Fig. 3. Decreases in the receptor D4 activation, under mesothalamic dopaminergic hypoactivity, turned the tonic state into the burst one in T_x.

In the case of mesothalamic hypoactivity, where the SN neuron spikes every 150ms, the constant activation of D4 as $\hat{g}_{d4}$ = 0.9 made the T_y neuron to spike through bursts - not T_x one. This occurs because the T_y activation is greater than the T_x one by an amount enough to trigger the LTS - after the hyperpolarization due to the high activity in the TRN. In Figure 4, we can observe the T_x and T_y behaviors. The receptor D4 activations imposed by $\hat{g}_{d4}$ = 1.0 or $\hat{g}_{d4}$ = 1.1 did not allow the TRN neurons to spike highly enough to start the necessary hyperpolarization that activates the calcium currents.

Another case of mesothalamic hypoactivity we simulate by fixing the SN frequency in one spike each 100ms. Compared to the previous experiment, the SN is slightly more active. This time, it is the T_x neuron that presents an oscillatory pattern, when $\hat{g}_{d4}$ = 0.9. In this case, the inhibition from TRN_x was not strong enough to hyperpolarize T_y. However, the less stimulated T_x neuron suffered the necessary inhibition that activated calcium currents, thus facilitating the consolidation of the burst mode of spiking. Figure 5 illustrates the distinct spiking modes of T_x and T_y.

Interval between Spikes in SN (ms)	Activity of Dopamine Receptor D_4^* ($\hat{g}_{d4}$)	Neurons	Spike Mode
150	0.9	T_y	Bursting
	1.0	all	Tonic
	1.1	all	Tonic
100	0.8	all	Tonic
	0.9	T_x	Bursting
	0.9 to 1.0	T_x and T_y	Bursting
5	1.1 to 0.8	TRN_x and TRN_y	Bursting

Table 6. Distinct dopaminergic activities in presence of different stimuli.

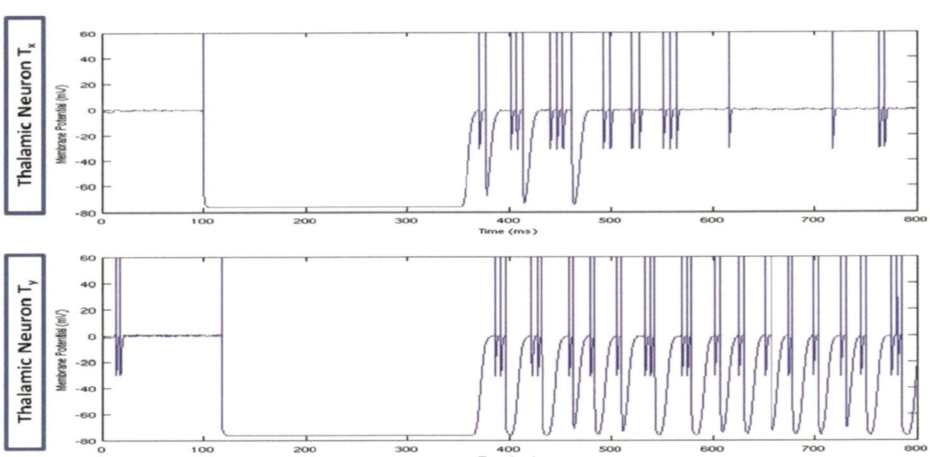

Fig. 4. Behaviors of T_x and T_y. Mesothalamic dopaminergic hypoactivity enables the oscillatory behavior of T_y. SN spikes every 150ms and $\hat{g}_{d4}$ = 0.9.

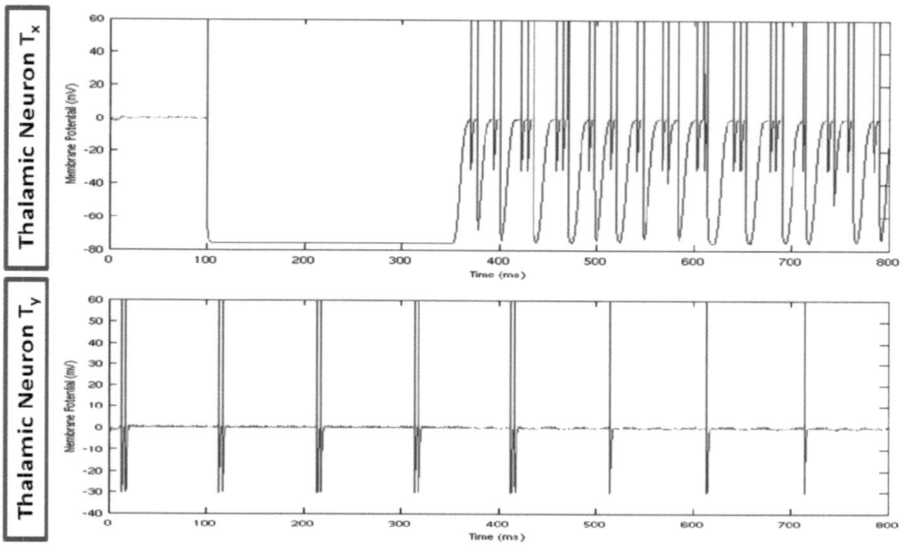

Fig. 5. The distinct spiking modes of T_x and T_y. When SN spikes every 100ms and $\hat{g}_{d4} = 0.9$, T_x presents the burst mode of spiking.

Also with the SN neuron set to spike each 100ms, we started a 800ms-experiment with the parameter $\hat{g}_{d4} = 0.9$. This time, however, we turned $\hat{g}_{d4}$ to 1.0 after 350ms. It is plausible to interpret such alteration in the $\hat{g}_{d4}$ value as a consequence of some increase in the dopaminergic level, due to an exogenous factor. In this case, both T_x and T_y start to oscillate. The last situation presented in Table 6 refers to the extreme case of mesothalamic hyperactivity. During a 800ms-experiment, the interval between spikes in the SN was set to 5ms. In addition, at the beginning we imposed a high activation in receptor D4 with $\hat{g}_{d4}$ = 1.1. This dopaminergic context inhibited the TRN neurons, which suffer even a hyperpolarization. It was, however, the imposed decrease of $\hat{g}_{d4}$ to 0.8, after 350ms, that starts the burst mode in both *TRN* neurons. In this case, the lowering in the dopaminergic receptor activity enables the *TRNs* membrane potential to reach a threshold value that triggered LTS in such neurons. Figure 6 illustrates such situation.

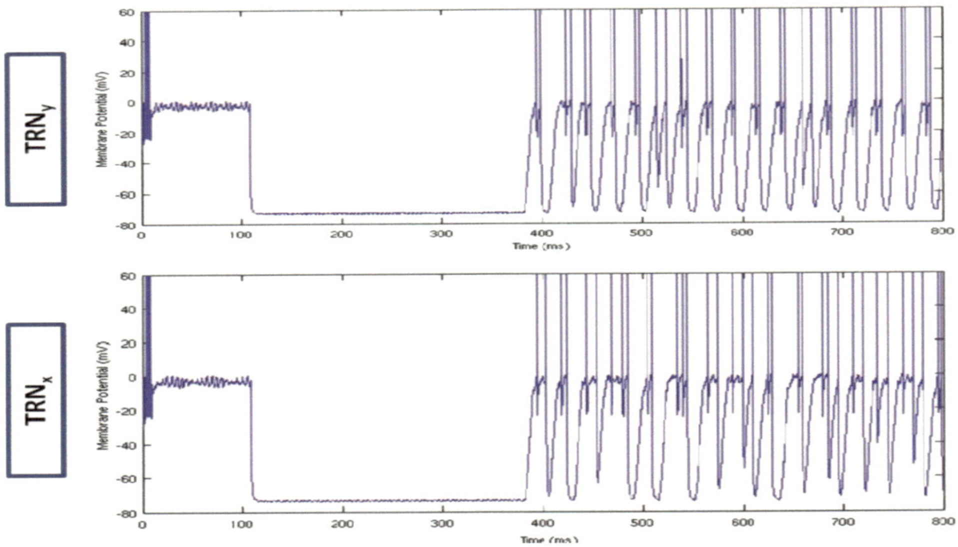

Fig. 6. Decrease in receptor D4 activation, under mesothalamic dopaminergic hyperactivity, originates the burst state in both TRN_x and TRN_y.

4. Discussion

Overall, the current knowledge in neuroscience conducts us through a multiscale world. The understanding of whatever peculiarity the human behavior exhibits requires us to travel throughout our brain's different levels of organization. In particular, this is the case with sleep neuroscience.

Here, we speculate the dopaminergic influence on neuron states associated to sleep and sleep alterations in PD. Our ideas, however, should be considered by keeping in mind the broad cascade of events that underlies the wake-sleep cycle.

Environmental as well as genetic factors trigger networks of intra and inter cellular signals, which promote the specific characteristics associated to wake or sleep states. For instance, due to the light impinging on the retina, signals from circadian oscillators reach specific hypothalamic regions. Such areas regulate the action of distinct brain systems associated to the different responses that an organism presents throughout the sleep-wake cycle. In this sense, the hypothalamus regulates wake-sleep switches through its suprachiasmatic, subparaventricular and dorsomedial nuclei; together with the basal forebrain, it controls ascending arousal systems, through its ventrolateral preopitic, lateral and tuberomammilary nuclei. The hypothalamus also regulates brainstem nuclei, as dorsal raphe and locus ceruleus, which control the cyclic transition between the rapid eye movement (REM) and non-REM (NREM) sleep phases. On the other hand, projections from such brainstem and diencephalon ascending arousal systems reach cortical and thalamic areas, known to be involved in the origin and maintenance of different brain rhythms that specifically underlie some sleep states (Pace-Schott & Hobson, 2002; Hobson & Pace-Schott, 2002).

Brain rhythms reflect the spike mode occurring in groups of neurons. And, as revealed by polysonographic recordings, the wake state as well as the NREM and REM sleep phases, are defined, each one, by characteristic field potential oscillations (Pace-Schott & Hobson, 2002;

Hobson & Pace-Schott, 2002). Accordingly, each behavioral state presents distinct cognitive activities and conscious experiences. Throughout the night, there is a cyclic occurrence of NREM and REM sleep phases, where the NREM stage is composed by the slow wave sleep (SWS) - that includes the sleep stages 3 and 4, besides the lighter sleep stages 1 and 2. In particular, the SWS is characterized by rhythms known as slow oscillations, spindles and sharp wave-ripples (Pace-Schott & Hobson, 2002; Hobson & Pace-Schott, 2002; Hobson, 2009; Diekelmann & Born, 2010).

Thalamocortical systems are highly involved in the achievement of oscillations associated to the SWS, in special, slow oscillations and spindles (Steriade et al., 1993; Steriade, 2006). Whereas slow oscillations originate at the cortex and propagate to the thalamus, the spindles have their origins in the thalamus and propagate to the cortex mediated by the TRN pacemaker (Steriade et al., 1993; Llinás & Steriade, 2006; Steriade, 2006). In both cases, however, the origin of the oscillatory pattern is associated to some strong inhibition leading to a consequent burst mode of spiking. More, according to (Steriade et al., 1993), different types of rhythms may appear depending on the magnitude of such inhibitory event.

Indeed, the cholinergic and noradrenergic neuromodulatory systems are known to regulate the neurophysiologic aspects underlying the brain rhythms in the NREM and REM sleep phases (Diekelmann & Born, 2010). However, the experiments revealing the existence of the mesothalamic dopaminergic pathway (Freeman et al., 2001) made it possible to hypothesize on the dopaminergic influence on neuron states associated to sleep (Pace-Schott & Hobson, 2002).

In this work, we propose that the mesothalamic dopamine action in the thalamocortical circuit is able of generating oscillatory patterns that are typical in sleep states, both in thalamic and TRN neurons, depending on the level of dopaminergic activity. In particular, we consider that the dopaminergic alteration in PD is an essential factor underlying the sleep problems observed in such disease. In this case, both the dopaminergic hypoactivity - due to the SN neurons degeneration -, and the increases in the dopaminergic activity due to the appliance of dopamine-related drugs, would contribute to the appearance of sleep alterations.

Basically, our computational simulations explore two ways by which mesothalamic dopamine may affect the thalamocortical dynamics: the SN activity and the dopamine receptor D4 activation. Overall, we conclude that an extreme dopaminergic mesothalamic hypoactivity favors the appearance of the burst mode in thalamic neurons. Conversely, a high degree of dopaminergic mesothalamic hyperactivity propitiates such an oscillatory rhythm in the TRN neurons. In addition, our simulations hint that, when the SN activity is markedly diminished, a slight factor inducing an increase in the receptor D4 activation triggers the bursting pattern in thalamic neurons. On the other hand, the application of some agent that lowers the D4 activation, under a situation of extreme mesothalamic dopamine hyperactivity, enables the burst mode in the TRN.

In the context of PD, such results point anomalous somnolence as a consequence of the lack of dopamine, due to the SN degeneration. More, neural sleep states may appear as a consequence of drugs administration to increase the dopamine action, when the SN activity is highly disrupted. Another situation we consider important to emphasize refers to the dopaminergic hyperactivity case. Due to the lifelong need of medication for equilibrating the nigral dopaminergic level, PD patients usually present symptoms related to excess of dopamine (March, 2005). We illustrate such situation by increasing the dopaminergic activity. We then observe that a slight diminishing in the receptor D4 activation induces the burst mode of spiking in the TRN. Since the TRN plays an essential role in the consolidation of brain rhythms associated to sleep states, it is plausible supposing that such unnatural dopaminergic hyperactivity underlies the emergence of some spurious sleep states, via TRN, in PD. On the other hand, with relation to the thalamic neurons, such dopaminergic hyperactivity prevents them from entering into an oscillatory state. It thus suggests that symptoms pointing to lack of sleep may have origins in the abnormal presence of high dopaminergic activity, due to drug administration. This situation would also contribute to the understanding of why, in PD, a night of sleep deprivation is commonly followed by a daytime of high alertness (Rye et al., 2000).

Our results agree with the striking ideas exposed in (Dzirasa et al., 2006), which shows that dopamine does play a role in the control of the sleep-wake cycle. Here, through a neurocomputational model, we indicate possible ways by which sleep-related states should emerge as a consequence of alterations in the mesothalamic dopamine activity.

Altogether, this work proposes a link between sleep neuroscience and PD. Through a mathematical and computational approach, we infer that the dopaminergic alterations in PD reach brain nuclei highly engaged in the control of rhythms that characterize different sleep states. Therefore, the presence of anomalous dopaminergic activities facilitate the appearance of spurious sleep states, not achieved in normal conditions through the brain systems directly associated to the circadian control of the sleep-wake cycle.

5. Acknowledgments

This work is kindly dedicated to the memory of Magdalena C. L. Madureira. The author thanks the Brazilian agency CNPq (PCI/LNCC, grants 560108/2010-9, 474218/2008) for the financial support.

6. References

Andrade LAF, Ferraz HB. Quadro clínico. In: Meneses MS, Teive HA (Eds). Doença de Parkinson. Rio de Janeiro: Guanabara Koogan, 2003:80-90.

Arnulf I and Leu-Semenescu S. Sleepiness in Parkinson's Disease. *Parkinsonism and Related Disorders* 1553, S101-S104 (2009).

Braak H, Rüb U, Sandmann-Keil D, Gai WP, de Vos RA, Jansen Steur EN, Arai K, Braak E. Parkinson's disease: affection of brain stem nuclei controlling premotor and motor neurons of the somatomotor system. *Acta Neuropathol* 99, 5:489-95 (2000).

Carvalho LAV. Modeling the Thalamocortical Loop. *International Journal of Bio-Medical Computing* 35, 267-296 (1994).

Carvalho LAV and Roitman VL. A Computational Model for the Neurobiological Substrates of Visual Attention. *International Journal of Bio-Medical Computing* 38, 33-45 (1995).

De Cock VC, Vidailhet M, Arnulf I. Sleep Disturbances in Patients with Parkinsonism. *Nature Clinical Practice Neurology* 4 (5), 254-266 (2008).

De Gennaro L and Ferrara M. Sleep Spindles: An Overview. *Sleep Medicine Reviews* 7, 5,432-440 (2003).

Diekelmann S and Born J. The Memory Function of Sleep. *Nature Reviews Neuroscience* 11, 114-126 (2010).

Dubois B, Pillon B. Cognitive deficits in Parkinson's disease. J Neurol. 1996;244:2–8.

Dzirasa K, Ribeiro S, Costa R, Santos LM, Lin S-C, Grosmark A, Sotnikova TD, Gainetdinov RR, Caron MG, Nicolelis MAL. Dopaminergic Control of Sleep-Wake States. *The Journal of Neuroscience* 26, 41, 10577-10589 (2006).

Florán B, Florán L, Erlij D, Aceves J. Activation of dopamine D4 receptors modulates [3H]GABA release in slices of the rat thalamic reticular nucleus. Neuropharmacology 2004;46:497-503.

Freeman A, Ciliax B, Bakay R, et al. Nigrostriatal collaterals to thalamus degenerate in parkinsonian animal models. Ann Neurol 2001;50:321-329.

Guillery RW, Harting JK. Structure and connections of the thalamic reticular nucleus: advancing views over half a century. J Comp Neurol 2003;463:360-371.

Hobson JA and Pace-Schott EF. The Cognitive Neuroscience of Sleep: Neuronal Systems, Consciousness and Learning. *Nature Reviews Neuroscience* 3, 679-693 (2002).

Hobson JA. REM Sleep and Dreaming: Towards a Theory of Protoconsciousness. *Nature Reviews Neuroscience* 10, 803-813 (2002).

Jankovic J. Emerging Views of Dopamine in Modulating Sleep/Wake State from an Unlikely Source: PD. *Neurology* 58 (3), 341-346 (2002).

Jeanmonod D, Magnin M, Morel A. Low-threshold Calcium Spike Bursts in the Human Thalamus: Common physiopatology for sensory, motor and limbic positive symptoms. *Brain* 119, 363-375 (1996).

Kandel, E.R., Schwartz, J.H. and Jessel, T.M., 2000, *Principals of neuroscience*. 4ed. International Edition: Mc-Graw Hill.

Llinás RR and Steriade M. Bursting of Thalamic Neurons and States of Vigilance. *Journal of Neurophysiology* 95, 3297-3308 (2006).

Llinás RR, Ribary U, Jeanmonod D, Kronberg E, Mitra PP. Thalamocortical Dysrhythmia: A Neurological and Neuropsychiatric Syndrome Characterized by Magnetoencephalography. *Proceedings of the National Academy of Science* 96, 26, 15222-15227 (1999).

Madureira DQM, Carvalho LAV, Cheniaux E. Attentional Focus Modulated by Mesothalamic Dopamine: Consequences in Parkinson's Disease and Attention Deficit Hyperactivity Disorder. *Cognitive Computation* 2, 1, 31-49. DOI 10.1007/s12559-009-9029-4 (2010).

Madureira DQM, Carvalho LAV, Cheniaux E. Modelagem Neurocomputacional do Circuito Tálamo-cortical: Implicações para Compreensão do Transtorno de Déficit de Atenção e Hiperatividade. *Arq. Neuro-Psiquiatr.* 65, 4a, 1043-1049 (2007).

March L. Psychosis in Parkinson's Disease. *Primary Psychiatry* 12, 7, 56-62 (2005).

McCormick, D.A., Connors, B.W., Lighthall, J.W. and Prince, D.A., 1985, Comparative electrophysiology of pyramidal and sparsely spiny stellate neurons of the neocortex. *Journal of Neurophysiology*, 54, 782-806.

Pace-Schott EF and Hobson JA. The Neurobiology of Sleep: Genetics, Cellular Physiology and Subcortical Networks. *Nature Reviews Neuroscience* 3, 591-605 (2002).

Rye DB, Bliwise DL, Dihenia B, Gurecki P. Daytime Sleepiness in Parkinson's Disease. *Journal of Sleep Research* 9, 63-69 (2000).

Rye DB. Parkinson's Disease and RLS: The Dopaminergic Bridge. *Sleep Medicine* 5, 317-328 (2004).

Steriade M, McCormick DA, Sejnowski TJ. Thalamocortical Oscillations in the Sleeping and Aroused Brain. *Science* 262, 679-685 (1993).
Steriade M. Grouping of Brain Rhythms in Corticothalamic Systems. *Neuroscience* 137, 1087-1106 (2006).

24

Pathophysiology of Non-Dopaminergic Monoamine Systems in Parkinson's Disease: Implications for Mood Dysfunction

Nirmal Bhide and Christopher Bishop
Department of Psychology, Binghamton University, Binghamton, NY USA

1. Introduction

Parkinson's disease (PD) is a neurodegenerative disorder affecting millions worldwide and is one of the most common diseases affecting the aging population (Delau et al., 2006). Clinical hallmarks of PD feature severe motor deficits characterized by bradykinesia, tremor, rigidity and postural instability. Though less recognized, PD symptoms also include psychiatric complications such as depression, anxiety and psychosis that deleteriously influence quality of life. While the origin of motor deficits is the progressive degeneration of nigrostriatal dopamine (DA) neurons, other monoamine neurons within the serotonin (5-HT) and norepinephrine (NE) system also degenerate, likely contributing to mood dysfunction. In this chapter the pathophysiology of non-dopaminergic monoamine systems, their contribution to PD-related mood dysfunction, and therapeutics targeting them will be discussed.

2. Norepinephrine system

In PD, the cardinal cell death of the dopaminergic substantia nigra pars compacta (SNpc) neurons is accompanied by deficits in other monoamine neurotransmitter systems. Of these, NE appears most most consistently affected. Numerous studies, both neuroanatomical and biochemical, have documented severe loss of NE neurons, originating from the locus coeruleus (LC), concomitant with or even preceding the loss of DA neurons (Mann and Yates, 1983; Marien et al., 2004; Schapira et al., 2006). The precise anatomical relationship between the LC and the SNpc and the striatum remains to be elucidated; however, evidence exists for a functional relationship between these brain regions (Fornai et al., 2007). Most notable, loss of NE may exacerbate damage to the DA nigrostriatal system, as NE is postulated to play a neuroprotective and neuromodulator role in the progression of PD (Rommelfanger and Weinshenker, 2007). The following sections will focus on the pathophysiology of NE, its relative contribution to the development of psychiatric symptoms of PD, and the treatment of these symptoms using noradrenergic drugs.

2.1 CNS pathophysiology of NE system in PD

2.1.1 Neuroanatomical evidence in PD patients

As early as 1917, noradrenergic neurons originating from the LC were reported to be severely deteriorated in patients suffering from PD (Tretiakoff et al., 1917; Fornai et al.,

2007). In a landmark study by Hornykiewicz et al., (1960), direct biochemical evidence supported these initial findings, by showing the loss of both NE neurons and NE content in several brain regions in PD, including the caudate nucleus and putamen (Ehringer and Hornykiewicz, 1960).

Neuropathological evidence in post-mortem tissue of PD patients ranges from observation of Lewy bodies (LB) within single NE cells and cytoplasmic neurofibrillary tangles (NT) to a loss of neurons in the LC (Mann, 1983). Patt and Gerhard (1993), using a variant of the Golgi method, found that medium-sized LC neurons containing neuromelanin granules were most affected in PD patients (Patt and Gerhard, 1993) correlating with loss of synaptic spines, a reduction in dendritic length, swollen perikarya and apoptosis. Bertrand et al., (1997) reported the presence of glial proliferation along with extracellular neuromelanin granules around dying NE neurons. Post-mortem studies carried out in PD patients have established a loss of approximately 70% of NE neurons when compared to age-matched controls (Bertrand et al., 1997; Zarow et al., 2003). Interestingly, the NE neuronal loss was greater in the LC compared to cholinergic loss in the nucleus basalis and dopaminergic loss in the SNpc in Alzheimer and PD patients, respectively (Zarow et al., 2003). Of note, the loss of LC neurons observed in PD patients is not homogenous as there appears to be a disease specific and regional pattern to degeneration in the LC. For example, German and co-workers (1992) observed that in PD patients with no dementia complications, the degeneration was consistent throughout the rostral and caudal portion of the LC, whereas, in PD patients with dementia, the cell loss occurred more severely in the rostral portion of the LC nucleus. These findings have led to the postulation that LC degeneration patterns could be used to classify and differentiate between various sub-groups of PD patients. Comprehensive evidence by Braak and colleagues have found that, in PD patients, the degeneration of NE neurons progressed from lower brain stem regions, like the LC, to more rostral areas, like the SNpc (Braak and Braak, 2000; Braak et al., 2003).

Biochemical evidence obtained from post-mortem and ante-mortem studies in PD patients suggests that NE levels in multiple brain regions, including the motor cortex, hippocampus, striatum, substantia nigra and hypothalamus, are significantly decreased (Gesi et al., 2000). Interestingly, brain regions that are innervated by NE nuclei other than LC are relatively spared from NE loss.

Accumulating evidence strongly suggests that the loss of NE neurons originating from the LC is a very important aspect of the pathophysiology of PD and contributes to the progression of PD, deleteriously affecting the survival of DA neurons. For example, various experimental studies have demonstrated that prior loss of NE innervation increases the vulnerability of the DA neurons to a further neurotoxic insult (Fornai et al., 1995; Mavridis et al., 1991). Conversely, it has been established that increased NE stimulation is neuroprotective against 1-methyl-4-phenyl-1,2,3,6-tetrahydropyridine (MPTP)-induced induced neurotoxicity (Kilbourn et al., 1998; Rommelfanger et al., 2004). Thus, it appears that NE may play a neurotrophic role acting as a neuroprotective mechanism for DA neurons. This was corroborated by Tong and colleagues (2006) who found an inverse relationship between intact NE innervation and DA loss in PD patients. Collectively, these findings suggest that the loss of LC neurons precedes and facilitates the subsequent damage to nigrostriatal DA neurons.

Therefore, since NE is known to act as a modulator of the dopaminergic system in various brain regions, the loss of NE appears to be a very critical event in the timeline of PD.

2.1.2 Mechanism(s) of NE loss

The mechanisms underlying NE loss like DA neurodegeneration remain to be elucidated. However, NE neurons are susceptible to the same insults that affect DA neurons such as oxidative stress, neuroinflammation, protein misfolding and neurotoxin-induced cell death. For example, Yavich et al. (2006) demonstrated that mice expressing a pathogenic mutation of α-synuclein have abnormal compartmentalization and metabolism of both DA and NE. In addition, it is well known that monoamines have a tendency to auto-oxidize leading to oxidative stress and neuronal cell loss (Chiueh et al., 2000; Maker et al., 1986); and the aforementioned abnormal compartmentalization of NE may make LC neurons vulnerable to oxidative stress. Genetic mutations in Parkin, a genotype found in PD, also make LC neurons vulnerable to cell death. Studies in mice have demonstrated that Parkin mutations lead to loss of LC neurons (Von Coelln et al., 2004) likely via protein misfolding and dysregulation of the ubiquitous-proteasome system. This is a compelling finding since alterations in the expression of proteasome activators have been shown to correlate with neuronal loss in SNpc and the LC. Poor expression of proteasome activators correlated with neuronal cell loss in the LC and regions expressing normal levels of the proteasome activators did not suffer from neuronal degeneration (McNaught et al., 2010). Finally, NE neurons are also susceptible to neurotoxin-induced apoptosis. For example, in the experimental 6-hydroxydopamine (6-OHDA) model of PD, administration of desipramine, a NE transporter (NET) inhibitor, infers protection to NE neurons. Since DA and NE transporters share homology in structure and display common affinity for several substrates, it is likely that NET takes up the same neurotoxins that affect DA neurons in sporadic PD. Collectively these factors could make the LC neurons vulnerable to damage in both genetic and sporadic models of PD. More studies that shed light on the neurodegenerative processes in the LC are necessary to better understand the progression of PD. Moreover, neuroprotective strategies directed toward LC neurons may be warranted since loss of LC neurons makes the DA neurons more vulnerable to neurodegeneration.

2.2 Non-motor symptoms

2.2.1 NE loss and non-motor symptoms

Although motor symptoms of PD are widely acknowledged hallmarks of this neurodegenerative disease, there exists compelling evidence for the presence of psychiatric complications, such as depression, anxiety and psychotic symptoms (Bosboom et al., 2004). Loss of dopaminergic and noradrenergic innervation has been associated with psychiatric complications such as depression (Remy et al., 2005) and anxiety (Stein et al., 1990; Lauterbach et al., 2003). Cognitive and mood dysfunction has been reported in >50% of PD patients. In patients with early PD, depression (40%), apathy (27%), and anxiety (27%) are widely reported (Aarsland et al., 2009) and it is notable that these non-motor symptoms are identified as the most important and devastating feature contributing towards poverty of quality of life (McKinlay et al., 2008; Schrag, 2006). Moreover, the incidence of depression and anxiety in PD exceeds not only rates within the normal population but also other neurological disorders (Weintraub et al., 2003), with anxiety disorders, such as off-period panic attacks and specific phobias, have been reported in nearly 40% of PD patients (Lauterbach, 2005). Collectively these findings lead to the important observation that depression and anxiety are likely a result of neuropathological processes rather than as a result of motor impairments.

The exact pathophysiology underlying these mood dysfunctions are unknown though given the role of NE in several of these symptoms, it is likely that NE loss in PD plays a critical role. As discussed earlier, neurodegeneration of LC neurons in PD is a well established phenomenon that precedes DA neuronal loss (Braak et al., 2003). It has been postulated that a compromised LC produces significant changes in NE receptors and transporters that may lead to the development or exacerbation of depression/anxiety (Eskow Jaunarajs et al., 2010). Additionally, Remy et al. (2005) have reported reduced binding for the DA/NE transporter, suggesting a loss of terminals, in the LC of PD patients suffering from anxiety and depression (Remy et al., 2005). In a rodent model of PD, alterations in DA and NE systems in the striatum have been reported to produce anxiety (Tadaiesky et al., 2008), consistent with findings in naïve rats that NE regulates anxiety behavior. Experimental studies have reported depression and anxiety-like behaviors in a 6-OHDA lesion model of PD (Branchi et al., 2010; Eskow Jaunarajs et al., 2010; Tadaiesky et al., 2008). Additionally, concomitant depletion of NE, 5-HT and DA in a unilateral rodent model of PD produced symptoms of depression, suggesting that loss of all three systems contribute to PD-like depression (Delaville et al., 2010). In an interesting study, Taylor et al. (2009) used a vesicular monoamine transporter-2 (VMAT-2) deficient mouse model to induce severe NE and DA loss thereby mimicking PD. VMAT-2 deficient mice exhibited severe depression and anxiety-like symptoms that worsened with advancing age (Taylor et al., 2009) highlighting a possible interplay between DA and NE. Histological studies have highlighted the fact that LC neuron morphology is more severely affected in PD with depression than in PD without depressio (Chan-Palay and Asan, 1989). While most of the evidence in clinical and experimental models correlating NE deficit with mood dysfunction is indirect, there exists evidence that noradrenergic drugs might provide relief in the treatment of these mood disorders.

2.2.2 Treatment of non-motor symptoms with NE drugs

The role for the NE system in affective disorders such as anxiety and depression has been partially implicated by the effectiveness of drugs that enhance NE levels. Reboxetine, a NET inhibitor, has been proven to be effective in the treatment of depression associated with PD (Pintor et al., 2006). In one of the largest Randomized Clinical Trials (RCT) to date Menza and colleagues (2009) found that Nortryptaline, a tricyclic antidepressant (TCA), with preferential actions as a NET inhibitor, was proven to be more effective in treating depression in PD patients compared to selective 5-HT reuptake inhibitors (SSRIs: Menza et al., 2009). In a similar placebo controlled study in PD patients, Desipramine, a NET inhibitor, was found to be effective in treating depression; however, these improvements were accompanied with mild adverse side effects (Devos et al., 2008). These therapeutic findings suggest a more prominent role for NE in the development of depression in PD. The few drugs that seem to be effective in treating depression likely act to elevate extracellular NE levels in the brain, by blocking NET (Dziedzicka-Wasylewska et al., 2006). Therefore, it seems feasible that drugs that mimic NE or elevate NE levels in the brain would be effective in treating NE-related non-motor symptoms in PD.

3. Serotonin system

The 5-HT system like the NE system undergoes significant, though more variable, neurodegeneration as PD progresses; a finding documented in various studies, both post-

and ante-mortem (Miyawaki et al., 1997; Scatton et al., 1983). Since the 5-HT system ubiquitously innervates and modulates basal ganglia nuclei, 5-HT loss likely affects both motor symptoms of PD and l-DOPA related side effects. In addition, given the role of 5-HT in mood, such alterations may also correlate with the preponderance of depression and anxiety seen in PD. Therefore, various treatment strategies have been developed that modulate the 5-HT system. In the following sections, we review the neuropathology of the 5-HT system in PD, the consequences of a damaged 5-HT system on non-motor aspects, and the line of experimental and clinical treatments targeting the 5-HT system to provide symptomatic relief for the PD patient.

3.1 CNS pathophysiology of 5-HT system in PD

3.1.1 Neuroanatomical evidence in PD patients

Even though degeneration of DA neurons in the SNpc remains the best identified neuropathological hallmark in PD, there exists increasing evidence suggesting PD-related pathology in the principle 5-HT cell bodies, the raphe nuclei and other regions innervated by raphe neurons (Braak et al., 2003).

Multiple studies have reported the presence of LB in the caudal group of raphe nuclei, like the raphe magnus and raphe pallidus, in early PD, sometimes occurring even before the onset of motor symptoms (Braak et al., 2003; Del Tredici et al., 2002; Parkkinen et al., 2008). It is interesting to note that these caudal raphe nuclei contain 5-HT neurons associated with functions like pain perception, and gastrointestinal motility that are manifest as early symptoms in PD patients prior to motor complaints (Chaudhuri and Schapira, 2009). The rostral raphe nuclei consisting of dorsal and medial raphe nuclei are equally affected in PD and according to Braak staging, are affected before the SNpc but after the caudal raphe nuclei (Braak et al., 2003).

Despite reports of raphe LB formation, evidence for the degeneration of 5-HT neurons in the rostral raphe nuclei is variable; post-mortem analysis of PD brains by Paulus and Jellinger (1991) revealed a profound loss of 5-HT neurons, however, other studies have not (Halliday et al., 1990; Mann and Yates, 1983). Several studies have employed transcranial sonography to study the midbrain raphe nuclei. This work has revealed abnormal pathology in the form of hypoechogenicity or an absence of sonographic signals in PD vs. control subjects. Interestingly, PD patients in one study also suffered from higher incidence of depression, reflecting a direct relationship between raphe nuclei loss and PD-related depression (Becker et al., 1997; Berg and Gaenslen, 2010; Walter et al., 2007b). MRI imaging studies carried out in depressed PD patients have also demonstrated a loss of homogeneity in the midbrain raphe consistent with neuronal compromise and/or cell loss (Berg et al., 1999).

PD-related pathology of the 5-HT system is not limited to the cell bodies of the raphe nuclei. Convincing evidence exists for damaged 5-HT projections and terminals as well. For example, post-mortem studies in PD patients have described significant loss of 5-HT markers, such as brain 5-HT concentrations. In cortical and the basal ganglia regions 5-HT content has been reported to be reduced by as much as 50% compared to controls (Birkmayer and Birkmayer, 1987). Kish and colleagues (2008) investigated the integrity of the forebrain 5-HT system. In contrast to DA loss, which was preferential to the putamen, 5-HT loss was more prominent in the caudate for all 5-HT markers including 5-HT (-66%), the 5-HT metabolite 5-HIAA (-42%), 5-HT transporter (SERT), (-56%) and the rate limiting enzyme in 5-HT synthesis tryptophan hydroxylase (-59%). These corroborated ante-mortem observations in PD patients that examined levels of 5-HIAA in cerebrospinal fluid and have found significant reductions when compared to control patients. Interestingly, the deficits in cerebrospinal fluid 5-HIAA levels were more pronounced in PD patients with depression in comparison to non-depressed PD patients, again supporting a relationship between decreased 5-HT function and depression in PD (Mayeux et al., 1984; Mayeux et al., 1986).

Development of additional imaging technologies, like PET and SPECT, has facilitated the measurement of SERT and thus the evaluation of the integrity of the 5-HT terminal (Meyer et al., 2007). In vivo SPECT studies, using non-specific ligands for SERT, found decreased binding in the cortex and hypothalamus of PD patients (Berding et al., 2003a; Berding et al., 2003b). However, these findings have been contradicted by studies that did not find any changes in the mid-brain but rather reduction in the thalamic nuclei of PD patients (Caretti et al., 2008; Kim et al., 2003; Roselli et al., 2010). Decreased SERT binding has been observed by use of PET imaging using more specific ligands. Under these circumstances reduced SERT was observed in the striatum, frontal cortex, caudate nucleus, putamen and the mid-brain raphe region of patients with PD (Albin et al., 2008; Guttman et al., 2007; Kerenyi et al., 2003). SERT binding is also labile, changing as PD progresses. For example, in the early stages of PD, SERT binding has been shown to be reduced in only in the striatum, thalamus and cingulate cortex. In later symptomatic stages of PD these alterations appear to extend to the prefrontal cortex and the raphe nuclei (Haapaniemi et al., 2001; Politis et al., 2010). Such findings suggest that a progressive reduction in SERT binding may serve as good a bio-marker for the diagnosis and development of treatment strategies for PD patients.

In addition to neuronal integrity, 5-HT receptors are also affected in PD. Modification of pre- and post-synaptic 5-HT receptors has been observed in various animal and human studies of PD. While it is not clear whether these compensatory changes are due to lost 5-HT input, DA innervation, or DA replacement, it is established that dopaminergic tone regulates the expression of several 5-HT receptors. 5-HT_{1A} receptor binding is not consistently affected in the 6-OHDA model of PD; however, studies in MPTP-treated macaques suggest increases in striatal and cortical binding (Frechilla et al., 2001; Huot et al., 2010b). 5-HT_{1B} receptor binding is significantly increased in the striatum (54%) and the globus pallidus (33%). Intranigral lesions have also been reported to increase 5-HT_4 receptor density in the caudate and the globus pallidus (Di Matteo et al., 2008). Studies using in situ hybridization and autoradiographic radioligand binding have revealed few changes in 5-HT_{1A} and 5-HT_{2B} receptor binding (Numan et al., 1995; Zhang et al., 2008); however, 5-HT_{2A} receptors have been shown to increase in the striatum (Zhang et al., 2008). The possibility exists that striatal 5-HT_{2A} and 5-HT_{2C} receptor are differentially regulated in 6-OHDA-lesioned animals and the changes observed in these receptors could be a reflection of the compensatory changes in the PD-afflicted brain. Some of the changes in 5-HT receptor binding are reversible after treatment with l-DOPA, Zhang and colleagues (2008) reported a reversal of increased striatal 5-HT_{2A} receptor mRNA in a 6-OHDA rodent model of PD after l-DOPA treatment. Interestingly, l-DOPA did not alter the changes in striatal 5-HT_{2C} receptor mRNA levels. It appears that changes in regulation of the 5-HT_{2A} receptor are dependent on striatal DA levels and the 5-HT_{2C} loss could be due to nigrostriatal loss, thus reflecting a difference in regulation between the two receptor sub-types. The 5-HT receptor changes seen in PD patients are partly similar to changes in the experimental PD models. Similar increases were seen in the density of 5-HT_{2A} and 5-HT_{2C} receptor in the striatum as well as other regions (Fox and Brotchie, 2000; Huot et al., 2010c; Radja et al., 1993). It is important to note that these changes may not be direct evidence of 5-HT neuropathology but definitely provide an insight into neuroplasticity of the 5-HT system that may unravel potential targets for therapeutic strategies in the treatment of PD.

An indirect marker for 5-HT alterations in PD is the assessment of responses to 5-HT challenge tests. Of these, the most common is the endocrine response to the 5-HT releasing agent, Fenfluramine. In normal subjects Fenfluramine produces robust increases in prolactin and corticosterone levels. However, in PD patients it was found that this endocrine response was impaired (Kostic et al., 1996; Volpi et al., 1997). Such effects may also correlate with non-motor symptoms since PD patients suffering from depression also displayed blunted prolactin responses in comparison to non-depressed PD patients (Kostic et al., 1996). Collectively these findings provide substantial evidence for neurochemical, neuroanatomical and functional alterations of the 5-HT system.

3.2 Non-motor symptoms

3.2.1 5-HT loss and non-motor symptoms

As previously mentioned depression and anxiety are some of the most common non-motor symptoms in PD and are even associated with an elevated risk towards the development of PD (Leentjens et al., 2003; Schuurman et al., 2002; Shiba et al., 2000). The underlying pathophysiological mechanisms remain to be completely understood; however, it is well established that 5-HT dysfunction plays an important role in several mood-disorders in non-PD patients (Michelsen et al., 2008). Depression not only reduces the quality of life for PD patients but has a negative effect on caregivers as well (Schrag et al., 2000; 2004).

During the progression of PD it has been observed that brain regions, like rostral raphe, thalamus and cortex, that mediate mood disturbances in PD are severely affected by the presence of Lewy bodies (Braak and Del Tredici, 2008). Currently, most evidence linking abnormal serotonergic neurotransmission to mood disturbances in PD is corroborative but points to a role for 5-HT pathology. For example, depressed PD patients display reduced brainstem raphe echogenicity, in comparison to non-depressed PD patients (Walter et al., 2007a). Post-mortem comparisons of neuronal density in the dorsal raphe nucleus between depressed and non-depressed PD patients found lower neuronal density in depressed PD patients (Paulus and Jellinger, 1991). In vivo studies measuring cerebrospinal fluid levels found lower levels of 5-HIAA in depressed PD patients indicating reduced 5-HT metabolism (Mayeux et al., 1986). Imaging studies have been less conclusive and have found either no change in SERT uptake (Kim et al., 2003) or reported elevated 5-HT receptor binding in depressed PD patients when compared to non-depressed PD patients (Boileau et al., 2008). Interestingly, acute tryptophan depletion in a small group of PD patients did not produce depression or anxiety in these patients (Leentjens et al., 2006). Another major non-motor symptom affecting PD patients is the development of psychosis that may lead to development of paranoid delusions in some PD patients (Ravina et al., 2007). The underlying cause remains to be elucidated and some investigators have postulated that there may be a serotonergic involvement. 5-HT_2 receptors, responsible for hallucinations and psychosis, are relatively intact or may even be upregulated in the cortex of PD patients suffering from psychosis compared to PD patients free from any psychotic disorder (Cheng et al., 1991; Huot et al., 2010a).

3.2.2 Treatment of non-motor symptoms with serotonergic drugs

Drugs acting on the serotonergic system are currently the standard of care for the treatment and management of psychiatric dysfunction, like anxiety, depression and psychosis in PD, despite causal evidence or 5-HT dysfunction in PD-related mood disorders. Most of the SSRIs currently used act by elevating the extracellular 5-HT levels and thus act indirectly on various post-synaptic 5-HT receptors, many of which have been implicated in mood disorders (Dobkin et al., 2011; Dobkin et al., 2010; Fox et al., 2009; Menza et al., 2009; Weintraub et al., 2006). The other potential side effects such as postural hypotension, sedation and 5-HT syndrome, due to 5-HT_1 receptor stimulation, continue to limit the use of these antidepressants in PD patients (Veazey et al., 2005). It is important to note that many PD patients suffer from orthostatic hypotension and tremors and these could get exacerbated. Nefazodone, a 5-HT_2 receptor antagonist/re-uptake inhibitor has been used as an antidepressant and to reduce extrapyramidal symptoms in PD patients (Avila et al., 2003).

Psychotic complications usually treated with drugs that have an anti-dopaminergic profile are not ideal for the PD patient since it can lead to worsening of motor symptoms. Therefore, atypical antipsychotics, like Clozapine and Quetiapine, have been found to be effective in treating psychosis in PD patients (Kurlan et al., 2007), an effect attributed to their 5-HT_2 receptor antagonistic properties. Another non-selective 5-HT_2 receptor antagonist Mianserin has been demonstrated to reduce visual hallucinations in a small group of PD patients without affecting the parkinsonian motor symptoms. Preliminary findings from a Phase II study evaluating Pimavanserin, a 5-HT2A receptor inverse agonist, are encouraging and show a trend in improving psychosis without affecting PD motor scores (Meltzer et al., 2010).

It is of interest to note that l-DOPA therapy has been traditionally assumed to improve affective symptoms, like depression and anxiety; however, emerging evidence suggests that chronic use of l-DOPA may aggravate mood problems (Eskow Jaunarajs et al., 2011). Preclinical investigations have reported that 6-OHDA-lesioned rats chronically treated with l-DOPA exhibit reduced 5-HT and 5-HIAA levels (Carta et al., 2007; Eskow Jaunarajs et al., 2011). Studies employing in vivo microdialysis have confirmed reductions in 5-HT levels, after acute l-DOPA, in the 6-OHDA-lesioned striatum as well as in non-motor affective sites (Navailles et al., 2010). Chronic l-DOPA treatment has been demonstrated to reduce expression of tryptophan hydroxylase within the dorsal raphe nucleus, which may lead to reduced 5-HT synthesis and release in efferent structures (Eskow Jaunarajs et al., 2011). l-DOPA uptake and release of DA by 5-HT terminals into the striatum may compete with native 5-HT function leading to an aggravation of affective disorders like depression and anxiety in PD patients undergoing chronic l-DOPA therapy (Eskow Jaunarajs et al., 2011) .

In sum, drugs acting on the serotonergic system provide some symptomatic relief for PD patients. However, l-DOPA therapy by itself has the potential to exacerbate mood disorders.

4. Conclusion

In conclusion, there exists convincing evidence that both 5-HT and NE systems are severely affected in PD and that they contribute towards PD progression and symptoms. Therapeutics targeting these systems appear beneficial; however, more research is necessary to develop more efficacious therapeutic targets and strategies.

5. References

Aarsland, D., Marsh, L., Schrag, A., 2009. Neuropsychiatric symptoms in Parkinson's disease. Movement disorders : official journal of the Movement Disorder Society. 24, 2175-86.

Albin, R.L., Koeppe, R.A., Bohnen, N.I., Wernette, K., Kilbourn, M.A., Frey, K.A., 2008. Spared caudal brainstem SERT binding in early Parkinson's disease. Journal of cerebral blood flow and metabolism : official journal of the International Society of Cerebral Blood Flow and Metabolism. 28, 441-4.

Avila, A., Cardona, X., Martin-Baranera, M., Maho, P., Sastre, F., Bello, J., 2003. Does nefazodone improve both depression and Parkinson disease? A pilot randomized trial. Journal of clinical psychopharmacology. 23, 509-13.

Becker, T., Becker, G., Seufert, J., Hofmann, E., Lange, K.W., Naumann, M., Lindner, A., Reichmann, H., Riederer, P., Beckmann, H., Reiners, K., 1997. Parkinson's disease and depression: evidence for an alteration of the basal limbic system detected by transcranial sonography. Journal of neurology, neurosurgery, and psychiatry. 63, 590-6.

Berding, G., Brucke, T., Odin, P., Brooks, D.J., Kolbe, H., Gielow, P., Harke, H., Knoop, B.O., Dengler, R., Knapp, W.H., 2003a. [[123I]beta-CIT SPECT imaging of dopamine and serotonin transporters in Parkinson's disease and multiple system atrophy. Nuklearmedizin. Nuclear medicine. 42, 31-8.

Berding, G., Schrader, C.H., Peschel, T., van den Hoff, J., Kolbe, H., Meyer, G.J., Dengler, R., Knapp, W.H., 2003b. [N-methyl 11C]meta-Hydroxyephedrine positron emission tomography in Parkinson's disease and multiple system atrophy. European journal of nuclear medicine and molecular imaging. 30, 127-31.

Berg, D., Supprian, T., Hofmann, E., Zeiler, B., Jager, A., Lange, K.W., Reiners, K., Becker, T., Becker, G., 1999. Depression in Parkinson's disease: brainstem midline alteration on transcranial sonography and magnetic resonance imaging. Journal of neurology. 246, 1186-93.

Berg, D., Gaenslen, A., 2010. Place value of transcranial sonography in early diagnosis of Parkinson's disease. Neuro-degenerative diseases. 7, 291-9.

Bertrand, E., Lechowicz, W., Szpak, G.M., Dymecki, J., 1997. Qualitative and quantitative analysis of locus coeruleus neurons in Parkinson's disease. Folia neuropathologica / Association of Polish Neuropathologists and Medical Research Centre, Polish Academy of Sciences. 35, 80-6.

Birkmayer, J.G., Birkmayer, W., 1987. Improvement of disability and akinesia of patients with Parkinson's disease by intravenous iron substitution. Annals of clinical and laboratory science. 17, 32-5.

Bosboom, J.L., Stoffers, D., Wolters, E., 2004. Cognitive dysfunction and dementia in Parkinson's disease. Journal of neural transmission. 111, 1303-15.

Braak, H., Braak, E., 2000. Pathoanatomy of Parkinson's disease. Journal of neurology. 247 Suppl 2, II3-10.

Braak, H., Del Tredici, K., Rub, U., de Vos, R.A., Jansen Steur, E.N., Braak, E., 2003. Staging of brain pathology related to sporadic Parkinson's disease. Neurobiology of aging. 24, 197-211.

Braak, H., Del Tredici, K., 2008. Invited Article: Nervous system pathology in sporadic Parkinson disease. Neurology. 70, 1916-25.

Branchi, I., D'Andrea, I., Armida, M., Carnevale, D., Ajmone-Cat, M.A., Pezzola, A., Potenza, R.L., Morgese, M.G., Cassano, T., Minghetti, L., Popoli, P., Alleva, E., 2010. Striatal 6-OHDA lesion in mice: Investigating early neurochemical changes underlying Parkinson's disease. Behavioural brain research. 208, 137-43.

Caretti, V., Stoffers, D., Winogrodzka, A., Isaias, I.U., Costantino, G., Pezzoli, G., Ferrarese, C., Antonini, A., Wolters, E.C., Booij, J., 2008. Loss of thalamic serotonin transporters in early drug-naive Parkinson's disease patients is associated with tremor: an [(123)I]beta-CIT SPECT study. Journal of neural transmission. 115, 721-9.

Carta, M., Carlsson, T., Kirik, D., Bjorklund, A., 2007. Dopamine released from 5-HT terminals is the cause of L-DOPA-induced dyskinesia in parkinsonian rats. Brain : a journal of neurology. 130, 1819-33.

Chaudhuri, K.R., Schapira, A.H., 2009. Non-motor symptoms of Parkinson's disease: dopaminergic pathophysiology and treatment. Lancet neurology. 8, 464-74.

Chaudhuri, K.R., Schapira, A.H., 2009. Non-motor symptoms of Parkinson's disease: dopaminergic pathophysiology and treatment. Lancet neurology. 8, 464-74.

Chan-Palay, V.,Asan, E., 1989. Alterations in catecholamine neurons of the locus coeruleus in senile dementia of the Alzheimer type and in Parkinson's disease with and without dementia and depression. Journal of comparative neurology. 287, 373-392.

Chiueh, C.C., Andoh, T., Lai, A.R., Lai, E., Krishna, G., 2000. Neuroprotective strategies in Parkinson's disease: protection against progressive nigral damage induced by free radicals. Neurotoxicity research. 2, 293-310.

Del Tredici, K., Rub, U., De Vos, R.A., Bohl, J.R., Braak, H., 2002. Where does parkinson disease pathology begin in the brain? Journal of neuropathology and experimental neurology. 61, 413-26.

Delaville, C., Chetrit, J., Abdallah, K., Morin, S., Cardoit, L., De Deurwaerdere, P., Benzazzouz, A. 2010. Involvement of monoamine deficiency in motor and nonmotor disabilities in Parkinson's disease: behavioral, bicochemical and electrophysiological studies. International Basal Ganglia Society abstract

Di Matteo, V., Pierucci, M., Esposito, E., Crescimanno, G., Benigno, A., Di Giovanni, G., 2008. Serotonin modulation of the basal ganglia circuitry: therapeutic implication for Parkinson's disease and other motor disorders. Progress in brain research. 172, 423-63.

Dobkin, R.D., Menza, M. Bienfait, K.L., Gara, M., Marin, H., Mark, M.H., Dicke, A., Troster, A. 2010. The impact of antidepressant treatment on cognitive functioning in depressed patients with Parkinson's disease. Joural of neuropsychiatry and neurological sciences. 22(2), 188-95.

Dobkin, R.D., Menza, M. Bienfait, K.L., Gara, M., Marin, H., Mark, M.H., Dicke, A., Friedman,J. 2011. Depression in Parkinson's disease: symptom improvement and residual symptoms after acute pharmacologic management. American joural of Geriatric Psychiatry. 19(3), 222-9.

Devos,D., Dujordin, K., Poirot, I., Moreau, C., Cottencin, O., Thomas, P., Destee, A., Bordet, R., Defebvre, L. 2008. Comparison of desipramine and citalopram treatments for depression in Parkinson's disease: a double-blind, randomized, placebo-controlled study. Movement Disorders.23 (6), 850-857.

Ehringer, H., Hornykiewicz, O., 1960. [Distribution of noradrenaline and dopamine (3-hydroxytyramine) in the human brain and their behavior in diseases of the extrapyramidal system]. Klinische Wochenschrift. 38, 1236-9.

Eskow Jaunarajs, K.L., Dupre, K.B., Ostock, C.Y., Button, T., Deak, T., Bishop, C., 2010. Behavioral and neurochemical effects of chronic L-DOPA treatment on nonmotor sequelae in the hemiparkinsonian rat. Behavioural pharmacology. 21, 627-37.

Eskow Jaunarajs, K.L., Angoa-Perez, M., Kuhn, D.M., Bishop, C., 2011. Potential mechanisms underlying anxiety and depression in Parkinson's disease: consequences of l-DOPA treatment. Neuroscience and biobehavioral reviews. 35, 556-64.

Fornai, F., Bassi, L., Torracca, M.T., Scalori, V., Corsini, G.U., 1995. Norepinephrine loss exacerbates methamphetamine-induced striatal dopamine depletion in mice. European journal of pharmacology. 283, 99-102.

Fornai, F., di Poggio, A.B., Pellegrini, A., Ruggieri, S., Paparelli, A., 2007. Noradrenaline in Parkinson's disease: from disease progression to current therapeutics. Current medicinal chemistry. 14, 2330-4.

Fox, S.H., Brotchie, J.M., 2000. 5-HT2C receptor binding is increased in the substantia nigra pars reticulata in Parkinson's disease. Movement disorders : official journal of the Movement Disorder Society. 15, 1064-9.

Fox, S.H., Chuang, R., Brotchie, J.M., 2009. Serotonin and Parkinson's disease: On movement, mood, and madness. Movement disorders : official journal of the Movement Disorder Society. 24, 1255-66.

Frechilla, D., Cobreros, A., Saldise, L., Moratalla, R., Insausti, R., Luquin, M., Del Rio, J., 2001. Serotonin 5-HT(1A) receptor expression is selectively enhanced in the striosomal compartment of chronic parkinsonian monkeys. Synapse. 39, 288-96.

German, D.C., Manaye, K.F., White, C.L., 3rd, Woodward, D.J., McIntire, D.D., Smith, W.K., Kalaria, R.N., Mann, D.M., 1992. Disease-specific patterns of locus coeruleus cell loss. Annals of neurology. 32, 667-76.

Gesi, M., Soldani, P., Giorgi, F.S., Santinami, A., Bonaccorsi, I., Fornai, F., 2000. The role of the locus coeruleus in the development of Parkinson's disease. Neuroscience and biobehavioral reviews. 24, 655-68.

Guttman, M., Boileau, I., Warsh, J., Saint-Cyr, J.A., Ginovart, N., McCluskey, T., Houle, S., Wilson, A., Mundo, E., Rusjan, P., Meyer, J., Kish, S.J., 2007. Brain serotonin transporter binding in non-depressed patients with Parkinson's disease. European journal of neurology : the official journal of the European Federation of Neurological Societies. 14, 523-8.

Haapaniemi, T.H., Ahonen, A., Torniainen, P., Sotaniemi, K.A., Myllyla, V.V., 2001. [123I]beta-CIT SPECT demonstrates decreased brain dopamine and serotonin transporter levels in untreated parkinsonian patients. Movement disorders : official journal of the Movement Disorder Society. 16, 124-30.

Halliday, G.M., Li, Y.W., Blumbergs, P.C., Joh, T.H., Cotton, R.G., Howe, P.R., Blessing, W.W., Geffen, L.B., 1990. Neuropathology of immunohistochemically identified brainstem neurons in Parkinson's disease. Annals of neurology. 27, 373-85.

Hein, L., Altman, J.D., Kobilka, B.K., 1999. Two functionally distinct alpha2-adrenergic receptors regulate sympathetic neurotransmission. Nature. 402, 181-4.

Huot, P., Johnston, T.H., Darr, T., Hazrati, L.N., Visanji, N.P., Pires, D., Brotchie, J.M., Fox, S.H., 2010a. Increased 5-HT(2A) receptors in the temporal cortex of parkinsonian patients with visual hallucinations. Movement disorders.25(10), 1399-1408.

Huot, P., Johnston, T.H., Koprich, J.B., Winkelmolen, L., Fox, S.H., Brotchie, J.M., 2010b. Regulation of cortical and striatal 5-HT(1A) receptors in the MPTP-lesioned macaque. Neurobiology of aging.

Huot, P., Johnston, T.H., Winkelmolen, L., Fox, S.H., Brotchie, J.M., 2010c. 5-HT(2A) receptor levels increase in MPTP-lesioned macaques treated chronically with L-DOPA. Neurobiology of aging.

Jackson, M.J., Al-Barghouthy, G., Pearce, R.K., Smith, L., Hagan, J.J., Jenner, P., 2004. Effect of 5-HT1B/D receptor agonist and antagonist administration on motor function in haloperidol and MPTP-treated common marmosets. Pharmacology, biochemistry, and behavior. 79, 391-400.

Kerenyi, L., Ricaurte, G.A., Schretlen, D.J., McCann, U., Varga, J., Mathews, W.B., Ravert, H.T., Dannals, R.F., Hilton, J., Wong, D.F., Szabo, Z., 2003. Positron emission tomography of striatal serotonin transporters in Parkinson disease. Archives of neurology. 60, 1223-9.

Kilbourn, M.R., Sherman, P., Abbott, L.C., 1998. Reduced MPTP neurotoxicity in striatum of the mutant mouse tottering. Synapse. 30, 205-10.

Kim, S.E., Choi, J.Y., Choe, Y.S., Choi, Y., Lee, W.Y., 2003. Serotonin transporters in the midbrain of Parkinson's disease patients: a study with 123I-beta-CIT SPECT. Journal of nuclear medicine : official publication, Society of Nuclear Medicine. 44, 870-6.

Kish, S.J., Tong, J., Hornykiewicz, O., Rajput, A., Chang, L.J., Guttman, M., Furukawa, Y., 2008. Preferential loss of serotonin markers in caudate versus putamen in Parkinson's disease. Brain : a journal of neurology. 131, 120-31.

Kostic, V.S., Lecic, D., Doder, M., Marinkovic, J., Filipovic, S., 1996. Prolactin and cortisol responses to fenfluramine in Parkinson's disease. Biological psychiatry. 40, 769-75.

Kurlan, R., Cummings, J., Raman, R., Thal, L., 2007. Quetiapine for agitation or psychosis in patients with dementia and parkinsonism. Neurology. 68, 1356-63.

Lauterbach, E.C.., Freeman, A., and Vogel, R.L. 2003. Correlates of generalized anxiety and panic attacks in dystonia and Parkinson's disease. Cognitive and behavioral neurology. 16, 225-233.

Lauterbach, E.C.., 2005. The neuropsychiatry of Parkinson's disease. Minerva medica. 96(3), 155-173.

Leentjens, A.F., Van den Akker, M., Metsemakers, J.F., Lousberg, R., Verhey, F.R., 2003. Higher incidence of depression preceding the onset of Parkinson's disease: a register study. Movement disorders : official journal of the Movement Disorder Society. 18, 414-8.

Leentjens, A.F., Scholtissen, B., Vreeling, F.W., Verhey, F.R., 2006. The serotonergic hypothesis for depression in Parkinson's disease: an experimental approach. Neuropsychopharmacology : official publication of the American College of Neuropsychopharmacology. 31, 1009-15.

Maker, H.S., Weiss, C., Brannan, T.S., 1986. Amine-mediated toxicity. The effects of dopamine, norepinephrine, 5-hydroxytryptamine, 6-hydroxydopamine, ascorbate, glutathione and peroxide on the in vitro activities of creatine and adenylate kinases in the brain of the rat. Neuropharmacology. 25, 25-32.

Mann, D.M., 1983. The locus coeruleus and its possible role in ageing and degenerative disease of the human central nervous system. Mechanisms of ageing and development. 23, 73-94.

Mann, D.M., Yates, P.O., 1983. Pathological basis for neurotransmitter changes in Parkinson's disease. Neuropathology and applied neurobiology. 9, 3-19.

Marien, M.R., Colpaert, F.C., Rosenquist, A.C., 2004. Noradrenergic mechanisms in neurodegenerative diseases: a theory. Brain research. Brain research reviews. 45, 38-78.

Marin, C., Aguilar, E., Rodriguez-Oroz, M.C., Bartoszyk, G.D., Obeso, J.A., 2009. Local administration of sarizotan into the subthalamic nucleus attenuates levodopa-induced dyskinesias in 6-OHDA-lesioned rats. Psychopharmacology. 204, 241-50.

Mavridis, M., Degryse, A.D., Lategan, A.J., Marien, M.R., Colpaert, F.C., 1991. Effects of locus coeruleus lesions on parkinsonian signs, striatal dopamine and substantia nigra cell loss after 1-methyl-4-phenyl-1,2,3,6-tetrahydropyridine in monkeys: a possible role for the locus coeruleus in the progression of Parkinson's disease. Neuroscience. 41, 507-23.

Mayeux, R., Williams, J.B., Stern, Y., Cote, L., 1984. Depression and Parkinson's disease. Advances in neurology. 40, 241-50.

Mayeux, R., Stern, Y., Williams, J.B., Cote, L., Frantz, A., Dyrenfurth, I., 1986. Clinical and biochemical features of depression in Parkinson's disease. The American journal of psychiatry. 143, 756-9.

McKinlay, A., Grace, R.C., Dalrymple-Alford, J.C., Anderson, T., Fink, J., Roger, D., 2008. A profile of neuropsychiatric problems and their relationship to quality of life for Parkinson's disease patients without dementia. Parkinsonism & related disorders. 14, 37-42.

McNaught, K.S., Jnobaptiste, R., Jackson, T., Jengelley, T.A., 2010. The pattern of neuronal loss and survival may reflect differential expression of proteasome activators in Parkinson's disease. Synapse. 64, 241-50.

Meltzer, H.Y., Mills, R., Revell, S., Williams, H., Johnson, A., Bahr, D., Friedman, J.H., 2010. Pimavanserin, a serotonin(2A) receptor inverse agonist, for the treatment of parkinson's disease psychosis. Neuropsychopharmacology : official publication of the American College of Neuropsychopharmacology. 35, 881-92.

Menza, M., Dobkin, R.D., Marin, H., Mark, M.H., Gara, M., Buyske, S., Bienfait, K., Dicke, A., 2009. A controlled trial of antidepressants in patients with Parkinson disease and depression. Neurology. 72, 886-92.

Meyer, J.S., Huang, J., Chowdhury, M.H., 2007. MRI confirms mild cognitive impairments prodromal for Alzheimer's, vascular and Parkinson-Lewy body dementias. Journal of the neurological sciences. 257, 97-104.

Michelsen, K.A., Prickaerts, J., Steinbusch, H.W., 2008. The dorsal raphe nucleus and serotonin: implications for neuroplasticity linked to major depression and Alzheimer's disease. Progress in brain research. 172, 233-64.

Miyawaki, E., Meah, Y., Koller, W.C., 1997. Serotonin, dopamine, and motor effects in Parkinson's disease. Clinical neuropharmacology. 20, 300-10.

Navailles, S., Bioulac, B., Gross, C., De Deurwaerdere, P., 2010. Serotonergic neurons mediate ectopic release of dopamine induced by L-DOPA in a rat model of Parkinson's disease. Neurobiology of disease. 38, 136-43.

Numan, S., Lundgren, K.H., Wright, D.E., Herman, J.P., Seroogy, K.B., 1995. Increased expression of 5HT2 receptor mRNA in rat striatum following 6-OHDA lesions of the adult nigrostriatal pathway. Brain research. Molecular brain research. 29, 391-6.

Parkkinen, L., Pirttila, T., Alafuzoff, I., 2008. Applicability of current staging/categorization of alpha-synuclein pathology and their clinical relevance. Acta neuropathologica. 115, 399-407.

Patt, S., Gerhard, L., 1993. A Golgi study of human locus coeruleus in normal brains and in Parkinson's disease. Neuropathology and applied neurobiology. 19, 519-23.

Paulus, W., Jellinger, K., 1991. The neuropathologic basis of different clinical subgroups of Parkinson's disease. Journal of neuropathology and experimental neurology. 50, 743-55.

Pintor, L., Bailles, E., Valldeoriola, F., Tolosa, E., Marti, M.J., de Pablo, J., 2006. Response to 4-month treatment with reboxetine in Parkinson's disease patients with a major depressive episode. General hospital psychiatry. 28, 59-64.

Politis, M., Wu, K., Loane, C., Turkheimer, F.E., Molloy, S., Brooks, D.J., Piccini, P., 2010. Depressive symptoms in PD correlate with higher 5-HTT binding in raphe and limbic structures. Neurology. 75, 1920-7.

Radja, F., Descarries, L., Dewar, K.M., Reader, T.A., 1993. Serotonin 5-HT1 and 5-HT2 receptors in adult rat brain after neonatal destruction of nigrostriatal dopamine neurons: a quantitative autoradiographic study. Brain research. 606, 273-85.

Ravina, B., Camicioli, R., Como, P.G., Marsh, L., Jankovic, J., Weintraub, D., Elm, J., 2007. The impact of depressive symptoms in early Parkinson disease. Neurology. 69, 342-7.

Remy, P., Doder, M., Lees, A., Turjanski, N., Brooks, D., 2005. Depression in Parkinson's disease: loss of dopamine and noradrenaline innervation in the limbic system. Brain : a journal of neurology. 128, 1314-22.

Richard, I.H., Schiffer, R.B., Kurlan, R., 1996. Anxiety and Parkinson's disease. The Journal of neuropsychiatry and clinical neurosciences. 8, 383-92.

Rommelfanger, K.S., Weinshenker, D., Miller, G.W., 2004. Reduced MPTP toxicity in noradrenaline transporter knockout mice. Journal of neurochemistry. 91, 1116-24.

Rommelfanger, K.S., Weinshenker, D., 2007. Norepinephrine: The redheaded stepchild of Parkinson's disease. Biochemical pharmacology. 74, 177-90.

Roselli, F., Pisciotta, N.M., Pennelli, M., Aniello, M.S., Gigante, A., De Caro, M.F., Ferrannini, E., Tartaglione, B., Niccoli-Asabella, A., Defazio, G., Livrea, P., Rubini, G., 2010. Midbrain SERT in degenerative parkinsonisms: a 123I-FP-CIT SPECT study. Movement disorders : official journal of the Movement Disorder Society. 25, 1853-9.

Scatton, B., Javoy-Agid, F., Rouquier, L., Dubois, B., Agid, Y., 1983. Reduction of cortical dopamine, noradrenaline, serotonin and their metabolites in Parkinson's disease. Brain research. 275, 321-8.

Schapira, A.H., Bezard, E., Brotchie, J., Calon, F., Collingridge, G.L., Ferger, B., Hengerer, B., Hirsch, E., Jenner, P., Le Novere, N., Obeso, J.A., Schwarzschild, M.A., Spampinato, U., Davidai, G., 2006. Novel pharmacological targets for the treatment of Parkinson's disease. Nature reviews. Drug discovery. 5, 845-54.

Schrag, A., Jahanshahi, M., Quinn, N., 2000. What contributes to quality of life in patients with Parkinson's disease? Journal of neurology, neurosurgery, and psychiatry. 69, 308-12.

Schrag, A., Morley, D., Quinn, N., Jahanshahi, M., 2004. Impact of Parkinson's disease on patients' adolescent and adult children. Parkinsonism & related disorders. 10, 391-7.

Schrag, A., 2006. Quality of life and depression in Parkinson's disease. Journal of the neurological sciences. 248, 151-7.

Schuurman, A.G., van den Akker, M., Ensinck, K.T., Metsemakers, J.F., Knottnerus, J.A., Leentjens, A.F., Buntinx, F., 2002. Increased risk of Parkinson's disease after depression: a retrospective cohort study. Neurology. 58, 1501-4.

Shiba, M., Bower, J.H., Maraganore, D.M., McDonnell, S.K., Peterson, B.J., Ahlskog, J.E., Schaid, D.J., Rocca, W.A., 2000. Anxiety disorders and depressive disorders preceding Parkinson's disease: a case-control study. Movement disorders : official journal of the Movement Disorder Society. 15, 669-77.

Stein,M.B., Heuser, I.J., Juncos, J.L., and Uhde, T.W. 1990. Anxiety disorders in patients with Parkinson's disease. American journal of pyschiatry. 41, 1086-1089.

Tadaiesky, M.T., Dombrowski, P.A., Figueiredo, C.P., Cargnin-Ferreira, E., Da Cunha, C., Takahashi, R.N., 2008. Emotional, cognitive and neurochemical alterations in a premotor stage model of Parkinson's disease. Neuroscience. 156, 830-40.

Taylor, T.N., Caudle, W.M., Shepherd, K.R., Noorian, A., Jackson, C.R., Iuvone, P.M., Weinshenker, D., Greene, J.G., Miller, G.W., 2009. Nonmotor symptoms of Parkinson's disease revealed in an animal model with reduced monoamine storage capacity. The Journal of neuroscience : the official journal of the Society for Neuroscience. 29, 8103-13.

Veazey, C., Aki, S.O., Cook, K.F., Lai, E.C., Kunik, M.E., 2005. Prevalence and treatment of depression in Parkinson's disease. The Journal of neuropsychiatry and clinical neurosciences. 17, 310-23.

Volpi, R., Caffarra, P., Boni, S., Scaglioni, A., Malvezzi, L., Saginario, A., Chiodera, P., Coiro, V., 1997. ACTH/cortisol involvement in the serotonergic disorder affecting the parkinsonian brain. Neuropsychobiology. 35, 73-8.

Von Coelln, R., Thomas, B., Savitt, J.M., Lim, K.L., Sasaki, M., Hess, E.J., Dawson, V.L., Dawson, T.M., 2004. Loss of locus coeruleus neurons and reduced startle in parkin null mice. Proceedings of the National Academy of Sciences of the United States of America. 101, 10744-9.

Walter, U., Dressler, D., Wolters, A., Wittstock, M., Benecke, R., 2007a. Transcranial brain sonography findings in clinical subgroups of idiopathic Parkinson's disease. Movement disorders : official journal of the Movement Disorder Society. 22, 48-54.

Walter, U., Hoeppner, J., Prudente-Morrissey, L., Horowski, S., Herpertz, S.C., Benecke, R., 2007b. Parkinson's disease-like midbrain sonography abnormalities are frequent in depressive disorders. Brain : a journal of neurology. 130, 1799-807.

Weintraub, D., Morales, K.H., Moberg, P.J., Bilker, W.B., Balderston, C., Duda, J.E., Katz, I.R., Stern, M.B., 2005. Antidepressant studies in Parkinson's disease: a review and meta-analysis. Movement disorders : official journal of the Movement Disorder Society. 20, 1161-9.

Zarow, C., Lyness, S.A., Mortimer, J.A., Chui, H.C., 2003. Neuronal loss is greater in the locus coeruleus than nucleus basalis and substantia nigra in Alzheimer and Parkinson diseases. Archives of neurology. 60, 337-41.

Zhang, X., Andren, P.E., Greengard, P., Svenningsson, P., 2008. Evidence for a role of the 5-HT1B receptor and its adaptor protein, p11, in L-DOPA treatment of an animal model of Parkinsonism. Proceedings of the National Academy of Sciences of the United States of America. 105, 2163-8.